MIDDLETON'S
ALLERGY ESSENTIALS

FIRST EDITION

MIDDLETON'S ALLERGY ESSENTIALS

Robyn E. O'Hehir, BSc, MBBS(Hons), FRACP, PhD, FRCP, FRCPath, FAHMS, FThorSoc

Professor and Director, Department of Allergy, Immunology, and Respiratory Medicine, Alfred Hospital and Monash University
Deputy Head, Central Clinical School, Monash University
Deputy Director Research, Alfred Health, Melbourne, Vic, Australia

Stephen T. Holgate, CBE, BSc, MBBS, MD, DSc, FRCP, FRCPath, FAAAAI, FERS, FMedSci, MEA MRC

Clinical Professor of Immunopharmacology and Honorary Consultant Physician, Clinical and Experimental Sciences Faculty of Medicine Southampton University and Hospital Trust, Southampton, United Kingdom

Aziz Sheikh, OBE, BSc, MBBS, MD, MSc, FRCGP, FRCP, FRCPE, FRSE, FFPH, FMedSci, FACMI

Professor of Primary Care Research & Development
Director, Asthma UK Centre for Applied Research
Co-Director, Centre of Medical Informatics, Usher Institute of Population Health Sciences and Informatics, The University of Edinburgh, Edinburgh, United Kingdom
Honorary Consultant in Paediatric Allergy, NHS, Lothian, Scotland, United Kingdom

For additional online content visit http://expertconsult.com

ELSEVIER

Edinburgh   London   New York   Oxford   Philadelphia   St Louis   Sydney   Toronto

ELSEVIER

ISBN: 978-0-323-37579-5
E-ISBN: 978-0-323-39273-0

Printed in China
Last digit is the print number: 9   8   7   6   5   4   3   2   1

Content Strategist: Belinda Kuhn
Content Development Specialists: Joanne Scott, Devika Ponnambalam
Project Manager: Anne Collett
Design: Miles Hitchen
Illustration Manager: Emily Costantino
Illustrators: Oxford Illustrators, Chartwell; Dartmouth Publishing, Inc., Graphic World Inc.
Marketing Manager(s) (UK/USA): Kristin Koehler

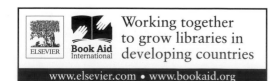

CONTENTS

Foreword vi

Preface vii

Contributors viii

Dedication.. x

1   Introduction to Mechanisms of Allergic Diseases 1
Terufumi Kubo, Hideaki Morita, Kazunari Sugita, and Cezmi A. Akdis

2   The Origins of Allergic Disease.. 29
John W. Holloway and Susan L. Prescott

3   Epidemiology of Allergic Diseases.. 51
Adnan Custovic

4   Indoor and Outdoor Allergens and Pollutants...................................... 73
Geoffrey A. Stewart and Clive Robinson

5   Principles of Allergy Diagnosis.. 117
Anca Mirela Chiriac, Jean Bousquet, and Pascal Demoly

6   Allergen-specific Immunotherapy 133
Anthony J. Frew and Helen E. Smith

7   Asthma.. 151
Stephen T. Holgate and Mike Thomas

8   Allergic Rhinitis and Conjunctivitis 205
Jonathan Corren

9   Drug Allergy 225
Oliver Hausmann

10   Urticaria and Angioedema without Wheals 249
Clive E. H. Grattan and Sarbjit S. Saini

11   Atopic Dermatitis and Allergic Contact Dermatitis 265
Donald Y. M. Leung and Mark Boguniewicz

12   Food Allergy and Gastrointestinal Syndromes 301
Anna Nowak-Węgrzyn, A. Wesley Burks, and Hugh A. Sampson

13   Anaphylaxis 345
Simon G. A. Brown and Paul J. Turner

14   Occupational Allergy 361
Catherine Lemière and Olivier Vandenplas

15   Insect Allergy 377
David B. K. Golden

APPENDIX A: Internet Resources 395

Index.. 397

FOREWORD

I am honored to provide this foreword to the Elsevier text *Middleton's Allergy Essentials,* edited by Professors O'Hehir, Holgate, and Sheikh. Not because I am an allergist or immunologist—I am a clinical informatician and academic general internist—nor because it will pad my *curriculum vitae* with another piece of writing. Rather, it gives me an opportunity to honor my father, Elliott Middleton Jr., M.D., and to share with readers of this text a glimpse into the man who inspired me and many others to pursue a career in medicine, and for his many fellows and trainees, a career in allergy and immunology. My dad had a passion both for life and for his work in clinical medicine, including research and teaching as well as a humility based upon a desire to help patients—those with asthma especially—and the myriad problems that may be associated with allergic disorders and the diseases of clinical immunology.

As I was growing up, my father always worked hard but always seemed to be having fun. There were frequent rounds in hospital early and late in the day, and extra time often spent in the lab Saturday mornings to 'catch up' after a busy week. Most nights were spent with the family for dinner, and then afterwards several hours on the living room couch editing one manuscript or chapter, or sorting slides on one of those now old-fashioned slide view-boxes, preparing for a lecture. For many years, it was a chapter for the text now known as *Middleton's Allergy: Principles and Practice.* He absolutely loved putting this text together: crafting the outline of chapters, meeting with the co-editors, and reviewing chapters and occasionally cajoling authors to get things done. It may be his proudest accomplishment.

On a couple of occasions we met at one of his national meetings, and I saw him in his element: gregarious, well known, interested in others, and respected. The passion my dad had about his work was infectious: he would always take the time to explain in simple terms what was going on with his laboratory and clinical investigations, whether it was the early work on mast cell functions and histamine release, leukotrienes, or bioflanonoids (we all came to recognize the terms *quercetin, rutin,* and others) and their impact on inflammation; the reverse transcriptase; or free radicals. Equally important, we came to know the good dietary sources for these compounds.

He instilled in me a sense of wonder, not only about the incredible processes of chemistry and biology that impact the human system and may manifest when aberrant as disease states or worse, but also about the human interaction with the natural world that seemed filled with potential allergens—pollen, grasses, sage, cat dander, **and more** (his fellows have told me his 'weed walks' were fun and informative). He viewed his research—whether it was basic laboratory investigation or clinical trials—from the patient's perspective and honored the patient as the center of his clinical attention.

One cannot really know the perception people have of one's parents as we as children are always too close, too intertwined with them, or even as adults as we try to both distance ourselves from them and take from them all that they have to offer that is good, as we come to define ourselves. In my training, I have been surprised to see people's faces light up and smile if the occasion ever arose for me to acknowledge that Elliott Middleton Jr. was my dad. It is a delight—he left an indelible mark on the world that I aspire to leave as well.

Blackford Middleton, MD, MPH, MSc

PREFACE

In 1978, the late Elliott Middleton Jr., along with founding editors Elliot Ellis and Charles Reed, published a landmark comprehensive book, *Middleton's Allergy: Principles and Practice*. This 2-volume set has been *the* definitive text on allergy practice and disease mechanisms worldwide, and, as a result, is now in its 8th edition. Over the last decade, the understanding of allergic diseases and their diagnosis, prevention, and management has advanced considerably. In addition, the prevalence, spectrum, and severity of allergy have increased so that allergic disorders have become a public health problem affecting a high proportion of the global population.

There is, in some quarters, a perception that allergy has little impact on the lives of sufferers, but nothing could be further from the truth. Diseases such as asthma, food allergy, drug allergy, and insect allergy can be life-threatening if not diagnosed and treated properly. Allergy often affects multiple organs in the same individual, magnifying the overall health burden that patients experience. Of note, allergy manifests in all age groups, being influenced by strong genetic, environmental, and epigenetic drivers.

Recognizing that most allergic disease is managed by busy clinicians in primary and secondary care settings, we have identified a need for a book that is both easily accessible and authoritative for the practitioner. The result is *Middleton's Allergy Essentials*.

In this first edition, we have extracted what we considered to be most useful to the healthcare practitioner in his or her daily practice, with a strong emphasis on disease diagnosis and management. Because the field is evolving so rapidly, we have also included some sections on mechanisms, but only when this adds value to each disease covered. In creating this text, the authors were asked to identify relevant sections in *Middleton's Allergy: Principles and Practice*, 8th edition, update these, and present the revised, abridged chapters with a generalist audience in mind. Naturally, such a text has to be selective, but we hope that the topics covered address the needs of both trainee and established practitioners across the healthcare sector, to enable them to access novel information to beneficially inform their practice.

The text portion of each section is relatively brief and easy to review, with illustrations and tables aimed at providing additional and more detailed information when considered informative. We have attempted to adopt a similar format for each chapter. Throughout, there is emphasis on a practical approach to evaluation, differential diagnosis, and treatment of allergic disorders, to maximize its use. To achieve this, we have called upon the same internationally outstanding authors of the original *Middleton's Allergy: Principles and Practice*, 8th edition, chapters. The editors wish to express their sincere thanks to all of our authors for the very considerable amount of work they have undertaken to produce this easily accessible book.

None of this would have been possible without Joanne Scott, Belinda Kuhn, and Devika Ponnambalam, who were the brainchildren and instigators of the project, and their team at Elsevier who have worked seamlessly with us throughout the commissioning and editorial process. As editors of this 'offspring' of *Middleton's Allergy: Principles and Practice*, 8th edition, we express our very sincere thanks to all the editors and authors of the parent publication but especially to its three founders, who had the vision to produce such a consistent beacon of success in the field of allergy. We are also indebted to Professor Blackford Middleton—son of Elliott Middleton, Jr.—for writing the Foreword to *Middleton's Allergy Essentials*. The best testament to Elliott and his coauthors would be its widespread use and impact across the way allergy treatment is delivered to our patients worldwide; after all, it is they who continue to motivate us to want to deliver ever better care.

Robyn E. O'Hehir

Stephen T. Holgate

Aziz Sheikh

CONTRIBUTORS

Cezmi A. Akdis, MD
Professor and Director, Swiss Institute of Allergy and Asthma Research University of Zürich; Director, Christine Kühne Center for Allergy Research and Education; President, European Academy of Allergy and Clinical Immunology, Zürich, Switzerland

Mark Boguniewicz, MD
Professor, Division of Allergy–Immunology, Department of Pediatrics, National Jewish Health University of Colorado School of Medicine, Denver, CO, USA

Jean Bousquet, MD
Professor of Pulmonary Medicine, CHRU Arnaud de Villeneuve, Montpellier, France

Simon G. A. Brown, MBBS, PhD, FACEM
Professor of Emergency Medicine. University of Western Australia, Royal Perth Hospital, Perth, WA, Australia

A. Wesley Burks, MD
Professor and Chair, Pediatrics; Physician-in-Chief, North Carolina Children's Hospital, University of North Carolina at Chapel Hill, Chapel Hill, NC, USA

Anca Mirela Chiriac, MD
Allergologist, Department of Respiratory Medicine and Addictology, Arnaud de Villeneuve Hospital, University Hospital of Montpellier, Montpellier, France

Jonathan Corren, MD
Associate Clinical Professor of Medicine, David Geffen School of Medicine, University of California, Los Angeles, Los Angeles, CA, USA

Adnan Custovic, MD, PhD
Professor of Allergy, Imperial College, London, United Kingdom

Pascal Demoly, MD, PhD
Professor of Respiratory Medicine, Department of Respiratory Medicine and Addictology, Arnaud de Villeneuve Hospital, University Hospital of Montpellier, Montpellier, France

Anthony J. Frew, MD, FRCP
Professor of Allergy and Respiratory Medicine, Department of Respiratory Medicine, Royal Sussex County Hospital, Brighton, United Kingdom

David B. K. Golden, MD
Associate Professor of Medicine, Division of Allergy and Clinical Immunology, Department of Medicine, Johns Hopkins University School of Medicine, Baltimore, MD, USA

Clive E. H. Grattan, MD
Consultant Dermatologist, Dermatology Centre, Norfolk and Norwich University Hospital, Norfolk, UK

Oliver Hausmann, MD
Specialist Consultant for Allergology and Immunology, Department of Rheumatology, Immunology and Allergology, Inselspital, University Hospital, Bern, Switzerland; Private Practice, Loewenpraxis, Lucerne, Switzerland

Stephen T. Holgate, CBE, BSc, MB BS, MD, DSc, FRCP, FRCPath, FAAAAI, FERS, FMedSci, MEA MRC
Clinical Professor of Immunopharmacology and Honorary Consultant Physician Clinical and Experimental Sciences Faculty of Medicine, Southampton University and Hospital Trust, Southampton, United Kingdom

John W. Holloway, PhD
Professor of Allergy and Respiratory
Genetics, Faculty of Medicine,
University of Southampton,
Southampton, United Kingdom

Terufumi Kubo, MD, PhD
Research Fellow, Swiss Institute of
Allergy and Asthma Research (SIAF),
Davos, Switzerland

Catherine Lemière, MD, MSc
Professor, Department of Medicine,
University of Montréal, Montréal,
QC, Canada; Department of Chest
Medicine, Hôpital du Sacré-Coeur de
Montréal

Donald Y. M. Leung, MD, PhD
Edelstein Family Chair of Pediatric
Allergy and Immunology, National
Jewish Health; Professor, Department
of Pediatrics, University of Colorado
School of Medicine, Denver, CO, USA

Hideaki Morita, MD, PhD
Research Fellow, Swiss Institute of
Allergy and Asthma Research (SIAF),
Davos, Switzerland

Anna Nowak-Węgrzyn, MD
Associate Professor, Department of
Pediatrics, Jaffe Food Allergy Institute,
Icahn School of Medicine at Mount
Sinai, New York, NY, USA

Susan L. Prescott, MD, PhD
Winthrop Professor, School of
Paediatrics and Child Health,
University of Western Australia;
Paediatric Allergist and Immunologist,
Princess Margaret Hospital, Perth,
WA, Australia

Clive Robinson, PhD, FHEA, FSB
Professor of Respiratory Cell Science,
Division of Biomedical Sciences,
St. George's University of London,
London, United Kingdom

Sarbjit S. Saini, MD
Associate Professor of Medicine,
Division of Allergy and Clinical
Immunology, Johns Hopkins
University School of Medicine,
Baltimore, MD, USA

Hugh A. Sampson, MD
Professor, Department of Pediatrics;
Dean for Translational Biomedical
Sciences, Icahn School of Medicine at
Mount Sinai, New York, NY, USA

Helen E. Smith, DM
Chair of Primary Care, Division of
Primary Care and Public Health,
Brighton and Sussex Medical School,
University of Sussex, Brighton, UK

Geoffrey A. Stewart, BSC, PhD
Professor, School of Pathology and
Laboratory Medicine, The University
of Western Australia, Perth, WA,
Australia

Kazunari Sugita, MD, PhD
Research Fellow, Swiss Institute of
Allergy and Asthma Research (SIAF),
Davos, Switzerland

Mike Thomas, MBBS, FRCP, PhD
Professor of Primary Care Research,
Primary Care and Population Sciences,
Faculty of Medicine, University of
Southampton, UK

Paul J. Turner, BMBCh, PhD, FRACP
MRC Clinician Scientist in Paediatric
Allergy and Immunology, Imperial
College London, United Kingdom;
Associate Clinical Professor in
Paediatrics, University of Sydney,
Sydney, NSW. Australia

Olivier Vandenplas, MD, PhD
Professor of Medicine, Department of
Chest Medicine, Centre Hospitalier
Universitaire de Mont-Godinne,
Université Catholique de Louvain,
Yvoir, Belgium

Robyn E. O'Hehir

This book is dedicated by Professor Robyn O'Hehir to two of the founders of the discipline of allergy, Professors Dan Czarny and Barry Kay, from whom so many learned so much.

Stephen T. Holgate

I dedicate this book to my Mentor and good friend, Dr. K. Frank Austen, who set me on a career in allergy and asthma that has been so enriching.

Aziz Sheikh

In loving memory of Tanveer Sheikh.

CHAPTER 1

Introduction to Mechanisms of Allergic Diseases

Terufumi Kubo, Hideaki Morita, Kazunari Sugita, and Cezmi A. Akdis

CHAPTER OUTLINE

INTRODUCTION

INNATE IMMUNITY

Microbial Pattern Recognition by the Innate Immune System

Pattern Recognition Receptors

Cellular Responses of Innate Immunity

Innate Instruction of Adaptive Immune Responses

Innate Immunity and Allergy

ADAPTIVE IMMUNITY

Adaptive Immune Response in Allergic Disease

Main Components of the Adaptive Immune System

Features of the Adaptive Immune Response

Mechanisms of Diseases Involving Adaptive Immunity

IMMUNOGLOBULIN STRUCTURE AND FUNCTION

B Lymphocytes and the Humoral Immune Response

Immunoglobulin Structure and Gene Rearrangement

Immunoglobulin Function

IMMUNOGLOBULINS AND HUMAN DISEASE

IMMUNE TOLERANCE

Introduction

Central and Peripheral Tolerance Mechanisms

Central Tolerance

Peripheral Tolerance

Immune Effector Cells and Molecules

   Regulatory T Cells

   Transforming Growth Factor-β (TGF-β)

   Interleukin-10 (IL-10)

CYTOKINES AND CHEMOKINES IN ALLERGIC INFLAMMATION

Cytokines in Allergic Inflammation

   Interleukin-4 (IL-4)

   Interleukin-5 (IL-5)

   Interleukin-9 (IL-9)

   Interleukin-13 (IL-13)

   Interleukin-25 (IL-25)

   Interleukin-33 (IL-33)

   Thymic Stromal Lymphopoietin (TSLP)

Chemokines in Allergic Diseases

   Asthma

   Atopic Dermatitis

BIOLOGY OF IMMUNE CELLS

T Lymphocytes

B Lymphocytes

Type 2 Innate Lymphoid Cells

Antigen-Presenting Dendritic Cells

Mast Cells

Basophils

Eosinophils

CONTRIBUTION OF STRUCTURAL CELLS TO ALLERGIC INFLAMMATIONS

   Introduction

   Airway Epithelial Cells

   Airway Smooth Muscle Cells

   Neuronal Control of Airway Function

CYTOKINE NETWORKS IN ALLERGIC INFLAMMATION

RESOLUTION OF ALLERGIC INFLAMMATION AND MAJOR PATHWAYS

SUMMARY OF IMPORTANT CONCEPTS

- Allergic inflammation is a result of a complex interplay amongst structural tissue cells and inflammatory cells, including mast cells, basophils, lymphocytes, dendritic cells, eosinophils, and sometimes, neutrophils.
- Cytokines are families of secreted proteins that mediate immune and inflammatory reactions at local or distant sites.
- The innate immune system first responds to early infectious and inflammatory signals, activates and instructs the adaptive immune system for antigen-specific T and B lymphocyte responses and the development of immunologic memory.

- Allergen recognition and uptake, allergic sensitization, inflammation, and disease originate in the innate immune system.
- Adaptive immune responses depend on activation of naive CD4$^+$ T cells and differentiation into effector cells. CD4$^+$ Th2 cells are critical mediators of allergic inflammation.
- Production of IgE antibody is regulated mainly by Th2 cells. Activated Th2 cells trigger IgE production in B cells through a combination of signals, including secreted cytokine (IL-4 or IL-13) and cell surface (CD40L).
- Better understanding of the pathophysiology of allergic inflammation will enable us to identify novel therapeutic targets in the treatment of chronic allergic inflammation.

INTRODUCTION

The inflammatory process has several common characteristics shared by various different allergic diseases, including asthma, allergic rhinitis or rhinosinusitis, and atopic dermatitis (eczema). Allergic inflammation is characterized by IgE-dependent activation of mucosal mast cells and an infiltration of eosinophils that is orchestrated by increased numbers of activated CD4$^+$ T helper type 2 (Th2) lymphocytes. In addition to these cells, various types of inflammatory cells produce multiple inflammatory mediators, including lipids, purines, cytokines, chemokines, and reactive oxygen species. Both innate and adaptive immune mechanisms and involvement of multiple cytokines and chemokines play roles.

INNATE IMMUNITY

Microbial Pattern Recognition by the Innate Immune System

Microbial recognition by the innate immune system is mediated by germline-encoded receptors with genetically predetermined specificities for microbial constituents. Natural selection has formed and refined the repertoire of innate immune receptors to recognize highly conserved molecular structures that distinguish large groups of microorganisms from the host. These microbe-specific structures are called *pathogen-associated molecular patterns* (PAMPs), and the *pattern recognition receptors* (PRRs) of the innate immune system recognize these structures (Table 1-1).

Pattern Recognition Receptors

PRRs of the innate immune system can be divided into two groups: secreted receptors and transmembrane signal-transducing receptors (Table 1-1). *Secreted PRRs* typically have multiple effects in innate immunity and host defense, including direct microbial killing, serving as helper proteins for transmembrane receptors, opsonization for phagocytosis, and chemoattraction of innate and adaptive immune effector cells. Antimicrobial peptides (AMPs) are secreted PRRs that are microbicidal and rapidly acting. When secreted onto skin and mucous membranes, they create a microbicidal shield against microbial attachment and invasion. *Transmembrane PRRs* are expressed on many innate immune cell types, including macrophages, dendritic cells (DCs), monocytes, and B lymphocytes (Fig. 1-1). These PRRs are exemplified by the Toll-like receptors and their associated recognition, enhancing, and signal transduction proteins (Fig. 1-1). Innate immune response at the epithelial cell- and DC-related processes are controlled by the activation of the epithelial PRR by pathogen-associated molecular patterns (PAMPS) found in the microorganisms as well as the host-derived damage-associated molecular patterns (DAMPs). Airway epithelial cells and dendritic cells express a wide range of Toll-like receptors (TLRs); NOD-like receptors (NLRs); RIG-I-like receptors (RLRs); AIM2-like receptors (ALRs); C-type lectin receptors (CLRs); protease-activated receptors (PAR); and others.[1]

TABLE 1-1 Innate Pattern Recognition Receptors in Humans

Pattern recognition receptors	PAMP structures recognized	Functions
Secreted		

Antimicrobial peptides
  α- and β-Defensins
  Cathelicidin (LL-37)
  Dermcidin
  RegIIIγ
	Microbial membranes (negatively charged)	Opsonization, microbial cell lysis, immune cell chemoattractant

Collectins Mannose-binding lectin	Microbial mannan	Opsonization, complement activation, microbial cell lysis, chemoattraction, phagocytosis
Surfactant proteins A and D	Bacterial cell wall lipids; viral coat proteins	Opsonization, killing, phagocytosis, proinflammatory and antiinflammatory mediator release
Pentraxins C-reactive protein	Bacterial phospholipids (phosphorylcholine)	Opsonization, complement activation, microbial cell lysis, chemoattraction, phagocytosis
Secreted and membrane bound		
CD14	Endotoxin	TLR4 signaling
LPS binding protein	Endotoxin	TLR4 signaling
MD-2	Endotoxin	TLR4 co-receptor
Membrane bound		
Toll-like receptors	Microbial PAMPs	Immune cell activation
C-type lectin receptors Mannose receptor (CD206)	Microbial mannan	Cell activation, phagocytosis, proinflammatory mediator release
DECTIN-1	β-1,3-Glucan	Cell activation, phagocytosis, proinflammatory mediator release
DECTIN-2	Fungal mannose	Cell activation, phagocytosis, proinflammatory mediator release
DC-SIGN	Microbial mannose, fucose	Immunoregulation, IL-10 production
Siglecs	Sialic acid containing glycans	Cell inhibition, endocytosis
Cytosolic		
NOD-like receptors NOD-1	Peptidoglycans from gram-negative bacteria	Cell activation
NOD-2	Bacterial muramyl dipeptides	Cell activation
NLRP1	Anthrax lethal toxin	PAMP recognition in inflammasome
NLRP3 (cryopyrin)	Microbial RNA	PAMP recognition in inflammasome
NLRC4	Bacterial flagellin	PAMP recognition in inflammasome
RIG-I and MDA5	Viral double-stranded RNA	Type 1 IFN responses

DC-SIGN, dendritic cell–specific intracellular adhesion molecule 3 (ICAM-3)–grabbing non-integrin; DECTIN, dendritic cell–specific receptor; IFN, interferon; IL, interleukin; LPS, lipopolysaccharide; MD-2, myeloid differentiation factor 2 (also called lymphocyte antigen 96 [LY98]); MDA5, melanoma differentiation-associated 5 (also called interferon induced with helicase domain 1 [IFIH1]); NLR, NOD-like receptor; NOD, nucleotide-binding oligomerization domain protein; PAMP, pathogen-associated molecular pattern; RegIIIγ, regenerating islet-derived 3 γ (REG3G); RIG-I, retinoic acid-inducible 1 (also called DDX58); Siglecs, sialic acid–binding immunoglobulin-like lectins; TLR, Toll-like receptor.

Cellular Responses of Innate Immunity

Microbial detection by PRRs activates the cells that express or bind them. Those in frontline positions for detection are the first responders of the innate immune system, such as tissue macrophages, fibrocytes, epithelial cells, and mast cells.

Innate immune activation also leads to multifaceted antimicrobial responses by tissue infiltrating immune cells (e.g., neutrophils, natural killer cells, dendritic cells, monocytes). These responses are potent antimicrobial effectors that usually are recruited by an innate immune intermediary to induce the full weight of their response, but they can respond directly to microbial stimuli through their own surface-expressed PRRs. On reaching the infected site, neutrophils phagocytose invading microorganisms that are opsonized by complement C3 fragments (e.g., C3b, iC3b) and immunoglobulin G (IgG).[2]

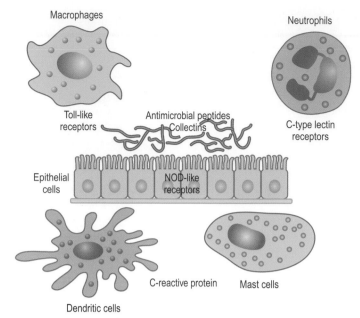

Figure 1-1 Main categories of pattern recognition receptors and the innate immune cell types that express them. NOD, nucleotide-binding oligomerization domain protein. *(Adapted from Liu AH. Innate microbial sensors and their relevance to allergy. J Allergy Clin Immunol 2008; 122:846–858.)*

Recruited and activated natural killer (NK) cells mediate antimicrobial activities by induction of apoptosis of cell targets and cytokine secretion that promote innate immune functions and contribute to adaptive immune responses.

Innate Instruction of Adaptive Immune Responses

The immediate and infiltrative responses of innate immunity activates and instructs the adaptive immune system for antigen-specific T and B lymphocyte responses and the development of immunologic memory. Because the adaptive immune system essentially has a limitless antigen receptor repertoire, instruction is necessary to guide adaptive antimicrobial immune responses toward pathogens and not self-antigens or harmless environmental antigens. Microbial pattern recognition by innate immune cells controls the activation of adaptive immune responses by directing microbial antigens linked to TLRs and other PRRs through the cellular processes leading to antigen presentation and the expression of costimulatory molecules (e.g., CD80 with CD86).

Innate Immunity and Allergy

The innate immune system of the airways, gastrointestinal tract, and skin, is continuously exposed to potential allergens. As with microbial antigens, allergens can engage innate PRRs, are processed through innate immune cells, and can lead to pathologic allergic/inflammatory immune responses. Although the circumstances leading to allergic immunity in humans are not clear, evidence suggests that allergic susceptibilities can originate in the innate immune system.

ADAPTIVE IMMUNITY

Adaptive Immune Response in Allergic Disease

A remarkable property of the adaptive immune system is its memory. Immunologic memory is made possible by the clonal expansion of T and B lymphocytes in response to antigen (including allergen) stimulation. From the time the human immune system begins to differentiate in fetal life, lymphocytes possessing unique reactivity are created by the recombination of genes encoding antigen receptors expressed on the lymphocyte cell membrane. Through the expression of these receptors, T and B lymphocytes have the ability to bind to and become activated by a specific antigen, which may be natural or artificial. Interaction with antigen activates the lymphocytes and generates long-lived, antigen-specific memory T and B cell clones. When the same antigen enters the body, there is immediate recognition by these memory cells. Cellular and humoral responses to the antigen are produced more rapidly than in the first encounter, and more memory cells are generated. This process of expansion of clonal populations of uniquely reacting lymphocytes first explained the B cell origin of antibody diversity and applies to cellular (T cell) immune responses.

Main Components of the Adaptive Immune System

All cells of the immune system are derived from the pluripotent hematopoietic stem cell found in the bone marrow. This pluripotential stem cell gives rise to lymphoid stem cells and myeloid stem cells. The lymphoid progenitor cell differentiates into three types of cell: *T cell, B cell, and NK cell*, and contributes to the development of subsets of DCs. The myeloid stem cell gives rise to dendritic cells, mast cells, basophils, neutrophils, eosinophils, monocytes, and macrophages, as well as megakaryocytes and erythrocytes. Differentiation of these committed stem cells depends on an array of cytokine and cell–cell interactions.

Features of the Adaptive Immune Response

Antigen-presenting cells (APCs), which include dendritic cells, monocytes or macrophages, process and present antigen within an antigen-binding cleft of major histocompatibility complex (MHC) molecules. These events start at the APC cell surface with the capture and endocytosis of antigens, followed by a complex sequence of enzymatic activities leading to the association of antigenic peptides with MHC molecules and expression back to the cell surface. CD4⁺ T cells recognize antigenic peptides when presented in the context of a class II MHC molecule (Fig. 1-2) together with the appropriate costimulatory signals, and become activated in response to monocyte-derived interleukin-1 (IL-1) and other cytokines, including autocrine stimulation by IL-2.

Subsets of helper T (Th) cells dictate the cytokine production involved in three types of immune responses. Th1 response, induced by IL-12 and interferon-γ (IFN-γ), is

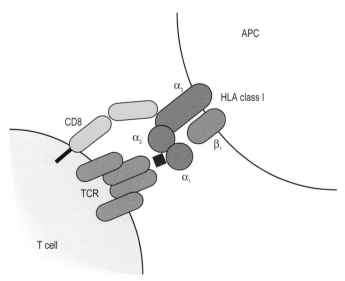

Figure 1-2 Interaction of a human leukocyte antigen (HLA) class I molecule on an antigen-presenting cell (APC) with a CD8⁺ T cell. The antigen receptor (i.e. T cell receptor, TCR) complex (purple) recognizes a combination of an antigen peptide (red) and an HLA molecule (brown and pink). The CD8 molecule (aqua blue) in the T cells interacts with the α₃ domain of the HLA molecule. HLA class II molecules present antigen peptides to CD4⁺ T cells in a similar manner, interacting with the TCR and the CD4 molecules.

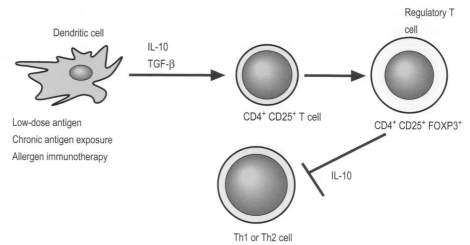

Figure 1-3 Regulatory T cells are generated by the interaction of antigen-presenting cells and T cells, mediated by the cytokines interleukin-10 (IL-10), transforming growth factor-β (TGF-β). These cytokines are secreted when the antigen is presented under certain conditions, such as when administering allergen immunotherapy at very low concentration. Regulatory T cells secrete IL-10 and inhibit effector T cells that share similar antigen specificity.

responsible for T cell-mediated cytotoxicity. Th2 response, induced by IL-4, IL-5, and IL-13, is responsible for development of immunoglobulin E (IgE)- and eosinophilia-mediated allergic disease. Th17 response leads to a characteristic neutrophilic inflammation and is pathogenic in some experimental models of autoimmunity. Transforming growth factor-β (TGF-β), IL-23, and IL-6 are essential cytokines for developing the Th17 response, which is mediated by IL-17A, IL-17F, IL-21, and IL-22.

The defensive capacity of the immune system needs a mechanism to counterbalance this proinflammatory response and to minimize unnecessary tissue damage. Several processes ensure that the different immune effector cells are not activated against host tissues and innocuous substances and that they can downregulate a response after the threat is resolved. All of these processes underlie *immune tolerance*, which is classified as central when occurring in primary lymphoid organs, or as peripheral when occurring in other tissues. Together with central and peripheral tolerance processes, a subset of T cells characterized by high levels of CD25 expression (IL-2R α chain) have been identified as regulatory T (Treg) cells because they were found to suppress the function of other T cells when present in the same site (Fig. 1-3).[3]

Mechanisms of Diseases Involving Adaptive Immunity

Distinct mechanisms of immune-mediated diseases are IgE-mediated hypersensitivity, antibody-mediated cytotoxicity, immune complex reaction, delayed hypersensitivity response, antibody-mediated activation or inactivation of biologic function, cell-mediated cytotoxicity, and granulomatous reaction.

IMMUNOGLOBULIN STRUCTURE AND FUNCTION

B Lymphocytes and the Humoral Immune Response

Engagement of the B cell receptor (BCR) by antigen initiates receptor aggregation at the cell surface followed by recruitment to lipid rafts. Lipid rafts are specialized membrane microdomains that facilitate assembly and activation of downstream signaling molecules.[4] This step places the complex in proximity to the LYN tyrosine kinase, which phosphorylates tyrosine residues in the Igα/Igβ ITAM motifs and triggers recruitment of spleen tyrosine kinase (SYK) and Bruton tyrosine kinase (BTK). Activated SYK phosphorylates and recruits the B cell linker (BLNK) protein, which provides binding sites for phospholipase Cγ2 (PLCγ2), BTK, and VAV proteins, which are guanine nucleotide exchange factors. PLCγ2 generates the second messengers inositol triphosphate and diacylglycerol, which are necessary for calcium release from intracellular stores and protein kinase C activation. BCR signal transduction also leads to activation of the mitogen-activated protein (MAP) kinase pathway. B cell activation is further aided by a co-receptor complex that amplifies signals delivered by the BCR. The members of this complex include CD19, the complement receptor type 2 (CR2 or CD21), and CD81. The CR2 enables the complement pathway to synergize with BCR signal transduction, which enhances B cell activation. Collectively, these signaling events lead to the activation of the transcription factors known as nuclear factor of activated T cells (NFAT), nuclear factor-κB (NF-κB), and activator protein 1 (AP-1). Activation of the BCR on naive and memory B cells results in their activation and migration to the draining lymph node or other lymphatic tissue. B cells can respond to three types of antigens, and the type of antigenic exposure dictates the quality of the ensuing response.

Immunoglobulin Structure and Gene Rearrangement

Immunoglobulins are composed of two identical heavy chains and two identical light chains (Fig. 1-4A). Light chains lack transmembrane domains and are anchored to heavy chains by disulfide bonds. The two heavy chains are linked to each other by a distinct set of disulfide bonds. Each heavy chain or light chain has two major domains referred to as the *constant region* (C) and the *variable region* (V), with each domain responsible for a specialized function. They are denoted as C_L and V_L for the light chains and as C_H and V_H for the heavy chains.

Heavy chain variable regions are encoded by one V gene, which encodes most V-region amino acids, as well as 1 of 23 diversity (D) and 1 of 6 joining (J) gene segments that are located 3′ of the V gene cluster. In contrast, light chain variable regions are encoded by only two types of genes: V genes and J genes. Whereas the $J_κ$ genes are organized in a cluster 3′ to the $V_κ$ gene cluster, $J_λ$ genes are interspersed with λ constant-region genes.

Immunoglobulin diversity has four sources: multiple V(D)J genes in the germline; random assortment of heavy chains and light chains; junctional nucleotide variability introduced during pre B cell immunoglobulin gene rearrangement; and somatic hyper mutation of immunoglobulin variable regions after encounters with antigens.

Immunoglobulin Function

The five classes of antibody molecules are designated IgM, IgD, IgG, IgA, and IgE. The IgG and IgA classes have more than one member. There are four IgG (γ) sub-classes, designated as IgG1, IgG2, IgG3, and IgG4, and their constant regions exhibit 90% homology with each other. However, because each IgG sub-class constant region is encoded by a separate constant-region gene, the IgG sub-classes are closely related isotypes that exhibit a similar overall structure. The two sub-classes of IgA are similarly related to each other. There are two types of light chains: κ and λ. There are four λ sub-types but only one form of κ. The nine class and sub-classes of antibody molecules have significantly different expression levels, anatomic locations, and effector functions (Table 1-2). The five antibody classes also display characteristic structural features (Fig. 1-4B).

IMMUNOGLOBULINS AND HUMAN DISEASE

Human conditions of dysregulated immunoglobulin production include antibody deficiencies and overproduction of specific antibodies. The most serious of the three major categories of antibody deficiencies result in reduced B cell numbers and a severe decrease in all isotypes of serum immunoglobulin, as in agammaglobulinemia. This type of immunodeficiency underscores the importance of tyrosine kinases in early B cell BCR signal transduction. The second category includes selective deficiencies of IgA or IgG2 production and various genetic mutations that result in hypogammaglobulinemia, such as deficiencies in transmembrane activator and calcium-modulating cyclophilin ligand

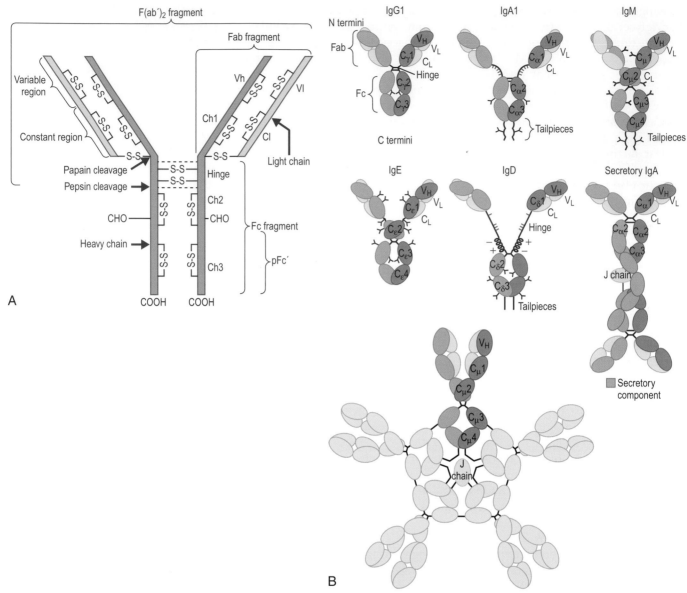

Figure 1-4 Basic structure of immunoglobulin molecules. **A.** In the monomeric structure of immunoglobulin molecules, disulfide bridges link the two heavy chains and the light chains with heavy chains. Enzymatic digestion with papain cleaves the immunoglobulin molecule into three fragments: two Fab fragments, each of which can bind a single antigen epitope, and the Fc fragment, which can bind to Fc receptors. Alternatively, pepsin digestion of immunoglobulins results in a single F(ab')₂ fragment, which remains capable of cross-linking and precipitating multivalent antigen. The Fc portion usually is digested into several smaller peptides by pepsin (pFc'). **B.** Schematic structures of the five classes of antibodies. IgG1 and IgA1 are shown as examples of the basic structure of the IgG and IgA classes of antibodies. The other IgG sub-classes differ primarily in the nature and length of the hinge, and the IgA2 hinge region is very short compared with IgA1. Although membrane IgM and IgA exist as monomers, secreted IgA can exist as dimers, and secreted IgM as pentamers, when linked by an extra polypeptide called the J chain. Both multimeric forms of antibodies can be transported across mucosal surfaces by binding to the polymeric immunoglobulin receptor. Dimeric IgA coupled to the J chain and secretory component, a part of the polymeric immunoglobulin (Ig) receptor remaining after transport through epithelial cells, is shown as an example of secretory Ig. *(From Delves PJ, Martin SJ, Burton DR, Roitt IM. Roitt's essential immunology. 12th ed. Oxford: Wiley-Blackwell; 2011. p. 56, 62.)*

interactor (TACI). The third category includes a number of mutations that give rise to hyper-IgM syndromes, which result from the failure of B cells to undergo class switch recombination. These disorders highlight the critical role that CD40–CD40L interaction plays in class switch recombination, as revealed by the lack of IgG, IgA, and IgE antibodies in these patients.

TABLE 1-2   Selected Biologic Properties of Human Immunoglobulin Isotypes

Characteristics	IgG1	IgG2	IgG3	IgG4	IgM	IgA1	IgA2	IgD	IgE
Physical properties									
Molecular weight (kD)	146	146	165	146	970*	160	160	170	190
Serum half-life (days)	29	27	7	16	5	6	6	–	2
Anatomic distribution									
Mean serum level (mg/mL)	5–12	2–6	0.5–1.0	0.2–1.0	0.5–1.5	0.5–2.0	0–0.2	0–0.4	0–0.002
Transport across placenta	+++	+	++	±	–	–	–	–	–
Transport across epithelium	–	–	–	–	+	+++[†]	+++[†]	–	–
Extravascular diffusion	+++	+++	+++	+++	±	++[‡]	++[‡]	+	+
Functional activity									
Antigen neutralization	++	++	++	++	++	++	++	–	–
Complement fixation	++	+	++	–	+++	+	+	–	–
ADCC	+	+	+	±	–	–	–	–	+
Immediate hypersensitivity	–	–	–	–	–	–	–	–	+++

ADCC, antibody-dependent cellular cytotoxicity; –, no effect; ±, no effect or negligible degree; +, small degree; ++, moderate degree; +++, large degree.
*Pentameric IgM plus J chain.
†Dimer.
‡Monomer.

IMMUNE TOLERANCE

Introduction

The physiopathology of immune tolerance–related diseases is complex and is influenced by factors, such as genetic susceptibility and route, dose, or time of the antigen exposure. Many common biologic mechanisms prevent immune responsiveness to innocuous environmental allergens and to self-antigens. Although most autoreactive T cells undergo selection and clonal deletion in the thymus, a small fraction of cells escape into the periphery. Additional immunologic control mechanisms eliminate or inactivate potentially hazardous effector cells that emerge from the thymus and move into the periphery (Fig. 1-5). Allergens enter the body through the respiratory and alimentary tract or injured skin, and the result usually is induction of tolerance.[5]

Central and Peripheral Tolerance Mechanisms

The processes that constitute immune tolerance normally ensure that immune effector cells are not activated against host tissues or innocuous agents. Immune tolerance is called *central* when the response occurs in primary lymphoid organs, such as thymus or *peripheral* when it occurs in peripheral lymph nodes, Peyer's patches, tonsils, or other tissues.

Central Tolerance

T cells experience the first step of tolerance during their maturation in the thymus. Prethymic T cells reach the subcapsular region of the thymus, where they proliferate. Maturing cells move deeper into the cortex and adhere to cortical epithelial cells. The T cell receptors (TCRs) on thymocytes are exposed to epithelial major histocompatibility complex (MHC) molecules through these contacts. Negative selection occurs by deletion of self-reactive T cells. Autoantigens are presented by medullary thymic epithelial cells, interdigitating cells, and macrophages at the corticomedullary junction. Cells expressing CD4 or CD8 subsequently exit to the periphery.

Cells that have escaped negative selection in the thymus are still subject to control in the periphery, because some self-reactive CD4+ T cells that are not deleted by negative

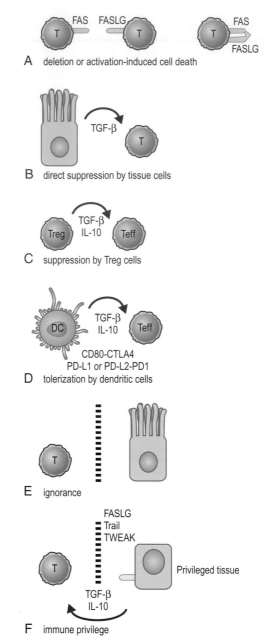

Figure 1-5 Multiple mechanisms of immune tolerance. **A.** Direct deletion of immune effector cell by expression of death-inducing ligands. **B.** Direct tolerization of effector T cells by suppressive cytokines released by tissue cells. **C.** Suppression of effector T cells by regulatory T cells. **D.** Tolerization of host T cells by tolerizing dendritic cells. **E.** Ignorance of effector mechanisms as a result of spatial separation of T cells and tissue cells, such as by basement membranes between the epithelium and immune cells in asthma. **F.** Immune privilege refers to certain sites in the body that can tolerate the introduction of antigen without eliciting an inflammatory immune response. These sites include the eyes, the placenta and fetus, and the testicles. Tissue cells in these organs use many mechanisms to suppress or delete highly activated effector cells that can damage these tissues. CTLA4, cytotoxic T lymphocyte–associated protein 4; DC, dendritic cell; FAS, member of the tumor necrosis factor receptor superfamily, member 6; FASLG, FAS ligand; IL, interleukin; PD-L1, programmed death-ligand 1; PD-L2, programmed death-ligand 2; PD-1, programmed cell death 1; T, T cell; Teff, effector T cell; TGF-β, transforming growth factor β; Trail, tumor necrosis factor (ligand) superfamily, member 10; TWEAK, tumor necrosis factor (ligand) superfamily, member 12; Treg, regulatory T cell.

selection develop into central regulatory T (Treg) cells. These central Treg cells circulate in the periphery as mature T cells, and inhibit immune or inflammatory responses against self-antigens.

Peripheral Tolerance

There are multiple mechanisms of peripheral immune tolerance (Fig. 1-5). These mechanisms prevent overactivation of immune system which cause intensive tissue inflammation. The fundamental strategy of immunotherapy for allergic diseases is to correct dysregulated immune responses by inducing peripheral allergen tolerance.

During inflammation, apoptosis of immune effector cells is induced by neighbor cells' death-inducing ligands. Immune effector cells can undergo apoptosis by expressing death receptors and ligands simultaneously. To keep tissue inflammation at low levels, effector T cells are directly tolerized by suppressive cytokines released by tissue cells. Treg cells suppress effector T cells. DCs induce tolerization of host T cells. In asthma, spatial separation of T cells and tissue cells, such as the presence of a basement membrane between the epithelium and immune cells, results in ignorance of effector mechanisms. Tissue cells in organs with immune privilege use many mechanisms to suppress or delete highly activated effector cells that could otherwise damage these tissues.

During an immune response, CD4$^+$ T cells normally receive signals activated through engagement of the TCR, which recognizes peptides of specific antigens presented on the surface of APCs by MHC class II molecules. Costimulatory receptors, such as CD28, CD2, and inducible costimulator (ICOS) recognize ligands, such as B7 proteins, CD80, CD86, lymphocyte function-associated antigen 3 (LFA-3), and ICOS ligand (ICOSL) expressed on the surface of APCs. These costimulatory receptors contribute to activation of the T cell. When T cells receive stimulus only through the TCR without any engagement of costimulatory receptors, they enter into a state of unresponsiveness. This state has been called *T cell anergy*.

Immune Effector Cells and Molecules

Regulatory T Cells

Although various types of cell contribute to establishing immune tolerance, CD4$^+$FOXP3$^+$ regulatory T (Treg) cells play a central role in immune control in the periphery. Two broad categories of Treg cells have been described: naturally occurring Treg cells and antigen-induced Treg cells that secrete inhibitory cytokines, such as IL-10 and TGF-β. In allergic disease, the balance between allergen-specific Treg cells and disease-promoting helper Th2 cells appears to determine whether an allergic or healthy immune response against allergen occurs. In healthy individuals, predominant Treg cells are specific for common environmental allergens, indicating a state of natural tolerance.

Transforming Growth Factor-β (TGF-β)

TGF-β is associated with the resolution of immune responses and the induction of Treg cell populations (Table 1-3). However, the effects of TGF-β in allergic disease are complex, with evidence of both disease inhibition and promotion. TGF-β can inhibit human Th2 responses in-vitro. In a murine model, overexpression of TGF-β1 in OVA-specific CD4$^+$ T cells abolished airway hyperresponsiveness and airway inflammation induced by OVA-specific Th2 cells.

On the other hand, in a mouse model exhibiting properties of chronic asthma, blockade of TGF-β significantly reduced peribronchiolar extracellular matrix deposition, airway smooth muscle cell proliferation, and mucus production in the lung without affecting established airway inflammation or Th2 cytokine production. TGF-β1 may be involved in a negative feedback mechanism to control airway inflammation and repair of asthmatic airways, inducing remodeling and fibrosis to exaggerate disease development in humans.

Interleukin-10 (IL-10)

IL-10 plays a role in the control of allergy and asthma. IL-10 inhibits many effector cells and disease processes, and its levels are inversely correlated with disease incidence

TABLE 1-3   Functions of Interleukin-10 and Transforming Growth Factor-β

Cell Type	IL-10	TGF-β
Dendritic cells	Inhibits DC maturation, reducing MHC class II and costimulatory ligand expression Inhibits proinflammatory cytokine secretion Inhibits APC function for induction of T cell proliferation and cytokine production (Th1 and Th2)	Promotes Langerhans cell development Inhibits dendritic cell maturation and antigen presentation Downregulates FcεRI expression on Langerhans cells
T cells	Suppresses allergen-specific Th1 and Th2 cells Blocks B7/CD28 costimulatory pathway on T cells	Promotes T cell survival Inhibits proliferation, differentiation, and effector function, including allergen-specific Th1 and Th2 cells Promotes the Th17 lineage
B cells and immunoglobulin E	Enhances survival Promotes Ig production, including IgG4 Suppresses allergen-specific IgE	Inhibits proliferation Induces apoptosis of immature or naïve B cells Inhibits most Ig class switching Switch factor for IgA Suppresses allergen-specific IgE
CD25$^+$ Tregs	Indirect effect on the generation	Upregulates FOXP3 Promotes generation in the periphery Potential effects on homeostasis
IL-10-secreting Tregs	Promotes induction of IL-10-secreting Tregs	Can promote IL-10 synthesis
Monocytes and macrophages	Inhibits proinflammatory cytokine production and antigen presentation	Inhibits scavenger and effector functions, including proinflammatory cytokine production and antigen presentation Promotes chemotaxis
Eosinophils	Inhibits survival and cytokine production	Chemoattractant
Mast cells	Inhibits mast cell activation, including cytokine production	Promotes chemotaxis Variable effects on other functions May inhibit expression of FcεR (receptor 1)
Neutrophils	Inhibits chemokine and proinflammatory cytokine production	Potent chemoattractant

APC, antigen-presenting cell; DC, dendritic cells; FcεR, Fc fragment of IgE receptor; FOXP3, Forkhead box P3 protein; Ig, immunoglobulin; IL, interleukin; MHC, major histocompatibility complex; TGF-β, transforming growth factor-β; Th, helper T cell subset; Treg, regulatory T cell.

and severity. IL-10 is synthesized by a wide range of cell types, including B cells, monocytes, DCs, NK cells, and T cells. It inhibits proinflammatory cytokine production and Th1 and Th2 cell activation, which is likely attributable to the effects of IL-10 on APCs and its direct effects on T cell function (Table 1-3).

IL-10 levels inversely correlate with the incidence and severity of asthmatic disease in the lung. In addition, the levels of IL-10 inversely correlate with skin-prick test reactivity to allergens. Beekeepers, who undergo multiple bee stings and are naturally tolerant to bee venom allergen have a high IL-10 response. IL-10 and IL-10-producing Treg and Breg cells play essential roles in immune tolerance to allergens. In addition, the roles of Treg and Breg cells and IL-10 have been shown in many autoimmune, organ transplantation, tumor tolerance conditions.[6]

CYTOKINES AND CHEMOKINES IN ALLERGIC INFLAMMATION

Cytokines in allergic inflammation

Interleukin-4 (IL-4)

In addition to T helper lymphocytes, IL-4 is derived from basophils, NK T cells, ILC2 mast cells, and eosinophils (Table 1-4). IL-4 induces immunoglobulin isotype switch from IgM to IgE. IL-4 has important influences on T lymphocyte growth, differentiation, and survival. As discussed later, IL-4 establishes the differentiation of naive Th0 lymphocytes into the Th2 phenotype.

TABLE 1-4   Sources of Interleukins IL-4 and IL-13

Cell source	IL-4	IL-13
T helper lymphocytes		
Naive T cells	No	No
T follicular helper (Tfh) cells	Yes	No
Th2 cells	Yes	Yes
Natural killer (NK) T cells	Yes	Yes
Basophils	Yes	Yes
Eosinophils	Yes	Yes
Mast cells	Yes	Yes
Type 2 innate lymphoid cells (ILC2)	Yes	Yes

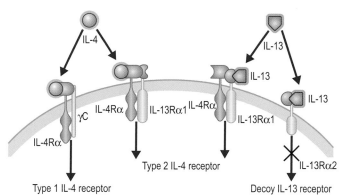

Figure 1-6 IL-4 and IL-13 receptors. Type 1 IL-4 receptors are heterodimers of IL-4Rα interacting with the shared γC chain and bind only IL-4. Their unique expression on most T helper cells and mast cells renders these cells only responsive to IL-4. Type 2 receptors can bind both IL-4 and IL-13. They are more widely expressed and consist of heterodimers of IL-4Rα and IL-13Rα1. In addition, IL-13 can bind to the IL-13Rα2, which lacks a cytoplasmic domain and thereby functions as a decoy receptor. IL, interleukin.

Another important activity of IL-4 is its ability to induce expression of vascular cell adhesion molecule-1 (VCAM-1) on endothelial cells. This enhances adhesiveness of endothelium for T cells, eosinophils, basophils, and monocytes, but not neutrophils, as a characteristic of allergic reactions. IL-4 receptors are present on mast cells, where they function to stimulate IgE receptor expression, along with the expression of the enzyme leukotriene C_4 (LTC$_4$) synthase. Functional IL-4 receptors are heterodimers consisting of the IL-4Rα chain interacting with either the shared γ chain or the IL-13Rα1 chain (Fig. 1-6). This shared use of the IL-4Rα chain by IL-4 and IL-13 and the activation by this chain of the signaling protein STAT6 serve to explain many of the common biologic activities of these two cytokines.

Interleukin-5 (IL-5)

IL-5 is the most important eosinophilopoietin and also can induce basophil differentiation. In addition to stimulating eosinophil production, IL-5 is chemotactic for eosinophils and activates mature eosinophils, inducing secretion and enhancing their cytotoxicity. IL-5 promotes accumulation of eosinophils through its ability to upregulate responses to chemokines and $\alpha_d\beta_2$ integrins on eosinophils, thereby promoting their adherence to VCAM-1-expressing endothelial cells. IL-5 prolongs eosinophil survival by blocking apoptosis.

Interleukin-9 (IL-9)

The primary source of IL-9 is the T helper lymphocyte population, including Th2 cells, with additional amounts coming from mast cells ILC2 and eosinophils. IL-9 contributes to mast cell–mediated allergic responses through its ability to stimulate production of mast cell proteases, inflammatory cytokines, and chemokines. Additionally, IL-9 primes mast cells to respond to allergens by increasing their expression of FcεRIα. IL-9 synergizes with IL-4 to enhance production of IgE and memory B cell differentiation. The same synergy leads to enhanced IL-5 production resulting in greater numbers and maturation of immature eosinophil precursors. IL-9 acts on airway epithelial cells by inducing T cell and eosinophil chemotactic factors, such as CCL11 (eotaxin), CCL2 (MCP-1), CCL3 (MIP-1α), and CCL7 (MCP-3).

Interleukin-13 (IL-13)

IL-13 is homologous to IL-4 and shares many of its biologic activities on mononuclear phagocytic cells, endothelial cells, epithelial cells, and B cells. Thus, IL-13 induces IgE isotype switch and VCAM-1 expression. Biologic activities of IL-4 and IL-13 are additionally distinguished by their distinct cellular sources (Table 1-4). IL-13, acting through this hormonal mechanism, causes mucus hypersecretion and non-specific airway hyperreactivity (AHR), and its expression results in the characteristic airway metaplasia of asthma, with the replacement of epithelial cells with goblet cells. The importance of IL-13 in presentations of asthma associated with a robust IL-13 signature is supported by the efficacy of IL-13–targeting therapies in this endotype.

Interleukin-25 (IL-25)

IL-25 is a member of the IL-17 family (IL-17E), but because of its unique spectrum of activities, it has been given this distinct nomenclature. Binding of IL-25 occurs via a heterodimer complex composed of IL-17RB and IL-17RA.[7] It is mainly derived from epithelial cells. The production of IL-25 by injured epithelial cells is an important innate immune signal driving Th2 immune deviation in the subsequent adaptive immune response. IL-25 stimulates release of IL-4, IL-5, and IL-13 from Th2 lymphocytes but, of note, also drives IL-5 and IL-13 secretion from type 2 innate lymphoid cells (ILC2).

Interleukin-33 (IL-33)

IL-33 is a member of the IL-1 superfamily (in which it is designated IL-1F11) that signals through an IL-1 receptor-related protein (originally termed ST2) and its co-receptor IL-1RAcP.[8]

IL-33 is primarily expressed by bronchial epithelial cells, with additional sources including fibroblasts and smooth muscle cells and it is also inducible in lung and dermal fibroblasts, keratinocytes, activated DCs, and macrophages. IL-33 receptors are expressed on T cells (specifically, Th2-like cells), macrophages, hematopoietic stem cells, eosinophils, basophils, mast cells, ILC2 and fibroblasts. As discussed, IL-33 enhances cytokine secretion by Th2 cells and, like IL-25, induces IL-5 and IL-13 secretion by ILC2.

Thymic Stromal Lymphopoietin (TSLP)

TSLP is another important contributor to Th2 immune deviation.[9] TSLP is expressed by epithelial cells of the skin, gut and lung, and primes resident DCs in such a way as to promote Th2 cytokine production by their subsequently engaged effector T cells. High levels of TSLP are found in the keratinocytes of patients with atopic dermatitis and in the lungs of asthmatic patients. The TSLP receptor is a heterodimer composed of a unique TSLP-specific receptor and the IL-7Rα chain (CD127). TSLP receptors are expressed primarily by DCs, but their expression by mast cells Th2 cells and ILC2 also promotes secretion of Th2 signature cytokines.

The role of IL-25, IL-33, and TSLP in promoting a Th2-associated milieu is summarized in Figure 1-7. In this model, injured epithelium has a central role in driving allergic inflammation through its ability to produce these cytokines. TSLP acts primarily on DCs to drive them to induce a Th2-like process. In addition, both IL-25 and IL-33 act directly on mast cells to drive their repertoire of Th2-associated cytokines. More

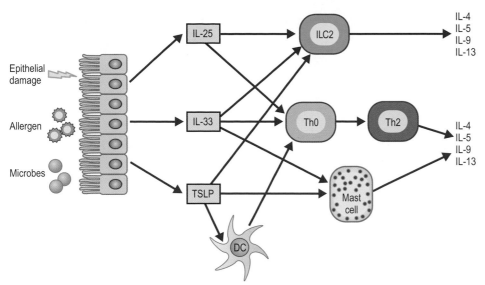

Figure 1-7 Epithelium-derived cytokines in Th2 differentiation and allergic inflammation. The interleukins IL-25 and IL-33 and thymic stromal lymphopoietin (TSLP) are produced by injured epithelium and play critical roles in driving expression of Th2 cytokines. TSLP acts on dendritic cells to direct them to promote the differentiation of naive T cells into Th2 cells. By contrast, IL-25 and IL-33 act directly on the naive T cells to promote Th2 immune deviation. In addition, these three cytokines can generate a Th2 cytokine milieu independent of the adaptive immune system. TSLP and IL-33 directly induce the full repertoire of Th2 cytokine secretion from mast cells. Similarly, IL-25, TSLP and IL-33 act on type 2 innate lymphoid cells (ILC2) to drive their more restricted secretion of IL-5 and IL-13.

important, IL-25, TSLP and IL-33 act on ILC2 to increase their selective production of IL-5 and IL-13. These actions on ILC2 and mast cells can occur independent of ongoing allergen exposure, suggesting a mechanism for allergen-independent perpetuation of allergic inflammation.

Chemokines in Allergic Diseases

Asthma

Asthma is a chronic inflammatory lung disease characterized by airway inflammation, mucus hypersecretion, and bronchial hyperresponsiveness. The cellular inflammatory infiltrate in asthma is composed of eosinophils, lymphocytes, mast cells, and to a varying extent, basophils and neutrophils.

Airway exposure to proteases from common allergens, such as mites and molds, disrupts airway epithelial integrity and induces epithelial TSLP production (Fig. 1-8). TSLP expands the number of basophils, prolongs eosinophil survival, and increases eosinophil production of CCL2, CXCL1, and CXCL8. Two other epithelial cytokines, IL-25 and IL-33, also are produced on allergen exposure or epithelial damage. IL-25 and IL-33 upregulate the production of TSLP by epithelial cells and mast cells; induce mast cell release of IL-4, IL-5, IL-13, CCL1 and CXCL8; promote eosinophil survival; and enhance eosinophil production of CCL2 and CCL3. Activated basophils release IL-4, IL-13, granulocyte-macrophage colony-stimulating factor (GM-CSF), and CCL3 as well as histamine and leukotriene C_4 (LTC$_4$), which causes vasodilation and increases vascular permeability. Activated eosinophils generate IL-3, IL-4, IL-5, tumor necrosis factor-α (TNF-α), LTC$_4$, platelet-activating factor (PAF), CCL3, CCL5, and CCL11. In addition to tryptase and chymase, activated mast cells are also a significant source of histamine, lipid mediators (LTB$_4$, PGD$_2$), cytokines (IL-3, IL-5, IL-13, IL-6, IL-10, TNF-α, GM-CSF), and chemokines (CCL1, CCL2, CCL3, CCL5, CCL17, CCL22, CXCL8).

Activation and differentiation of naive T cells into Th2 cells are marked by downregulation of L-selectin and CCR7 and appearance of CCR4, CCR8, CRTh2, and the

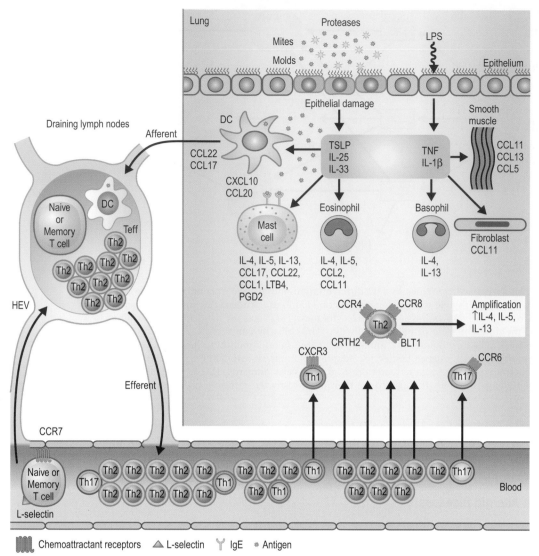

Figure 1-8 Chemokines and asthma. Asthma is characterized by the infiltration of lung tissue with T helper type 2 (Th2) cells producing IL-4, IL-5, and IL-13. Allergen proteases disrupt airway epithelial integrity and induce thymic stromal lymphopoietin (TSLP), IL-25, and IL-33, whilst epithelial TLR activation leads to IL-1β and TNF production. These cytokines upregulate CC chemokine and Th2 cytokine production and release by smooth muscle cells, fibroblasts, mast cells, eosinophils, and basophils. Activated antigen-presenting cells travel to the draining lymph nodes and promote the generation of Th2 cells, which enter the lung and release more Th2 cytokines, thus amplifying the allergic response in the lung. LPS, lipopolysaccharide.

BLT1 receptor for leukotriene B_4 (LTB_4). These receptors enable Th2 cells to move down the concentration gradient in response to CCL17, CCL22, CCL1, prostaglandin D_2 (PGD_2), and LTB_4, mediators released by DCs and activated mast cells. IL-4 and IL-13 induce lung-residing macrophages, DCs, epithelial cells, and endothelial cells to produce CCL11, CCL24, CCL26, CCL1, CCL17, and CCL22, thus amplifying the allergic inflammatory response by attracting more eosinophils and Th2 cells.

Atopic Dermatitis

Atopic dermatitis is a pruritic chronic inflammatory disease of the skin in which CD4+ memory T lymphocytes, dendritic cell (DC) subsets, eosinophils, and mast cells infiltrate the perivascular, subepidermal, and intraepidermal areas. A number of chemokines are aberrantly expressed in the skin of patients with atopic dermatitis and help recruit the inflammatory infiltrate in this disorder. These include CCR2 and CCR3 ligands (CCL13, CCL11, and CCL26) for eosinophil and mast cell recruitment, CCR4 and CCR8 ligands

(CCL22 and CCL1) for Th2 cell recruitment, CCR10 ligand (CCL27) for T cell entry into the epidermis, and CCL18.

The pathophysiology of atopic dermatitis begins with intense pruritus and the mechanical injury that results from chronic scratching (Fig. 1-9). Mechanical trauma can directly activate mast cells, which release histamine, neuropeptides, proteases, kinins, and cytokines, many of which further exacerbate pruritus. Furthermore, TSLP levels increase acutely in the skin after mechanical trauma. TSLP induces DC activation and DC production of CCL17 and CCL22.

The trafficking of memory T cells into the skin requires cutaneous lymphocyte antigen (CLA), which interacts with E-selectin on inflamed endothelium, and initiates rolling. The trafficking molecules most highly expressed by T cells isolated from healthy skin are CLA, CCR4, and CCR6 (>80–90%) and to a lesser extent CCR8 (50%). Whereas

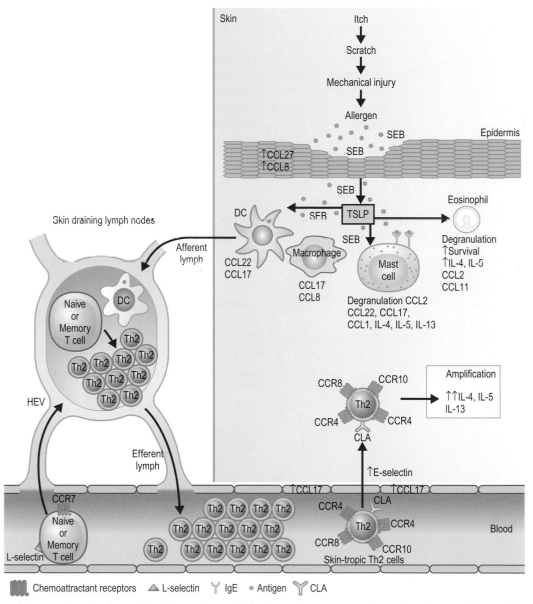

Figure 1-9 Chemokines and atopic dermatitis. Atopic dermatitis begins with intense pruritus, chronic scratching, and mechanical injury to the skin. Mechanical trauma leads to mast cell release of Th2 cytokines and CC chemokines and upregulates local TSLP production, whilst loss of normal barrier function increases exposure to allergens and SEB. TSLP-activated dendritic cells travel to the draining lymph nodes and promote Th2 cell differentiation. Th2 cells enter the skin and release Th2 cytokines, thus amplifying the allergic response in the skin.

the ligands for CCR6 and CCR8 are upregulated in inflammation, skin endothelial cells and keratinocytes constitutively express CCL17 (one of the ligands for CCR4) and CCL27 (only known ligand for CCR10), respectively.

Eczema lesions as the hallmark of atopic dermatitis and allergic contact dermatitis lesions are induced by keratinocyte apoptosis, related to IFN-γ, Fas-Fas-ligand interaction, TNF-α, TNF-related weak inducer of apoptosis (TWEAK) and IL-32.[10,11]

BIOLOGY OF IMMUNE CELLS

T Lymphocytes

Two classes of α/β T lymphocytes that bear the co-receptors CD4 or CD8 are involved in adaptive immune responses. CD4$^+$ T cells are traditionally called helper T (Th) cells, because they activate and direct other immune cells. There are also populations of CD4$^+$ regulatory T (Treg) cells that modulate immune responses. CD4$^+$ T cells recognize antigen presented by class II MHC molecules on APCs, including dendritic cells, B cells, and macrophages. Exogenous protein antigens are taken up by APCs and processed into peptides in endocytic vesicles, which are presented on the cell surface bound to class II MHC molecules. The CD8$^+$ cytotoxic T cells (CTLs) recognize antigen presented on MHC class I molecules. Class I MHC molecules are present on the surface of all nucleated cells. Their cytotoxic functions are carried out by release of preformed effector molecules and by interactions of cell surface molecules.

Antigen-activated CD4$^+$ T cells have the potential to differentiate into effector cells, each with distinct functional properties conferred by the pattern of cytokines they secrete (Fig. 1-10).[12] *Helper T type 1* (Th1) cells are a subset of CD4$^+$ T cells that secrete IFN-γ, whereas *helper T type 2* (Th2) cells produce IL-4, IL-5, IL-9, IL-10, and IL-13. *Helper T type 17* (Th17) cells produce IL-17A, IL-17F, and IL-22. Treg cells produce IL-10 and transforming TGF-β1, are naturally occurring and induced, suppress T cell differentiation and APC activation, and are not considered effector cells. Th1 cells stimulate strong cell-mediated immune responses, particularly against intracellular pathogens. Th2 cells

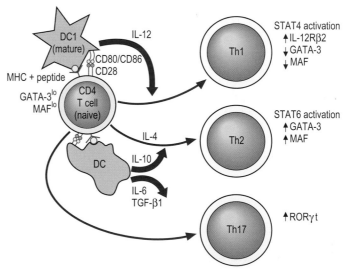

Figure 1-10 Generation of helper T cell types 1, 2, and 17 (Th1, Th2, and Th17) from a naive CD4$^+$ T cell. A naive CD4$^+$ T cell does not secrete cytokines and has low expression levels of transcription factors GATA-3 and MAF. Differentiation along the Th1, Th2, or Th17 pathway is triggered by stimulation by antigen presented to the T cell receptor in the context of the major histocompatibility complex (MHC) by the appropriate antigen-presenting cell (APC) and a second signal imparted by ligation of costimulatory molecules CD80/CD86 and CD28. Dendritic cells (DCs) represent the key APCs for naive T cells. Those that produce interleukin-10 (IL-10) favor Th2 differentiation, and those that produce interleukin-12 (IL-12) stimulate Th1 differentiation. Th17 cells can be generated in the presence of interleukin-6 (IL-6) and transforming growth factor-β1 (TGF-β1), presumably produced by DCs.

are elicited in immune responses that require a strong humoral component and in anti-parasitic responses. Th17 serve critical host defense functions at mucosal surfaces.

Cytokines are the primary factors that influence the CD4+ Th cell generation and are considered the third signal in CD4+ T cell differentiation.[6] IFN-γ and IL-12 stimulate the induction of Th1 cells. IL-4 drives Th2 cell generation by direct action on CD4+ T cells. IL-13 is involved in the induction of Th2 cells by an unknown mechanism, although not through direct effects on CD4+ T cells. IL-6, IL-1β, TGF-β1, and in some situations, IL-23 promote Th17 development.

In the secondary lymphoid tissue, a naive T cell differentiates into an effector cell. Compared with naive T cells, effector cells do not require costimulation to be activated, allowing these cells to respond to antigen with hair-trigger rapidity to produce high levels of cytokines and chemokines, which then direct the immune response. Most activated effector CD4+ T cells die subsequent to an immune response through the process of activation-induced cell death, but a subset of CD4+ T cells will persist as memory cells for the life of the host. CD4+ memory T cells persist in lymphoid organs as central memory cells and in non-lymphoid tissues as effector memory cells. The effector memory T cells respond rapidly to repeat exposures to antigen, whereas central memory T cells are slower to be mobilized.

B Lymphocytes

The humoral immune response is generated by B cells. Mature B cells express immunoglobulin on its cell surface, which constitutes the antigen-specific B cell receptor (BCR). BCR is a molecular complex made up of antigen-binding or variable (V) regions. This region of the protein varies amongst immunoglobulins, allowing each antibody to bind to any foreign structure that the individual may encounter. To generate this diverse immunoglobulin repertoire, during development in the bone marrow, B cells undergo somatic deoxyribonucleic acid (DNA) recombination of the variability (V), diversity (D), and joining (J) regions of the immunoglobulin heavy and light chains. The invariant or constant region of the antibody is specialized for different effector functions in the immune system after antibody is secreted. There are five main constant-region forms: IgM, IgD, IgG, IgE, and IgA. The BCR in the membrane-bound form recognizes and binds antigen and transmits activation signals into the cell.

Naive B cells recirculate through peripheral lymphoid tissues until it binds specific antigen through surface immunoglobulin and is activated (i.e., signal 1). Most antibody responses, including antibody responses to protein antigens, require antigen-specific T cell help. Antigen bound to surface immunoglobulin is internalized, processed, complexed with MHC class II molecules, and displayed on the cell surface. Previously primed CD4+ T cells that recognize the peptide-MHC class II complex on the B cell provide the second signal for activation. The cytokines secreted by CD4+ helper T cells during B cell activation regulate, which immunoglobulin heavy-chain constant regions will be selected during class-switch recombination to best serve the functions of the specific immune response. Th2 responses to allergens stimulate B cell activation and result in elevated levels of allergen-specific IgE.

Type 2 Innate Lymphoid Cells

Populations of lymphoid cells that lack rearranged antigen receptors, which were called *innate lymphoid cells* (ILC), have been recently identified. These ILC populations can be divided into three groups, based on shared phenotypic and functional properties like T cells. Type 1 ILC (ILC1) constitutively express T-bet and are able to produce IFN-γ upon activation. Type 2 ILC (ILC2) constitutively express GATA-3 and in response to IL-25, IL-33 and TSLP stimulation produce IL-5 and IL-13. Type 3 ILC (ILC3) constitutively express ROR-γ and in response to IL-1β and IL-23 produce IL-17, IL-22 and IFN-γ.[13] ILC2 appear to control the mucosal environment through production of cytokines and induction of chemokines that recruit suitable cell populations to promote Th2 development.

Antigen-Presenting Dendritic Cells

Dendritic cells (DCs) are the most important antigen-presenting cells found throughout the body and are mainly recognized for their exceptional potential to generate a primary immune response and sensitization to allergens. DCs determine the T cell polarization process that produces Th1 cells (generating mainly IFN-γ), Th2 cells (generating mainly IL-4, IL-5, and IL-13), Th17 cells (generating mainly IL-17), and regulatory T (Treg) cells (generating mainly IL-10 and TGF-β). These cells are also recognized for their ability to produce ongoing effector responses that are crucial in maintaining allergic inflammation. In humans, circulating DCs can be broadly divided into two groups: (1) myeloid dendritic cells (mDCs) and (2) plasmacytoid dendritic cells (pDCs). Both subsets express a different repertoire of TLRs and display a diverse cytokine signature after microbial stimulation. mDCs selectively express TLR2-6 and -8 and respond to bacterial and viral infections by producing large amounts of IL-12. In contrast, pDCs constitutively express the endosome-associated TLR7 and TLR9, and they are the main producers of type 1 interferons in humans.[14]

Mast Cells

Mast cells are present throughout connective tissues and mucosal surfaces and are especially prominent at the interface with the external environment, such as the skin, respiratory tract, conjunctiva, and gastrointestinal tract. Mast cells contribute to the maintenance of tissue homeostasis, with important roles in wound repair, revascularization, and protective responses to bacterial infection and envenomation. Their 'misguided' activation by allergens contributes to the development of allergic symptoms.

The best-studied mechanism of mast cell activation, and the one considered most relevant to allergic disease, is activation mediated through the high-affinity IgE receptor FcεRI. IgE-dependent signaling in vivo is initiated when multivalent allergen binds to allergen-specific IgE bound to the FcεRIα chain. IgE-dependent activation of the mast cell induces granule swelling, crystal dissolution, and granule fusion. This sequence is followed by exocytosis with release of mediators into the extracellular space—a process termed anaphylactic degranulation. In addition to the stored granule-derived mediators, newly formed metabolites of arachidonic acid also are released from mast cells after IgE-dependent activation (Table 1-5).

Basophils

Basophil granulocytes develop in the bone marrow and are released into the circulation as mature end-stage cells representing less than 1% of blood leukocytes. Basophils play a critical role in allergic disease by infiltrating sites of allergic inflammation and releasing mediators and cytokines that perpetuate type I (immediate) hypersensitivity reactions. Degranulation events resulting in the release of these mediators are preceded by the interaction of allergen with specific IgE molecules bound to the high-affinity IgE receptors on the surface of these cells. This IgE-dependent activation also leads to the production of immunomodulatory cytokines. In particular, basophils are a significant source of IL-4 and IL-13, two Th2 cytokines, whose expression is characteristic of allergic lesions and which are now considered critical components in the pathogenesis of allergic disease.

Eosinophils

Eosinophils are bone marrow–derived granulocytes that play an important pathophysiologic role in a wide range of conditions, including asthma and related allergic diseases and parasitic helminth infections. Eosinophils are unique amongst circulating leukocytes in their prodigious capacity to produce a variety of mediators, including granule proteins, cytokines, lipids, oxidative products, and enzymes (Table 1-6). Eosinophils express receptors recognizing the Fc portion of various immunoglobulins (FcR). Beads coated with IgA or secretory IgA (sIgA) induce degranulation of eosinophils, and

TABLE 1-5 Classical Preformed and Newly Generated Human Mast Cell Autacoid Mediators and Proteases with Examples of their Biologic Effects

Mediator	Activity
Histamine (stored)	Bronchoconstriction; tissue edema; ↑vascular permeability; ↑ mucus secretion; ↑ fibroblast proliferation; ↑ collagen synthesis; ↑ endothelial cell proliferation, dendritic cell differentiation and activation
Heparin (stored)	Anticoagulant; mediator storage matrix; sequesters growth factors; fibroblast activation; endothelial cell migration
Tryptase (stored)	Degrades respiratory allergens and cross-linked IgE; generates C3a and bradykinin; degrades neuropeptides; TGF-β activation; increases basal heart rate and ASM contractility; ↑ fibroblast proliferation and collagen synthesis; epithelial ICAM-1 expression and CXCL8 release; potentiation of mast cell histamine release; neutrophil recruitment
Chymase (stored)	↑ mucus secretion; ECM degradation, type I procollagen processing; converts angiotensin I to angiotensin II; ↓ T cell adhesion to airway smooth muscle; activates IL-1β, degrades IL-4, releases membrane-bound SCF
PGD$_2$ (synthesized)	Bronchoconstriction; tissue edema; ↑ mucus secretion; dendritic cell activation; chemotaxis of eosinophils, Th2 cells, and basophils via the CRTH2 (CD294) receptor
LTC$_4$/LTD$_4$ (synthesized)	Bronchoconstriction; tissue edema; ↑ mucus secretion; enhances IL-13-dependent airway smooth muscle proliferation; dendritic cell maturation and recruitment; eosinophil IL-4 secretion; mast cell IL-5, IL-8, and TNF-α secretion; tissue fibrosis

ASM, airway smooth muscle; CRTH2, chemoattractant receptor of Th2 cells; ECM, extracellular matrix; ICAM-1, intercellular adhesion molecule 1; IgE, immunoglobulin E; IL, interleukin; LTC$_4$, leukotriene C$_4$; LTD$_4$, leukotriene D$_4$; PAF, platelet-activating factor; PGD$_2$, prostaglandin D$_2$; SCF, stem cell factor; TGF-β, transforming growth factor-β; TNF-α, tumor necrosis factor-α.

TABLE 1-6 Eosinophil Mediators

Granule proteins	Cytokines*
Major basic protein (MBP)	IL-1α
MBP homolog (MBP2)	IL-2
Eosinophil cationic protein (ECP)	IL-3
Eosinophil-derived neurotoxin (EDN)	IL-4
Eosinophil peroxidase (EPX)	IL-5
Charcot–Leyden crystal (CLC) protein	IL-6
Secretory phospholipase A$_2$ (sPLA$_2$)	IL-9
Bactericidal/permeability-inducing protein (BPI)	IL-10
Acid phosphatase	IL-11
Arylsulfatase	IL-12
β-Glucuronidase	IL-13
	IL-16
Lipid mediators	Leukemia inhibitory factor (LIF)
	Interferon-γ (IFN-γ)
Leukotriene B$_4$ (negligible)	Tumor necrosis factor-α (TNF-α)
Leukotriene C$_4$	GM-CSF
5-HETE	APRIL
5,15- and 8,15-diHETE	
5-oxo-15-hydroxy-6,8,11,13-ETE	**Chemokines**
Platelet-activating factor (PAF)	
Prostaglandin E$_1$ and E$_2$	CXCL8 (IL-8)
Thromboxane B$_2$	CCL2 (MCP-1)
	CCL3 (MIP-1α)
Oxidative products	CCL5 (RANTES)
	CCL7 (MCP-3)
Superoxide radical anion (OH$^-$)	CCL11 (eotaxin)
Hydrogen peroxide (H$_2$O$_2$)	CCL13 (ECP-4)
Hypohalous acids	
	Growth factors
Enzymes	
	Nerve growth factor (NGF)
Collagenase	Platelet-derived growth factor (PDGF)
Metalloproteinase-9	Stem cell factor (SCF)
Indoleamine 2,3-dioxygenase (IDO)	Transforming growth factor (TGF-α, TGF-β)

APRIL, a proliferation-inducing ligand; ETE, eicosatetraenoic acid; GM-CSF, granulocyte-macrophage colony-stimulating factor; HETE, hydroxyeicosatetraenoic acid; IL, interleukin.
*Physiologic significance of these cytokines needs to be confirmed.

eosinophils from allergic individuals display enhanced FcαR expression. However, most reports suggest that ligation of FcεRI does not result in measurable eosinophil degranulation. Exposure of eosinophils ex vivo to various cytokines mimics in vivo primed eosinophils. IL-5 activates LTC_4 and O_2^- generation, phagocytosis, and helminthotoxic activity, as well as Ig-induced degranulation. Both TSLP and IL-33 activate eosinophil effector functions, such as adhesion to matrix proteins, cytokine production, and degranulation.

CONTRIBUTION OF STRUCTURAL CELLS TO ALLERGIC INFLAMMATIONS

Introduction

Whilst structural cells, such as epithelial, bone, smooth muscle cells or fibroblast, have their proper function, they produce cytokines, chemokines, lipid mediators, and growth factors which control mobility of immune cells and local inflammatory milieu. Symptoms of allergic airway disease, such as sneezing, rhinorrhea, unproductive coughing, episodic bronchospasm, and sensations of breathlessness, are neuronally mediated in response to inflammation. Accordingly, these structural cells play crucial roles in the pathogenesis and symptoms of allergic disease and asthma in concert with immune cells.

Airway Epithelial Cells

The epithelium constitutes the interface between the external environment and the internal milieu of the lung. It is the site of first contact with inhaled particles, pollutants, respiratory viruses, and airborne allergens. Consequently, the epithelium plays an important role as a physical and immune barrier. The epithelium senses pathogen-associated molecular patterns (PAMPs) on inhaled foreign substances via their PRRs and regulates airway homeostasis through the production of a multitude of mediators, such as GM-CSF, TSLP, IL-25, and IL-33, which promote a Th2 bias in dendritic cell precursor (Fig. 1-11). In other words, epithelial cells bridge the innate and adaptive immune responses by translating environmental exposures into disease phenotypes.

Epithelial cell structure and function are abnormal in patients with asthma. At a gross level, the composition of the asthmatic airway epithelium is different from that of the non-asthmatic population. For example, goblet cell hyperplasia and excessive mucus production are common features of asthma that contribute significantly to morbidity and mortality. Moreover, epithelial cells isolated from patients who have asthma have a deficient innate immune response from type I antiviral interferons, particularly of

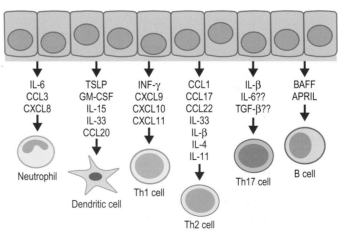

Figure 1-11 Interaction between airway epithelial cell–derived cytokines and inflammatory cells. APRIL, A proliferation-inducing ligand; BAFF, B cell–activating factor of the TNF family; GM-CSF, granulocyte-macrophage colony-stimulating factor; IFN-γ, interferon-γ; IL, interleukin; TGF-β, transforming growth factor-β; Th, helper T cell subset; TSLP, thymic stromal lymphopoietin.

IFN-β release during rhinovirus infection. Changes of epithelial cell structure and function occur early in disease pathogenesis. These findings place the epithelium at the forefront of asthma pathogenesis, and understanding the mechanisms that underlie these abnormalities will have short- and long-term clinical significance for the treatment of this disease.

Epithelial tight junctions (TJ) seal the epithelia and form an essential part of the barrier between the inner tissues and the external environment. They control the paracellular flux and epithelial permeability, and prevent the entrance of foreign particles, such as allergens and toxins to subepithelial tissues. They form complexes with members of the claudin family, the marvel family, and the junctional adhesion molecule (JAM) family spanning the membrane and forming homo- and heterodimeric connections between adjacent cells. Scaffold proteins, such as the zonula occludens (ZO) family link the TJ complex to the actin cytoskeleton. Epithelial barrier TJ defects are reported in several allergic and inflammatory disorders, such as atopic dermatitis, asthma, and chronic rhinosinusitis, and a role for TJ in smooth muscle cells is described in asthma pathogenesis.[15–22]

Airway Smooth Muscle Cells

In asthma, the airway smooth muscle (ASM) contracts in response to multiple stimuli, but it also produces extracellular matrix (ECM) proteins, proteases that modulate these proteins, and myriad growth factors and cytokines. These collectively lead to airway remodeling—the pathology that characterizes asthma and consists of thickening of the airway wall, increased angiogenesis, mucous cell hyperplasia, thickening of the basement membrane, and increased bulk of muscle. It was previously thought that remodeling was a response to chronic airway inflammation, but it seems more likely that inflammation and remodeling develop along separate pathways. This is consistent with the finding that bronchoconstriction alone in the absence of an inflammatory or allergic stimulus can lead to airway remodeling.

ASM is a functional part of the innate immune system. It expresses messenger RNAs (mRNAs) for TLR1 through TLR10 and functional TLR2 and TLR3, indicating ASM can respond to bacterial and viral infections. ASM modulates leukocyte trafficking and function in asthma by activating cell adhesion molecules and secretion of chemokines and cytokines. When the response from cells obtained from people with asthma and people without asthma were compared, higher levels of cytokines and profibrotic factors were observed in the asthma-derived cells.

Neuronal Control of Airway Function

Both the immune system and the nervous system are critical to host defense within the airways. The immune system uses cellular and humoral mechanisms to protect the peripheral air spaces from invasion and colonization by microorganisms. The nervous system protects the airways by orchestrating reflexes, such as sneezing, coughing, mucus secretion, and bronchospasm in response to inflammation. Therefore, the nervous system serves as the principal transducer between immunologic aspects of allergic inflammation and the symptomatology of immediate hypersensitivity.

Nerve-immune interactions can be inappropriate and deleterious, as with allergy; the immune response triggered by allergen exposure can recruit the nervous system in a way that is not beneficial to the host and causes or exacerbates the symptoms of allergic disease: irritation, pruritus, sneezing, coughing, hypersecretion, reversible bronchospasm, and dyspnea. Relatively little is known about the specific pharmacology of allergen-immune-nerve interactions, but the mediators likely include histamine, arachidonic acid metabolites, tryptase, neurotrophins, chemokines, and cytokines. In addition, the allergic reaction in the respiratory tract is associated with overt activation, increases in electrical excitability, as well as phenotypic changes in sensory, central, and autonomic neurons. Future research into the mediators and mechanisms of allergen-induced neuromodulation will not only increase our basic understanding of the pathophysiology of allergic disease, but will also suggest novel therapeutic strategies.

CYTOKINE NETWORKS IN ALLERGIC INFLAMMATION

Cytokines play a key role in the orchestration and perpetuation of allergic inflammation and are now targeted in therapy (Fig. 1-12).[23] Allergic inflammation is characterized by the secretion of Th2 cytokines, including IL-4, IL-5, IL-9, and IL-13, which are secreted mainly by Th2. The use of biologic immune response modifiers that target and neutralize cytokines is beginning to shed new light on the role of individual Th2 cytokines. IL-4 and IL-13 play a key role in IgE synthesis through isotype switching of B cells and appear to play a critical role in animal models of asthma. Thus far, blocking IL-4 and IL-13 or their common receptor IL-4Rα has not yet been shown to be of clinical benefit in asthma, but many clinical trials are currently under way. IL-5 is of critical importance in the differentiation, survival, and priming of eosinophils. A humanized monoclonal IL-5 neutralizing antibody, mepolizumab, induced a profound decrease in eosinophils in the blood and in induced sputum in patients with mild asthma but had no effect on the response to inhaled allergen. Clinical trials of anti-IL-5 in unselected symptomatic asthmatic patients showed no overall clinical improvement. Yet in highly selected patients with severe asthma and sputum eosinophilia, despite high doses of inhaled or oral corticosteroids, mepolizumab decreased the frequency of exacerbations and reduced requirements for oral corticosteroids, although it did not lessen symptoms or AHR. This observation suggests that blockade of individual cytokines may provide clinical benefit only in carefully selected patients.

Several proinflammatory cytokines have been implicated in allergic diseases, including IL-1β, IL-6, TNF-α, and GM-CSF, which are released from a variety of cells, including

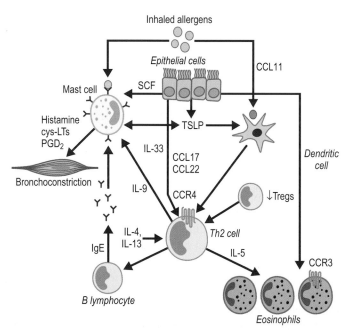

Figure 1-12 Inflammation in allergy. Inhaled allergens activate sensitized mast cells by cross-linking surface-bound immunoglobulin E (IgE) molecules to release several bronchoconstrictor mediators, including cysteinyl leukotrienes (cys-LTs) and prostaglandin D$_2$ (PGD$_2$). Epithelial cells release stem cell factor (SCF) (i.e. Kit ligand), which is important for maintaining mucosal mast cells at the airway or skin surface. Allergens are processed by myeloid dendritic cells, which are conditioned by thymic stromal lymphopoietin (TSLP) secreted by epithelial cells and mast cells to release the chemokines CCL17 and CCL22, which act on CCR4 to attract T helper 2 (Th2) cells. Th2 cells have a central role in orchestrating the inflammatory response in allergy through the release of interleukin (IL)-4 and IL-13 (which stimulate B cells to synthesize IgE), IL-5 (which is necessary for eosinophilic inflammation), and IL-9 (which stimulates mast cell proliferation). Epithelial cells release CCL11, which recruits eosinophils via CCR3. Patients with allergic disease may have a defect in regulatory T cells (Tregs), which may favor further Th2 cell activation. CCL, C-C chemokine ligand; CCR, C-C chemokine receptor.

macrophages and epithelial cells, and may be important in amplifying the allergic inflammatory response. Although available evidence is persuasive that TNF-α may be important in patients with severe asthma, and earlier small clinical studies with anti-TNF-α therapies were promising, a large placebo-controlled trial of an anti-TNF antibody (golimumab) in severe asthma showed no overall benefit. Some of the subjects may have been responders, however, and patients with greater bronchodilator reversibility showed an apparent reduction in exacerbations. IL-17 also is increased in severe asthma, but anti-IL-17 antibodies have not yet been tested in asthma patients.

Interest has now focused on upstream regulatory cytokines in the pathogenesis of asthma because it is thought that they may have greater therapeutic potential. TSLP is an upstream IL-7-like cytokine that may initiate and propagate allergic immune responses and plays an important role in immune responses to helminths. TSLP is produced predominantly by airways and nasal epithelial cells and by skin keratinocytes and also stimulates immature myeloid dendritic cells, which express the heterodimeric TSLP receptor to differentiate into mature dendritic cells. TSLP-activated dendritic cells promote naïve CD4+ T cells to differentiate into a Th2 phenotype and promote the expansion of Th2 memory cells through the release of Th2 chemotactic cytokines CCL17 and CCL22 and expression of the costimulatory molecule OX40 ligand. In addition, TSLP suppresses the IL-12 p40 receptor in dendritic cells and, by suppressing Th1 responses, further enhances Th2 responses. TSLP also promotes allergic inflammation by activating the differentiation IL-4 gene transcription in Th2 cells and the production of IL-13 from mast cells, by recruiting eosinophils and by amplifying responses of basophils. TSLP may therefore play a pivotal role in the initiation of allergic asthma, rhinitis, and atopic dermatitis. It is highly expressed in the airways of asthmatic patients, and its expression is correlated with disease severity and the expression of CCL17. TSLP is also expressed in epithelial cells of patients with allergic rhinitis and atopic dermatitis. Overexpression of TSLP in skin keratinocytes of mice amplifies the inflammatory response of inhaled allergen in sensitized animals, thus providing a mechanism for the 'allergic march' whereby atopic dermatitis commonly precedes the development of asthma in children.

IL-25 (IL-17E) is a member of the IL-17 family of cytokines and induces allergic inflammation through increased production of Th2 cytokines. Although originally shown to be produced by Th2 cells, it is now known to be released from many different cells, including mast cells, basophils, eosinophils, macrophages, and epithelial cells. Blockade of IL-25 is effective in animal models of allergic disease, and blocking antibodies are now in clinical development. IL-33 is another upstream cytokine and a member of the IL-1 family of cytokines, which is unusual in its localization within the nucleus, where it may regulate chromatin structure and gene expression. It appears to be released only on damage to epithelial or endothelial cells, presumably acting as an alarmin, and is constitutively expressed at mucosal surfaces such as the airways. It signals through a receptor, ST2, that activates NF-κB and mitogen-activated protein kinase (MAPK) pathways. Its relevance to allergic inflammation is that it enhances ILC2 and Th2 cell function, leading to eosinophilia, mast cell activation, and mucus hypersecretion, potentially acting as a bridge between innate and adaptive immunity in allergic inflammation. It also directly activates eosinophils, mast cells, epithelial cells, and dendritic cells. It appears to switch alveolar macrophages to the alternatively activated form (M2) that has been found in animal models of asthma with increased secretion of CCL17, although whether this association is relevant to human allergic disease is uncertain. IL-33 shows increased expression in airway epithelium of asthmatic patients, and level of expression is related to disease severity. IL-33 is increased in the skin of patients with atopic dermatitis and is released into the circulation during as well as mediating anaphylactic shock. IL-33 also is expressed in mast cells after activation through IgE receptors and also activates mast cells, providing a means of maintaining mast cell activation. Antibodies that block IL-33 or ST2 are now in clinical development.

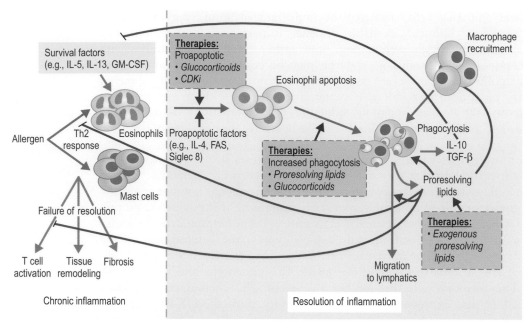

Figure 1-13 Inflammation resolution and therapeutic opportunities. After the initial Th2-mediated proinflammatory events that occur in allergic inflammation and that are characterized by increased eosinophil recruitment, activation, and survival along with mast cell degranulation, progression to the resolution phase of inflammation allows return of normal tissue structure and function. Increasing proapoptotic factors drive eosinophil apoptosis for their timely clearance by macrophages, a process that is controlled by and increases the production of proresolving lipids. Apoptosis can be enhanced through the use of glucocorticoids, which can also increase the phagocytic capacity of macrophages and a variety of proresolving lipids. IL-10 released from a variety of cell types, including macrophages, can indirectly attenuate eosinophil survival and promote resolution. CDKi, cyclin-dependent kinase inhibitor; GM-CSF, granulocyte-macrophage colony-stimulating factor; IL, interleukin; Siglec, sialic acid–binding immunoglobulin-like lectin; TGF-β, transforming growth factor-β; Th2, helper T cell type 2.

RESOLUTION OF ALLERGIC INFLAMMATION AND MAJOR PATHWAYS

Inflammation resolution is a tightly regulated and active process essential for the restoration of tissue homeostasis after an inflammatory insult. Dysregulated resolution results in chronic inflammation, tissue remodeling and fibrosis. Granulocyte apoptosis mediated caspase family proteins is essential for the clearance of these infiltrating inflammatory cells; cell survival is increased during inflammation, and apoptosis is accelerated during the resolution phase.

Phagocytosis of apoptotic cells by macrophages ensures the safe disposal of dead and dying cells without release of toxic intracellular mediators. Engulfment of apoptotic cells signals to the phagocytosing macrophage that inflammation is coming to an end and alters macrophage mediator production from predominantly proinflammatory to pro-resolution, with enhanced production of cytokines with antiinflammatory properties, including IL-10 and TGF-β. This pattern contrasts with macrophage phagocytosis of necrotic eosinophils, which leads to enhanced proinflammatory mediator production such as GM-CSF.

Several proresolving lipids promote and control the resolution phenotype. The delivery of exogenous protectins, lipoxins, and resolvins has increased inflammation resolution and improved clinical outcomes in a variety of allergic murine models. Advances in our understanding of proresolving lipids, granulocyte apoptosis, and phagocytic clearance of dead and dying cells are creating new avenues for generation of novel proresolving agents with which to tackle allergic inflammation (Fig. 1-13).

REFERENCES

1. *Lambrecht BN, Hammad H. The airway epithelium in asthma. Nat Med 2012;18(5):684–92.
2. Joiner KA, Brown EJ, Frank MM. Complement and bacteria: chemistry and biology in host defense. Annu Rev Immunol 1984;2:461–91.

3. Mellor AL, Munn DH. Physiologic control of the functional status of Foxp3+ regulatory T cells. J Immunol 2011;186(8):4535–40.

4. *Pierce SK, Liu W. The tipping points in the initiation of B cell signalling: how small changes make big differences. Nat Rev Immunol 2010;10(11):767–77.

5. Macaubas C, DeKruyff RH, Umetsu DT. Respiratory tolerance in the protection against asthma. Curr Drug Targets Inflamm Allergy 2003;2(2):175–86.

6. *Akdis M, Akdis CA. Mechanisms of allergen-specific immunotherapy: multiple suppressor factors at work in immune tolerance to allergens. J Allergy Clin Immunol 2014;133(3):621–31.

7. Fort MM, Cheung J, Yen D, et al. IL-25 induces IL-4, IL-5, and IL-13 and Th2-associated pathologies in vivo. Immunity 2001;15(6):985–95.

8. *Schmitz J, Owyang A, Oldham E, et al. IL-33, an interleukin-1-like cytokine that signals via the IL-1 receptor-related protein ST2 and induces T helper type 2-associated cytokines. Immunity 2005; 23(5):479–90.

9. *Wang YH, Ito T, Wang YH, et al. Maintenance and polarization of human TH2 central memory T cells by thymic stromal lymphopoietin-activated dendritic cells. Immunity 2006;24(6):827–38.

10. Klunker S, Trautmann A, Akdis M, et al. A second step of chemotaxis after transendothelial migration: keratinocytes undergoing apoptosis release IFN-gamma-inducible protein 10, monokine induced by IFN-gamma, and IFN-gamma-inducible alpha-chemoattractant for T cell chemotaxis toward epidermis in atopic dermatitis. J Immunol 2003;171(2):1078–84.

11. Rebane A, Zimmermann M, Aab A, et al. Mechanisms of IFN-gamma-induced apoptosis of human skin keratinocytes in patients with atopic dermatitis. J Allergy Clin Immunol 2012;129(5):1297–306.

12. *Zhu J, Yamane H, Paul WE. Differentiation of effector CD4 T cell populations (*). Annu Rev Immunol 2010;28:445–89.

13. Sonnenberg GF, Mjosberg J, Spits H, et al. SnapShot: innate lymphoid cells. Immunity 2013;39(3): 622, e1.

14. Palomares O, Ruckert B, Jartti T, et al. Induction and maintenance of allergen-specific FOXP3+ Treg cells in human tonsils as potential first-line organs of oral tolerance. J Allergy Clin Immunol 2012;129(2):510–20, e1–9.

15. Schulzke JD, Gunzel D, John LJ, et al. Perspectives on tight junction research. Ann N Y Acad Sci 2012;1257(1):1–19.

16. Matter K, Balda MS. SnapShot: epithelial tight junctions. Cell 2014;157(4):992.e1.

17. De Benedetto A, Rafaels NM, McGirt LY, et al. Tight junction defects in patients with atopic dermatitis. J Allergy Clin Immunol 2011;127(3):773–86, e1–7.

18. de Boer WI, Sharma HS, Baelemans SM, et al. Altered expression of epithelial junctional proteins in atopic asthma: possible role in inflammation. Can J Physiol Pharmacol 2008;86(3):105–12.

19. *Fujita H, Chalubinski M, Rhyner C, et al. Claudin-1 expression in airway smooth muscle exacerbates airway remodeling in asthmatic subjects. J Allergy Clin Immunol 2011;127(6):1612–21, e8.

20. *Holgate ST. Epithelium dysfunction in asthma. J Allergy Clin Immunol 2007;120(6):1233–46.

21. Soyka MB, Wawrzyniak P, Eiwegger T, et al. Defective epithelial barrier in chronic rhinosinusitis: The regulation of tight junctions by IFN-gamma and IL-4. J Allergy Clin Immunol 2012;130(5):1087–96, e10.

22. Xiao C, Puddicombe SM, Field S, et al. Defective epithelial barrier function in asthma. J Allergy Clin Immunol 2011;128(3):549–56, e1–12.

23. *Barnes PJ. The cytokine network in asthma and chronic obstructive pulmonary disease. J Clin Invest 2008;118(11):3546–56.

Key references are preceded by an asterisk.

CHAPTER 2

The Origins of Allergic Disease

John W. Holloway and Susan L. Prescott

CHAPTER OUTLINE

INTRODUCTION

GENETICS OF ALLERGIC DISEASE

Evidence for a Genetic Component in Allergic Disease

  Heritability Studies

Finding Genes for Allergic Disease

  Approaches to the Study of the Genetics of Allergic Disease

CURRENT UNDERSTANDING OF ALLERGIC DISEASE GENETICS

Atopy

Asthma

  Genetic Studies Increase the Understanding of Asthma Pathogenesis

  Early Life Development and Asthma

Atopic Dermatitis

Rhinitis

Food Allergy and Anaphylaxis

GENE–ENVIRONMENT INTERACTION

PHARMACOGENETICS OF ALLERGIC DISEASE

EPIGENETICS AND ALLERGIC DISEASE

POTENTIAL FOR CLINICAL APPLICATION OF GENETICS IN ALLERGIC DISEASE

DEVELOPMENTAL ORIGINS OF ALLERGIC DISEASE

Maternal Environmental and in-Utero Programming of Allergic Disease

  Evidence for Developmental Programming

  Maternal Environmental Exposures during Pregnancy and Allergic Disease Risk in Offspring

Postnatal Immune Development and Allergic Disease

  T Regulatory Cells

  Innate Immune System and Postnatal Immune Development

  Gut Microbiome and Postnatal Immune Development

CONCLUSIONS

SUMMARY OF IMPORTANT CONCEPTS

- Susceptibility to and severity of allergic disease have a genetic basis.
- Allergic disease has its origins in early life as the result of the interaction between inherited susceptibility and environmental exposure.
- Multiple genes, each with a modest effect, and environmental influences combine to produce the phenotypes of allergic diseases.
- Identification of genetic susceptibility factors through genome-wide association studies has provided novel insights into the pathogenesis of atopy and allergic disease.
- Pharmacogenetic analysis of genes in pathways relevant to a given therapy has the potential to allow treatment to be tailored to the patient.
- Modern environmental changes are increasing predisposition to allergic disease and many other immune-mediated diseases, with evidence that some lifestyle risk factors can modify events in gene expression through epigenetic changes.
- In the context of rising rates of allergic disease, perinatal differences in immune function, including effector T cell, Treg, and innate responses, are likely to reflect changing maternal environmental influences, as well as genetic risk. In addition, differences in other organs, such as lung and skin, are evident at birth in those who subsequently go on to develop asthma and atopic dermatitis.
- Infants who subsequently develop allergic disease show age-related differences in the postnatal immune development, including the pattern and trajectory of effector T cell and innate responses, with emerging differences in Treg function.

- Recent findings suggest that engagement of pathogen-associated molecular patterns (PAMPs) receptors, such as the Toll-like receptors (TLRs), in prenatal and early postnatal life is critical for shaping the immune system, and differences in microbial exposure, including the microbiota within the gastrointestinal tract, influence development of allergic disease.

INTRODUCTION

It has long been recognized that allergic disease runs in families and that genetic factors are important in determining individual susceptibility. At the same time, the early environment plays a critical role in shaping early development and modifying risk through effects on both the immune system and the developing organ systems (Fig. 2-1). This is reflected in the recent and dramatic increase in infant allergies, which can only be explained in terms of recent environmental change. However, genetic variants are also likely to play a role in individual vulnerability to a range of environmental risk factors and myriad phenotypic consequences. The added potential for transgenerational influences underscores the complexity of gene–environment interactions.

Whilst allergy is a 'systemic' immune disease, it is largely manifest in specific organs, particularly those that interface with the environment, such as the skin, the respiratory tract, and the gastrointestinal tract. These are also the sites where mucosal tolerance is initiated and regulated, to determine patterns of systemic immunity. For this reason, organ development and early events at mucosal surfaces may have a pivotal role in programming systemic profiles of both mucosal and systemic immunity and susceptibility to inflammation and immune disease.

Environmental exposures, including maternal diet, nutrient balance, microbial colonization, toxin exposures, and other factors inducing oxidative stress and inflammation, interact with inherited genetics and epigenetic factors to directly and indirectly influence organ development and immune programming—in both pregnancy and the postnatal period. In this chapter, we summarize our understanding of how inherited genetic factors contribute to individual susceptibility, severity and response to treatment in allergic disease and the evidence that allergy is a consequence of intrauterine and early life dysregulation of the immune system and organ development, with specific focus on contributing environmental risk factors occurring preconception, in-utero and in the early postnatal period. The understanding of both of these factors is essential in identifying at-risk individuals and the possible therapeutic interventions for primary prevention of allergic disease.

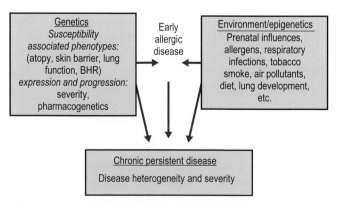

Figure 2-1 Allergic disease such as asthma, is due to a combination of both genetics and environmental exposures leading to early disease. Additional gene variants and further environmental exposures lead to chronic persistent disease with heterogeneous subtypes (e.g., mild vs severe asthma). *(Adapted from Meyers DA, Bleecker ER, Holloway JW, et al. Asthma genetics and personalized medicine. Lancet Respir Med 2014; 2(5):405–415.)*

GENETICS OF ALLERGIC DISEASE

There is a genetic basis to susceptibility for most common diseases, and individual susceptibility depends on the interaction between both inherited factors and multifaceted environmental exposures.[1] In addition, it is widely recognized that variation in individual response to therapy and risk of adverse reactions also has, in part, a genetic basis.[2] Heritability is the proportion of observed variation in a particular trait that can be attributed to inherited genetic factors in contrast to environmental ones. Heritability studies have shown heritable risk to both atopy (the propensity for allergen-specific IgE production) and asthma, but that many of these genetic risk factors are independent. For example, asthma can manifest in the absence of atopy, and heritability studies have shown that there are genetic factors that determine susceptibility to allergic disease that are independent of atopy. Similarly, atopy is frequently present in the absence of clinical disease. Thus, whilst atopy is a risk factor for asthma, studies have now confirmed that major genetic susceptibility factors for allergic disease, such as asthma and eczema, are not related to atopy susceptibility *per se*.

In the main, susceptibility to allergic disease results from the inheritance of many genetic susceptibility factors, each with a small effect. As for many common diseases, the specific biochemical defect(s) at the cellular level and environmental exposures that trigger initiation of allergic disease are unclear, even though considerable knowledge has accrued on the molecular pathways involved in pathogenesis. The study of the genetics of these conditions provides an opportunity to identify novel factors in allergic disease etiology, providing a greater understanding of the fundamental mechanisms of these disorders (Box 2-1).

Evidence for a Genetic Component in Allergic Disease

Heritability Studies

In familial aggregation and twin studies, a significant familial aggregation of atopy, allergic disease and related intermediate phenotypes, such as bronchial hyperresponsiveness (BHR) and total serum IgE levels, has been described. For example, if an individual has a sibling with asthma, the likelihood of the individual developing asthma is 3 to 4 times greater than that of the general population.[3] Higher concordance rates for a disease phenotype in monozygotic twins (who share 100% of their genes) compared with dizygotic twins (who share 50% of their genes identical by descent) also provide important evidence of a genetic component to allergic disease. For example, an increased correlation of serum total IgE levels and a higher concordance of asthma is seen in monozygotic twins compared with dizygotic twins.[4,5]

A key observation from heritability studies of allergic disease is the issue of 'end-organ susceptibility,' i.e. which allergic disease an atopic individual will develop is controlled by specific genetic factors, differing from those that determine susceptibility to atopy

---

Box 2-1   **Key Concepts**

How do Genetics Studies of Allergic Disease Improve Knowledge and Treatment of Disease?
- Greater understanding of disease pathogenesis
  - Identification of specific genetic variants that are associated with disease susceptibility, highlights the role for novel genes and biochemical and cellular pathways in which they lie in disease. This can lead to new pharmacologic targets for developing therapeutics
- Identification of environmental factors that interact with an individual's genetic make-up to initiate disease
  - Prevention of disease by environmental modification
- Identification of susceptible individuals
  - Early-in-life screening and targeting of preventative therapies for at-risk individuals to prevent disease
- Targeting of therapies
  - Sub-classification of disease (endotypes) on the basis of genetics and targeting of specific therapies based on this classification
  - Determination of the likelihood of an individual responding to a particular therapy (pharmacogenetics) and individualized treatment plans

per se. For example, in a study of 176 normal families, Gerrard and co-workers found a striking association between asthma in the parent and asthma in the child, between hay fever in the parent and hay fever in the child, and between eczema in the parent and eczema in the child.[6] Such observations from heritability studies have since been confirmed by molecular genetic studies of allergic disease, which show that there is only a small degree of overlap between the genetic variants predisposing to different allergic diseases.

Finding Genes for Allergic Disease

Variation in DNA sequences occurs once in approximately every 200 to 500 base pairs in the human genome. Sequence variation (mutations) occurring in over 1% of the population are termed 'polymorphisms' and those that occur in less than 1% are rare 'alleles'. Polymorphisms in DNA sequences between individuals can take many forms including differences at a single base pair involving substitution, insertion, or deletion of a single nucleotide (commonly termed 'single nucleotide polymorphisms' or 'SNPs'), and repetition, insertion, or deletion of longer stretches of DNA ranging from a few base pairs to many thousands of base pairs, often termed 'copy number variations' or 'CNVs'. The different versions of the nucleotide sequence present at any one location in the genome (locus) are termed 'alleles'. Polymorphisms form the basis of human diversity, including our responses to environmental stimuli. Genetic epidemiology has provided statistical methods for measuring the association of gene polymorphisms with a clinical phenotype through assessing the difference in frequency of the variant between cases of controls and inheritance of a variant with the phenotype in families. There have been a number of approaches utilized to identify genetic factors that contribute to allergic disease susceptibility.

Approaches to the Study of the Genetics of Allergic Disease

Two general approaches have been widely used to study the genetics of allergic disease: candidate gene association studies, usually performed in unrelated cases and controls, and hypothesis-independent approaches that involve the study of genetic variation genome-wide, such as genome-wide association studies (GWAS) in large case–control cohorts.[1]

Candidate Gene Association Studies. Candidate gene association studies evaluate genetic variation in the region of genes that are physiologically suggested (candidates) to be involved in disease pathogenesis. For example, genes, such as those encoding cytokines, chemokines, and their receptors, as well as transcription factors, high affinity IgE receptor (FcεR1), etc. are plausible candidate genes for allergic disease. The data for this type of study are usually obtained from unrelated individuals (cases and controls). Polymorphisms within the gene that are believed to be functional (i.e. affecting gene expression or encoded protein function) are then tested for association with the disease or phenotype in question. The advantage of the candidate approach is that candidate genes have biologic plausibility and often display known functional consequences that have potentially important implications for the disease of interest. Disadvantages are the limitation to genes of known or postulated involvement in the disease, thereby excluding the discovery of novel genes that influence the disease.

Genome-wide Association Studies (GWAS). Although genes have been identified for common diseases, such as asthma and allergy, from studies of candidate or pathway genes in cases and controls, it is now possible due to both the mapping of polymorphisms in the genome and the advances in genotyping technology, to scan the whole genome in a hypothesis-independent manner in cases versus controls, to identify multiple susceptibility genes, each alone contributing a small effect.[7] Chips are now available for genotyping millions of SNPs/person at once. The cost has progressively decreased and the accuracy rates have increased, making this a powerful approach for studying the genetics of common diseases. The first GWAS for complex diseases were reported in 2005 and have now transformed the study of genetic factors in complex common disease. For hundreds of phenotypes, from common diseases to physiological measurements, e.g., height and body mass index and biologic measurements, e.g., circulating lipid and eosinophil levels, GWAS have provided compelling statistical associations for hundreds of different loci in the human genome, giving new insight into the biologic processes that underlie these phenotypes and diseases.[8]

Interpreting Results of Genetic Studies. It is important to remember with association studies, that there are a number of reasons which can lead to an observation of association between a phenotype and a particular allele. A positive association between the phenotype and the allele will occur if the allele is the cause of, or contributes to, the phenotype. This association would be expected to be replicated in other populations with the same phenotype, unless there are several different alleles at the same locus contributing to the same phenotype, in which case association would be difficult to detect, or if the trait was predominantly the result of different genes in the other population (genetic heterogeneity) or depended on interaction with an environmental exposure not present in the replication population. Another reason for non-replication could be different phenotype definition between studies. For example, the phenotype 'atopy' has been defined as a positive skin-prick test (SPT), a positive radioallergosorbent test (RAST), high serum total IgE, or a combination of these tests. Although these phenotypes are clearly related, it is likely that some genes that influence total IgE levels do not influence specific IgE response to allergens, and vice versa. Finally, positive associations may not be replicated because the true model of genetic susceptibility for diseases, such as asthma and atopy, is complex. It is highly possible that any particular susceptibility variant has a relatively minor effect on the phenotype and that the magnitude of its effect will be influenced by genes at other loci (gene–gene interactions, epistasis) and by environmental exposures (gene–environment interactions).[9–12] As a result of background genes and environmental factors differing between populations, it would not be surprising if associations with single SNPs or haplotypes differed between populations.

Positive associations may also be identified between an allele and a phenotype for a number of reasons other than a true effect of the variant in question on disease susceptibility. Linkage disequilibrium (LD) is the correlation between nearby variants such that the alleles at neighboring polymorphisms (observed on the same chromosome) are associated within a population more often than if they were unlinked. Thus, an allele may show positive association with disease if the allele tends to occur on the same parental chromosome that also carries the trait-causing mutation more often than would be expected by chance. For example, the SNP most strongly associated with the disease phenotype at a particular locus in a GWAS is unlikely to be the true casual polymorphism, rather it is marking a region of LD containing one or more genes in which the causal polymorphism(s) lie. An association may not be replicated in subsequent studies because of different patterns of LD in different populations. A positive association between an allele and a trait can also be artifactual as a result of recent population admixture. In a population of mixed ancestry, any trait present in a higher frequency in a subgroup of the population (e.g., a particular ethnic group) will show positive association with an allele that also happens to be more common in that population subgroup. To avoid spurious association arising through admixture, studies should be performed in large, relatively homogeneous populations. Positive association between polymorphisms and phenotype can reflect type I error or false-positive results. The main source for type I error is multiple comparisons in studies of multiple polymorphisms in the same gene, polymorphisms in multiple genes, or multiple phenotypes.

CURRENT UNDERSTANDING OF ALLERGIC DISEASE GENETICS

Atopy

Genetic studies using phenotypes relevant to atopy, such as specific-IgE responses and total serum IgE levels, have identified a number of genetic variants associated with atopy.

For example, initial candidate gene studies in obvious functional candidate genes, e.g. the Th2 cytokine signaling pathway, have shown consistent association with atopy.[1] More recently, the use of the genome-wide association approaches has provided significant insights into the genetic basis of atopic predisposition. This has identified a number of gene variants associated with atopy phenotypes in genes, such as the alpha chain of the high affinity receptor for IgE (*FCER1A*), the transcription factor that regulates Th2 responses *STAT6*, and the genetic region on chromosome 5q31 that contains the genes encoding the typical Th2 cytokines IL-4 and IL-13.

As might be expected, some of the loci identified in these studies are also associated with allergic diseases such as asthma. For example, variation within the Th2 cytokine cluster on chromosome 5 has also been shown to be associated with asthma. This overlap between genetic variation identified as predisposing to atopy and that underlying asthma is not surprising, given the current understanding of the role played by IgE and Th2-mediated immune responses in the pathogenesis of allergic disease, and studies of heritability that have suggested that genes that predispose to atopy overlap with those that predispose to asthma. However, what is remarkable is that the overlap between loci identified as predisposing to serum IgE levels and allergic disease is so small. For example, in a large GWAS study of 10 365 European subjects with physician-diagnosed asthma and 16 110 controls, loci strongly associated with IgE levels were not associated with asthma with the exception of IL-13 and the HLA region, suggesting that the genetic determinants of atopy are largely distinct from those that predispose to specific clinical manifestations of atopy such as asthma.[13]

Asthma

Asthma has been the most extensively studied allergic disease with respect to genetics. Genetic variants in many genes have been associated with asthma and related phenotypes, such as airway hyperresponsiveness, bronchodilator response, and lung function both using candidate gene and genome-wide approaches, as described above.

Genetic Studies Increase the Understanding of Asthma Pathogenesis

The study of the genetic basis of asthma has revealed astonishing insights into the pathogenesis of this complex condition. Initially, as for atopy, most candidate gene studies of asthma were focused on association of functional polymorphisms in components of Th2-mediated immune responses. For example, the gene encoding the Th2 effector cytokine, IL-13, is one of the most consistently associated genes with asthma and related phenotypes. Polymorphisms of a number of other genes encoding either proteins regulating Th2 T cell production such as GATA-binding protein 3 (*GATA3*), T-bet, the transcription factor necessary for Th1 cell development (encoded by the gene *TBX21*), and the cytokine IL-4, its receptor IL-4Rα, and downstream signal transducer *STAT6* have also all been repeatedly associated with increased susceptibility to asthma and related phenotypes, and there is evidence that there may be a synergistic effect on disease risk in inheriting more than one of these variants.[10]

Whilst studies of these, and other, biologic candidate genes have increased the understanding of the genetic basis of asthma susceptibility, they have not given new insights into the biologic mechanisms important in asthma, as the role of the proteins encoded by these genes was already, in general, well established in asthma in the absence of genetic studies. However, the startling observation from genetic studies of asthma, especially genes identified through hypothesis-independent genome-wide approaches, is that genes encoding proteins involved in Th2-mediated immune responses are not the only, or even the most important, factors underlying asthma susceptibility. It is clear from heritability studies of allergic disease that the propensity to develop atopy is influenced by factors different from those that influence clinical manifestations of allergic diseases such as asthma. However, these disease factors require interaction with atopy (or something else) to trigger disease. For example, in asthma, bronchoconstriction is triggered mostly by an allergic response to inhaled allergen, accompanied by an eosinophilic inflammation in the airways, but in some people who may have 'asthma susceptibility genes' but not atopy, asthma is triggered by other exposures, such as toluene diisocyanate. It is possible to segregate the genes identified as contributing to asthma, into five broad groups[1]:

1. *Genes involved in directly modulating a response to environmental exposures.* These include genes encoding components of the innate immune system that interact with levels of microbial exposure to alter the risk of developing allergic immune responses, such as the genes encoding components of the LPS response pathway, for example CD14 and TLR4, highlighting the importance of innate immunity in asthma. Other environmental response genes include detoxifying enzymes, such as the glutathione *S*-transferase (GST) genes that modulate the effect of exposures involving oxidant stress, such as tobacco smoke and air pollution, and the gene *CDHR3* that is an epithelial expressed rhinovirus receptor, identified as being associated with severe asthma exacerbations in early childhood.

2. *Genes involved in maintaining the integrity of the epithelial barrier at the mucosal surface* and which cause the epithelium to signal the immune system following environmental exposure. For example, the gene *PCDH1*, encoding protocadherin-1, a member of a family of cell adhesion molecules and expressed in the bronchial epithelium, has also been identified as a susceptibility gene for BHR. Interleukin 33, identified by both candidate gene and genome-wide approaches, is produced by the airway epithelial in response to damage, and drives production of Th2-associated cytokines, such as IL-4, IL-5, and IL-13.

3. *Genes that regulate the immune response*, including those such as regulating Th1/Th2 differentiation and effector function as discussed above, but also others, such as the *IL6R*, identified recently in a GWAS study in an Australian population, and may regulate the level of inflammation that occurs in the lung.

4. *Genes involved in determining the tissue response to chronic inflammation*, such as airway remodelling. They include genes such as *SMAD3*, an intracellular signaling protein that is activated by the profibrotic cytokine TGF-β.

5. *Disease-modifying genes* that, rather than determine susceptibility of asthma *per se*, alter phenotypes related to disease progression such as exacerbation frequency, disease severity and development of fixed (irreversible) airflow obstruction. For example, studies have shown that genetic factors can modify the effect of environmental exposures, such as vitamin D or particulate air pollutant (PM_{10}) exposure on exacerbation frequency. The advent of genome-wide association studies in populations of severe asthma and asthma exacerbations may aid in better prediction of exacerbation phenotypes and the sub-classification of patients into sub-phenotypes that may reflect differing pathogenicity and response to treatment, allowing for better targeting of therapeutics.[2]

Early Life Development and Asthma

Another area in which genetic studies of asthma have reinforced observations from traditional epidemiology is in the importance of early life events in determining asthma susceptibility. A number of genetic studies have now provided evidence to support a role for early life developmental effects in allergic disease.[14] For example, a large proportion of genetic variants associated with measures of adult lung function in a GWAS study, showed consistent effects on lung function in children (7–9 years of age), and some have been shown to be associated with infant lung function. This suggests that genetic determinants of lung function in adults may in part act via effects on lung development, or alternatively, that some genetic determinants of lung growth and lung function decline are shared.

In summary, genetic studies have shown that variation in genes regulating atopic immune responses are not the only, or even the major, factor in determining susceptibility to asthma. This has provided strong additional evidence as to the importance of local tissue response factors and epithelial susceptibility factors in the pathogenesis of both asthma and other allergic diseases.

Atopic Dermatitis

As with asthma, a genetic basis for atopic dermatitis (AD, eczema) has long been known to be a complex trait, with disease susceptibility involving the interactions between multiple genes and environmental factors.[15] Heritability studies support a role for both genetic factors related to atopy in general and also for disease-specific AD genes, with the risk of AD in a child much greater if one or both parents have AD, compared with one or both parents having asthma or allergic rhinitis.[6] Whilst the majority of candidate gene studies have examined polymorphisms in genes related to atopic immune responses, more recently a number of studies have investigated genes encoding proteins involved in the epidermal barrier. This has been prompted by the identification of the filaggrin (*FLG*) gene, which has a key role in epidermal barrier function, and is one of the strongest genetic risk factors for AD.[16]

Filaggrin (a filament-aggregating protein) is a major component of the protein-lipid cornified envelope of the epidermis, important for water permeability and blocking the entry of microbes and allergens. In 2006, it was recognized that loss of function mutations in the *FLG* gene caused *ichthyosis vulgaris*, a skin disorder characterized by dry, flaky skin and a predisposition to AD and associated asthma. Subsequently, it was recognized that individuals heterozygous (carrying 1 copy) for these null alleles had a significantly increased risk of AD. It has been estimated that although *FLG* null alleles are relatively rare in the Caucasian population (combined carrier frequency of null filaggrin mutations is approximately 9%), they nonetheless account for up to 15% of the population attributable risk of AD, with penetrance estimated to be between 40% and 80%; suggesting that between 40% and 80% of subjects carrying one or more *FLG* null mutations will develop AD. The increased risk of atopic sensitization and atopic asthma in the presence of AD suggests that by conferring a deficit in epidermal barrier function, *FLG* mutation could initiate systemic allergy by allergen exposure through the skin and start the 'atopic march' in susceptible individuals.[16]

Rhinitis

At the present time, little is known about the genetics of atopic rhinitis. Familial aggregation has been observed in genetic epidemiology studies but genetic studies are limited. It remains to be conclusively demonstrated whether genetic susceptibility to rhinitis involves specific genetic factors that are distinct from those underlying susceptibility to atopy.

Food Allergy and Anaphylaxis

Heritability studies indicate that propensity to allergic reactions to food has a heritable component. However, the precise genetic factors underlying this have been comparatively under-researched compared with studies of other allergic diseases. A recent GWAS study of peanut allergy identified an association within the HLA gene region on chromosome 6, common to many other studies of immune-mediated diseases. It is also possible that *FLG* polymorphism may increase susceptibility to food allergy by increasing sensitization, as recent temporal sequence analyses of initially eczema-free participants has shown that in *FLG* deficient individuals, sensitization precedes development of clinical manifestation of AD. The same may indeed hold true for food allergy, especially to allergens, such as peanut, where transcutaneous exposure in the environment or in topical preparations plays an important role. Recent observations that *FLG* mutations are associated with peanut allergy support this theory. Whilst these observations await replication in other cohorts, they do show that it may be possible to predict those atopic subjects at risk of developing severe reactions to allergens in the future, allowing targeting of preventative treatments, such as allergen immunotherapy, before development of sensitization.

GENE–ENVIRONMENT INTERACTION

The evidence for the increased prevalence of allergic disease in the last decades is strongly suggestive of an important environmental component in its pathogenesis, with the onset of the disease and its clinical course determined by gene–environment interactions. Among affected individuals in the population, the relative influence of genetic and environmental factors probably varies and individuals with different allergy-related genotypes have different sensitivities to environmental exposures. Several possible patterns for gene–environment interaction have been suggested. For example, both the presence of a given disease-susceptibility gene and an environmental exposure may be necessary to produce excess risk of a disease.

With regards to asthma, there are extensive data showing that passive tobacco smoke increases airway responsiveness and incident asthma, especially in prenatal exposure, and that this interacts with genetic susceptibility to determine disease onset. Analysis of the effect of a number of asthma-susceptibility genes has now shown interaction with tobacco smoke exposure and genetic variation determines disease susceptibility.

Another example on gene–environment interaction, is the interaction between polymorphisms in components of the innate immune response, such as CD14 and TLR4 involved in the recognition and clearance of bacterial endotoxin (LPS), by activating a cascade of host innate immune responses. Single nucleotide polymorphisms that alter the biology of these receptors could influence the early life origins of allergic disease, by modifying the effect of microbial exposure on the developing immune system. A number of studies have now shown interaction between polymorphism of CD14 and measures of microbial exposure, such as living on a farm, consumption of farm milk, and household dust endotoxin levels in determining serum IgE levels, sensitization and asthma (Fig. 2-2). In the future, identification of the factors that influence variability to environmental exposure could improve allergic disease management. Interactions between SNPs in a causal pathway and a relevant environmental exposure (e.g., innate immunity SNPs and farm living) would help to provide additional proof that the environmental exposure is truly causal and not confounded. This could lead to primary prevention by environmental modification. Furthermore, better characterization of gene–environment interactions would help to identify at-risk groups who would benefit

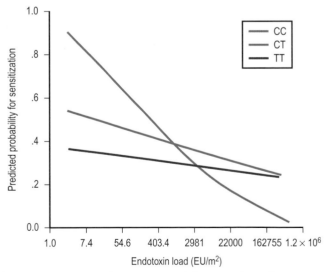

Figure 2-2 The effect of genotype on disease susceptibility may depend on environmental exposure. For example, a promoter polymorphism of the CD14 gene can produce an opposing effect on allergic sensitization depending on the level of endotoxin exposure. The graph shows fitted predicted probability curves for allergic sensitization at 5 years of age in relation to environmental endotoxin load in children with CC, CT, and TT genotypes in the promoter region of the CD14 gene (CD14/-159 C to T). *(From Simpson A, John SL, Jury F, et al. Endotoxin exposure, CD14, and allergic disease: an interaction between genes and the environment. Am J Respir Crit Care Med 2006; 174(4):386–392.)*

most from preventive strategies. This identification of at-risk groups, the degree of their sensitivity to exposure and their frequency in the population, will aid in the cost–benefit analysis of 'safe' exposure levels in the public health setting.

PHARMACOGENETICS OF ALLERGIC DISEASE

Pharmacogenetics refers to the relationship between genotype (genetic variation) and drug response. Essentially, pharmacogenetics represents a further example of gene–environment interaction, in which the environment is the exposure to a pharmacologic agent/biologic and the outcome is a therapeutic drug response (including adverse events). For example, short-acting β2-adrenoceptor agonists (SABA) and long-acting β2-adrenoceptor agonists (LABA) are the most commonly prescribed medications for treating bronchoconstriction and are controllers for long-term symptom relief in asthma. Pharmacogenetic studies have shown coding variants in the β2-adrenergic receptor gene (ADRB2) are associated with short-term bronchodilator response (i.e. bronchodilator responsiveness performed in a clinical setting) and identify a subgroup of patients with worsening symptoms during long-term regular SABA therapy. Other pharmacogenetic studies have also identified genetic variants associated with responses to drugs, such as corticosteroids and antileukotrienes.[2] However, the size of the effects of these genetic variants on treatment response tend to be small and there are no ready alternatives for therapy. Thus, whilst personalizing therapies based on genotypic profiling are now becoming a reality for some diseases, especially cancers, they are not yet applicable to allergic diseases such as asthma. However, multiple studies of new targeted therapies are currently underway in asthma and hold the promise of advancing personalized medicine approaches, including responder analyses based on pharmacogenetic parameters. For example, in a dose-ranging study of a biologic (pitrakinra, a recombinant human IL-4 variant) inhibiting the IL4/13 pathway, there was a significant dose–response effect on the primary endpoint of asthma exacerbation, observed only in individuals with a specific IL4R genotype representing approximately one third of the patient population (Fig. 2-3). Given that the targeted biologic therapies that are being developed will be expensive, biomarkers such pharmacogenetic predictors of response

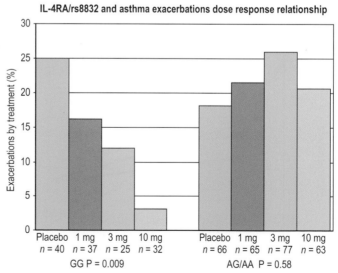

Figure 2-3 ILRA polymorphisms and reduced asthma exacerbations in response to treatment with an anti-interleukin 4 receptor antagonist (pitrakinra). Subjects with the rs8832 GG genotype demonstrated a significant dose-dependent reduction (placebo/1 mg/3 mg/10 mg) in exacerbations. There was no dose-dependent relationship with exacerbations for subjects with the AG/AA genotypes. *(Adapted from Slager RE, Otulana BA, Hawkins GA, et al. IL-4 receptor polymorphisms predict reduction in asthma exacerbations during response to an anti-IL-4 receptor [alpha] antagonist. J Allergy Clin Immunol 2012; 130: 516–22, e4.)*

could improve targeting of therapy to those who would most benefit, increasing efficacy and reducing the cost of prescribing to individuals who will not benefit.

EPIGENETICS AND ALLERGIC DISEASE

Epigenetics refers to biochemical changes to DNA that do not alter the DNA sequence but may be induced by environmental factors and transmitted mitotically and meiotically (i.e. through generations). Epigenetic factors include modification of histones by acetylation and methylation, and DNA methylation (Fig. 2-4). Modification of histones, around which the DNA is coiled, alters the rate of transcription-altering protein expression. DNA methylation involves adding a methyl group to specific cytosine bases in the DNA to suppress gene expression. Importantly, both changes to histones and DNA methylation can be induced in response to environmental exposures, such as tobacco smoke, and alterations in the early life environment, e.g., maternal nutrition, and these changes can last decades.[17]

There is evidence that epigenetic factors are important in allergic disease. Epigenetic profiles differ between individuals with and without allergic disease, though it is important to note that in most cases, these epigenetic changes could either be the cause or consequence of allergic disease. Importantly, changes to histone modifications and DNA methylation can be induced by risk factors for allergy, such as tobacco smoke, cesarean birth, and maternal nutrition in early life. This evidence strongly supports epigenetics as a mechanism by which the environment affects allergic disease risk and a mechanism by which gene–environment interaction can occur. However, in itself, environmentally induced epigenetic change to an individual's epigenome cannot explain the observed heritability of allergic disease—this would require the epigenetic change to be inherited through meiosis and the effect of exposure in one generation could lead to increased risk in subsequent generations. In humans, transgenerational effects have been observed where the initial environmental exposure occurred in F0 generation and changes in disease susceptibility were still evident in F2 (grandchildren). In mouse models, ancestral folate deprivation causes congenital malformations that persist for five generations, most

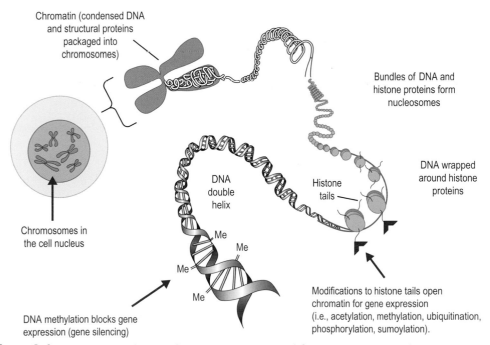

Figure 2-4 Epigenetic regulation of gene expression. Modifications to DNA and DNA-associated packaging proteins (histones) control the patterns of gene expression in each cell. *(From Prescott SL. The allergy epidemic: a mystery of modern life. Crawley, Western Australia: UWA; 2011. ©Susan L. Prescott.)*

likely via epigenetic mechanisms. Observations, such as grandmaternal smoking increasing the risk of childhood asthma in their grandchildren, support the concept that transgenerational epigenetic effects may be operating in allergic disease. This is further supported by the study of animal models, for example in one model where mice were exposed to in-utero supplementation with methyl donors and exhibited enhanced airway inflammation following allergen challenge, a phenotype persisted in their daughters, despite the absence of exposure in the second generation. It is probable in the near future, that the study of large prospective birth cohorts with information on maternal environmental exposures during pregnancy, will provide important insights into the role of epigenetic factors in the heritability of allergic disease.[17]

POTENTIAL FOR CLINICAL APPLICATION OF GENETICS IN ALLERGIC DISEASE

The varying and sometimes conflicting results of studies to identify allergic disease susceptibility genes, reflect the genetic and environmental heterogeneity seen in allergic disorders and illustrate the difficulty of identifying susceptibility genes for complex genetic diseases. However, despite this, there is now a rapidly expanding list of genes robustly associated with a wide range of allergic disease phenotypes. It is still however, not possible to predict the likelihood an individual will develop allergic disease based on genetics alone. This simply reflects the complex interactions between different genetic and environmental factors required both to initiate disease and determine progression to a more severe phenotype in an individual, meaning that the predictive value of variation in any one gene is low, with a typical genotype relative risk of 1.1–1.5. It is possible that genetic studies combined with more sophisticated patient characterization to define sub-phenotypes of allergic disease may lead to predictive genetic tests for disease in the future (Box 2-2).

Whatever the future value of genetic studies of allergic disease in predicting risk, it is unlikely that this will be the area of largest impact of genetics studies on the treatment and prevention of these conditions. Rather, it is the insight the genetic studies have provided, and undoubtedly will continue to provide, into disease pathogenesis. In conclusion, whilst genetic studies of allergic disease have led to the identification of many

---

Box 2-2   Key Concepts

How does Inherited Genetic Variability Affect Allergic Disease?

- Determine susceptibility atopy
  - 'Th2' or 'IgE switch' genes
    e.g., the α-chain of the high affinity IgE receptor (FCER1A) associated with sensitization and serum IgE levels
- Determine specific target-organ disease in atopic individuals
  - Asthma susceptibility genes
  - 'Lung-specific factors' that regulate susceptibility of lung epithelium/fibroblasts to remodeling in response to allergic inflammation, such as *ADAM33*
  - Atopic dermatitis susceptibility genes
  - Genes that regulate dermal barrier function, such as *FLG*
- Influence the interaction of environmental factors with atopy and allergic disease
  - Determining immune responses to factors that drive Th1/Th2 skewing of the immune response, such as *CD14* and *TLR4* polymorphism and early childhood infection
  - Modulating the effect of exposures involving oxidant stress, such as tobacco smoke and air pollution on asthma susceptibility, e.g., glutathione *S*-transferase genes
  - Altering the response to environmental factors that play a role in the initiation of disease in susceptible individuals, e.g., ORMDL3 and CDHR3 and rhinovirus infection
  - Altering interaction between environmental factors and established disease, such as genetic polymorphism regulating responses to respiratory virus infection and asthma symptoms
- Modify severity of disease
  - Examples are tumor necrosis factor α polymorphisms and asthma severity
- Regulate response to therapy
  - Pharmacogenetics
  - Examples are β$_2$-adrenergic receptor polymorphism and response to β$_2$-agonists

loci that alter the susceptibility of an individual to allergic disease, further research is needed to translate statistical significance from genetic and genomic studies to biologic and clinical impact.

DEVELOPMENTAL ORIGINS OF ALLERGIC DISEASE

The concept that early life events and environmental exposures play a critical role in determining the predisposition to future disease has been gathering momentum across all medical disciplines, even those where disease is not manifest until adult life. This is based on the inextricable link between maternal and early life influences on many aspects of development and is grounded in evidence that structural, physiologic, metabolic, immune and even behavioral patterns of response are programmed to a significant degree in the formative stages of life (Fig. 2-5). Rising rates of a wide range of non-communicable diseases (NCDs), including autoimmune, metabolic, cardiovascular and degenerative disorders, implicate common environmental and lifestyle risk factors associated with progressive modernization. The very fact that inflammation is a common feature in many of these conditions highlights a central role of immune effects.[18]

For allergic diseases, which frequently become evident in infancy and early childhood, the implications of early events are even more obvious. Together with the unparalleled rise in virtually all immune diseases in the last 50 years, this clearly highlights the specific vulnerability of the developing immune system to modern environmental changes. The same modern lifestyle changes are associated with a much wider range of NCDs, suggesting common risk factors that may be promoting chronic inflammatory disorders

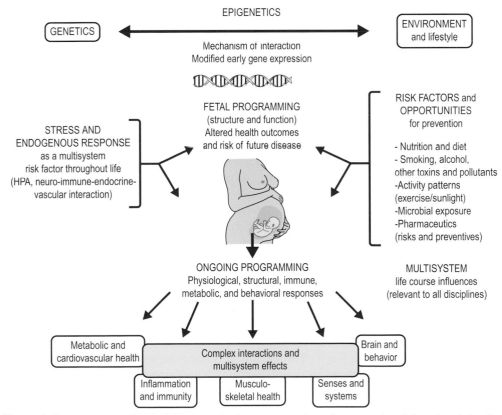

Figure 2-5 Importance of early life events in the programming of structural and functional development. Physiologic, immune, metabolic, and behavioral patterns of response are determined early in development and may be modified by events and exposures early in life. Epigenetic effects provide a mechanism for gene–environment interactions, which may alter future disease risk with potentially greater effects in early life, when systems. *(Adapted from the University of Western Australia Developmental Origins of Health and Disease [DOHaD] Consortium, Perth, Australia, 2012.)*

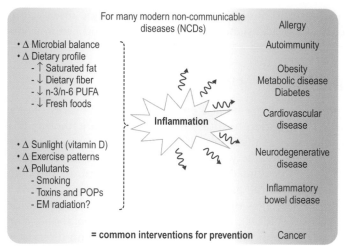

Figure 2-6 Common risk factors for many non-communicable diseases (NCDs); inflammation a common element. Lifestyle changes are associated with an increase in inflammatory diseases, suggesting common risk factors and a central role for the immune system. Many risk factors for allergic disease are also implicated in many other NCDs, highlighting the need for a multidisciplinary approach to disease prevention. EM, electromagnetic; POPs, persistent organic pollutants; PUFA, polyunsaturated fatty acid.

(Fig. 2-6). This in turn suggests that reducing the burden of all NCDs will be considerably advanced by identifying common risk factors for inflammation and giving greater emphasis to the prevention strategies in early life.

The developmental plasticity inherent in these observations also provides opportunities to utilize the same pathways to prevent disease. Immune development is under epigenetic control and there is growing evidence that a number of these environmental exposures can induce stable epigenetic changes in gene expression, which could foreseeably be passed to offspring and subsequent generations.[17] These emerging epigenetic paradigms provide a new mechanism for long observed gene–environment interactions, which may be utilized in primary prevention strategies. Furthermore, it is likely that the preventive strategies that target common risk factors for inflammation effects and many other NCDs, may have more wide-ranging multisystem benefits for human health. Our current health problems are global, interrelated, and part of the other global challenges our planet is facing. This highlights the need for a coordinated interdisciplinary approach to prevent a wide range of NCDs, especially as the more populous regions of the world undergo the same environmental and lifestyle changes. An understanding of the developing immune system is a key element in defining the multisystem effects of environmental change.

Maternal Environmental and in-Utero Programming of Allergic Disease

Evidence for Developmental Programming

The strongest evidence for the importance of developmental programming in allergic disease is the observation that that there are marked phenotypic differences already apparent at the time of birth between individuals who do, or do not, go on to develop allergic conditions later in life.[19] For example, measurements of lung function have shown that children who go on to develop asthma have impaired lung function shortly after birth in comparison with healthy children. In the skin, reduced barrier function at both 2 days and 2 months of age—as measured by transepidermal water loss—has been shown to precede the development of eczema at 1 year of age, independently of filaggrin loss-of-function genetic variants.

Neonates with allergic predisposition have recognized differences in many aspects of immune function at birth, including effector T cells, Treg cells, hematopoietic progenitor populations and innate cells (Table 2-1). These altered patterns of immune function

TABLE 2-1 Differences in Aspects of Neonatal Immune Function Based on Allergic Risk/Allergic Outcomes

	Based on allergic risk	Based on allergic outcomes
	'High-risk' neonates based on maternal family history	Neonates who develop subsequent allergy
Effector T cell responses		
Proliferation response at birth	Several studies report higher proliferative responses to various stimuli (evidence of altered T Cell signaling patterns)	Trends for higher proliferative responses (evidence of reduced gene expression following activation)
Neonatal cytokine responses	Reduced Th1 IFN-γ responses (multiple studies) Mixed findings for other cytokines: some reporting higher Th2 cytokine production	Reduced Th1 IFN-γ responses (multiple studies) Mixed findings for other cytokines: some reporting higher Th2 cytokine production
Innate responses		
Neonatal TLR expression	Reduced TLR2 and TLR4 expression on monocytes, and progenitor cells	Increased TLR2 on pDC in one study, no other differences in TLR expression
Cytokine responses at birth	One study showed reduced IL-10 to TLR2 activation, others showed increased inflammatory cytokine production (IL-6, IL1β, TNF-α to multiple TLR ligands)	One study demonstrated increased inflammatory cytokine production (IL-6, IL1β, TNF-α to multiple TLR ligands)
Regulatory function		
% Treg cells	Reduced proportion of Treg cells in HR neonates	Trends for lower % Treg cells at birth (inconclusive)
Neonatal *Foxp3* expression	Reduced *Foxp3* expression (inconclusive, more studies needed)	Trends for lower *Foxp3* expression at birth (inconclusive, more studies needed)
Suppressive capacity	Reduced suppressive capacity (inconclusive, more studies needed)	Trends for reduced suppressive (inconclusive, more studies needed)

reflect inherited epigenetic programs as a result of modifications by in-utero events and exposures. Persistent Th2 skewing to polyclonal activators and vaccine antigens during the first year of life is observed in infants at high risk for developing allergic disease and are associated with the subsequent expression of allergic disease. It is important to emphasize that diminished Th1 cytokine production is not a persistent finding in infants at high risk for developing allergic disease, or who subsequently develop allergic disease, but rather this appears to be a maturational lag that is likely influenced by genetic and environmental factors and may be necessary at the inception of allergen sensitization.

Significant differences in magnitude and relative maturity of effector T cell responsiveness have been associated with the subsequent development of allergic disease. Of these, reduced Th1 function (IFN-γ production) has been the most consistent observation; however, reduced production of other T cell cytokines has also been noted, suggesting that allergy-prone individuals may have more extensive differences in T cell function. Collectively, these observations suggest that early functional differences may affect the developmental transition of T cell phenotypes in the periphery shortly after birth, and increase the risk of early allergic disease.

Maternal Environmental Exposures during Pregnancy and Allergic Disease Risk in Offspring

That differences are already evident at birth in organ and immune function between those who do and do not go on to develop allergic disease, suggests that genetic and environmental factors during pregnancy and development have a critical influence on allergic disease risk. A wide range of environmental exposures during pregnancy have been shown to influence the subsequent development of allergy in the offspring (Fig. 2-7; Table 2-2).

Whilst parental allergic disease is one of the strongest risk factors for allergy in the child, reflecting the effect of inherited genetic factors (as discussed above), it is clear that maternal allergy—and hence presumably an altered in-utero environment—has an additional effect on risk of allergy in the child. Besides allergic disease status, other

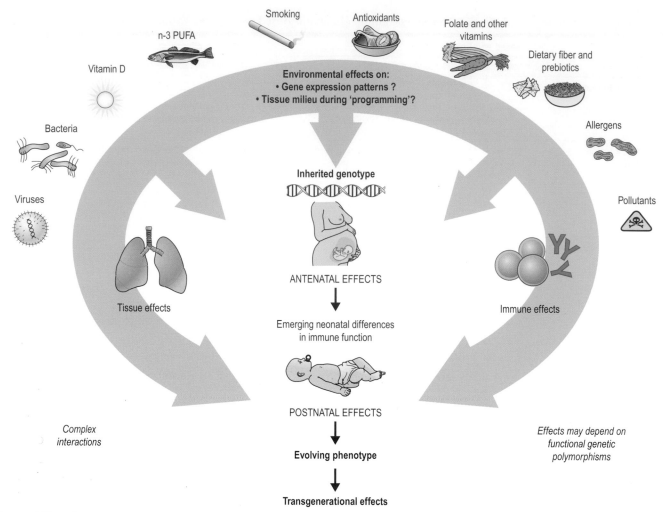

Figure 2-7 Early gene–environment interactions in the pathogenesis of allergic disease. A wide range of environmental factors, acting antenatally or postnatally, influence the maturation of immunologic competence and thus modulate risk for development of allergic diseases. In addition to effects on early gene expression patterns, some of these factors could modify local tissue milieu during early immune programming. *(From Holt PG, Sly PD, Prescott SL. Early life origins of allergy and asthma. In: Holgate ST, Church MK, Broide DH, Martinez FD, eds. Allergy: principles and practice. 4th edn. London: Elsevier; 2012.)*

maternal characteristics also influence the offspring's risk of allergy. Maternal obesity (a body mass index of at least 35) and greater weight gain during pregnancy (at least 25 kg gained) both increase the child's risk of asthma, but not eczema or rhinitis. Maternal obesity also results in fewer eosinophils and CD4+ T helper cells in the baby's cord blood, as well as altering cord blood cell innate immune responses.

Maternal smoking during pregnancy is one of the most well studied in-utero exposures, and has been known for decades to increase the risk of multiple allergic diseases. Grandmaternal smoking during pregnancy has also been shown to increase the risk of asthma in grandchildren, although data are conflicting. Other maternal exposures, such as airborne pollutant chemicals, have been suggested to influence the child's allergy risk. Higher levels of exposure to nitrogen dioxide, soot, and particulate matter of diameter ≤2.5 μm ($PM_{2.5}$) at the child's birth address, have been associated with increased risk of asthma, and increased maternal exposure levels to PM_{10} during late pregnancy have been shown to be associated with increased inflammation and decreased regulatory cytokine levels in cord blood.

It is increasingly likely that the importance of microbial biodiversity in pregnancy has been underestimated. Whilst the maternal gut microbiome is an important determinant of postnatal infant colonization, it also has newly recognized antenatal effects

TABLE 2-2   Early Environmental Factors Associated with Variations in Immune Development and Allergy Risk

	Reported effects and associations
Environmental pollutants	
Maternal cigarette smoking (and passive exposure)	Effects on neonatal T cell proliferation, cytokine responses, innate (TLR) mediated responses (and subsequent asthma risk)
Diesel exhaust particles	Effects on T cell cytokine expression in animal models (associated with epigenetic effects). Associations with asthma risk in humans and epigenetic variations)
Persistent organic pollutants	PCB and/or pesticide exposure in pregnancy and lactation associated with increased cord blood IgE levels and increased allergen-specific IgE in later childhood (and asthma risk). Evidence of epigenetic effects
Dietary factors	
Maternal n-3 PUFA intake	Effects on neonatal T cell proliferation, T cell signaling, TLR-mediated cytokine responses. Effects appear more significant in pregnancy than in the postnatal period, with some protection from asthma, eczema and sensitization in intervention studies
Maternal antioxidant intake	Some associations between vitamin E and reduced neonatal proliferation, and reduced risk of some allergic outcomes (but other studies showing no effects). In-vitro studies and animal studies suggest 'redox' status can alter T cell differentiation
Vitamin D	Preliminary reports suggest increased neonatal expression of tolerogenic genes (ILT3 and ILT4) and IFN-γ responses. However, other studies suggest lower Treg numbers. Levels in pregnancy associated with reduced wheeze, asthma and allergic rhinitis, and eczema, although not in all studies. Recognized immunomodulatory properties on epithelial cell, B cell, T cell, and DC functions. Awaiting results of several ongoing intervention studies
Folate	Effects on immune development in humans not clear. Animal studies demonstrate epigenetic changes in pregnancy associated with atopic immune effects and increased risk of 'asthma' phenotype. Human observational studies show some association between maternal supplements and allergic outcomes (not consistent or conclusive)
Prebiotics (soluble dietary fiber)	Some evidence of direct anti-inflammatory effects of short chain fatty acids (SCFA) and allergy protective effects in several randomized controlled trials. May also have effects by promoting 'favorable' gut colonization
Microbial factors	
Maternal microbial exposure in pregnancy	Neonates of mothers in high microbial (farming) environments have increased TLR expression and increased Treg cell activity, associated with subsequent allergy protective effects. Preliminary evidence of epigenetic associations. Animal studies also show immunomodulation and allergy protective effects of antenatal microbial exposure
Postnatal/perinatal microbial exposure	Some studies show protective effects of probiotic supplements on eczema (depending the strain and other host factors). Various immune effects of probiotics reported

on multiple aspects of fetal development. Contrary to the long-standing belief that the womb is 'sterile', maternal microbial transfer to the offspring begins during healthy pregnancy, with microbes detected in normal amniotic fluid placental and fetal membranes, cord blood, and meconium. The maternal microbiome adapts during pregnancy to modulate both metabolism and immune function[20] and this is highly responsive to dietary changes (discussed further below), providing important metabolic and immune influences on the fetus. Modern, refined low-fiber diets are a major determinant of disruptions in 'gut homeostasis' and immune maturation.[21,22] Changes in diet lead to rapid changes in microbiome composition, even within a single day,[23] making this an important target in improving gut biodiversity. This essentially means there are both *direct* immunomodulatory effects of microbial exposure, as well as the *indirect* effects mediated by their metabolites released into the systemic circulation from the mother.

There is significant interest in whether sufficiency of or supplementation with dietary micronutrients and their timings influence allergic disease outcomes.[24] Potential detrimental effects of folate were first highlighted in a mouse model exploring the effects of maternal supplementation with a variety of methyl donors, including folate, on the development of lung disease in the offspring. In humans, several observational studies have associated folic acid supplements in late pregnancy with an increased risk of childhood asthma and eczema. Again, exposure timing appears important, as a recent meta-analysis found no evidence of increased asthma risk with early periconceptional folic acid supplementation used to prevent neural tube defects (NTD).

Animal models suggest a key role for vitamin A in development of antibody responses and Treg cells, and human studies, suggesting important effects on lung development. In-vitro vitamin D has relevant immunomodulatory effects, but there are many contradictory reports on allergy and asthma outcomes related to insufficiency of vitamin D. In general, observational cohort and cross-sectional studies, which have reported an association between low maternal vitamin D and increased infant atopy (including eczema, wheeze and allergen sensitization), have been based on estimates of vitamin D by dietary questionnaires, whereas those studies that have measured maternal serum vitamin D levels in late pregnancy or in cord blood, have generally not reported the same association. Two large RCTs are underway to investigate the potential for vitamin D supplementation in pregnancy to influence atopic outcomes (VDAART and ABCvitD, NCT00920621 and NCT00856947). Other nutritional exposures, such as dietary n-3 PUFA, have favorable effects on the developing immune system both in-utero and in the postnatal period, but achieving favorable n-3/n-6 PUFA balance earlier in development might have greater potential to reduce the burden and risk of allergic disease.

Finally, there is growing interest in the role of dietary fiber as an important immunomodulatory factor, principally because of emerging appreciation of the potent anti-inflammatory effects of short-chain fatty acid metabolites. Colonic microflora ferment dietary fiber to produce SCFA (acetate, and butyrate and propionate), which have been shown in a series of landmark studies to mediate the protective immunomodulatory effects of the commensal bacteria.[25-27] A high-fiber diet significantly increases SCFA metabolites in both feces and serum,[22] with systemic suppression of allergic airways responses.[28] Seminal studies have shown that these microbial-derived dietary fiber metabolites (butyrate) induce tolerogenic dendritic cells (DC) and Treg differentiation, mediating these effects through epigenetic changes, including chromatin modification at the Foxp3 locus.[25,27] In both adults and infants, prebiotic oligosaccharides selectively stimulate growth of immunomodulatory gut microbiota, with favorable effects on colonization, metabolic and immune parameters.[22,29] So far, most human intervention studies have focused on improving *postnatal* infant colonization, and these have not generally examined the metabolic effects of SCFA. It has been proposed that the effects of modulating the maternal microbiome with prebiotic fiber begin in-utero, and that effects on the developing immune system are mediated, at least in part, by SCFA and associated metabolic changes. There may be additional postnatal effects through breast milk and infant colonization. One recent study shows that prebiotic supplements (8 g/day in pregnancy and lactation) alters gene expression in breast milk and significantly increases immune-modulatory cytokines (IL-27) in both colostrum and breast milk.[30] Thus, intervention to increase dietary fiber earlier in pregnancy, when fetal responses are first initiated, is likely to be more effective—given the importance of the maternal microbiome in pregnancy for both immune and metabolic homeostasis.

Postnatal Immune Development and Allergic Disease

Perinatal differences in allergy prone individuals appear to amplify with age with clear differences in postnatal developmental patterns as allergic disease becomes established in children as summarized in Table 2-3. The postnatal development of Th1 immune function appears to proceed more slowly in children who develop subsequent allergic disease. Reduced capacity for Th1 responses in children at risk of allergic diseases is also implicated in attenuated responsiveness to vaccine antigens and greater susceptibility to respiratory infections, which in conjunction with atopic sensitization, appears to be an important risk factor in asthma pathogenesis. Thus, an early relative 'Th2 bias' appears to consolidate in early childhood, and by 5 years of age the production of Th2 cytokines to both allergens and mitogens is significantly higher in allergic children, suggesting this bias influences overall adaptive immune function. Newer approaches utilizing more comprehensive comparisons of differential gene expression in T cells during

TABLE 2-3   Differences in Ontogeny of Immune Responses in Allergic and Non-allergic Infants in the Postnatal Period

	Based on allergic outcomes
	Children who develop subsequent allergy
Antibody responses	
IgE	Progressive increase in allergen-specific IgE titers with age (often will increases in total IgE levels)
IgG	Some studies have shown higher allergen-specific IgG1 and IgG4 sub-classes in young children developing allergic disease, although the significance is not clear
Effector T cell responses	
Proliferation	Several studies report higher frequency and magnitude of proliferative responses to allergens compared with aged-matched non-allergic children
Cytokine responses	Early (pre-symptomatic) increase in allergen-specific Th2 cytokine production (often detected by 6 months of age in children who develop subsequent allergic disease. Slower rate of postnatal Th1 IFN-γ maturation with age (several studies) compared with non-allergic children, however once allergic disease is established some studies show higher production of both Th2 and Th1 cytokine (in what has been described as a Th0 pattern)
Innate responses	
TLR expression	Several studies suggest dysregulated expression of TLR on monocytes of children with established allergic disease. One study also suggested reduced TLR2 expression on pDC.
Cytokine responses	Several studies suggest that children with established allergic disease show reduced TLR responsiveness (with reduced innate cytokine production). Further studies are needed.
Regulatory function	
% Treg cell and *Foxp3* expression	Preliminary studies suggest reduced thymic Treg, *Foxp3* expression and suppressive function in children with atopy, but more studies are needed. In allergic children (e.g., food allergy) there is some evidence that a higher proportion of peripheral allergen-specific Treg is associated with resolution.

stimulation using microarray technology have identified evidence of pre-symptomatic differences in the early T cell. Ongoing investigations are now exploring differences in the epigenetic regulation of early T cell development in allergic and non-allergic children. This approach will identify novel pathways that may shed further light on disease pathogenesis and may also provide early predictors of allergic propensity.

T Regulatory Cells

The dramatic recent rise in such a broad range of immune-mediated disorders has drawn speculation that environmental changes may be having effects on common 'regulatory' immune pathways. A wide range of cells have been designated as regulatory T cells, according to their various abilities to suppress an effector response or to induce tolerance. These include the thymically derived Treg cells or naturally occurring Treg cell, which constitutively express CD25 (the α-chain of the IL-2 receptor) along with other suppressive molecules including CTLA-4. Treg cells can also be generated in the periphery from either CD4+ or CD8+ T cells under specific conditions dictated by ambient cytokine production by other cells. Treg cells undoubtedly play an important role in tolerance. Allergic disease can be viewed as a breakdown in tolerance, and their importance in allergic disease is illustrated by the allergic manifestations disorders in which Tregs are absent or non-functional. Infants with mutations in the FOXP3 gene (IPEX syndrome) develop neonatal onset severe atopy and autoimmune disease requiring bone marrow transplant for survival. Similarly, infants with dedicator of cytokinesis 8

(*DOCK8*) deficiency, who also manifest in infancy with severe eczema and anaphylaxis to food allergens (in addition to their immunocompromise), have impaired suppressive activity of circulating Treg cells.[24]

Studies of human newborn Treg function generally support an association between reduced function at birth and allergic outcomes. For example, suppressor function of newborn Treg cells, who developed egg allergy are reduced and postnatal changes in Treg numbers and/or immunosuppressive function are inversely related to allergy phenotypes in infancy. Whereas the turnover and suppressor function of non-atopic infant's Treg cells appears to increase with age, there is a delay in this process in atopic infants. Lower frequency of circulating Treg cells at birth have been linked to environmental exposures, such as maternal smoking and maternal allergy, and these low numbers are associated with increased risk of atopic sensitization and the development of atopic dermatitis in early childhood.

Innate Immune System and Postnatal Immune Development

Recent findings suggest that engagement of pathogen-associated molecular patterns (PAMPs) receptors, such as the Toll-like receptors (TLRs), in prenatal and early postnatal life is critical for shaping the immune system, and is inversely correlated with the development of allergic disease; this is termed the 'hygiene hypothesis'. In tandem with the emergence of the hygiene hypothesis, there was obvious speculation that early deficiencies in Th1 function of allergic infants may be due to underlying deficiencies in innate immune activation. Microbial products are arguably the most powerful immunostimulants in the early environment and are likely to play a key role in the maturation of innate pathways, Treg cell, and Th1 responses, which may all act together to prevent inappropriate allergic Th2 responses.

Whilst allergic individuals appear to have increased inflammatory responses to microbial products during the early perinatal period, this does not result in sufficient Th1 maturation to suppress allergen-specific Th2 responses. This focuses attention on the role of inflammatory cytokines, such as IL-6, in unfavorably altering the early balance between tolerance and inflammation. Although innate immune responses are important for host defense, excessive inflammatory responses are maladaptive and can lead to unwanted tissue damage. It is possible that the early propensity for innate inflammatory responses is a driver for Th2 cytokine production, potentially 'tipping the balance' during this critical period of T cell development. What role these cytokines then have in the declining innate responses of allergic children is as yet unknown.

Gut Microbiome and Postnatal Immune Development

The mucosal immune system must coordinate and integrate environmental signals to determine immunologic or tolerogenic outcomes upon antigen exposure. This is arguably the dominant factor driving maturation of Th1 and regulatory immune responses in the postnatal period. Declining biodiversity globally has been postulated as a contributing factor to the increasing prevalence of allergic and other chronic inflammatory NCDs. Observations of altered gut microbiota composition in infants who developed allergic disease spawned numerous studies of the use of probiotics and prebiotics to 'restore' an evolutionary normal allergy-protective gut microbiota, and these have been of variable success. However, emerging evidence suggests that it is the immune system, especially within the gastrointestinal tract, that determines the composition of the local commensal flora. For example, Treg cells can facilitate this through inflammation and regulation of IgA to control host–microbiota symbiosis. Therefore, differences in microbiota that are reported to be associated with the development of allergic disease might reflect pre-existing differences in gut mucosal immune function programmed via environmental and genetic interactions during perinatal development. The exogenous supply of various immunomodulatory molecules, first via the amniotic fluid and then postnatally via the breast milk might be critical determinants of immune function and thereby the composition of the microbiota within the gastrointestinal tract. In addition, there is growing awareness of the interplay between nutrition and the microbiome, particularly the effects of specific nutrients, such as vitamin D and soluble dietary fiber

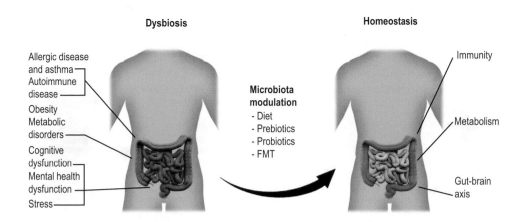

Figure 2-8 Dysbiosis, an imbalance in the structure and/or function of the microbiota that leads to disruption of host–microorganism homeostasis, has been implicated in a broad range of inflammatory disease states including allergic disease. There is also suggestive evidence that changes in gut microbiota have implications for cognitive and mental health dysfunction and stress responses. These diverse multisystem influences have sparked interest in strategies to favorably modulate the gut microbiota to attain homeostasis. *(From West CE, Renz H, Jenmalm MC, Kozyrskyj AL, Allen KJ, Vuillermin P, Prescott SL; in-FLAME Microbiome Interest Group. The gut microbiota and inflammatory non-communicable diseases: associations and potentials for gut microbiota therapies. J Allergy Clin Immunol 2015; 135(1):3–13.)*

(oligosaccharides). In addition to their direct immunomodulatory effects, these nutrients also appear to modulate the microbiome.

Despite emerging data on the role of maternal commensal flora composition during pregnancy in shaping immune function of the offspring, we are far from fully understanding the complexity of this interplay in humans. However, given the clear role for the microbiome in shaping immune development and risk of a range of non-communicable disease including allergies, interventional strategies for modulation of the gut microbiotas, such as prebiotics and probiotics and even fecal transplants, are being actively investigated for the treatment and prevention of NCDs (Fig. 2-8).[24,31]

CONCLUSIONS

The origins of allergic disease lie in early life, involving the complex interaction between inherited genetic susceptibility and early environmental exposures. Allergy-associated genetic variants, along with the uterine environment—influenced by maternal exposures and experiences—produce phenotypic differences, already visible at birth, between those who go on to develop allergic disease and those who do not. Our current best predictors of childhood asthma retain a degree of inaccuracy, suggesting we have not yet captured the full range of variations, exposures, and interaction effects that explain allergy risk. However, in the future, a more complete understanding of the genetic variants that underlie susceptibility and more precise delineation of environmental factors determining developmental trajectories will potentially allow interventions very early in life, perhaps even in-utero, offering the greatest opportunity for primary prevention of allergic disease.

REFERENCES

1. *Holloway JW, Yang IA, Holgate ST. Genetics of allergic disease. J Allergy Clin Immunol 2010; 125(2 Suppl. 2):S81–94.
2. *Meyers DA, Bleecker ER, Holloway JW, et al. Asthma genetics and personalised medicine. Lancet Respir Med 2014;2(5):405–15.
3. Hemminki K, Li X, Sundquist K, et al. Familial risks for asthma among twins and other siblings based on hospitalizations in Sweden. Clin Exp Allergy 2007;37(9):1320–5.
4. Duffy DL, Martin NG, Battistutta D, et al. Genetics of asthma and hay fever in Australian twins. Am Rev Respir Dis 1990;142(6 Pt 1):1351–8.
5. Hopp RJ, Bewtra AK, Watt GD, et al. Genetic analysis of allergic disease in twins. J Allergy Clin Immunol 1984;73(2):265–70.

6. Gerrard JW, Vickers P, Gerrard CD. The familial incidence of allergic disease. Ann Allergy 1976; 36(1):10–15.
7. International HapMap Consortium. A haplotype map of the human genome. Nature 2005; 437(7063):1299–320.
8. Hindorff LA, Sethupathy P, Junkins HA, et al. Potential etiologic and functional implications of genome-wide association loci for human diseases and traits. Proc Natl Acad Sci U S A 2009;106(23):9362–7.
9. Ege MJ, Strachan DP, Cookson WO, et al. Gene-environment interaction for childhood asthma and exposure to farming in Central Europe. J Allergy Clin Immunol 2011;127(1):138–44.
10. Kabesch M, Schedel M, Carr D, et al. IL-4/IL-13 pathway genetics strongly influence serum IgE levels and childhood asthma. J Allergy Clin Immunol 2006;117(2):269–74.
11. Howard TD, Koppelman GH, Xu J, et al. Gene-gene interaction in asthma: IL4RA and IL13 in a Dutch population with asthma. Am J Hum Genet 2002;70(1):230–6.
12. Simpson A, John SL, Jury F, et al. Endotoxin exposure, CD14, and allergic disease: an interaction between genes and the environment. Am J Respir Crit Care Med 2006;174(4):386–92.
13. *Lockett GA, Holloway JW. Genome-wide association studies in asthma; perhaps, the end of the beginning. Curr Opin Allergy Clin Immunol 2013;13(5):463–9.
14. *Martino D, Prescott S. Epigenetics and prenatal influences on asthma and allergic airways disease. Chest 2011;139(3):640–7.
15. Bussmann C, Weidinger S, Novak N. [Genetics of atopic dermatitis]. J Dtsch Dermatol Ges 2011;9(9): 670–6.
16. Irvine AD, McLean WH, Leung DY. Filaggrin mutations associated with skin and allergic diseases. N Engl J Med 2011;365(14):1315–27.
17. *Lockett GA, Patil VK, Soto-Ramírez N, et al. Epigenomics and allergic disease. Epigenomics 2013;5(6):685–99.
18. *Prescott SL. Early-life environmental determinants of allergic diseases and the wider pandemic of inflammatory non-communicable diseases. J Allergy Clin Immunol 2013;131(1):23–30.
19. *Lockett GA, Huoman J, Holloway JW. Does allergy begin in-utero? Pediatr Allergy Immunol 2015;[Epub ahead of print].
20. Koren O, Goodrich JK, Cullender TC, et al. Host remodeling of the gut microbiome and metabolic changes during pregnancy. Cell 2012;150(3):470–80.
21. Nauta AJ, Garssen J. Evidence-based benefits of specific mixtures of non-digestible oligosaccharides on the immune system. Carbohydr Poly 2013;93(1):263–5.
22. *Thorburn AN, Macia L, Mackay CR. Diet, metabolites, and 'Western-lifestyle' inflammatory diseases. Immunity 2014;40(6):833–42.
23. David LA, Maurice CF, Carmody RN, et al. Diet rapidly and reproducibly alters the human gut microbiome. Nature 2014;505(7484):559–63.
24. *Campbell DE, Boyle RJ, Thornton CA, et al. Mechanisms of allergic disease – environmental and genetic determinants for the development of allergy. Clin Exp Allergy 2015;45(5):844–58.
25. Arpaia N, Campbell C, Fan X, et al. Metabolites produced by commensal bacteria promote peripheral regulatory T-cell generation. Nature 2013;504(7480):451–5.
26. Fukuda S, Toh H, Hase K, et al. Bifidobacteria can protect from enteropathogenic infection through production of acetate. Nature 2011;469(7331):543–7.
27. Furusawa Y, Obata Y, Fukuda S, et al. Commensal microbe-derived butyrate induces the differentiation of colonic regulatory T cells. Nature 2013;504(7480):446–50.
28. Trompette A, Gollwitzer ES, Yadava K, et al. Gut microbiota metabolism of dietary fiber influences allergic airway disease and hematopoiesis. Nat Med 2014;20(2):159–66.
29. Slavin J. Fiber and prebiotics: mechanisms and health benefits. Nutrients 2013;5(4):1417–35.
30. Kubota T, Shimojo N, Nonaka K, et al. Prebiotic consumption in pregnant and lactating women increases IL-27 expression in human milk. Br J Nutr 2014;111(4):625–32.
31. *West CE, Renz H, Jenmalm MC, et al. The gut microbiota and inflammatory non-communicable diseases: associations and potentials for gut microbiota therapies. J Allergy Clin Immunol 2015;135(1):3–14.

Key references are preceded by an asterisk.

CHAPTER 3

Epidemiology of Allergic Diseases

Adnan Custovic

CHAPTER OUTLINE

INTRODUCTION

DEFINITIONS

Asthma

Allergic Rhinitis

Atopy and Atopic Sensitization

Food Allergy

ESTIMATES OF WORLDWIDE PREVALENCE OF ASTHMA, RHINITIS, ATOPIC SENSITIZATION, AND FOOD ALLERGY

Asthma

Geographical Variations in the Prevalence of Asthma

   Childhood Asthma

   Adult Asthma

Allergic Rhinitis

Food Allergy

TRENDS IN PREVALENCE OVER TIME

Asthma, Allergic Rhinitis and Atopic Sensitization

Food Allergy

RISK FACTORS FOR ASTHMA AND ALLERGIC DISEASES

The 'Hygiene Hypothesis'

Protective Exposures in Rural Areas

Timing of Exposure

Urban Lifestyle and Air Pollution

Allergens

The Interaction between Environmental Exposures and Genetic Predisposition

CONCLUDING REMARKS: EPIDEMIOLOGY IN THE 21ST CENTURY

'Team Science' to Solve the Puzzle of Asthma and Allergies

SUMMARY OF IMPORTANT CONCEPTS

- Epidemiology is the study of the distribution of disease and, by extension, its causes and consequences, mostly in general populations.
- The rates of allergic sensitization and allergic diseases have been increasing, although the increase in prevalence of asthma may have slowed amongst children in some parts of the developed world.
- Allergic disease is less common in rural parts of low-income countries, although allergic sensitization can be common in these areas.
- There has been very little success in explaining the increased prevalence of allergic disease. The great changes observed in prevalence and distribution strongly suggest a major role for the environment.
- Factors that initiate allergy and allergic diseases should be differentiated from factors that exacerbate these after they have been established.
- Allergies are affected by environmental factors, including diet; exposure to a normal, diverse microflora; infections; exposure to air pollutants; and occupational exposures.
- Outcomes for asthma can be considerably improved by good management.

INTRODUCTION

Epidemiology studies the distribution of disease in populations and addresses the issues related to the definition of disease(s), overall morbidity and mortality in the community, factors that may cause or predispose to the development of disease(s), and the effect of interventions (such as therapeutic and preventative strategies). Thus, the focus is on populations rather than individual patients. At the simplest level, this involves surveys that measure disease frequency at a single time point within a given population. Such studies may also identify factors that are associated with disease and that can be quantified in terms of risk.

In the area of allergic disease, a large number of cross-sectional studies have been carried out, both in adults and in children, to ascertain the prevalence of these conditions and explore their associated risk factors. Some of these crucially important studies, such as the International Study of Asthma and Allergies in Childhood (ISAAC; http://isaac.auckland.ac.nz/) and the European Community Respiratory Health Survey (ECRHS; http://www.ecrhs.org/), are reviewed in this chapter. This chapter does not offer a complete overview of the epidemiology of allergic diseases, but focuses on examining the definitions of the relevant clinical outcomes, the estimates of prevalence (including changes in prevalence over time and the differences by geographical area/place), and the association between IgE-mediated sensitization and symptomatic allergic disease (asthma, allergic rhinitis, and IgE-mediated food allergy). Some of the major risk factors are examined, including a brief discussion on some of the intervention studies aiming at primary (preventing disease development) and secondary prevention (reducing morbidity or severity).

DEFINITIONS

One of the challenges to understanding the epidemiology, pathophysiology, and etiology of allergic diseases is the lack of consensus in defining these conditions. Here, we use 'asthma' as an example, but also briefly discuss the definitions of allergic rhinitis, atopy, and food allergy.

Asthma

There have been many attempts to reach a consensus definition of 'asthma,' both for clinical practice and epidemiologic studies (Table 3-1). However, despite such efforts, a recent systematic review showed that in 122 publications investigating the risk factors associated with childhood asthma, 60 different definitions of 'asthma' were used.[9] Whilst many of these definitions were similar (with only subtle differences between them), the overall impact of such heterogeneity in defining the primary outcome on the reported prevalence and on our understanding of the risk factors associated with asthma, is unclear. When four of the most commonly used definitions of 'asthma' were applied to a high-risk population of children, the overall agreement was 61%, suggesting that 39% of the subjects in a study could move from being assigned as 'asthma' to 'no asthma' depending on which definition of asthma was used.[9] Throughout the remainder of this chapter, evidence is provided to support the view that 'asthma' is not a single disease entity, but rather an umbrella term to describe a syndrome encompassing a collection of several diseases, each with unique underpinning pathophysiologic mechanisms, and environmental and genetic associates.[10,11] Some have proposed abolishing the term 'asthma' altogether, proposing that asthma symptoms reflect a similar clinical manifestation of several distinct diseases.[12] Identification and adequate description of these separate disease entities (sometimes referred to as 'asthma endotypes'[10,13]) is crucial for the advancement of personalized medicine in asthma.[11] In this context, 'asthma phenotype' can be considered to be an observable characteristic, which can be shared between several diseases within the asthma syndrome, whilst 'asthma endotype' is a unique disease with clearly defined pathophysiologic mechanisms, pathology, and genetic and environmental risk factors. However, because true asthma 'endotypes' have not as yet been identified with absolute certainty (aspirin-sensitive asthma and occupational asthma probably being the closest to the definition of endotype), it has to be emphasized that, currently, 'asthma endotype' is primarily a hypothetical construct, which has value in helping us to better understand the frequency of asthma-related diseases within the population, their risk factors, and underlying pathophysiologic mechanisms.[14] Unless epidemiologic studies find better ways to distinguish between different endotypes at a population level, it will be difficult to discover their underlying genetic risk factors,

TABLE 3-1 Asthma Definitions

Source	Year	Definition
CIBA Foundation[1]	1959	Condition of subjects with widespread narrowing of the bronchial airways, which changes its severity over short periods spontaneously or during treatment
American Thoracic Society[2]	1962	Disease characterized by increased responsiveness of the trachea and bronchi to various stimuli and manifested by widespread narrowing of the airways that changes in severity spontaneously or as a result of therapy
World Health Organization (WHO)[3]	1975	Chronic condition characterized by recurrent bronchospasm resulting from a tendency to develop reversible narrowing of the airway lumina in response to stimuli of a level or intensity not inducing such narrowing in most individuals
American Thoracic Society[4]	1987	Clinical syndrome is characterized by increased responsiveness of the tracheobronchial tree to a variety of stimuli. Major symptoms are paroxysms of dyspnea, wheezing, and cough, which may vary from mild and almost undetectable to severe and unremitting (i.e. status asthmaticus). Primary physiologic manifestation of this hyperresponsiveness is variable airway obstruction, occurring in the form of fluctuations in the severity of obstruction after bronchodilator or corticosteroid use, or increased obstruction caused by drugs or other stimuli, as well as evidence of mucosal edema of bronchi, infiltration of bronchial mucosa or submucosa with inflammatory cells (especially eosinophils), shedding of epithelium, and obstruction of peripheral airways with mucus
NHLBI/NIH[5]	1991	Lung disease with the following characteristics: (1) airway obstruction that is reversible (but not completely in some patients) spontaneously or with treatment; (2) airway inflammation; and (3) increased airway responsiveness to a variety of stimuli
NHLBI/NIH[6,7]	1993 1995 1997	Chronic inflammatory disorder of the airways in which many cells play a role, particularly mast cells, eosinophils, and T lymphocytes. In susceptible individuals, this inflammation causes recurrent episodes of wheezing, breathlessness, chest tightness, and cough in early morning. Symptoms are usually associated with widespread but variable airflow limitation that is at least partly reversible spontaneously or with treatment. Inflammation also causes an increase in airway responsiveness that is associated with a variety of stimuli
NIH/NHLBI[8]	2002	Chronic inflammatory disorder of the airways, in which many cells and cellular elements play a role. The chronic inflammation causes an increase in airway hyperresponsiveness that leads to recurrent episodes of wheezing, breathlessness, chest tightness, and coughing, particularly at night or in the early morning. These episodes are usually associated with widespread but variable airflow obstruction that is often reversible spontaneously or with treatment.

NHLBI/NIH, National Heart, Lung, and Blood Institute/National Institutes of Health.

pathophysiologic processes, or identify novel therapeutic targets for stratified treatment, as any signal will be diluted by phenotypic heterogeneity.[11] The phenotypic heterogeneity of asthma may result in difficulties in the interpretation of the findings across different populations, and in discrepancies between different studies investigating asthma epidemiology (e.g., when estimating asthma prevalence and associated risk factors). Further problems for asthma epidemiology arise from the difficulties in distinguishing the disease state (i.e. the presence or absence of the disease), from triggers of acute asthma attacks.

Allergic Rhinitis

Epidemiologic studies of rhinitis have been undertaken less frequently, but are arguably as problematic and difficult to interpret as those of asthma. It is likely that phenotypic heterogeneity in rhinitis mirrors that of asthma, with the existence of a number of different but as yet poorly defined endotypes of rhinitis.[15] Most studies rely only on reported symptoms, and most questionnaires collect self-reports of responders, confirming that they have 'allergic rhinitis' or 'hay fever'. Symptoms suggestive of rhinitis include nasal blockage and/or itching, runny nose (rhinorrhea) and sneezing, which may be seasonal (e.g., related to pollen exposure in hay fever), or perennial. In the case of rhino-conjunctivitis, symptoms also include ocular involvement such as conjunctival irritation and lachrymation. However, these symptoms are relatively non-specific, and when using only questionnaire surveys, they may be confused with viral upper respiratory tract infections. Acknowledging all of the above potential pitfalls, epidemiologic studies reported to date show that allergic rhinitis is amongst the most common chronic diseases, particularly amongst school-age children and young adults in developed countries.

Atopy and Atopic Sensitization

A large number of epidemiologic studies have indicated that atopic sensitization is a strong risk-factor for asthma and rhinitis/conjunctivitis.[16] However, in different parts of the world, there is considerable variability in the strength of this association.[17,18] Furthermore, most sensitized subjects (i.e. those producing IgE antibodies towards common inhalant and food allergens) do not have symptoms of asthma or any other allergic disease, and many sensitized individuals will remain asymptomatic throughout their lives. One of the reasons for the inconsistencies of findings on the association between atopic sensitization and asthma may be due to phenotypic heterogeneity in the definition of asthma, which is outlined above. However, similar concerns can be raised about the current definitions of 'atopy' and 'atopic sensitization' used in epidemiology and clinical practice. It is often assumed that 'atopy' can be relatively easily assessed and confirmed by skin-prick tests or measurement of serum-specific IgE. Similar to clinical practice, most epidemiologic studies define atopic sensitization as a positive allergen-specific serum IgE (most commonly specific IgE level $>0.35\,\mathrm{kU_A/L}$) or a positive skin-prick test (usually, but not exclusively, a wheal diameter ≥ 3 mm) to any common food or inhalant allergen. However, positive 'allergy' tests indicate only the presence of allergen-specific IgE (either in serum or bound to the membrane of mast cells in the skin), and are not necessarily related to the development of clinical symptoms upon allergen exposure. Indeed, a sizeable proportion of individuals with positive allergy tests have no evidence of allergic disease.[19] A number of studies have shown that the level of specific IgE antibodies and the size of skin test wheal diameter predict the presence and severity of allergic diseases (both respiratory and food allergies) much better than the presence of a positive 'allergy test'.[20–22] It is now recognized that quantification of allergen-specific serum IgE amongst young wheezy children is likely the best predictor to help identify those who are at high risk of subsequent development of persistent asthma.[23] In addition, the level of IgE antibodies and the size of skin test wheal diameter to inhalant allergens are associated with an increased risk of hospital admission with acute asthma attacks in both adults and children.[24,25]

A stratification of atopic sensitization into several subtypes has recently been demonstrated by using a data driven machine learning approach with Bayesian inference to cluster 'allergy tests' (skin-prick tests and allergen-specific IgE antibody measurements), which were longitudinally collected in a population-based birth cohort study from birth to school-age.[26] This analysis took into account the timing of the onset of sensitization, its progression and/or remission, and the type of allergens causing sensitization. Most of the children who would be considered 'atopic' using conventional epidemiologic and clinical definitions were clustered into four distinct subtypes of atopic sensitization. Based on their characteristics, these subtypes were named: 'Multiple Early,' 'Multiple Late,' 'Predominantly Dust Mite,' and 'Non-Dust Mite' atopic vulnerabilities.[26] This data-driven approach to stratification of atopy uncovered an unexpected, but very strong risk factor for asthma; although less than one third of the children considered to be sensitized using conventional definitions clustered to the 'Multiple Early' class, the risk of asthma was highly and significantly increased amongst the children in this class (with an odds ratio of 29.3), but not amongst those in other subtypes (Fig. 3-1). In addition, children in the 'Multiple Early' atopy subtype had significantly lower lung function and were at high risk of severe asthma exacerbations compared with all other classes (subtypes).[26,27]

In this chapter, atopic sensitization will not be referred to as a simple yes/no phenomenon in relation to presence, onset, progression, and severity of allergic diseases. The emerging data suggest that not only 'asthma' but also 'atopy' is an umbrella term encompassing several different subtypes that differ in their association with allergic disease.[28] In this conceptual framework, detectable serum IgE or positive skin-prick tests alone do not define atopic sensitization. Rather, these tests should be viewed as intermediate phenotypes of a true latent allergic vulnerability[29]—thus, similar to asthma, atopy may not be a single phenotype, but rather a sum of several atopic vulnerabilities, which differ in their relationship with clinical allergy.[26,30]

Food Allergy

The focus in this chapter is on IgE-mediated food allergy. Diagnosis of food allergy is based on clinical history and diagnostic test results, and the gold standard test to confirm or refute the diagnosis is a double-blind, placebo-controlled oral food challenge.[20] However, many reported food allergies are not confirmed using such a thorough diagnostic evaluation. As a result, conducting large epidemiologic surveys that rely only on questionnaires may not provide accurate data on true prevalence, and estimates of prevalence obtained from questionnaires are likely to be inflated. It is therefore not surprising that systematic reviews of the literature on the prevalence of food allergies have reported considerable heterogeneity between different studies, and confirmed that the prevalence estimates based on self-reported symptoms tend to be higher than those based on objective assessments.[31,32]

To facilitate the conduct of future studies, it would be useful to develop simpler tests that discriminate accurately food-allergic from food-tolerant subjects, without the need to perform placebo-controlled oral food challenges.[32]

ESTIMATES OF WORLDWIDE PREVALENCE OF ASTHMA, RHINITIS, ATOPIC SENSITIZATION, AND FOOD ALLERGY

Most of the studies collected data using standardized questionnaires enquiring about the symptoms, usually assessing point prevalence (the proportion of individuals in a population with a disease at a particular time point) of allergic diseases, or their lifetime prevalence (the proportion of individuals in a population who have had a disease at some point in their life up to the time of assessment). For children, the most widely used questionnaire was developed for the International Study of Asthma and Allergies in Childhood (ISAAC).[33–35] For studies in adults, the questionnaire developed for the International Union against Tuberculosis and Lung Disease (IUATLD)[36] was adapted for use in the European Community Respiratory Health Survey (ECRHS)[37] and the World Health Survey.[38] Studies using these tools have reported that across the world, there is a large variability in the prevalence of asthma (Figs. 3-2–3-4), upper airway allergic disease (such as allergic rhinitis), atopic sensitization, and food allergy.[39,40] Generally low rates have been reported from developing countries, with much higher prevalence in the developed 'Western' countries. Furthermore, within the same ethnic group, there is considerable variation in the prevalence over time and across different geographical areas.[18,41–45] In general, allergic sensitization and allergic diseases increase with affluence, both at a country and the individual level.[41] Today, high socioeconomic status as assessed by parental education remains a strong risk factor for atopy, even in affluent countries such as Germany. In contrast, in inner city areas of the USA, increased rates of allergic sensitization and asthma are related to poverty.[46] These observations are further proof that there is a strong environmental component to the causation of these conditions, and that the recent epidemic of allergic diseases in the developed countries is

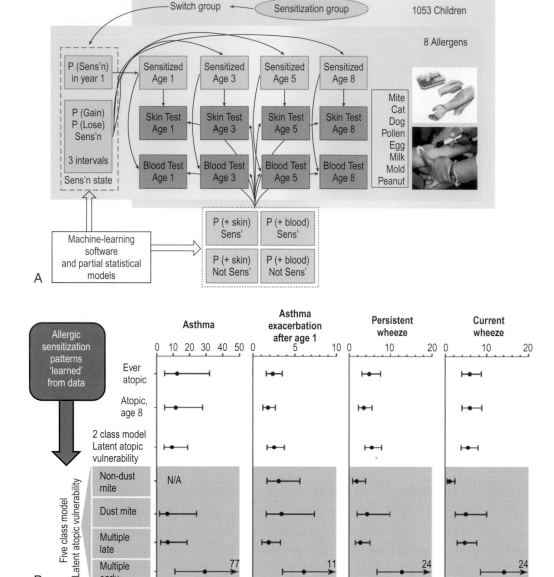

Figure 3-1 A. Hypothesizing with data revealed a stratification of atopy. **B.** An unexpected risk factor for asthma discovered. Sens'n, sensitization; Sens', sensitized. *(Adapted from: Simpson A, Tan VY, Winn J, Svensen M, Bishop CM, Heckerman DE, et al. Beyond atopy: multiple patterns of sensitization in relation to asthma in a birth cohort study. Am J Respir Crit Care Med 2010; 181(11):1200–1206.)*

predominantly caused by the changes in environment. On the other hand, genetic studies have demonstrated a clear familial aggregation, and several genetic loci have been reproducibly linked to asthma, atopy, and total IgE in genome-wide association studies and linkage analyses,[47,48] suggesting an additional and important genetic component (for details see Ch. 2).

Asthma

Asthma is one of the most common chronic diseases globally, and individuals of all ages throughout the world are affected by this disorder, which can be severe and sometimes fatal. It is estimated that approximately 300 million people worldwide have asthma, and by 2025, a further 100 million will likely be affected. Deaths from asthma are relatively rare and do not correlate well with prevalence; annual worldwide mortality from asthma has been estimated at 250 000.

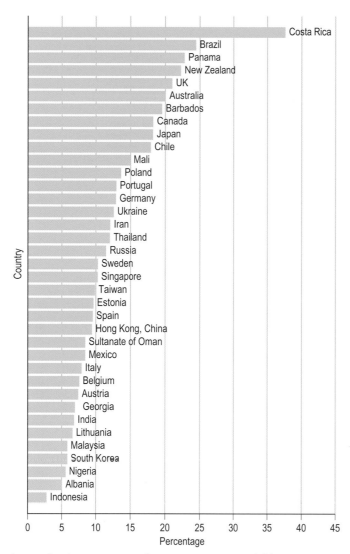

Figure 3-2 Prevalence of asthma symptoms by country amongst children 6–7 years of age, according to the 1999–2004 International Study of Asthma and Allergies in Childhood (ISAAC) III study. *(From Asher MI, Montefort S, Bjorksten B, et al. Worldwide time trends in the prevalence of symptoms of asthma, allergic rhinoconjunctivitis, and eczema in childhood: ISAAC Phases One and Three repeat multicountry cross-sectional surveys. Lancet 2006; 368:733–743.)*

Geographical Variations in the Prevalence of Asthma

Data from standardized, multicenter international studies have shown striking geographical variations in the prevalence of asthma symptoms throughout the world, with the highest prevalence rates observed in English-speaking countries (UK, Australia, New Zealand, Ireland, USA) and Latin America, and the lowest in the Mediterranean, Eastern Europe and rural areas of Africa and China.[17,34,36,39,44] These patterns appear comparable between children and adults, and the global asthma prevalence seems to range from 1% to 18%.

Childhood Asthma

The International Study of Asthma and Allergies in Childhood[33–35,39] was established in 1991 and used a global and standardized approach to address the perceived increase in prevalence of asthma and allergies worldwide and the paucity of reliable and comparable data to measure the scale of the problem. ISAAC Phase One was conducted between 1992 and 1998 and used a simple validated questionnaire to measure worldwide prevalence of asthma, rhinitis, and hay fever in 56 countries in a study involving

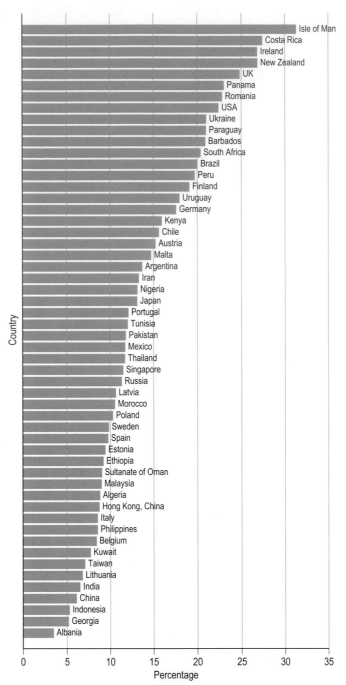

Figure 3-3 Prevalence of asthma symptoms by country amongst children 13–14 years of age, according to the 1999–2004 International Study of Asthma and Allergies in Childhood (ISAAC) III study. *(From Asher MI, Montefort S, Bjorksten B, et al. Worldwide time trends in the prevalence of symptoms of asthma, allergic rhinoconjunctivitis, and eczema in childhood: ISAAC Phases One and Three repeat multicountry cross-sectional surveys. Lancet 2006; 368:733–743.)*

~700 000 children aged 6 to 7 years and 13 to 14 years.[35] Asthma was defined as a positive answer to the question "Have you (has your child) had wheezing or whistling in the chest in the last 12 months?". There was a staggering 20-fold variation worldwide in the prevalence of asthma, with the highest prevalence rates reported in the UK, Australia, New Zealand, and Ireland, and the lowest in Eastern Europe, Indonesia, Greece, China, Taiwan, India, and Ethiopia. Wide variations in asthma prevalence were observed in populations that appeared genetically similar, leading to a series of follow-up studies in ISAAC Phase Two, which investigated a range of environmental factors that could

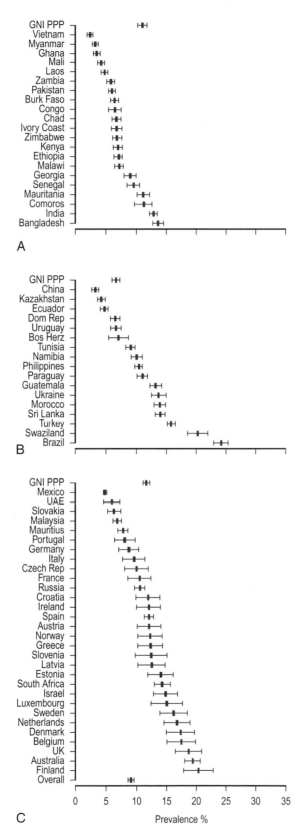

Figure 3-4 A–C. Estimates of adult asthma prevalence from the World Health Survey by country and gross national income. Bos Herz, Bosnia Herzegovina; Burk Faso, Burkina Faso; Dom Rep, Dominican Republic; GNI PPP, gross national income per capita at purchasing power parity rates; Rep, Republic; UAE, United Arab Emirates; UK, United Kingdom. *(From Sembajwe G, Cifuentes M, Tak SW, et al. National income, self-reported wheezing and asthma diagnosis from the World Health Survey. Eur Respir J 2010; 35:279–286.)*

contribute to disease risk (including diet, infection, indoor and outdoor environment, climate, and allergens).[34] These studies investigated variations in prevalence, which emerged from Phase One, amongst children aged 10 to 12 years. Comparisons between populations in different centers have been undertaken using objective measures of disease and assessment of environment, lifestyle, and clinical management. However, no single unifying factor has emerged to account for the observed differences.

Adult Asthma

The European Community Respiratory Health Survey (ECRHS) is a multicenter study designed to estimate geographical variation in the prevalence, management, and determinants of asthma and allergy amongst 140 000 adults aged 22 to 44 years from 22 countries, using standardized instruments and definitions.[37] This study used a validated questionnaire to assess the prevalence of asthma and allergic diseases and to collect information on possible risk factors. 'Diagnosed current asthma' was defined as a positive answer to either having had an attack of asthma in the previous 12 months or being on current medication for asthma. This study also aimed to assess the prevalence of airway hyperresponsiveness, and to estimate variations in exposures to known or suspected risk factors for asthma, and assess their contribution in explaining the variations in the prevalence of disease. A smaller random sample of participants from multiple centers was selected for more detailed questionnaires, skin-prick testing, blood tests for the measurement of total and specific IgE, spirometry and methacholine challenge during Stage II, which took place from 1991 to 1993. ECRHS II was conducted subsequently, directed towards assessment of the incidence and risk factors for the development of allergic disease, atopy and rapid loss of lung function in middle-aged adults (with collection of dust samples and air pollution data). ECRHS III is a follow-up survey of more than 10 000 adults, who were first recruited in 1992–1994, aiming (amongst other things) to describe the change in the prevalence of respiratory symptoms and IgE sensitization in adults as they age.

The ECRHS reported a six-fold variation in the prevalence of current asthma between different countries.[37] There was a large variation in self-reported asthma symptoms; for example, from 4.1% (95% CI 3.1–5.2) in India to 32.0% (95% CI 30.1–33.9) in Dublin, for recent wheeze. The prevalence of respiratory symptoms and asthma tended to be low in Western Europe (Belgium, France, Germany, Switzerland, Austria, and Iceland); in Mediterranean countries (Greece, Italy, Spain Portugal, and Algeria); and in India. In Australia, New Zealand, Ireland, the UK, and the single center sampled in the USA, prevalence rates of asthma symptoms were high. The geographical distribution of airway hyperresponsiveness fitted well with that for symptoms and asthma. A high prevalence of atopic sensitization was found in English-speaking countries (Australia, New Zealand, USA, and the UK), whilst it was low in Iceland, Greece, Norway, and parts of Spain.

Allergic Rhinitis

In ISAAC, allergic rhino-conjunctivitis was defined, based on questionnaire responses, as sneezing or a runny or a blocked nose without a cold or flu, accompanied by itchy, watery eyes. There was a 30-fold variation in the prevalence rate amongst children aged 13–14 years between different sites from 56 countries (from 1.4% to 39.7%). Estimates for adults obtained in the ECRHS suggested median prevalence of nasal allergies of approximately 21%, with a range from 9.5% (95% CI 8.5–10.6) in Algeria to 40.9% (95% CI 39.2–42.7) in Australia. Countries with high prevalence rates included the Netherlands, Belgium, France, Switzerland, the UK, New Zealand, Australia, and the USA.

Food Allergy

Most of the estimates on the prevalence of food allergy to date, are based on data from telephone surveys and cross-sectional surveys. A telephone survey administered in 2002 in the USA reported that 2.3% of the general population reported allergy to fish or shellfish.[49] Another telephone survey estimated the prevalence rate of peanut or tree nut allergy to be ~1.4% amongst adults, and ~2.1% amongst children.[50] A school-based survey in Singapore and the Philippines estimated a prevalence rate of peanut and tree nut allergy to be <1%.[51] In Australia, the prevalence of food allergy may be higher than that observed in the USA or the UK, and the prevalence of peanut allergy amongst 1-year-old children was estimated to be ~3%.[52]

In contrast to the above data, a report from the UK general practices, which interrogated a large health database on almost 3 million patients registered with 422 general practices, suggested a much lower prevalence rate of peanut allergy of 0.05%.[53] This reported prevalence rate was markedly lower than the estimates derived from other reports from England, such as findings from unselected birth cohorts from Southampton and Manchester, which corroborated questionnaire data with detailed objective assessment such as skin tests, peanut-specific IgE measurement, and oral peanut challenges, and estimated the prevalence of peanut allergy amongst school-age children to be ~2%.[19,32] These data suggest a worrying possibility that in the UK (and probably in many other countries), a considerable proportion of children with peanut allergy are not diagnosed by their primary care physicians and consequently, are not appropriately managed. This alarming suggestion underpins the urgent need to tackle this problem. A meta-analysis of studies that used objective measures (such as peanut sensitization or food challenge) reported little heterogeneity between different studies in children aged 0 to 4 years and 5 to 16 years, with the estimates of prevalence of peanut allergy based on oral peanut challenge ranging from 0.2% to 1.6% in different countries.[54]

Our current knowledge about the epidemiology of food allergies resembles that of respiratory allergies before the conduct of large standardized international studies (such as ISAAC and ECRHS). One such effort to address this problem is the EuroPrevall study, which aims to characterize the patterns and prevalence of food allergies across Europe. As part of the project, a multicenter birth cohort study recruited more than 12000 newborn babies in nine European countries, between 2005 and 2009, and all children with a suspected food allergy are being evaluated in detail, including double-blind, placebo-controlled oral food challenge tests. It would be important for similar endeavors using standardized methodology and accurate phenotyping (including oral food challenges) to follow across the USA and the rest of the world because an increasing body of evidence suggests that peanut allergy and other food allergies represent a significant health concern. The pressing need to address this issue is further emphasized by the evidence, which suggests that the prevalence of IgE-mediated food allergy amongst children may be increasing at an alarming rate.

TRENDS IN PREVALENCE OVER TIME

There has been a steep rise in the prevalence of asthma and allergic diseases in the last century, which has been documented in a number of repeated cross-sectional surveys[55] (Fig. 3-5). This increasing prevalence of symptomatic allergic diseases has been accompanied by the rising trends in IgE-mediated sensitization.[42] It appears that since the 1990s, the prevalence of some allergic diseases (e.g., asthma) may have peaked in regions with previously documented high prevalence, whereas an increase was recorded in several centers with presumed lower prevalence, mostly in low- and mid-income countries.[39] It is of note that the increases in different allergic diseases may not have occurred contemporaneously; there are some data to suggest that hay fever increased in the USA as early as the mid-20th century, followed by an increase in asthma between 1960s and 1990s, whilst the rise in food allergies may be a phenomenon that started in the late 20th century, with this trend continuing into the first decades of the current century.

Asthma, Allergic Rhinitis and Atopic Sensitization

ISAAC Phase Three (conducted 1999–2004) was broadly a repetition of Phase One, with an approximately 7-year interval to investigate the differences in time trends

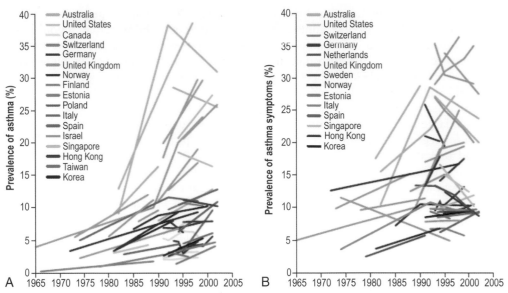

Figure 3-5 Changes in the prevalence of diagnosed asthma and asthma symptoms over time in children and young adults. *(From: Eder W, Ege MJ, von Mutius E. The asthma epidemic. N Engl J Med 2006; 355(21):2226–2235, with permission.)*

internationally.[39] When all the results are pooled together, it can be seen that there has been an overall increase in the prevalence of asthma and rhinitis in both age groups from 13.2% to 13.7% in the 13–14 years age group, and from 11.1% to 11.6% in the 6–7 years age group.[39] However, wide variations were observed between centers, and different patterns were noted in different regions. For example, increases were seen in Asia-Pacific, India, North America, Eastern Mediterranean, and Western Europe in the younger age group, and Africa, Asia Pacific, India, Latin America, and Northern and Eastern Europe amongst children in the older age group. The most marked reduction in current asthma symptoms was observed in English-speaking countries (0.5% reduction at age 13–14 years, and 0.1% reduction at age 6–7 years). A similar effect was seen for severe asthma symptoms. Overall, the global burden of allergic airway diseases and atopic sensitization has likely increased, and the geographical differences in prevalence globally appear to have decreased.

Other investigators have studied the variation in asthma prevalence in different communities that live within the same country. For example, in Ghana, the prevalence of exercise-induced bronchospasm (objective marker of airway hyperreactivity and asthma) was found to be significantly higher amongst urban affluent children (4.7%) compared with urban poor children (2.2%) and children living in rural communities (3.8%).[41] Similar differences were observed for atopic sensitization (determined objectively using skin-prick tests). A subsequent study using identical methodology demonstrated that the prevalence of both atopic sensitization and exercise-induced bronchospasm doubled over a 10-year period, between 1993 and 2003.[42]

The proportion of patients consulting their primary care physicians for asthma has also changed over time, with an eight-fold increase for children aged up to 14 years between 1960 and 1990, and a three- to four-fold increase amongst adults (but notably with fewer consultations per patient). Asthma prevalence recorded by the general practice research databases increased from 3% to 5% from 1990–1998 in all age groups; however, the rates of incident asthma recorded in the same database fell during the same period of time. Rates of hospital admissions have possibly shown the most dramatic trends, with a steady and significant increase in all age groups between 1960 and 1985 (especially for children under the age of 4 years),[56] after which time a steady fall has occurred. Death from asthma is a relatively rare event and overall has fallen steadily (e.g., for young adults, the rate has approximately halved, to 1 per 100 000 per annum), likely reflecting improvements in the provision of medical care.

Food Allergy

In the USA, three nationwide telephone surveys suggested that the prevalence of self-reported peanut allergy in children in 2008 was 1.4%, compared with 0.8% in 2002 and 0.4% in 1997. In the UK, reported rates of peanut allergy in three cohorts of 3- to 5-year-old children born in 1989, 1994–1996, and 2001–2002 in the same geographical area were 0.5%, 1.4%, and 1.2%, respectively. These trends have been indirectly confirmed in a recent report from ECRHS on the prevalence of sensitization to foods in a sample of young adults from Western Europe, the USA, and Australia, which reported that prevalence of sensitization to peanut was highest in the USA center in Portland.[57] Unfortunately, the data to provide accurate estimates on time-trends of food allergies are lacking, and we have to fill this knowledge gap as a matter of urgency.

To summarize, the prevalence rates of asthma, atopic sensitization, and other allergic diseases vary considerably throughout the world, and are highest in the English-speaking nations, higher in western than eastern parts of Europe, and higher in urban than rural parts of Africa. Overall, the evidence suggests that there has been a marked increase (two- to three-fold) in the prevalence of asthma in the latter part of the last century, seen across all grades of severity of symptoms and all ages. Evidence collected more recently suggests that the increase is asthma may have flattened off, and that at least in some age groups, asthma prevalence may be decreasing. However, ISAAC Phase Three suggests that in many parts of the world, asthma prevalence continues to increase, and that the global differences may be shrinking in magnitude.

The sharp increase in the prevalence of asthma and allergic diseases observed since the mid-20th century has occurred in a timeframe that is too short for the increase to be attributable to genetic factors alone. The explanation for the increasing trends therefore must lie in the influences brought about by environmental exposures and associated lifestyle, both of which have undergone rapid and profound changes in the last half of the century. Numerous environmental changes have occurred in parallel during this period, including changes in diet and exercise, patterns of microbial exposure in early life, family size and childcare arrangements, changes to housing design, and environmental exposure to a number of pollutants. It is important to emphasize that the increase in the prevalence of asthma and allergic diseases is likely a consequence of environmental factors increasing the risk in genetically susceptible individuals mediated through gene–environment interactions, and that the effect of environmental exposures is usually context-dependent.[58]

RISK FACTORS FOR ASTHMA AND ALLERGIC DISEASES

In general, risk factors for asthma and allergic diseases can be divided into those that cause their development and those that trigger symptoms amongst patients with established disease (although some do both, and the mechanisms by which this happens are complex and interactive). For example, multiple genes interact with each other and with the environment in determining individual susceptibility. In addition to gene–environment interactions, environmental factors may also interact with each other (e.g., some air pollutants may increase the allergenicity of pollen grains). There is a wealth of information about the putative risk factors for asthma development in children, coming mainly from a number of birth cohort studies; however, there is a relative paucity of data for adult-onset disease. Numerous environmental exposures, such as exposure to indoor and outdoor allergens, tobacco smoke, air pollution, viral and bacterial infections, and diet (especially obesity) are important in the etiology and severity of asthma, and we will briefly discuss some of these.

In the developed world, where the prevalence of allergic diseases is high, the general trend is to have smaller family size, cleaner living conditions, and highly processed and often sterilized food, with additives and altered nutrient content. A proportion of the population in the developing countries (particularly in the urban areas) is following this pattern and adopting certain aspects of the 'Westernized' lifestyle, and this may be associated with an increase in allergic disease. Similarly, migration from developing to developed countries may result in an increased risk for allergies amongst migrants.

The 'Hygiene Hypothesis'

The 'hygiene hypothesis' for allergic diseases took shape following a seminal publication by David Strachan on the inverse association between family size and the development of hay fever,[59] with a suggestion that infections in early life may be an underlying protective factor against allergies. A decrease in infections during childhood consequent to the cleaner living conditions and less contact with other children may constitute a loss of a protective factor, leading to the increased risk for the development of allergies.[60] Following this initial observation, a number of studies have reported an inverse relation between atopic diseases and overcrowding, contact with other children (which has been studied using day-care attendance as proxy of exposure) and other markers of affluence,[61] but the underlying mechanisms have not been elucidated. In most studies, day-care attendance during the first year of life was associated with decreased rates of allergic sensitization and atopic asthma (but in some studies, day-care increased the risk of early childhood wheezing).[62–65] Similarly, contact with domestic pets early in life (in particular dogs) has been shown to be protective against the development of allergic sensitization.[66] Overcrowding, day-care attendance, and dog ownership may be associated with higher environmental exposure to microbial compounds such as endotoxins,[67,68] and may be the markers of increased microbial diversity in the environment.[69] Whether high and diverse exposures to microbial compounds account for the protective effect associated with large sibship size, exposure to other children in early life and dog ownership remains to be determined.

Experimental animal studies have shown that gut microbiota may also play an important role.[70] In mouse experiments, colonization of the gastrointestinal tract by bacteria is a prerequisite for the normal development of systemic and local mucosal immune responses, the absence of bacteria is associated with impaired immune responses and a predominance of Th2 type responses, and introduction of a gastrointestinal (GI) microflora has a protective effect and allows the development of tolerance. Although differences in GI flora have been observed between allergic and non-allergic children,[71,72] conclusive evidence to confirm the role of gut microbiota in the development of allergies in humans is lacking. Several intervention studies using different probiotics and prebiotics (and the combinations thereof) have reported conflicting results.[73–75] In general, reported intervention studies indicate some benefit for the prevention of eczema, but the effect on allergic sensitization, asthma and rhinitis remain unclear.

Protective Exposures in Rural Areas

Numerous studies have reported a marked difference in the prevalence of allergic sensitization and allergic diseases between urban and rural areas within the same country (e.g., Ghana, China, Mongolia, Germany, Greece, Poland, Canada, etc.),[41,42,76–79] with some studies suggesting that individuals who move from rural areas into cities may in part retain this protection. Studies from rural areas in Europe reported a considerably lower prevalence of hay fever and atopic sensitization amongst individuals living on farms compared with those living in the same rural area, but not on farms.[80,81] Some, but not all, studies reported a similar protective effect of living in a farming environment, on asthma.[82–84] In a longitudinal study of >13 000 children without asthma in Canada, the cumulative incidence of doctor-diagnosed asthma over a 2-year period was 2.3%, 5.3% and 5.7% amongst children living in farming, rural non-farming, and non-rural environments, respectively.[85] Similar observations have been reported from studies in adults (e.g., the prevalence of allergic rhinitis in subjects aged 20 to 44 years in ECRHS was 20.7%, with a considerably lower rate of 14.0% found amongst animal farmers of the same age).[86] This raises an important question as to what may be the sources of protective exposures in farming environments. Some studies suggested that an important protective component of the farm environment may be exposure to livestock (e.g., keeping pigs in addition to dairy farming),[87-93] and/or consumption of unpasteurized milk.[93] One could argue that children exposed to livestock are likely to encounter very high levels of allergens, bacteria, and fungi, but a specific 'protective factor' in the farming environment that could be used in primary prevention studies has not as yet been identified.

Timing of Exposure

There is increasing evidence that the effect of any environmental exposures (including farming) is strongly dependent on the timing of exposure. The overall evidence suggests that there may be windows of opportunity and vulnerability towards external exposures during certain developmental stages. For example, the protective effect of farming environments on allergic diseases appears largest when the farm contact started during childhood, and that of day-care, when the attendance started in the first year of life. Evidence to date suggests that early childhood exposures seem to be of greatest importance in the life course of sensitization and allergic diseases.

Prenatal factors may also play a significant role, either through mechanisms acting in-utero, or as epigenetic modulation of subsequent developmental trajectories. For example, the PARSIFAL Study has demonstrated that the risk of atopic sensitization was not only influenced by a child's exposure to the farming environment, but also by maternal exposure to stables during pregnancy.[94]

Urban Lifestyle and Air Pollution

In addition to microbial exposures, other environmental exposures may also be associated with urban living (e.g., air pollution and sedentary lifestyle). These have been scrutinized over the last decades, with no unequivocal conclusions. The evidence about the association of obesity, increasing body mass index, sedentary lifestyle and asthma is conflicting. Some studies suggest a positive relationship between obesity and asthma, with gender-specific effects of obesity being reported in some of the studies.[95] Most studies have not found an effect of obesity on atopy.

Whilst the evidence is conclusive that air pollution (e.g., short-term exposure to elevated levels of O_3, particulate matter, NO_2, and SO_2) is associated with worsening of asthma symptoms, decline in lung function, and increasing medication and healthcare use amongst patients with established disease, the role of air pollution in the development of asthma and allergic diseases, is unclear. The body of evidence generally suggests that the adverse effect of traffic exposure appears more pronounced for the incidence of asthma than for allergic sensitization. Indoor pollutants, particularly indoor environmental tobacco smoke exposure, also contribute to asthma-associated morbidity.

Allergens

Our understanding of the importance and the role of allergen exposure in the development of allergic disease has changed considerably over the last 25 years.[96] Both observational and primary prevention studies have investigated these relationships, and different studies reported inconsistent and sometimes contradictory findings, resulting in a considerable debate in the research community. We wish to note here, that currently we lack a clear understanding of how and when aeroallergen exposure occurs, and what is the relative importance of the timing of exposure (e.g., early-life exposure vs exposure in later life) and the route of exposure (e.g., inhaled vs oral vs transcutaneous).[96] A body of available evidence suggests that the dose–response relationship between allergen exposure and allergic disease may differ between different allergens, dose ranges, and exposure patterns, and that these relationships may further differ between different populations and geographical areas.

Several primary prevention studies investigate whether reduction in allergen exposure in early life can reduce the risk of the development of sensitization and asthma. However, the clinical outcomes reported to date are inconsistent and often confusing. For example, in the UK Isle of Wight study, house-dust mite sensitization and asthma were significantly reduced from early childhood to age 18 years,[97] whilst in the Manchester study, stringent mite allergen avoidance resulted in the increase in mite-specific sensitization.[98–100] The reported effect of intervention often differed depending on the age when outcomes were measured, and some of the intervention trials (e.g., in the Netherlands and Australia) reported no observable effect of allergen avoidance. Given this heterogeneity, longer follow-ups and more detailed analyses will be required before we can draw any conclusions.

It is likely that the effect of allergens and other environmental exposures (and their interactions) differ between individuals with different genetic predispositions, but the precise nature of these complex relationships remains unclear.

The Interaction between Environmental Exposures and Genetic Predisposition

The relationship between genetic predisposition and environmental exposures in the development of asthma and allergic diseases has received increasing attention over the last decade.[58] One of the most replicated examples to date, is the interaction between endotoxin exposure and variants in *CD14* gene. Several studies have confirmed that high endotoxin exposure is protective against the development of allergic sensitization amongst individuals with a specific genotype (C allele homozygotes of *CD14/-159*, rs2569190), but not in those with other genetic variants (e.g., T allele homozygotes).[101,102] A further level of complexity is added by the interactions with other environmental exposures (such as dust-mite allergen), resulting in a complex gene (*CD14*) by environment (endotoxin exposure) by environment (house-dust mite allergen exposure) interactions.[101] In this example, increasing mite allergen exposure increases the risk of sensitization in a simple dose–response manner, but the effect of dust mite allergen exposure is further modulated by endotoxin exposure amongst children with specific genotype (CC homozygotes at *CD14/-159*, Fig. 3-6), but not amongst those with other *CD14/-159* variants.[101]

Further examples of gene–environment interactions include the observation that the effect of early-life day-care attendance on asthma development differs between children with different variants in the *TLR2* gene (with day-care being protective in some, but

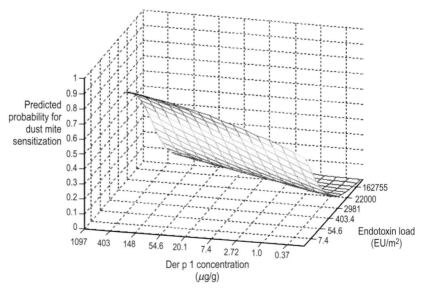

Figure 3-6 Fitted predicted probability for sensitization to mite at age 5 years in relation to environmental endotoxin load and Der p 1 exposure in children with CC genotype in the promoter region of the CD14 gene (CD14/-159 C to T) derived from the logistic regression analysis. *(From Simpson A, John SL, Jury F, Niven R, Woodcock A, Ollier WE, Custovic A, Endotoxin exposure, CD14, and allergic disease: an interaction between genes and the environment. Am J Respir Crit Care Med 2006; 174:386–392, with permission.)*

increasing the risk in others).[103] *Filaggrin* has been another gene of interest, and it has been demonstrated that in children who carry *filaggrin* loss of function mutations, cat ownership increases the risk of eczema,[104] and exposure to peanut allergens in household dust increases the risk of peanut allergy.[105] No such effects of environmental exposures were observed amongst children without *filaggrin* mutations. The Gabriel Consortium study investigated the effects of farming on genome wide genetic variation in relation to asthma, and whilst failing to replicate previously published associations, the genome wide gene by environment analysis identified some novel associations with rare variations (of note, these findings should be interpreted with caution because of a limited statistical power).[106]

Another level of complexity when investigating risk factors for asthma and allergic diseases may arise through gene–environment correlations (in that the effects, which are often attributed to environmental exposures may be a reflection of genetic predisposition). A recent example of gene–environment correlations is the finding that the association between antibiotic use and childhood asthma (which was often explained within the context of hygiene hypothesis, with the effect being attributed to antibiotics changing the host microbiome), may actually arise as a result of a complex confounding by indication.[107] The hidden factors, which increase the likelihood of both early-life antibiotic prescription and later asthma, appear to be impaired antiviral immunity and increased susceptibility to virus infections, and genetic variants on 17q21 (with the same variants being associated with both early-life antibiotic prescription and subsequent asthma).[107]

The important conclusion that can be drawn from these studies, is that the same environmental exposure may be protective in some individuals, but may increase the risk in others, and that the effect of environmental exposures depends on genetic predisposition. The lesson for primary prevention and intervention studies is that when identifying environmental protective and susceptibility factors, which are amenable to intervention, genetic predisposition of the individual will have to be taken into account to enable the development of genotype-specific strategies for prevention using different environmental interventions.[108]

CONCLUDING REMARKS: EPIDEMIOLOGY IN THE 21st CENTURY

'Team Science' to Solve the Puzzle of Asthma and Allergies

The prevalence rates of atopy, asthma, and other allergic diseases vary throughout the world, and are the highest in English speaking nations, higher in western than eastern parts of Europe, and higher in urban than rural parts of Africa. In the last several decades, there has been a marked increase in the prevalence of these disorders across all ages and ranges of disease severity. More recent evidence suggests that this increase may have reversed for some of the outcomes (such as asthma) in some developed countries and in certain age groups. However, in developing parts of the world, the prevalence continues to increase, and global differences may be getting smaller. The fundamental role of the environment in the allergy epidemic is suggested by the relatively short timeframe within which the increase in allergies and asthma has occurred. Numerous environmental changes have occurred at the same time as the increase in allergies, and amongst many factors, these include changes in the family size and childcare arrangements, pattern of microbial exposures, housing design, exposure to a number of pollutants, exercise, diet, etc. It is likely that the increase in allergic diseases is a consequence of numerous different environmental factors increasing the risk in genetically susceptible individuals, mediated through gene–environment interactions. However, all this effort has as yet failed to identify a single intervention that could be used to prevent the development of asthma, and at the present time, we cannot give any meaningful advice on primary prevention. The only exceptions are the recent findings that early introduction of peanuts significantly decreases the frequency of the development of peanut allergy in high-risk children with severe eczema, egg allergy, or both in early life.[109]

Epidemiology of asthma and allergic diseases has made a major contribution to our understanding of the worldwide prevalence and environmental risk and protective factors, and has informed numerous basic science studies aiming to discover the underlying pathophysiologic mechanisms of these disorders. However, due to the many factors discussed above, which include residual confounding, heterogeneity in the definition of primary outcomes, multiple influences of modest effect size, and lack of statistical power to detect interactions between numerous factors, traditional epidemiology may be reaching the limit of what can be achieved through conventional hypothesis-driven research. The evidence is mounting that asthma is not a single disease, but a collection of several diseases. Different manifestations of asthma symptom profiles over time may be a reflection of distinct causes and underlying biologic mechanisms, and may help in identification of different asthma subtypes. However, the proposed subtypes (or endotypes) of asthma remain as yet ill-defined hypothetical constructs, and unless epidemiology finds better ways of distinguishing between different diseases under this umbrella diagnosis, it will be difficult to identify their unique risk and protective factors, and discover their underlying pathophysiologic processes, as any signal is likely to be diluted by phenotypic heterogeneity.

The ability to generate new data in research studies has increased exponentially over a short period of time, resulting in a vast amount of collected data. We seek to use this information to predict disease outcomes and understand their causes, so that we can design personalized prevention strategies and targeted treatments. To map a way forward in the areas of asthma and allergic diseases, the enormous body of evidence, which has been generated on these topics needs to be harnessed in an iterative way to inform next steps. For example, in most patients asthma starts early in life, and may progress, remit or relapse over time. Different temporal patterns of various symptoms, physiologic measurement and biomarkers may reflect different pathophysiologic processes underpinning the subtypes (or endotypes) of allergic diseases. Temporal analysis may therefore be crucial for distinguishing between different endotypes, and the population-based birth cohorts may provide a framework for investigating the development of these diseases. A major challenge facing epidemiology in the 21st century is how best to utilize a vast amount of available data; how to integrate different scales of data (spanning from molecular-level, genetic and epigenetic, to population-level variables, including symptoms and objective measures of lung function and atopy); and different levels of directness of measurement of the many variables of interest (including multiple environmental exposures). Ideally, one would want to use all available data (e.g., multiple questions, directly observed and/or measured environmental exposures, outcome measures and laboratory readouts at multiple time points, genetic information, etc.) to identify the structure within the data that may arise as a consequence of different pathophysiologic processes. Such models would need to be tailored to individual datasets, and be able to scale-up to very large volumes of data, and would have to take into account the time course of developmental profiles at an individual level. Instead of using a 'black box' or 'data-mining' approach, this process should be informed by and capitalize on the current and future biologic and clinical knowledge about asthma and allergies. To do this effectively, it is essential to integrate the data with models/methods that can be tailored in full to the problem space of asthma, *and* the human expertise to make sense of the results.[14] This can be achieved through pooling resources and multidisciplinary expertise from different disciplines and centers of excellence to maximize the potential of existing and newly collected data. The future of research in asthma and allergic diseases should be a genuine iterative interdisciplinary dialogue between epidemiologists, clinicians, statisticians, computer scientists, mathematicians, geneticists and basic scientists, all working on a common problem—to solve the puzzle of asthma and allergies.[14]

REFERENCES

1. Fletcher CM, Gilson J, Hugh-Jones P, et al. Terminology, definitions, and classification of chronic pulmonary emphysema and related conditions: a report of the conclusions of a CIBA guest symposium. Thorax 1959;14:286–99.
2. American Thoracic Society. Chronic bronchitis, asthma, and pulmonary emphysema. Am Rev Respir Dis 1962;85:762–8.

3. World Health Organization. Epidemiology of chronic non-specific respiratory diseases. Bull World Health Organ 1975;52:251–9.
4. American Thoracic Society. Standardization of spirometry—1987 update. Am Rev Respir Dis 1987; 136:1285–98.
5. National Institutes of Health (NIH). Expert panel report on guidelines for diagnosis and management of asthma. Bethesda, MD: National Heart, Lung, and Blood Institute Information Center; 1991.
6. National Heart, Lung, and Blood Institute/World Health Organization. Global Initiative for Asthma. Washington, DC: US Government Printing Office; 1993.
7. US Department of Health and Human Services (USDHHS), Public Health Service, National Institutes of Health (NIH), et al. Practical guide for the diagnosis and management of asthma. Publication no. 97-4053. Bethesda, MD: National Institutes of Health; 1997.
8. National Institutes of Health (NIH), National Heart, Lung, and Blood Institute. Global initiative for asthma. Global strategy for asthma management and prevention. Publication no. 02-3659. 2002. Bethesda, MD: National Institutes of Health; 2002.
9. Van Wonderen KE, Van Der Mark LB, Mohrs J, et al. Different definitions in childhood asthma: how dependable is the dependent variable? Eur Respir J 2010;36(1):48–56.
10. Lotvall J, Akdis CA, Bacharier LB, et al. Asthma endotypes: a new approach to classification of disease entities within the asthma syndrome. J Allergy Clin Immunol 2011;127(2):355–60.
11. Belgrave DC, Custovic A, Simpson A. Characterizing wheeze phenotypes to identify endotypes of childhood asthma, and the implications for future management. Expert Rev Clin Immunol 2013; 9(10):921–36.
12. A plea to abandon asthma as a disease concept. Lancet 2006;368(9537):705.
13. Anderson GP. Endotyping asthma: new insights into key pathogenic mechanisms in a complex, heterogeneous disease. Lancet 2008;372(9643):1107–19.
14. *Custovic A, Ainsworth J, Arshad H, et al. The Study Team for Early Life Asthma Research (STELAR) consortium 'Asthma e-lab': team science bringing data, methods and investigators together. Thorax 2015;doi: 10.1136/thoraxjnl-2015-206781.
15. Papadopoulos NG, Bernstein JA, Demoly P, et al. Phenotypes and endotypes of rhinitis and their impact on management: a PRACTALL report. Allergy 2015;70(5):474–94.
16. Custovic A, Lazic N, Simpson A. Pediatric asthma and development of atopy. Curr Opin Allergy Clin Immunol 2013;13(2):173–80.
17. Weinmayr G, Weiland SK, Bjorksten B, et al. Atopic sensitization and the international variation of asthma symptom prevalence in children. Am J Respir Crit Care Med 2007;176(6):565–74.
18. Pekkarinen PT, von Hertzen L, Laatikainen T, et al. A disparity in the association of asthma, rhinitis, and eczema with allergen-specific IgE between Finnish and Russian Karelia. Allergy 2007; 62(3):281–7.
19. Nicolaou N, Poorafshar M, Murray C, et al. Allergy or tolerance in children sensitized to peanut: prevalence and differentiation using component-resolved diagnostics. J Allergy Clin Immunol 2010; 125(1):191–7.
20. Sicherer SH, Sampson HA. Food allergy: Epidemiology, pathogenesis, diagnosis, and treatment. J Allergy Clin Immunol 2014,133(2).291–307, quiz 8.
21. Yunginger JW, Ahlstedt S, Eggleston PA, et al. Quantitative IgE antibody assays in allergic diseases. J Allergy Clin Immunol 2000;105(6 Pt 1):1077–84.
22. Simpson A, Soderstrom L, Ahlstedt S, et al. IgE antibody quantification and the probability of wheeze in preschool children. J Allergy Clin Immunol 2005;116(4):744–9.
23. Sly PD, Boner AL, Bjorksten B, et al. Early identification of atopy in the prediction of persistent asthma in children. Lancet 2008;372(9643):1100–6.
24. Murray CS, Poletti G, Kebadze T, et al. Study of modifiable risk factors for asthma exacerbations: virus infection and allergen exposure increase the risk of asthma hospital admissions in children. Thorax 2006;61(5):376–82.
25. Green RM, Custovic A, Sanderson G, et al. Synergism between allergens and viruses and risk of hospital admission with asthma: case-control study. BMJ 2002;324(7340):763.
26. *Simpson A, Tan VY, Winn J, et al. Beyond atopy: multiple patterns of sensitization in relation to asthma in a birth cohort study. Am J Respir Crit Care Med 2010;181(11):1200–6.
27. Lazic N, Roberts G, Custovic A, et al. Multiple atopy phenotypes and their associations with asthma: similar findings from two birth cohorts. Allergy 2013;68(6):764–70.
28. Simpson A, Tan VYF, Winn J, et al. Beyond atopy: multiple patterns of sensitization in relation to asthma in a birth cohort study. Am J Respir Crit Care Med 2010;181(11):1200–6.
29. Custovic A, Sonntag HJ, Buchan IE, et al. Evolution pathways of IgE responses to grass and mite allergens throughout childhood. J Allergy Clin Immunol 2015;doi: 10.1016/j.jaci.2015.03.041.
30. Simpson A, Lazic N, Belgrave DC, et al. Patterns of IgE responses to multiple allergen components and clinical symptoms at age 11 years. J Allergy Clin Immunol 2015;doi: 10.1016/j.jaci.2015.03.027.
31. *Zuidmeer L, Goldhahn K, Rona RJ, et al. The prevalence of plant food allergies: a systematic review. J Allergy Clin Immunol 2008;121(5):1210–18.
32. Custovic A, Nicolaou N. Peanut allergy: overestimated in epidemiology or underdiagnosed in primary care? J Allergy Clin Immunol 2011;127(3):631–2.
33. Ellwood P, Asher MI, Beasley R, et al. The international study of asthma and allergies in childhood (ISAAC): phase three rationale and methods. Int J Tuberc Lung Dis 2005;9(1):10–16.
34. Weiland SK, Bjorksten B, Brunekreef B, et al. Phase II of the International Study of Asthma and Allergies in Childhood (ISAAC II): rationale and methods. Eur Respir J 2004;24(3):406–12.
35. Asher MI, Keil U, Anderson HR, et al. International Study of Asthma and Allergies in Childhood (ISAAC): rationale and methods. Eur Respir J 1995;8(3):483–91.
36. Burney PG, Chinn S, Britton JR, et al. What symptoms predict the bronchial response to histamine? Evaluation in a community survey of the bronchial symptoms questionnaire (1984) of the International Union Against Tuberculosis and Lung Disease. Int J Epidemiol 1989;18(1):165–73.

37. *Variations in the prevalence of respiratory symptoms, self-reported asthma attacks, and use of asthma medication in the European Community Respiratory Health Survey (ECRHS). Eur Respir J 1996; 9(4):687–95.

38. Sembajwe G, Cifuentes M, Tak SW, et al. National income, self-reported wheezing and asthma diagnosis from the World Health Survey. Eur Respir J 2010;35(2):279–86.

39. *Asher MI, Montefort S, Bjorksten B, et al. Worldwide time trends in the prevalence of symptoms of asthma, allergic rhinoconjunctivitis, and eczema in childhood: ISAAC Phases One and Three repeat multicountry cross-sectional surveys. Lancet 2006;368(9537):733–43.

40. *Upton MN, McConnachie A, McSharry C, et al. Intergenerational 20 year trends in the prevalence of asthma and hay fever in adults: the Midspan family study surveys of parents and offspring. BMJ 2000;321(7253):88–92.

41. Addo Yobo EO, Custovic A, Taggart SC, et al. Exercise induced bronchospasm in Ghana: differences in prevalence between urban and rural schoolchildren. Thorax 1997;52(2):161–5.

42. Addo-Yobo EO, Woodcock A, Allotey A, et al. Exercise-induced bronchospasm and atopy in Ghana: two surveys ten years apart. PLoS Med 2007;4(2):e70.

43. von Mutius E, Martinez FD, Fritzsch C, et al. Prevalence of asthma and atopy in two areas of West and East Germany. Am J Respir Crit Care Med 1994;149(2 Pt 1):358–64.

44. Wong GW, Ko FW, Hui DS, et al. Factors associated with difference in prevalence of asthma in children from three cities in China: multicentre epidemiological survey. BMJ 2004;329(7464): 486.

45. Vartiainen E, Petays T, Haahtela T, et al. Allergic diseases, skin prick test responses, and IgE levels in North Karelia, Finland, and the Republic of Karelia, Russia. J Allergy Clin Immunol 2002; 109(4):643–8.

46. Lewis SA, Weiss ST, Platts-Mills TA, et al. Association of specific allergen sensitization with socioeconomic factors and allergic disease in a population of Boston women. J Allergy Clin Immunol 2001;107(4):615–22.

47. Koppelman GH, Stine OC, Xu J, et al. Genome-wide search for atopy susceptibility genes in Dutch families with asthma. J Allergy Clin Immunol 2002;109(3):498–506.

48. Castro-Giner F, Bustamante M, Ramon Gonzalez J, et al. A pooling-based genome-wide analysis identifies new potential candidate genes for atopy in the European Community Respiratory Health Survey (ECRHS). BMC Med Genet 2009;10:128.

49. Sicherer SH, Munoz-Furlong A, Sampson HA. Prevalence of seafood allergy in the United States determined by a random telephone survey. J Allergy Clin Immunol 2004;114(1):159–65.

50. Sicherer SH, Munoz-Furlong A, Sampson HA. Prevalence of peanut and tree nut allergy in the United States determined by means of a random digit dial telephone survey: a 5-year follow-up study. J Allergy Clin Immunol 2003;112(6):1203–7.

51. Shek LP, Cabrera-Morales EA, Soh SE, et al. A population-based questionnaire survey on the prevalence of peanut, tree nut, and shellfish allergy in 2 Asian populations. J Allergy Clin Immunol 2010; 126(2):324–31.

52. Osborne NJ, Koplin JJ, Martin PE, et al. Prevalence of challenge-proven IgE-mediated food allergy using population-based sampling and predetermined challenge criteria in infants. J Allergy Clin Immunol 2011;127(3):668–76.

53. Kotz D, Simpson CR, Sheikh A. Incidence, prevalence, and trends of general practitioner-recorded diagnosis of peanut allergy in England, 2001 to 2005. J Allergy Clin Immunol 2011;127(3):623–30.

54. *Rona RJ, Keil T, Summers C, et al. The prevalence of food allergy: a meta-analysis. J Allergy Clin Immunol 2007;120(3):638–46.

55. *Eder W, Ege MJ, von Mutius E. The asthma epidemic. N Engl J Med 2006;355(21):2226–35.

56. Mitchell EA. International trends in hospital admission rates for asthma. Arch Dis Child 1985; 60(4):376–8.

57. Woods RK, Abramson M, Bailey M, et al. International prevalences of reported food allergies and intolerances. Comparisons arising from the European Community Respiratory Health Survey (ECRHS) 1991–1994. Eur J Clin Nutr 2001;55(4):298–304.

58. Custovic A, Marinho S, Simpson A. Gene-environment interactions in the development of asthma and atopy. Expert Rev Respir Med 2012;6(3):301–8.

59. *Strachan DP. Hay fever, hygiene, and household size. BMJ 1989;299(6710):1259–60.

60. Gore C, Custovic A. Protective parasites and medicinal microbes? The case for the hygiene hypothesis. Prim Care Respir J 2004;13(2):68–83.

61. von Mutius E. The influence of birth order on the expression of atopy in families: a gene-environment interaction? Clin Exp Allergy 1998;28:1454–6.

62. Celedon JC, Litonjua AA, Ryan L, et al. Day care attendance, respiratory tract illnesses, wheezing, asthma, and total serum IgE level in early childhood. Arch Pediatr Adolesc Med 2002;156(3):241–5.

63. Celedon JC, Wright RJ, Litonjua AA, et al. Day care attendance in early life, maternal history of asthma, and asthma at the age of 6 years. Am J Respir Crit Care Med 2003;167(9):1239–43.

64. Ball TM, Castro-Rodriguez JA, Griffith KA, et al. Siblings, day-care attendance, and the risk of asthma and wheezing during childhood. N Engl J Med 2000;343(8):538–43.

65. Nicolaou NC, Simpson A, Lowe LA, et al. Day-care attendance, position in sibship, and early childhood wheezing: a population-based birth cohort study. J Allergy Clin Immunol 2008;122(3):500–6.

66. Chen CM, Tischer C, Schnappinger M, et al. The role of cats and dogs in asthma and allergy – a systematic review. Int J Hyg Environ Health 2010;213(1):1–31.

67. Wickens K, Douwes J, Siebers R, et al. Determinants of endotoxin levels in carpets in New Zealand homes. Indoor Air 2003;13(2):128–35.

68. Rullo VE, Rizzo MC, Arruda LK, et al. Daycare centers and schools as sources of exposure to mites, cockroach, and endotoxin in the city of Sao Paulo, Brazil. J Allergy Clin Immunol 2002;110(4): 582–8.

69. Maier RM, Palmer MW, Andersen GL, et al. Environmental determinants of and impact on childhood asthma by the bacterial community in household dust. Appl Environ Microbiol 2010;76(8): 2663–7.

70. Troy EB, Kasper DL. Beneficial effects of Bacteroides fragilis polysaccharides on the immune system. Front Biosci 2010;15:25–34.

71. Gore C, Munro K, Lay C, et al. Bifidobacterium pseudocatenulatum is associated with atopic eczema: a nested case-control study investigating the fecal microbiota of infants. J Allergy Clin Immunol 2008;121(1):135–40.

72. Murray CS, Tannock GW, Simon MA, et al. Fecal microbiota in sensitized wheezy and non-sensitized non-wheezy children: a nested case-control study. Clin Exp Allergy 2005;35(6):741–5.

73. Osborn DA, Sinn JK. Probiotics in infants for prevention of allergic disease and food hypersensitivity. Cochrane Database Syst Rev 2007;(4):CD006475.

74. Lee J, Seto D, Bielory L. Meta-analysis of clinical trials of probiotics for prevention and treatment of pediatric atopic dermatitis. J Allergy Clin Immunol 2008;121(1):116–21.

75. Gore C, Custovic A, Tannock GW, et al. Treatment and secondary prevention effects of the probiotics Lactobacillus paracasei or Bifidobacterium lactis on early infant eczema: randomized controlled trial with follow-up until age 3 years. Clin Exp Allergy 2012;42(1):112–22.

76. Viinanen A, Munhbayarlah S, Zevgee T, et al. Prevalence of asthma, allergic rhinoconjunctivitis and allergic sensitization in Mongolia. Allergy 2005;60(11):1370–7.

77. Viinanen A, Munhbayarlah S, Zevgee T, et al. The protective effect of rural living against atopy in Mongolia. Allergy 2007;62(3):272–80.

78. Wong GW, Hui DS, Chan HH, et al. Prevalence of respiratory and atopic disorders in Chinese school-children. Clin Exp Allergy 2001;31(8):1225–31.

79. Ogbuanu IU, Karmaus W, Arshad SH, et al. Effect of breastfeeding duration on lung function at age 10 years: a prospective birth cohort study. Thorax 2009;64(1):62–6.

80. Naleway AL. Asthma and atopy in rural children: is farming protective? Clin Med Res 2004;2(1): 5–12.

81. von Mutius E, Radon K. Living on a farm: impact on asthma induction and clinical course. Immunol Allergy Clin North Am 2008;28(3):631–47, ix–x.

82. Ernst P, Cormier Y. Relative scarcity of asthma and atopy among rural adolescents raised on a farm. Am J Respir Crit Care Med 2000;161(5):1563–6.

83. Omland O, Sigsgaard T, Hjort C, et al. Lung status in young Danish rurals: the effect of farming exposure on asthma-like symptoms and lung function. Eur Respir J 1999;13(1):31–7.

84. von Mutius E, Illi S, Nicolai T, et al. Relation of indoor heating with asthma, allergic sensitisation, and bronchial responsiveness: survey of children in south Bavaria. BMJ 1996;312(7044):1448–50.

85. Midodzi WK, Rowe BH, Majaesic CM, et al. Reduced risk of physician-diagnosed asthma among children dwelling in a farming environment. Respirology 2007;12(5):692–9.

86. Radon K, Danuser B, Iversen M, et al. Respiratory symptoms in European animal farmers. Eur Respir J 2001;17(4):747–54.

87. Ege MJ, Frei R, Bieli C, et al. Not all farming environments protect against the development of asthma and wheeze in children. J Allergy Clin Immunol 2007;119(5):1140–7.

88. Downs SH, Marks GB, Mitakakis TZ, et al. Having lived on a farm and protection against allergic diseases in Australia. Clin Exp Allergy 2001;31(4):570–5.

89. Wickens K, Lane JM, Fitzharris P, et al. Farm residence and exposures and the risk of allergic diseases in New Zealand children. Allergy 2002;57(12):1171–9.

90. Riedler J, Braun-Fahrlander C, Eder W, et al. Early life exposure to farming environment is essential for protection against the development of asthma and allergy: A cross-sectional survey. Lancet 2001;358:1129–33.

91. Von Ehrenstein OS, Von Mutius E, Illi S, et al. Reduced risk of hay fever and asthma among children of farmers. Clin Exp Allergy 2000;30:187–93.

92. Remes ST, Iivanainen K, Koskela H, et al. Which factors explain the lower prevalence of atopy amongst farmers' children? Clin Exp Allergy 2003;33(4):427–34.

93. Perkin MR, Strachan DP. Which aspects of the farming lifestyle explain the inverse association with childhood allergy? J Allergy Clin Immunol 2006;117(6):1374–81.

94. *Ege MJ, Bieli C, Frei R, et al. Prenatal farm exposure is related to the expression of receptors of the innate immunity and to atopic sensitization in school-age children. J Allergy Clin Immunol 2006;117(4):817–23.

95. Murray CS, Canoy D, Buchan I, et al. Body mass index in young children and allergic disease: gender differences in a longitudinal study. Clin Exp Allergy 2011;41(1):78–85.

96. Custovic A. To what extent is allergen exposure a risk factor for the development of allergic disease? Clin Exp Allergy 2015;45(1):54–62.

97. Scott M, Roberts G, Kurukulaaratchy RJ, et al. Multifaceted allergen avoidance during infancy reduces asthma during childhood with the effect persisting until age 18 years. Thorax 2012;67(12):1046–51.

98. Custovic A, Simpson BM, Simpson A, et al. Effect of environmental manipulation in pregnancy and early life on respiratory symptoms and atopy during first year of life: a randomised trial. Lancet 2001;358(9277):188–93.

99. Simpson A, Simpson B, Custovic A, et al. Stringent environmental control in pregnancy and early life: the long-term effects on mite, cat and dog allergen. Clin Exp Allergy 2003;33(9):1183–9.

100. Woodcock A, Lowe LA, Murray CS, et al. Early life environmental control: effect on symptoms, sensitization, and lung function at age 3 years. Am J Respir Crit Care Med 2004;170(4):433–9.

101. Simpson A, John SL, Jury F, et al. Endotoxin exposure, CD14, and allergic disease: an interaction between genes and the environment. Am J Respir Crit Care Med 2006;174(4):386–92.

102. Simpson A, Martinez FD. The role of lipopolysaccharide in the development of atopy in humans. Clin Exp Allergy 2010;40(2):209–23.

103. Custovic A, Rothers J, Stern D, et al. Effect of day care attendance on sensitization and atopic wheezing differs by Toll-like receptor 2 genotype in 2 population-based birth cohort studies. J Allergy Clin Immunol 2011;127(2):390–7.
104. Bisgaard H, Simpson A, Palmer CN, et al. Gene-environment interaction in the onset of eczema in infancy: filaggrin loss-of-function mutations enhanced by neonatal cat exposure. PLoS Med 2008;5(6):e131.
105. Brough HA, Simpson A, Makinson K, et al. Peanut allergy: effect of environmental peanut exposure in children with filaggrin loss-of-function mutations. J Allergy Clin Immunol 2014;134(4):867–75.
106. Ege MJ, Strachan DP, Cookson WO, et al. Gene-environment interaction for childhood asthma and exposure to farming in Central Europe. J Allergy Clin Immunol 2011;127(1):138–44.
107. Semic-Jusufagic A, Belgrave D, Pickles A, et al. Assessing the association of early life antibiotic prescription with asthma exacerbations, impaired antiviral immunity, and genetic variants in 17q21: a population-based birth cohort study. Lancet Respir Med 2014;2(8):621–30.
108. Custovic A, Simpson A. Environmental allergen exposure, sensitisation and asthma: from whole populations to individuals at risk. Thorax 2004;59(10):825–7.
109. Du Toit G, Roberts G, Sayre PH, et al. Randomized trial of peanut consumption in infants at risk for peanut allergy. N Engl J Med 2015;372(9):803–13.

Key references are preceded by an asterisk.

CHAPTER 4

Indoor and Outdoor Allergens and Pollutants

Geoffrey A. Stewart and Clive Robinson

CHAPTER OUTLINE

INTRODUCTION

ALLERGENS AND ALLERGENICITY

INDOOR AND OUTDOOR ALLERGEN SOURCES

AEROBIOLOGY OF INDOOR AND OUTDOOR ALLERGEN SOURCES

OUTDOOR ALLERGEN MONITORING

INDOOR ALLERGEN MONITORING

THE CHEMICAL NATURE OF ALLERGENS

ALLERGEN NOMENCLATURE AND ALLERGEN DATABASES

OUTDOOR ALLERGENS

Outdoor Allergen Sources – Pollen

Pollen Structure and Allergen Release

Pollen Allergens

Cell Wall Modifying Allergens

Allergens Involved in Defense

Ligand Binding Pr-10 Allergens

Non-specific Lipid Transfer Proteins (Pr-14)

Non-PR Defense-related Pollen Allergens

Profilins and Polcalcins

Outdoor Allergen Sources – Fungi

Fungal Allergens

Alternaria, *Aspergillus*, and *Cladosporium*

Penicillium, *Candida*, and *Trichophyton*

INDOOR ALLERGENS

Indoor Allergen Sources – Non-mammalian

Acaridae

Mite Allergens

Insecta

Cockroach Allergens

Indoor Allergen Sources – Mammalian

Cats, Rabbits, and Dogs

Cat and Dog Allergens

Rodents and Rodent Allergens

ALLERGENS AND ALLERGENICITY

ENVIRONMENTAL MODIFIERS OF ALLERGIC SENSITIZATION AND DISEASE

Avoidance Measures for Indoor Allergens

House-dust Mites

Domestic Animals

Cockroaches and Other Allergens

AIR POLLUTION, ALLERGIC SENSITIZATION, AND DISEASE

Sources of Air Pollution

Biomass

Environmental Tobacco Smoke (ETS)

Lipopolysaccharide (LPS)

TYPES OF POLLUTANT AND THEIR EFFECTS ON ALLERGENS, ALLERGIC SENSITIZATION, AND ASTHMA

Particulates

Gaseous Pollutants

Sulfur Dioxide (SO_2)

Nitrogen Dioxide (NO_2)

Ozone (O_3)

CONCLUSIONS

ACKNOWLEDGMENTS

SUMMARY OF IMPORTANT CONCEPTS

- Allergens in and outside the home are primarily proteins, capable of stimulating IgE synthesis in genetically susceptible people.
- Subsequent exposures to allergen may precipitate diseases such as rhinitis, asthma, conjunctivitis, and urticaria.
- The major route of exposure, both inside and outside the home, is by inhalation, and the size of allergen-containing particles will influence both sensitization and symptoms, with submicronic particles likely to be associated with asthma rather than rhinitis.
- The main sources of outdoor allergen exposure are pollens and fungi.
- In the home, the most significant allergen sources are mites, cockroaches, and pets such as cats and dogs.

- Methods exist to monitor allergen exposure, and sensitization thresholds for a few allergen sources established.
- Allergic symptoms may occur in patients due to cross-reactivity between aeroallergens and certain foods, giving rise to oral allergic syndromes or pollen-food syndromes.
- That indoor and outdoor air pollution exacerbates asthma symptoms is established but, with the exception of tropospheric ozone, the evidence that pollution causes new asthma is less convincing.
- Pollutant exposure can induce allergic and/or non-allergic inflammation in people with asthma.
- Air pollution can modify the allergen exposure of allergic persons.
- Rising carbon dioxide levels and increasing surface temperatures affect plant pollination in ways that might affect pollination and pollen potency.

INTRODUCTION

Individuals are exposed to a range of potentially allergenic sources in both domestic and work settings. Certain allergen sources are associated with different clinical presentations reflecting the associated portal of entry into the host. Thus, atopic dermatitis and anaphylaxis are associated with food allergen sources such as peanuts, milk, and fish, whereas rhinitis and asthma are associated with aeroallergens such as pollens and house-dust mites. Each source will contain a variety of proteins, and the term *allergen* is used to describe any of those that are capable of stimulating the production of specific immunoglobulin E (IgE) in a genetically predisposed individual. This term, together with the term *allergy* was introduced in 1906 by Clemens von Pirquet (1874–1929) to describe the body's hyperreactivity to a foreign substance, and over time, these terms have been appropriated by those interested in immediate hypersensitivity.

The production of allergen-specific IgE will rise after exposure to an allergen source, such as pollen in the pollen season, and the percentage specific IgE may represent a significant proportion (e.g., 13–50%) of total IgE in a patient's serum. There has been much interest in defining the allergens contained within a particular source over several decades, a process driven by the desire to prepare better diagnostic reagents, produce more effective immunotherapies, and determine whether they possess unique properties that differentiate them from other immunogens. This chapter is devoted to describing the clinically important indoor and outdoor allergens, their aerobiology (including the effects of climate change and pollution), their biological function, and the potential for this to impact on the process of sensitization.

ALLERGENS AND ALLERGENICITY

Allergens are described in a number of ways and the terms *indoor* and *outdoor* are commonly used to describe those entering the body via the respiratory tract in the home or at work, or outside, respectively. However, allergens such as foods can enter the body via the gastrointestinal tract, be absorbed percutaneously or be injected naturally (envenomation and insect bites) and iatrogenically (biologics, antibiotics, anesthetics) (Fig. 4-1). The route of allergen exposure will influence the types of allergic symptoms subsequently experienced, with exposure to aeroallergens giving rise to respiratory symptoms, in contrast with those ingested, injected, or absorbed, which cause localized gastrointestinal or dermal symptoms or more generalized systemic symptoms. In this regard, the most clinically significant route of exposure is via the respiratory tract (Fig. 4-1).

The term *allergenic* is used to describe the IgE-inducing property of an allergen, and *allergen*, *allergenic*, and *allergenicity* are synonymous with the terms *antigen*, *antigenic*, and *antigenicity*, respectively, which are routinely used to describe immunogens generating IgG, IgM, or IgA responses. However, in addition to IgE, allergens also stimulate

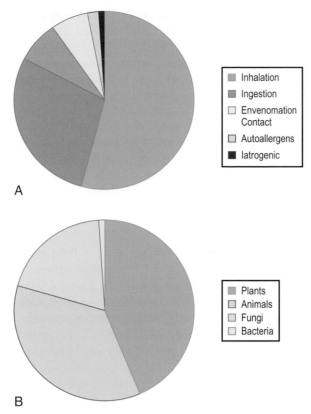

Figure 4-1 Percentage distribution of allergens present in the Allergome database, based on route of exposure and origin. *(From Radauer C, Bublin M, Wagner S, Mari A, Breiteneder H. Allergens are distributed into few protein families and possess a restricted number of biochemical functions. J Allergy Clin Immunol 2008; 121:847–852.)*

the induction of other immunoglobulin isotypes but this is most evident in those already allergic. In addition, a source may contain several allergens, and each one may possess a number of potential epitopes, i.e., areas of a protein that interact with the B and T cell receptors on lymphocytes, which stimulate their own specific IgE. Thus, IgE in a patient's serum is polyclonal and will reflect that produced to different allergens, as well as to different parts of an individual allergen.

In addition to these distinctions, allergens may also be described as *cross-reactive* allergens. This means that a patient may produce IgE to an allergen, which will not only react with the primary sensitizing allergen but, because of significant sequence homology and hence common epitopes, it will also react with a related one. This situation may occur, for example, with allergens from phylogenetically related species, such as house-dust mites and grass pollens, but cross-reactivity may also be evident between allergens from phylogenetically dissimilar species. They include, for example, the tropomyosins in mites, snails, cockroaches, and shellfish, and the profilins from physiologically dissimilar tissues such as pollens and more distantly related fruits.[1] These allergens are known as *pan-allergens* and respiratory sensitization can give rise to *oral allergy syndrome* (OAS) (also known as pollen–food syndrome) in patients eating food containing these allergens.

INDOOR AND OUTDOOR ALLERGEN SOURCES

The majority of the clinically important allergens are derived from plant, fungal, and animal sources. With plant and fungal sources, both with inhaled and ingested allergens, most will be associated with or contained within structures designed for the dispersal of genetic material such as pollen, spores, seeds, nuts, and fruits, or in flours derived from them. Indoors, allergens will be secreted and deposited onto danders or into saliva and urine, or into fecal pellets, for example, in mite and cockroach feces as part of their digestive processes. Thus, most individuals are exposed to particulates, and all the potential allergens associated with them.[2]

Clinically important allergen sources will often contain mixtures of (glyco)proteins unless exposure occurs in occupational settings. The most complex of these sources are pollens, fungal spores, seeds, and mites, with the least complex being animal danders and urine and those from occupational sources, where one or two pure proteins are used in a particular manufacturing process. Patients usually produce IgE to more than one protein present in any given source, and a spectrum of reactivities in an individual serum will exist. In addition, individuals can be monosensitized, i.e., they are sensitized to a single allergen source (e.g., house-dust mites) or polysensitized to multiple allergen sources (e.g., pollen, house dust mite and danders). Polysensitization is common (>70% of allergic individuals) and data suggest that monosensitization often precedes polysensitization; patients who are polysensitized manifest more severe clinical symptoms.

Within a single source, some constituent allergens will be recognized by a greater percentage of the members of an exposed population than others, and some will stimulate significantly more IgE than others. Allergens in a particular source that are recognized by 50% or more of allergic individuals are termed *major*, with the remaining ones being referred to as *minor*. More recently, other criteria that might be used to define a major allergen have been promulgated (Box 4-1) and include reference to the percentage specific IgE, as a proportion of total IgE to that allergen. However, some allergens considered to be *minor* on a population basis may be clinically significant for a particular individual. Similarly, some allergens considered to be *major* ones within a particular allergic population in a specific geographical location may not be so dominant in another location, indicating that local environmental, cultivar, or genetic factors may influence specific allergen production.

AEROBIOLOGY OF INDOOR AND OUTDOOR ALLERGEN SOURCES

Sensitization to outdoor and indoor allergen sources is dependent upon inhalation which, in turn, will require allergen aerosolization. This process will be influenced by a variety of factors such as climate, humidity, seasonality, and other ecological factors that

---

Box 4-1   International Union of Immunologic Societies (IUIS) Allergen Nomenclature Criteria and Criteria for Defining a Major Allergen

PHYSICOCHEMICAL REQUIREMENTS
- It is of proven homogeneity
- Its molecular weight, isoelectric point (pI), and carbohydrate composition have been determined
- Its nucleotide sequence and/or amino acid sequence has been determined
- Specific antisera (mono- or polyclonal) are available

ALLERGENICITY REQUIREMENTS
- It demonstrates allergenicity using a biological assay such as skin testing, or basophil histamine release
- A reduction in allergenic activity can be demonstrated after its removal from an allergen extract
- The allergenic activity of a recombinant protein is comparable to that of the native allergen

MAJOR ALLERGEN DESIGNATION REQUIREMENTS
- It sensitizes >80% of a predisposed and exposed population
- A significant proportion of total specific serum IgE is directed to the allergen (>10%)
- Removal of the allergen from the source material greatly reduces the biological and immunochemical (IgE) activity of the extract
- The allergen represents a significant proportion of the total extractable protein in the extract
- The allergen may be used as a marker of environmental exposure
- Both humoral (IgE) and cellular (T cell/basophil) responses to the allergen can be measured in a high proportion of a sensitized population
- The allergen, its cDNA or its constituent peptides can be shown to be effective in an allergy vaccine

(Modified from Chapman, M. D. (2008). Allergen Nomenclature. Allergens and Allergen Immunotherapy. R. F. Lockey and D. K. Ledford. Boca Raton: CRC Press; 47–58.)

impact on the allergen source and allergen concentrations within it and in reservoirs but, particularly for indoor allergens, aerosolization will depend on anthropogenic factors such as bed-making, vacuuming, animal husbandry practices, and industrial processes. The aerodynamic (rather than absolute) size of the aerosolized particles generated is significant, as it will influence the site of deposition in the respiratory tree and, therefore, symptoms. For example, large particles (>10 μm) are trapped in the nose giving rise to nasal symptoms, whereas submicronic particles enter the bronchi giving rise to lower airways inflammation, resulting in asthma rather than rhinitis.

In addition to influencing deposition characteristics, size will influence the length of time particles remain suspended in the atmosphere and, therefore, exposure. Thus, smaller-sized allergenic particles will remain airborne for extended periods and patients may inhale relatively high concentrations, in contrast to larger-sized particles, which fall rapidly. In the context of allergy, these considerations form part of the science of aerobiology, which is concerned with the study of outdoor allergen sources such as pollens and fungal spores, their fragments, submicronic particles and specific outdoor and indoor allergens. Such studies have enabled the mapping of allergenic plants and associated pollen distributions and the development of methods for quantifying atmospheric allergen concentrations and allergen size distributions.

OUTDOOR ALLERGEN MONITORING

Being able to measure and/or identify allergen sources and specific allergens is paramount in aerobiology, not just from an academic point of view but also from a clinician's and patient's perspective, as it may provide a means of forecasting when outdoor allergens are expected to precipitate symptoms of rhinitis and conjunctivitis, predicting when increased emergency room visits for asthma are likely, and establishing concentration thresholds for sensitization and how reductions might be achieved in the home and workplace. The first aerobiological study of an allergen source was performed by the pioneering English physician Charles Blackley (1820–1900) and described in his book *Experimental Researches on the Causes and Nature of Catarrhus Aestivus (Hay Fever or Hay Asthma)* in 1873. He was the first to scientifically demonstrate that pollen was the cause of rhinitis and, in so doing, developed gravitational methods to detect pollen in the atmosphere; studied the heights to which pollen might be found using pollen capture devices attached to kites; produced the first pollen calendar; performed the first skin test; and studied the link between pollen concentrations and symptoms.

Various methods are available to monitor allergens including methods for counting morphologically distinct allergen sources such as pollens, fungal spores in the atmosphere and whole mites in house dust, or for determining allergen concentrations using specific immunoassays. The techniques used for counting whole pollen and fungal spores or allergen-containing particles include gravimetric devices (e.g., Durham gravity-sampling device), impaction devices (Rotorod Sampler, Anderson Cascade Impactor), and suction and trapping devices (Hirst and Burkard traps) (Fig. 4-2) in combination with microscopy. Whole pollen and fungal spore results can be expressed either as the number of grains or spores/m^3 per 24 h or as an index representing the potential risk (pollen index) of developing symptoms using the terms "low," "moderate," "high," "very high," and "extreme," terms which also take into consideration the known allergy-provoking potential of the pollen species identified. The public dissemination of pollen data is often supported by national allergy organizations and public and commercial broadcasting organizations via the Internet (e.g., https://www.aaaai.org/global/nab-pollen-counts.aspx; http://www.weatherzone.com.au/pollen-index/).

INDOOR ALLERGEN MONITORING

As indoor allergen-containing particles in air or reservoir dusts are difficult to identify due to their amorphous nature or size, a number of immunochemical assays have been developed to measure individual allergens in the indoor environment. Their availability

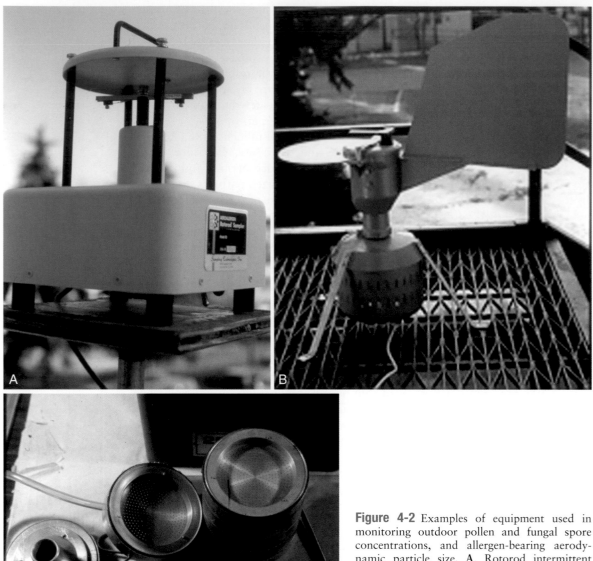

Figure 4-2 Examples of equipment used in monitoring outdoor pollen and fungal spore concentrations, and allergen-bearing aerodynamic particle size. **A.** Rotorod intermittent rotary impactor sampler. **B.** Burkard suction drum Hirst-type spore trap, with rain guard and large weather vane. **C.** Disassembled Andersen multistage cascade impactor.

make it possible to correlate allergen exposure with sensitization, and a number of threshold concentrations have been determined, above which sensitization may occur in susceptible individuals (Table 4-1). In establishing these concentrations, it is assumed that there will be a linear relationship between exposure, sensitization, and induction of symptoms. However, accumulating data indicate that the concentration of allergen required to cause sensitization will often be lower than that required for induction of symptoms, and that dose–response relationships may be bell-shaped, with very high exposure inducing tolerance.

THE CHEMICAL NATURE OF ALLERGENS

Most allergens (and antigens) are proteins of varying sizes, and may exist as monomers or dimers (either hetero- or homo-). However, certain low molecular weight chemically reactive compounds may also be allergenic, but only so when they have reacted, and thus modified, host proteins; these are known as *haptens*. The most common haptenic compounds in clinical practice are the beta-lactam antibiotics such as the benzyl

TABLE 4-1   Allergen Exposure Concentrations Regarded as Risk Factors for Sensitization

Allergen	Threshold concentration	Industry/Source
Air (ng/m³)		
Subtilisin (bacterial)	15–60	Detergent
Lipase (fungal)	5–20	Detergent
Cellulase (fungal)	8–20	Baking
Amylase (fungal)	<0.25	Baking
Latex proteins (*Hevea brasiliensis*)	0.6	Latex glove manufacturing
Mouse urinary allergens	<5	Laboratory animal housing
Air (mg/m³)		
Flour	0.5–1	Baking
Grain dust	1–1.5	Baking, grain handling
Reservoir dust (μg allergen/g dust/m²)		
Fel d 1	8	Domestic dust
Bla g 2	10	Domestic dust
Bos d 2	1–20	Farming
Can f 1	10	Domestic dust
Der p 1/Der f 1	<2–20	Domestic dust
Reservoir dust (/g dust/m²))		
House-dust mites	100–1000	Domestic dust

penicillins. Every protein allergen contains a number of potential *epitopes*, which are also known as *antigenic determinants*, and represent linear amino acid sequences or adjacent sections of a sequence that engage with either the B cell receptor or its soluble antibody form or the T cell receptor sitting on the surface of a lymphocyte.

The number of amino acid residues comprising a B cell epitope that interact with the actual binding site of a B cell receptor or allergen-specific IgE is about five amino acid residues (Fig. 4-3). In contrast, T cell epitopes are larger (13–17 amino acid residues) and are allergen-derived peptides presented to the T cell receptor in the groove of an MHC class I or II molecule. Some epitopes may stimulate a stronger immune response than others for a variety of reasons, and these are termed *immunodominant*. An individual may also recognize epitopes that are different to those recognized by other individuals because of differences in MHC haplotype.

Lipids do not appear to be allergenic, although the lipid content of some sources such as pollens may play an adjuvant role in sensitization. However, IgE may be produced against glycan structures present on some glycoprotein allergens, and approximately 15–30% of allergic patients, particularly teenagers, may produce IgE. Whether the IgE is specific for a particular glycoprotein allergen is unclear because glycoproteins from diverse sources possess immunochemically similar glycan moieties and are referred to as *cross-reacting carbohydrate determinants* (CCDs).[3]

A number of CCDs have been described but recent data indicate that glycosylation patterns on allergens are far more complex than previously understood. In general, CCDs are not particularly important, but the β1–6 linked fucose and β1–2 linked xylose and the Galα1–3Galβ1–4GlcNAc-R (α-Gal) epitope are immunogenic. In this regard, the presence of IgE to the α-Gal moiety on animal serum immunoglobulins, red meat proteins, and on therapeutic murine monoclonal antibody (Cetuximab) may cause immediate anaphylaxis in certain patients given Cetuximab and delayed anaphylaxis (3–6 h) in some patients after ingesting red meat.[4] This IgE is thought to be stimulated

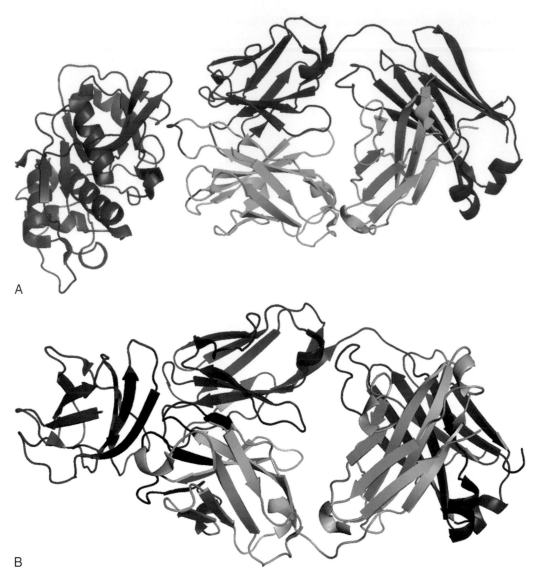

Figure 4-3 The 3-dimensional (3D) structure of allergenic B cell epitopes on a mite (Der p 1) and grass pollen allergen (Phl p 2). **A.** Binding of the Fab fragment of a genetically engineered IgE antibody molecule to a conformational B cell epitope on the timothy grass pollen allergen Ph1 p 2. **B.** Binding of the Fab fragment of a mouse IgG monoclonal antibody to Der p 1. Both allergens are shown in *red*, whereas the light and heavy chains of the Fab portions are shown in *blue* and *green*, respectively. The actual amino acid residues comprising each of the two epitopes binding to the hypervariable regions of the Fab fragments are shown in black, as are the interacting amino acid residues of the hypervariable regions of the antibody combining sites in the Fab fragments (the paratope). The images were constructed with the PyMOL molecular graphics system using Worldwide Protein Data Bank (PDB) entries 2VXQ and 3RVX. *IgE*, *IgG*, Immunoglobulins E, G.

by a prior exposure to tick bite salivary proteins, and its presence in these individuals may give rise to false-positive results when using certain allergen extracts in skin testing, for example, cat extracts. In addition to being potentially important in certain clinical situations, allergen glycosylation patterns may be very important in antigen presentation, given the diverse array of receptors in the innate immune system that have evolved to differentiate pathogen from host.

ALLERGEN NOMENCLATURE AND ALLERGEN DATABASES

One of the main drivers for the denomination of allergens has been the desire to describe a specific allergen and its source in a precise and consistent manner. The study of allergens at the molecular level started in the 1960s and a number of clinically important proteins from pollens, cat and fish were then identified, aided by the development of highly resolving purification techniques. It soon became apparent that some allergens were more important than others and that allergen sources possessed multiple allergens. Although allergens were denominated, the ad hoc and idiosyncratic method of denomination in use at the time was not particularly informative. This problem was addressed and, under the auspices of the World Health Organization (WHO) and the International Union of Immunologic Societies (IUIS), an Allergen Nomenclature Subcommittee was established in 1984,[5] which introduced a systematic nomenclature system, based on a set of specific criteria as shown (see Box 4-1).

The Subcommittee's systematic naming of purified allergens is based on using the first three letters of the genus (e.g., *Dermatophagoides*) combined with the first one or two letters of the species name (e.g., *pteronyssinus*) and an Arabic numeral reflecting either the order in which the allergen was isolated or its clinical importance, or both. In order to avoid confusion where such abbreviations of the genus are identical, four letters rather than three may be used, for example, Cand and Can for *Candida* and *Canis*, respectively). To differentiate the recombinant from the native form, the prefixes 'r' and 'n', respectively, are used (e.g., rDer p 1, nDer p 1).

Similar allergens from related species use the same nomenclature. For example, the house-dust mite cysteine protease allergens from the species *Dermatophagoides pteronyssinus*, *D. farinae*, *Euroglyphus maynei*, and *Blomia tropicalis* are individually referred to as Der p 1, Der f 1, Eur m 1, and Blo t 1, respectively, and collectively as the group 1 mite allergens or as the mite cysteine proteases. As allergens are proteins demonstrating allelic variation (isoforms, isoenzymes), the term *isoallergen* was introduced to describe closely related allergens. Those allergens from the same species demonstrating >67% sequence identity are denominated using a suffix (e.g., Amb a 1.01, Amb a 1.02) but for multiple isoallergens in the same source and differing by only a few residues, an additional two digits are added (e.g., Amb a 1.0101). The Subcommittee also created the first official allergen database but other allergen databases have been established, with different emphases (Table 4-2). On the basis of these databases, predictive algorithms now make it possible (with caveats) to determine whether a newly described protein is likely to be allergenic based on sequence similarity alone, as well as developing expert systems for automated allergy diagnosis.

OUTDOOR ALLERGENS

Outdoor allergens constitute one of the most common causes of allergic disease, and are typically derived from pollens and fungal spores. A high proportion of individuals that are exposed become sensitized (30–40%) depending on the community. Allergic reactions to outdoor allergens are usually seasonal rather than perennial, and for example, tree pollen exposure may occur during spring, and grass and herbaceous dicotyledon pollen exposure may occur in summer through to autumn. Both pollen and fungal spore concentrations in the atmosphere will also be influenced by microclimatic conditions such as temperature, wind, or rain. Symptoms generally (but not always) correspond to atmospheric pollen and fungal spore concentrations or, in their absence, submicronic allergenic particles (fragmented pollen or fungal spores or released starch granules). Similarly, the age of the pollen will also influence manifestations, as immature and aging pollens are not as potent as mature pollen. Exposure to outdoor allergens may also occur in the home as outdoor allergen sources may enter and become deposited in house dust and become amenable to aerosolization. In normal circumstances, concentrations of fungal spores in the home are also influenced by those outside, but in damp rooms such as basements, the presence of spores will be influenced by inherent fungal growth.

Outdoor Allergen Sources – Pollen

Pollen (derived from the Latin word for 'flour' or 'fine dust') from allergenic plants arises predominantly from wind-pollinated (anemophilous) angiosperms and

TABLE 4-2   Various Databases Containing Information on Allergen Structure and Function, and Allergen Prediction Software

Database/Software	Content	Web address: http://www.
Non–allergen-specific*		
GenBank	Nucleotide sequences	ncbi.nlm.nih.gov/genbank/
Universal Protein Resource (UniProt)	Protein sequences and function	ebi.ac.uk/uniprot/
European Nucleotide Archive (ENA)	Nucleotide sequences	ebi.ac.uk/ena/
Worldwide Protein Data Bank (wwPDB)	3-dimensional protein structures	wwpdb.org/
Pfam	Protein structures and domain architectures	pfam.sanger.ac.uk/
MEROPS	Peptidases and peptidase inhibitors	merops.sanger.ac.uk/
Allergen-specific		
International Union of Immunologic Societies (IUIS) Allergen Nomenclature Subcommittee	A curated database of all officially recognized allergens	allergen.org
Allergome	Similar to the IUIS database but contains other information, as well as data on allergens yet to be denominated by the IUIS Subcommittee	allergome.org
AllFam	A database of allergens curated on basis of information contained in Allergome and Pfam	meduniwien.ac.at/allergens/allfam/
Food Allergy Research and Resource Program Allergen Database	A database of allergens relevant to the food industry	allergenonline.com
InFormAll	A database of allergens relevant to the food industry	allergens.ifr.ac.uk/
Structural Database of Allergenic Proteins (SDAP)	An allergen database including epitope data, together with a collection of bioinformatic tools for their analysis	fermi.utmb.edu/SDAP/index.html
Immune Epitope Database and Analysis Resource	A database of epitopes of both antigens and allergens	IEDB.org
Allergenicity prediction servers		
AllerTOP	*In silico* prediction of allergenicity and route of exposure	pharmfac.net/allertop/
AllerHunter	*In silico* prediction of allergen cross-reactivity	http://tiger.dbs.nus.edu.sg/AllerHunter
AlgPred	*In silico* prediction of allergenicity and epitopes	http://imtech.res.in/raghava/algpred

*Although not allergen-focused *per se*, these databases may cross-reference structure and sequence data with allergenicity data.

gymnosperms, including trees, herbaceous dicotyledons (weeds), and grasses (Fig. 4-4). They carry the male gametophyte and interact with the stigma in angiosperms, and with the pollen drop in the stigma-less gymnosperms, to fertilize the plant ovum via the micropyle. Exposure to pollens usually reflects the types of plants growing in a particular location, since most pollen settles close to their origin. However, pollen-specific characteristics such as size, buoyant density and profusion can mean that pollens may travel many hundreds of kilometers from their original source and reach heights of several hundred meters. Pollen grains vary in shape according to species, and were observed in detail for the first time by Nehemiah Grew (1641–1712) and Marcello Malpighi (1628–1694), using the newly discovered microscope. They range in size from approximately 5 μm to >200 μm, and examples of allergenic pollens are shown in Figure 4-5. A concentration of 20–100 pollen grains/m³ is sufficient to provoke disease, but the concentrations of specific pollen-derived allergens required to initiate symptoms are unknown, as are those that could be considered threshold levels.

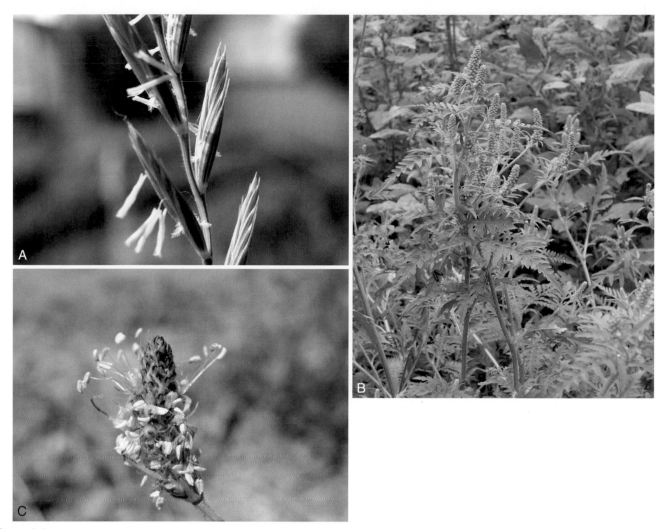

Figure 4-4 Photographs of clinically important sources of pollen producing plants. **A.** Rye grass. **B.** Short ragweed. **C.** English plantain.

Pollen Structure and Allergen Release

Pollen comprise a cytoplasmic core, a multilayered, tough, sporopollenin-containing external wall layer (exine), with various apertures including microchannels and germination pores through which the pollen tube emerges, and an internal wall, the intine (Fig. 4-5). The exine comprises three layers and provides the pollen with strong, mechanical resistance, enabling it to survive for long periods in the atmosphere. It is covered with a pollen coat containing a variety of proteins, lipids, and pigments, which have important functions in pollen-stigma interactions. Beneath the exine is the intine layer wall and then the cytoplasm, which contains a variety of components, including the generative cell (gametophyte) and the tube cell that grows into the pollen tube, and various carbohydrate-containing particles, enzymes and various other biochemicals. The main pollen-derived particles include starch granules (i.e., amyloplasts; approximately 700–1000/pollen grain, each approximately 3 μm in diameter), which act as a metabolic substrate for the pollen, and polysaccharide (pectin)-containing wall precursor bodies termed *P-particles* that move along the growing pollen tube to supply building material for tube tip growth, which emerges through the exine via a germination pore (operculum).

Prior to release, allergens may be found within the pollen cytoplasm, on starch granules and in the exine, intine, and pollen coat layers and, in some instances, in the orbicles

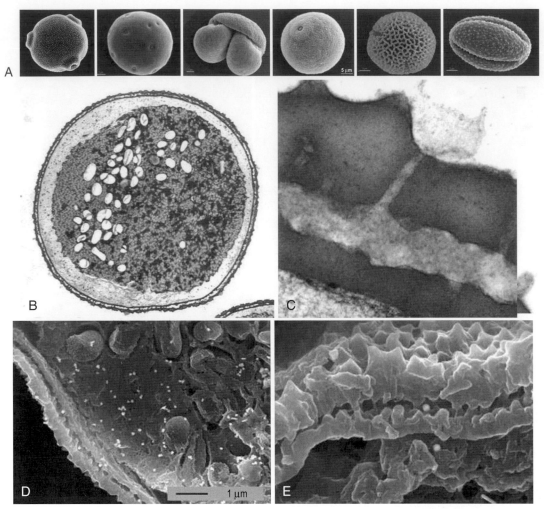

Figure 4-5 Scanning and transmission electron microscopy of pollens, their internal structures and allergen location. **A.** Varieties of grass pollen that carry allergens. **B.** As shown by transmission electron microscopy, a pollen has an inner, cellulose-rich layer, the intine, which encloses the cytoplasm and organelles, and an outer wall, the exine, which is composed mostly of sporopollenin. **C.** Apertures form in the exine through which cytoplasmic material can be transported to the pollen surface. **D.** Location of allergens in the cytoplasm. **E.** Location of allergens between the exine and intine. The presence of allergen in D and E is indicated by the colloidal gold particles bound to secondary antibody attached to IgE. *(B from Behrendt H, et al. Timothy grass (Phleum pratense L.) pollen as allergen carriers and initiators of an allergic response. Int Arch Allergy Immunol 1999; 118:414–418.)*

of some but not all grass, herbaceous dicotyledon, and tree species. Knowledge of this distribution has recently assumed some diagnostic relevance, since the usual practice of allergen-extract manufacturers is to remove the water impermeable pollen coat, and thus allergens, using organic solvents before making an aqueous extract of the remaining, intact pollen. Studies now show that up to 25% of pollen-allergic patients may respond preferentially to allergens in this coat.

When pollens land on the stigma, they adhere and then hydrate through the microchannels in the exine or across the intine, which results in their expansion and activation. As they hydrate, proteins (allergens) and other biochemicals are rapidly released, which usually occurs within minutes, as it does when they land on moist mucosal tissues. However, in hypotonic conditions such as rain, pollen cytoplasmic contents, including allergen-containing starch granules may be rapidly discharged, particularly from grass and ragweed pollen, a phenomenon first reported by Charles Blackley. However, in angiosperm Fagales tree pollens (e.g., birch), the expulsion mechanism differs in that pollen landing in water will release submicronic particles through the rupturing of the tips of pollen tubes that are induced to grow, although abortively.[6] In contrast to angiosperms, in gymnosperms (e.g., *Cupressus* and *Juniperus* spp.) pollen is trapped by a pollination drop and immediately hydrate through a pore. The intine rapidly expands and the exine layer is discarded.

Pollen Allergens

Most of our knowledge of pollen allergens arises from the study of clinically important species of grasses, herbaceous dicots, and trees in mainly temperate climates including the USA, Europe, and Australia (Table 4-3). At the molecular level, the first structural information on pollen allergens was obtained using ragweed and rye pollens in the late 1970s and early 1980s by conventional Edman amino acid sequencing, which was then followed by an exponential increase in our understanding of allergen structure due to the application of molecular biologic techniques. The first pollen allergens to be cloned were the Dac g 2, Amb a 1, and Bet v 1 from orchard grass, ragweed, and birch, respectively, and data from related disciplines have greatly facilitated the determination of pollen allergen function. Pollen allergens can be divided into three types: those that are ubiquitous; those that are present in a limited number of plant families; and those that are restricted to a single plant family or order (Tables 4-4–4-6).[7] Most allergens fall into a small number of protein groups that include plant cell wall modifying proteins,

TABLE 4-3   Common Allergenic Pollens and Sources

Cross-reacting groups	Representative genera*
Grasses	
Pooideae	*Poa* (bluegrass), *Dactylis* (orchard), *Festuca* (fescue), *Lolium* (perennial rye), *Agrostis* (redtop), *Anthoxanthum* (vernal), *Phleum* (timothy)
Chloridoideae	*Cynodon* (Bermuda)
Panicoideae	*Paspalum* (Bahia), *Sorghum* (Johnson)
TREES	
Aceraceae	*Acer* (maples, box elder)
Betulaceae	*Alnus* (alder), *Betula* (birches), *Corylus* (hazelnut)
Cupressaceae	*Cupressus* (cypress), *Juniperus* (junipers, cedars), *Taxodium* (bald cypress)
Fabaceae	*Acacia* (mimosa), *Robinia* (locust), *Prosopis* (mesquite)
Fagaceae	*Quercus* (oaks), *Fagus* (beech)
Juglandaceae	*Carya* (hickory, pecan), *Juglans* (walnut)
Moraceae	*Morus* (mulberry)
Oleaceae	*Olea* (olive), *Fraxinus* (ash), *Ligustrum* (privet)
Pinaceae	*Pinus* (pines)
Platanaceae	*Platanus* (sycamore)
Salicaceae	*Populus* (cottonwood, poplars), *Salix* (willows)
Ulmaceae	*Ulmus* (elms)
Herbaceous dicotyledons	
Chenopodiaceae	*Atriplex* (scales, saltbush), *Chenopodium* (lamb's quarter), *Salsola* (Russian thistle), *Kochia* (firebush)
Asteraceae	*Artemisia* (mugworts, wormwood, sages), *Ambrosia* (ragweeds), *Xanthium* (cocklebur)
Amaranthaceae	*Amaranthus* (careless weed, pigweeds), *Acnida* (Western water hemp)
Plantaginaceae	*Plantago* (plantain)
Polygonaceae	*Rumex* (dock, sorrel)

*Representative genera are members of the same botanical family or subfamily. Manufacturers currently offer allergen products derived from one or more species of each listed genus.

TABLE 4-4 Physicochemical and Biochemical Characteristics of Grass Pollen Aeroallergens

Allergen	Frequency of reactivity* (%)	Mol. size (kDa)	Function
Poaceae and Panicoideae[†]			
Example species: *Phleum pratense, Lolium perenne, Cynodon dactylon, Oryza sativa, Secale cereal, Triticum aestivum*			
Group 1 (e.g., Lol p 1)	>90	30	β-Expansin; involved in cell wall loosening; shows homology with group 2 and group 3 allergens
Group 2 (e.g., Lol p 2)	>60	11	Shows homology with the C-terminal half of group 1 allergens; shows homology with group 3 allergens
Group 3 (e.g., Lol p 3)	70	11	Shows homology with group 1 and group 2 allergens
Group 4 (e.g., Lol p 4)	50–88	57	Berberine bridge enzyme
Group 5 (e.g., Lol p 5)	>90	29–31	Single-stranded nuclease with topoisomerase-like activity
Group 6 (e.g., Phl p 6)	76	11	Shows homology with group 5 allergens; associated with P-particles
Group 7 (e.g., Phl p 7)	>10	6	Polcalcin; shows homology with Bet v 4, Ole e 3, Aln g 4, Jun o 2
Group 10 (e.g., Lol p 10)	?	12	Cytochrome *c*
Group 11 (e.g., Lol p 11)	65	16	Function unknown; shows homology with tree allergen Ole e 1 and soybean trypsin inhibitor
Group 12 (e.g., Phl p 12)	14–93	14	Profilin
Group 13 (e.g., Phl p 13)	50	55–60	Polygalacturonase
Group 15 (e.g., Phl p 15)	?	9	Function unknown
Group 22 (e.g., Phl p 22)	?	?	Enolase
Group 23 (e.g., Phl p 23)	?	9	Function unknown
Cyn d CP	63	23	Cysteine protease; also found in Johnson grass and Timothy, shows homology with enzymes from maize and rice
Cyn d EXY	75	30	Endoxylanase; shows homology with enzymes from maize and rice

Data obtained from original references and from http://www.allergen.org and http://www.allergome.org.

*Frequency data presented in these tables are indications only, because they will vary with the population studied and geographic location. In addition, the data presented may reflect immediate hypersensitivity diseases, including atopic dermatitis and allergic bronchopulmonary aspergillosis, as well as delayed-type hypersensitivity disease. '?' Indicates lack of data at the time of the publication. When frequency data are shown for allergens described in groups, the data refer to the example in parentheses.

[†]Classification of species throughout table is derived from the Catalogue of Life (www.catalogueoflife.org).

(All allergen data tables adapted from Stewart GA, Peden DP, Thompson PJ, Ludwig M. Allergens and air pollutants. In: Holgate ST, Church MK, Broide DH, Martinez FD, eds. Allergy. 4th edn. Edinburgh: Saunders; 2012.)

proteins associated with abiotic and biotic stressors, actin cytoskeleton associated proteins, and calcium-binding proteins.

Cell Wall Modifying Allergens

Breaching of the pellicle and cuticle of the stigma in dry stigma angiosperms by the pollen tube requires enzymes to gain entry to the style, and pollens from all plant types produce proteins that facilitate this, although the biochemistry involved will vary. Most are major allergens and include the β-expansins and endoxylanases in grass pollens, and the pectin degrading allergens (polygalacturonases, pectin methylesterases, pectin lyases) present in all pollen. In grass pollens, the β-expansins loosen cell wall structures rather than hydrolyzing these, and account for approximately 4% of extractable protein. The pectin-associated enzymes fulfill the same role as the β-expansins and are either hydrolases or lyases. All pollens contain proteases, which may be involved in degrading the pellicle that covers the stigma.

Allergens Involved in Defense

Some pollen proteins are produced to deal with pathogens, and are grouped into families because of their sequence homology with the constitutive or inducible

TABLE 4-5 Physicochemical and Biochemical Characteristics of Pollen-derived Aeroallergens from Herbaceous Dicotyledon Species

Allergen	Frequency of reactivity (%)	Mol. size (kDa)	Function
Asteraceae			
Short ragweed (*Ambrosia artemisiifolia, Ambrosia elatior, Ambrosia psilostachya, Ambrosia trifida*)			
Group 1 (e.g., Amb a 1)*	>90	38	Pectate lyase, cleaved into two chains by protease by pollen trypsin-like protease
Group 3 (e.g., Amb a 3)	51	11	Plastocyanin, a copper containing protein
Group 4 (e.g., Amb a 4)	20–39	30	Defensin-like protein with a proline-rich C-terminal domain; shows homology with Art v 1
Group 5 (e.g., Amb a 5)	10–15	5	Secreted basic protein
Group 6 (e.g., Amb a 6)	21	11	Non-specific lipid transfer protein
Group 7 (e.g., Amb a 7)	15–20	12	Plastocyanin, possible isoallergen of Amb a 3
Group 8 (e.g., Amb a 8)	25–56	14	Profilin
Group 9 (e.g., Amb a 9)	10–15	10	Polcalcin, 2EF-hand binding protein
Group 10 (e.g., Amb a 10)	9–26	10	Polcalcin, 3EF-hand binding protein
Group 11	53	37	Cysteine protease
Mugwort (*Artemisia vulgaris*)			
Art v 1	95	28	Plant defensin-like domain and a hydroxyproline/proline-rich domain; shows homology with Amb a 4, PR-12
Art v 2	33	20	Pathogenesis-related protein PR-1
Art v 3	25–56	12	Non-specific lipid transfer protein
Art v 4	36	14	Profilin
Art v 5	10	10	Polcalcin
Art v 6	89	44	Pectate lyase; shows homology with Amb a 1
Feverfew (*Parthenium hysterophorus*)			
Par h 1	>90	31	β-Extensin
Sunflower (*Helianthus annuus*) (Insect pollinated)			
Hel a 1	65	34	Function unknown
Hel a 2	31	14	Profilin
Urticaceae			
Wall pellitory (*Parietaria judaica/officinalis*)			
Group 1 (e.g., Par o 1)	95	15	Non-specific lipid transfer protein, Par j 1.0101 isoform with a 37 amino acid extension possess LPS binding activity
Group 2 (e.g., Par o 2)	82	10–14	Non-specific lipid transfer protein
Group 3 (e.g., Par j 3)	100	14	Profilin
Group 4 (e.g., Par j 4)	6	9	Polcalcin, 2EF-hand calcium binding protein
Bra n PG	28	43	Polygalacturonase
Euphorbiaceae			
Mercurialis annua			
Mer a 1	59	14	Profilin
Chenopodiaceae			
Chenopodium album			
Che a 1	77	17	Trypsin inhibitor; shows homology with Ole e 1
Che a 2	50–60	14	Profilin
Che a 3	46	10	Polcalcin

Continued on following page

TABLE 4-5   Physicochemical and Biochemical Characteristics of Pollen-derived Aeroallergens from Herbaceous Dicotyledon Species (Continued)

Allergen	Frequency of reactivity (%)	Mol. size (kDa)	Function
Amaranthaceae			
Russian thistle (*Salsola kali*)			
Sal k 1	65	38	Pectin methylesterase
Sal k 2	?	36	Protein kinase homolog
Sal k 3	67	45	Methionine synthase
Sal k 4	46	14.4	Profilin
Sal k 5	34–64	18.2	Ole e 1-like protein

*Amb a 2 is now considered to be an isoallergen of Amb a 1 and is designated Amb a 1.05.

TABLE 4-6   Physicochemical and Biochemical Characteristics of Tree Pollen Aeroallergens

Allergen	Frequency of reactivity (%)	Mol. size (kDa)	Function
Angiosperms			
Fagales			
Birch, alder, hornbeam, oak, chestnut, hazel			
Group 1 (e.g., Bet v1)	>95	17	Plant steroid carrier; shows homology with pathogenesis-related proteins (e.g., PR-10)
Group 2 (e.g., Bet v 2)	5–37	15	Profilin
Group 3 (e.g., Bet v 3)	<10	24	Polcalcin
Group 4 (e.g., Bet v 4)	20	9	Polcalcin; shows homology with Aln g 4, Ole e 3, Syr v 3
Group 6 (e.g., Bet v 6)	32	35	Isoflavone reductase
Group 7 (e.g., Bet v 7)	21	18	Cyclophilin
Group 8 (e.g., Bet v 8)	66	65	Pectin methylesterase
Group 10 (e.g., Bet v 10)	?	70	Luminol-binding protein
Bet v GST	13	27	Glutathione-*S*-transferase
Lamiales			
Olive, lilac, privet, ash			
Group 1 (e.g., Ole e 1)	>90	20	Shows limited homology with soybean trypsin inhibitor and Lol p 11
Group 2 (e.g., Ole e 2)	61–91	15	Profilin
Group 3 (e.g., Ole e 3)	20->50	9	Polcalcin
Group 5 (e.g., Ole e 5)	35	16	Cu/Zn superoxide dismutase
Group 6 (e.g., Ole e 6)	5–20	10	Cysteine rich protein
Group 7 (e.g., Ole e 7)	>60	10	Lipid transfer protein
Group 8 (e.g., Ole e 8)	8	21	Polcalcin
Group 9 (e.g., Ole e 9)	65	45	1,3-β-Glucanase, shows homology with peptide originally designated Ole e 4
Group 10 (e.g., Ole e 10)	55	11	Shows homology with the C-terminal domain of Ole e 9, carbohydrate-binding module CBM 43
Group 11 (e.g., Ole e 11)	56–76	39	Pectin methylesterase
Group 12, e.g, Ole e 12			Isoflavone reductase

TABLE 4-6 Physicochemical and Biochemical Characteristics of Tree Pollen Aeroallergens (Continued)

Allergen	Frequency of reactivity (%)	Mol. size (kDa)	Function
Hamamelidales			
London plane tree (*Platanus acerifolia*)			
Pla a 1	84	18	Invertase inhibitor
Pla a 2	83	43	Polygalacturonase
Pla a 3	51	10	Ns Lipid transfer protein
Pla a 8	90	15	Profilin
Gymnosperms (conifers)			
Cupressaceae			
Japanese cedar (*Cryptomeria japonica*)			
Cry j 1	>85	41–45	Pectate lyase; shows homology with bacterial pectate lyase and Amb a 1 and 2
Cry j 2	76	45	Polygalacturonase
Cry j 3	27	27	Shows homology with thaumatin, osmotin, and amylase/trypsin inhibitor; PR-5–related
Cry j AP	58	52	Aspartate protease
Cry j Chitinase	100	34	Chitinase
Cry j LPT	37	10	ns Lipid transfer protein
Cry j CPA9	89	?	Plant subtilisin-like serine protease
Cry j IFR	76	34	Isoflavone reductase; shows homology with Bet v 5
Juniper species (e.g., *Juniperus ashei, Juniperus rigida, Juniperus virginiana, Juniperus oxycedrus, Juniperus communis*)			
Group 1 (e.g., Jun a 1)	71	43	Pectate lyase
Group 2 (e.g., Jun a 2)	100	43	Polymethylgalacturonase
Group 3 (e.g., Jun a 3)	33	30	Shows homology with thaumatin, osmotin, and amylase/trypsin inhibitor; PR-5–related
Group 4 (e.g., Jun o 4)	15	29	Polcalcin
Cypress (e.g., *Cupressus sempervirens, Cupressus arizonica, Chamaecyparis obtusa*)			
Group 1 (e.g., Cup s 1)	50–81	38–42	Pectate lyase
Group 2 (e.g., Cha o 2)	83	45	Polygalacturonase
Group 3 (e.g., Cup a 3)	63	34	Shows homology with thaumatin, osmotin, and amylase/trypsin inhibitor; PR-5–related
Group 8 (e.g., Cup s 8)	?	14	Profilin

pathogenesis-related proteins (PR) previously demonstrated in tissues other than pollen.[8] Some 17 PR families have been identified, and pollen-derived allergens belonging to six have been identified (eight, if latex, fruit, and seed allergens are included). Tree pollens are associated with the PR-2, -5, -10, and -14 families, whereas herbaceous dicotyledon allergens are associated with the PR-1, and -12 families (Tables 4-4–4-6) but none of the grass pollen allergens are members. In general, pollen PR family members are usually minor allergens, although some are clinically important.

Ligand Binding PR-10 Allergens

The major group 1 Fagales allergens belong to the PR-10 family and are protease-resistant allergens, which may comprise >20% of the total extractable pollen protein. They possess a seven-stranded β-sheet structure together with a large hydrophobic cavity. Grass, herbaceous dicotyledons, or gymnosperm pollens do not express any homologues, but they are found in fruits, carrots, celery, nuts, and soybeans. Whilst their true physiological function remains to be determined, they possess ligand binding activity for the naturally occurring, yellow-colored glycosylated flavonoid, quercetin-3-O-sophoroside and may help protect pollen from ultraviolet (UV) damage.

Non-specific Lipid Transfer Proteins (PR-14)

The nsLTP proteins are a ubiquitous group of small cationic proteins that bind a variety of ligands in their hydrophobic pocket, such as palmitic acid and L-α-myristoyl-phosphatidylcholine. There are two main types but it is the 9 kDa form that is linked with allergy, not only in pollen but also in seeds, latex, fruits, and vegetables. They are generally considered to be minor allergens but in *Pellitory* and mugwort pollen, they are major ones, particularly in Mediterranean countries, and in northern and central Europe. Some nsLTP are larger than the normal members of this family because of a 37 residue extension that binds to bacterial lipopolysaccharide (LPS). In the minority of individuals allergic to the nsLTP, initial sensitization results from ingestion of nsLTP-containing fruits but where they are major allergens, the pollen form is the true sensitizer. The function of these proteins in pollen is unclear, although they are grouped as members of the PR-14 family due to a body of data showing killing effects on bacteria and fungi, although this has not been demonstrated with pollen allergens.

Non-PR Defense-related Pollen Allergens

A variety of non-PR related pollen allergens may also play a defense function because of their association with secondary metabolite function such as phytoalexin and alkaloid synthesis, for example, the group 4 berberine bridge enzymes in grass pollen and the isoflavone reductases in tree pollen. Similarly, group 11 grass and tree pollen allergens share sequence homology with soybean trypsin inhibitor, suggesting a protease inhibitory role, although no such activity has been demonstrated. The function of the major group 5 and related group 6 allergens is unknown and pollens from trees and herbaceous dicotyledons do not contain a homologue. Phl p 5 was reported to possess single-stranded ribonuclease and topoisomerase-like activity, and given that PR-10 family members in other tissues possess ribonuclease activity, it is possible they could play some defensive function in grasses, However, given the lack of sequence homology with known ribonucleases, it has been suggested that they are not ribonucleases unless they represent a unique family of enzymes.

Profilins and Polcalcins

The profilins and polcalcins are ubiquitous proteins found in all pollens, and profilins are present in most cells of eukaryotes. Both are low molecular weight proteins that are usually minor pan-allergens involved in OAS or food cross-activity syndrome (Table 4-7), although they may be major ones in certain species. The profilins represent a group of proteins involved in actin polymerization in the microtubule cytoskeleton, as well as playing other roles such as signaling. However, their function when released onto the stigma is unknown. The polcalcin allergens are also thought to play a role in modulating pollen tube growth because of the importance of Ca+ ions in this process but may also be involved in signaling. They bind metal ions using a characteristic structural motif consisting of an ion-binding peptide loop sequence flanked by a small helical sequence; an arrangement classified as an 'EF' hand. This group of proteins may contain two, three, or four such ion-binding structures, but in pollens, the two-handed version predominates.

Outdoor Allergen Sources – Fungi

Fungi are significant sources of allergens, and of the more than 180 fungal species shown to produce allergenic proteins, those of the *Ascomycota* and *Basidiomycota* phyla are clinically important (Table 4-8).[9] All use airborne conidia (spore) dispersal for reproduction and spores are often produced in concentrations exceeding those seen with pollens. In addition, allergens are found in mycelia, fragmented hyphae, and yeast forms. The majority of fungal allergens are proteins or glycoproteins, but mannans from *C. albicans* and *M. furfur* may also be allergenic.

TABLE 4-7 Examples of Indoor and Outdoor Allergens Involved in Oral Allergy or Food Cross-reactivity Syndromes

Syndrome/Sensitizing source	Provoking source – food	Cross-reacting indoor or outdoor allergen(s) in sensitizing source
Outdoor allergens – pollens/food		
Grass pollen	Melon, tomato, watermelon, orange, cherry, potato	Profilin (Grass group 12)
Mugwort pollen	Celery, carrot, spices, melon, apple, chestnut, camomile, watermelon, hazelnut	Lipid transfer protein (Art v 3), profilin (Art v 4), PR-12 (Art v 1)
Ragweed pollen	Melon, camomile, honey, banana, sunflower seeds	Pectate lyase (Amb a 1)
Fagales tree pollen	Apple, carrot, cherry, pear, peach, plum, fennel, walnut, potato, spinach, wheat, buckwheat, peanut, honey, celery, kiwifruit, persimmon	Pathogenesis-protein PR-10 (Bet v 1), related profilin (Bet v 2), and Bet v 6 homologues
Japanese cedar pollen	Melon, apple, peach, kiwifruit	Pectate lyase (Cry j 1), thaumatin-like PR proteins (Cry j 3)
Indoor allergens – arthropods/snails/shellfish/parasites		
Mites	Shellfish, snails	Tropomyosin (Der p 10)
Mites	*Anisakis simplex*	Tropomyosin (Der p 10)
Cockroach	Shellfish, snails	Tropomyosin (Per a 7)
Indoor allergens – pork/cat		
Animal danders	Meat	Serum albumin (Bos d 6)
Animal danders	Meat	α-Gal epitope on serum IgA, IgM

OAS or pollen–food syndrome is due to the cross-reactivity between proteins in the respiratory allergen source and pan-allergens in food. The condition is associated predominantly with uncooked food, because processing and cooking generally result in protein denaturation. Clinical manifestations range from mild oropharyngeal symptoms to severe, systemic reactions. Such reactions are often classified by reference to the respiratory sensitizer and oral elicitors. The allergens associated with latex–fruit allergies are PR family proteins, and those associated with arthropod–crustaceans are tropomyosins but are not included here.

Although fungal allergens can be found in both mycelia and spores, some of the spore-derived allergens may be absent in mycelial extracts. At present, it is not clear whether atopic individuals are initially sensitized to spore- or to mycelium-derived allergens, but sensitization may occur with exposure to fragmented spores or hyphae, rather than to intact structures. This process is clearly different from that seen with pollen and mite fecal pellets, both of which quickly release their contents—through the operculum in pollen and through the peritrophic membrane in mites. With regard to spore release, fungi can be classified into two groups: those that release spores during dry, windy conditions (e.g., *Alternaria* and *Cladosporium*) and those that release spores when ambient humidity is high (e.g., when it is raining [ascomycetes and basidiomycetes]).

Fungal Allergens

Fungi of clinical importance include *Aspergillus*, *Penicillium*, *Cladosporium*, and *Alternaria* species (Fig. 4-6; Table 4-8), and the allergens may be cell wall- or cytoplasm-derived. Many are involved in protein synthesis or energy metabolism, although secretory (e.g., proteases) allergens also may be involved. As with pollens, allergens common across allergenic fungal species (of both *Ascomycota* and *Basidiomycota*) exist, as well as species-specific allergens. For example, enolases, heat shock proteins (HSPs), aldehyde dehydrogenases, thioredoxins, proteases, and cyclophilins (peptidyl-prolyl isomerase) are common allergens, although they may be minor or major, depending on species.

Alternaria, Aspergillus, and Cladosporium

The major allergens from the three clinically important species include Alt a 1, and 13, Asp f 1, 2, and 4, and Cla h 1, respectively (Table 4-8), although the functions of several are unknown. In this regard, the heat stable Alt a 1, is released from spores prior to

TABLE 4-8   Physicochemical and Biochemical Characteristics of Fungi-derived Aeroallergens

Allergen	Frequency of reactivity (%)	Mol. size (kDa)	Function
Ascomycota			
Alternaria alternata			
Alt a 1	>80	14	Function unknown
Alt a 2	0–61	20	EIF-2α kinase
Alt a 3	5	70	HSP70
Alt a 4	42	57	Protein disulfide isomerase
Alt a 5	8	11	Ribosomal P_2 protein; shows homology with Cla h 4
Alt a 6	50	45	Enolase
Alt a 7	7	22	1,4-Benzoquinone reductase; shows homology Cla h 5
Alt a 8	41	29	Mannitol dehydrogenase
Alt a 10	2	54	Aldehyde dehydrogenase; shows homology with Cla h 3
Alt a 12	?	11	Acid ribosomal P1 protein
Alt a 13	82	26	Glutathione *S*-transferase
Aspergillus fumigatus			
Asp f 1	85	17	Ribonuclease; ribotoxin shows homology with mitogillin
Asp f 2	96	37	Shows homology with *Candida albicans* fibrinogen-binding protein
Asp f 3	84	19	Peroxisomal membrane protein; belongs to the peroxiredoxin family; thiol-dependent peroxidase
Asp f 4	78–83*	30	Shows homology with bacterial ABC transporter–binding protein; associated with peroxisome
Asp f 5	74	40	Metalloprotease
Asp f 6	42–56*	27	Manganese superoxide dismutase; shows homology with Mal s 11 and Hev b 10
Asp f 7	29	12	Shows homology with fungal riboflavin, aldehyde-forming enzyme
Asp f 8	8–15	11	Ribosomal P_2 protein
Asp f 9	31	34	Shows homology with plant and bacterial endo-β1,3; 1,4-glucanases
*Asp f 10	3–28	34	Aspartic protease
Asp f 11	90	24	Cyclophilin
Asp f 12	?	90	HSP90
Asp f 13	79	34	Alkaline serine protease
Asp f 15	?	16	Shows homology with a serine protease antigen from *Coccidioides immitis*; also designated Asp f 13
Asp f 16	70	43	Shows homology with Asp f 9
Asp f 18	79	34	Vacuolar serine protease
Asp f 22	30	46	Enolase, shows homology with Pen c 22
Asp f 23	?	44	L3 ribosomal protein
Asp f 27	75	18	Cyclophilin
Asp f 28	30	13	Thioredoxin
Asp f 29	50	13	Thioredoxin
Asp f 34	93	20	Phi A cell wall protein

TABLE 4-8   Physicochemical and Biochemical Characteristics of Fungi-derived Aeroallergens (Continued)

Allergen	Frequency of reactivity (%)	Mol. size (kDa)	Function
Cladosporium herbarum			
Cla h 1	>60	13	Function unknown
Cla h 2	43	45	Function unknown
Cla h 3	36	53	Aldehyde dehydrogenase
Cla h 4	22	11	Ribosomal P_2 protein
Cla h 5	22	22	1,4-Benzoquinone reductase; shows homology with Cla h 5
Cla h 6	20	46	Enolase
Cla h 8	57	28	NaDP-dependent mannitol dehydrogenase
Cla h 9	16	38	Vacuolar serine protease; shows homology with Pen ch 18 and Asp f 18
Cla h 12	?	11	Ribosomal P1 protein
Cla h HSP70	?	70	HSP, previously denominated Cla h 4
Cla h TCTP	50	19	Shows homology with human translationally controlled tumor protein (TCTP)
Penicillium chrysogenum/notatum			
Pen ch 13	>80	34	Alkaline serine protease
Pen ch 18	77	32	Vacuolar serine protease
Pen ch 20	56	68	β-N-acetylglucosaminidase from *Candida albicans*
Penicillium citrinum			
Pen c 3	46	18	Peroxisomal membrane protein; belongs to the peroxiredoxin family; thiol-dependent peroxidase
Pen c 13	100	33	Alkaline serine protease
Pen c 19	41	70	Show homology with HSP70
Pen c 22	30	46	Enolase
Pen c 24	7.6	?	Elongation factor 1β
Pen c 30	?	97	Catalase
Pen c 32	?	40	Pectate lyase
Penicillium oxalicum			
Pen a 18	89	34	Vacuolar serine protease
Candida albicans/boidinii			
Cand a 1	77	40	Alcohol dehydrogenase
Cand b 2	100	20	Peroxisomal membrane protein A
Cand a 3	56	20	Peroxisomal protein
Cand a FPA	?	37	Aldolase
Cand a PGK	?	43	Phosphoglycerate kinase
Cand a Enolase	50	46	Enolase
Cand a CAAP	75	35	Aspartate protease
Trichophyton tonsurans			
Tri t 1	54	30	Function unknown
Tri t 2	42	30	Subtilisin-like protease; shows homology with Pen ch 13, Pen c 13
Tri t 4	61	83	Dipeptidyl peptidase

Continued on following page

TABLE 4-8 Physicochemical and Biochemical Characteristics of Fungi-derived Aeroallergens (Continued)

Allergen	Frequency of reactivity (%)	Mol. size (kDa)	Function
Trichophyton rubrum			
Tri r 1/2	43	30	Subtilisin-like protease; shows homology with Pen ch 13, Pen c 13
Tri r 4	44	83	Dipeptidyl peptidase
Curvularia lunata			
Cur l 1	80	31	Serine protease
Cur l 2	75	48	Enolase
Cur l 3	?	54	Cytochrome *c*
Cur l 4	81	54	Vacuolar serine protease
Basidiomycota			
Malassezia furfur			
Mala f 1	61	35	Function unknown; cell wall protein
Mala f 2	72	21	Peroxisomal membrane protein; belongs to the peroxiredoxin family, thiol-dependent peroxidase; shows homology with Asp f 3
Mala f 3	70	20	Peroxisomal membrane protein; belongs to the peroxiredoxin family, thiol-dependent peroxidase; shows homology with Asp f 3, Mala f 2
Mala f 4	83	35	Mitochondrial malate dehydrogenase
Mala f 5	?	18	Peroxisomal membrane protein; belongs to the peroxiredoxin family, thiol-dependent peroxidase; shows homology with Mala f 2/3, Asp f 3
Mala f 6	?	17	Cyclophilin
Mala f 7	89	16	Function unknown
Mala f 8	?	19	Shows homology with immunoreactive mannoprotein from *Cryptococcus neoformans*
Mala f 9	44	14	Function unknown
Malassezia sympodialis			
Mala s 10	69	86	HSP70
Mala s 11	75	23	Manganese superoxide dismutase; shows homology with Asp f 6
Mala s 12	?	67	Glucose-methanol-choline (GMC) oxidoreductase
Mala s 13	50	13	Thioredoxin
Coprinus comatus			
Cop c 1	34	11	Leucine zipper protein
Cop c 2	19	12	Thioredoxin
Cop c 3	?	37	Function unknown
Cop c 5	?	16	Function unknown
Cop c 7	?	16	Function unknown
Psilocybe cubensis			
Psi c 1	>50	46	Function unknown
Psi c 2	>50	16	Cyclophilin
Rho m 1	21	47	Enolase
Rho m 2	?	31	Vacuolar serine protease

HSP, Heat shock protein; NaDP, nicotinamide-adenine dinucleotide phosphate.
*Higher frequency determined in patients with allergic bronchopulmonary aspergillosis.

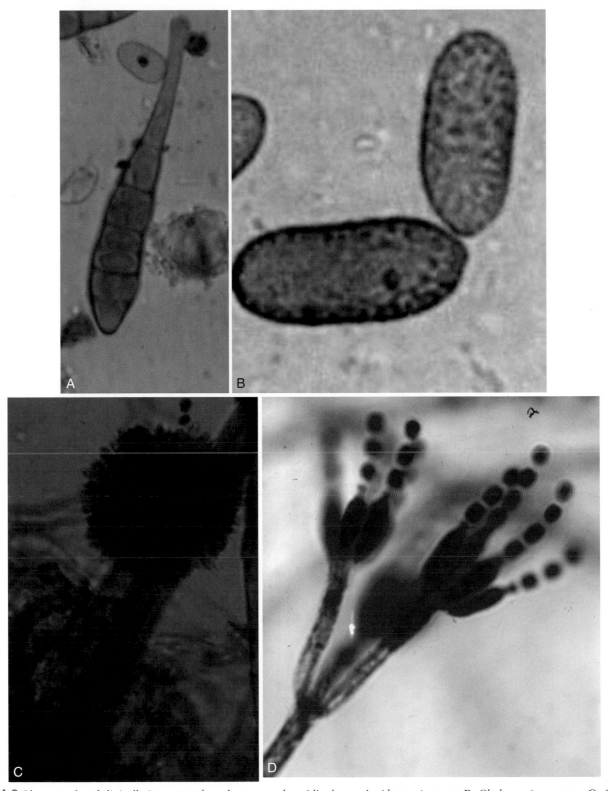

Figure 4-6 Photographs of clinically important fungal spores and conidiophores. **A.** *Alternaria* spore. **B.** *Cladosporium*, spore. **C.** *Aspergillus* conidiophore. **D.** *Penicillium* conidiophore.

hyphal growth when invading fruit and bind to the fruit PR-5 thaumatin-like protein. Alt a 13 is a glutathione-*S*-transferase and this enzyme is produced by a number of allergenic fungi and is a cross-reactive allergen. Asp f 1 is homologous with the fungal cytotoxin mitogillin from *Aspergillus restrictus* and α-sarcin from *Aspergillus giganteus*. These are cytotoxic low molecular weight, non-glycosylated purine-specific ribonucleases and are found in both spores and mycelium. The Asp f 2 allergen is a protein showing homology with the *C. albicans* 54-kDa mannoprotein, which has been shown to bind to human fibrinogen. The Asp f 4 is a binding protein associated with peroxisomes, self-replicating organelles that undertake metabolic detoxification in cells.

Penicillium, *Candida*, and *Trichophyton*

Major allergens from *Penicillium*, *Candida*, and *Trichophyton* species include serine proteases, dipeptidyl peptidases, aspartic proteases, enolases, and peroxisomal membrane proteins or are of unknown function (Table 4-8). With regard to proteases, the serine proteases are similar to the bacterial subtilisins and two types have been identified, namely, the secreted 33 kDa alkaline proteases (e.g., Asp f 13) and the 39 kDa vacuolar proteases (e.g., Asp f 18) involved in protein processing within vacuoles. The dipeptidyl peptidase from *Trichophyton* species (e.g., Tri t 4) is a secretory protein and shares sequence similarity with enzymes from *Aspergillus* species implicated in aspergilloma. The function of the 30 kDa *Trichophyton* Tri t 1 allergen is unknown, although it may be an exo-β-1,3-glucanase. The peroxisomal membrane protein allergens possess thiol-dependent peroxidase activity. The enolases, glycolytic enzymes involved in the dehydration of glycerate-2-phosphate to produce phosphoenolpyruvate, represent a major group of cross-reacting allergens from a variety of fungal species.

INDOOR ALLERGENS

House dust is a complex mixture of biochemically diverse components from various sources (mites, mammals, insects, fungi, and materials introduced from the outside world) (Box 4-2). The significance of house dust as a cause of allergic disease was first recognized by Kern in 1921 who observed that many patients with rhinitis or asthma had positive skin responses to an extract of dust from their own homes. A major advance in our understanding of the allergenicity of house dust was the discovery in 1967 by Voorhorst and Spieksma, which established that the house-dust mite (HDM), *Dermatophagoides pteronyssinus*, was an important source of indoor allergens. In temperate climates, which provide significant humidity, dust mites trigger the development of high allergen-specific IgE titers and form the single most important allergen source associated with asthma. Given the largely sedentary, indoor lifestyle in affluent countries and the creation of warm, draught-free and increasingly humid living and working conditions, human exposure to dust mites is extreme—up to 23 h/day—with important consequences for allergic disease.

Population-based, cross-sectional and prospective studies show that individuals with specific IgE to one or more major allergens, are significantly more likely to have asthma than non-sensitized individuals (Table 4-9).[9–14] Historically, chronic rhinitis, asthma and atopic dermatitis and, only rarely, conjunctivitis, urticaria and anaphylaxis have been associated with exposure to HDM or other indoor allergens. Recently, however, a significant positive association between glaucoma and IgE to cockroach and cat, and a negative association with dog has been reported. In the case of atopic dermatitis, the epidemiologic evidence is mainly from HDM sensitization, with high IgE (>30 IU/mL) strongly associated with the condition. A common finding in surveys of allergic sensitization is that up to 15% of asymptomatic individuals are sensitized to an indoor allergen. This raises questions about why and how individuals become sensitized and why only some develop frank symptoms.

Mammalian allergens are also a feature of indoor domestic or occupational dusts and are encountered in the form of cat, dog, rat, and mouse proteins from pets, and from domestic rodent infestations or in animal rearing institutions (Table 4-10). The nature

---

Box 4-2   Sources of Allergens in House Dust

ACARIDS

- Dust mites/domestic mites
  - *Dermatophagoides pteronyssinus*
  - *Dermatophagoides farinae*
  - *Euroglyphus maynei*
  - *Blomia tropicalis*
  - Storage mites
- Others
- Spiders

MAMMALS

- Cats (*Felis domesticus*)
- Dogs (*Canis familiaris*)
- Rabbits
- Ferrets
- Rodents
- Pets (mice, gerbils, guinea pigs, chinchilla, others)
- Pests
- Mice (*Mus musculus*)
- Rats (*Rattus norvegicus*)

INSECTS

- Cockroaches
  - *Blattella germanica* (German cockroach)
  - *Periplaneta americana* (American cockroach)
  - *Blatta orientalis* (Oriental cockroach)
- Others
  - *Harmonia axyridis* – Asian lady beetle
  - Crickets

- Flies
- Fleas
- Moths
- Midges
- *Lepisma saccharina* – silverfish

FUNGI

DERIVED FROM INSIDE HOUSE

- *Penicillium*
- *Aspergillus*
- *Cladosporium* (growing on surfaces of rotting wood)
- Other species

DERIVED FROM OUTSIDE HOUSE

- Multiple species from entry with incoming air

POLLENS

DERIVED FROM OUTSIDE HOUSE

- Multiple plant species

MISCELLANEOUS

- Horse hair in furniture
- Kapok (insulation, filling; silky fibers from ceiba tree)
- Food dropped by residents

---

of the airborne particles that carry cat and dog allergens differs from that associated with mite and cockroach allergens and confers on these greater airborne persistence. This results in cat and dog allergens becoming widely distributed by passive carriage on people.[15] Domestic pets, especially dogs, may bring significant LPS and bacteriologic diversity into the home, and there are reasons to think this may further influence the development of allergy.

Indoor Allergen Sources – Non-Mammalian

The main non-mammalian sources of indoor allergens are those from arthropods, particularly from the *Insecta* and *Arachnida* classes. Of the arthropods, house-dust mites (HDMs) and cockroaches are clinically important, and allergens are derived from whole bodies, salivary secretions, and fecal pellets accumulating in house dust or in dust generated by the rearing of insects. Many such allergens are gut-derived and are, therefore, present in fecal pellets, although other sources such as saliva, body debris, and secretions may contain allergens. The spectra of allergens in these two allergen sources are similar, but allergens may be specific to either.

Acaridae

Mites are small arthropods of the class Arachnida, and are eight-legged, sightless creatures living on a diet of skin and other debris such as bacteria shed from human bodies. The most clinically important species belong to the Pyroglyphidae, Acaridae, Glycyphagidae, and Echimyopodidae families. Many mite species are found in house dust but, in most parts of the world, the Pyroglyphidae family (e.g., *Dermatophagoides pteronyssinus*, *D. farinae*, and *Euroglyphus maynei*) dominates (Fig. 4-7).[16] In tropical or semi-tropical climates, allergy to *Blomia tropicalis* may also be prevalent. Domestic dwellings can also contain storage mites (e.g., *Lepidoglyphus destructor*, *Tyrophagus putrescentiae*), and large predator mites of the family Cheyletidae or the smaller *Tarsonemus* spp.

TABLE 4-9 Physicochemical and Biochemical Characteristics of Arthropod-derived Indoor Allergens

Allergen	Frequency of reactivity (%)	Mol. size (kDa)	Function
Chironomidae (midges)			
Chironomus thummi			
Chi t 1 to 5	>50	15	Hemoglobin
Cladotanytarsus lewisi			
Cla l 1	>50	17	Hemoglobin
Polypedilum nubifer			
Pol n 1	>50	17	Hemoglobin
Chironomus kiiensis			
Chi k 10	81	33	Tropomyosin
Blattidae and Blattellidae			
German cockroach (*Blattella germanica*), American cockroach (*Periplaneta americana*)			
Group 1 (e.g., Bla g 1)	1–77	46	Nitrile-specifier protein
Group 2 (e.g., Bla g 2)	7–62	36	Aspartate protease (inactive); shows homology with pepsin
Group 3 (e.g., Per a 3)	26–95	78	Arylphorins/TO Arthropod hemocyanins
Group 4 (e.g., Bla g 4)	5–53	21	Lipocalin, male cockroach allergen, binds tyramine and octopamine, involved in pheromone transport
Group 5 (e.g., Bla g 5)	7–72	23	Glutathione S-transferase
Group 6 (e.g., Bla g 6)	50	21	Troponin C
Group 7 (e.g., Per a 7)	2–31	31	Tropomyosin
Group 8 (e.g., Bla g 8)	?	20	Myosin
Group 9 (e.g., Per a 9)	34–100	45	Arginine kinase
Group 10 (e.g., Per a 10)	82	80	Trypsin
Group 11		57	Amylase
Bla g Enolase	25	45	Enolase
Vitellogenin	47	50	Shows homology with Der p 14
Pyralidae			
Indianmeal moth (*Plodia interpunctella*)			
Plo i 1	25	40	Arginine kinase
Bombycidae			
Silkworm larvae (*Bombyx mori*)			
Bom m 1	>90	42	Arginine kinase; shows homology with cockroach enzyme Per a 9
Pyroglyphidae/Glycyphagidae/Acaridae/Echimyopodidae			
Various mite species			
Group 1 (e.g., Der p 1)	>90	25	Cysteine protease
Group 2 (e.g., Der p 2)	>90	14	MD-2–related protein family, lipid binding, binds LPS
Group 3 (e.g., Der p 3)	90	25	Trypsin
Group 4 (e.g., Der p 4)	25–46	60	Amylase
Group 5 (e.g., Der p 5)	9–70	14	Function unknown; possible ligand-binding protein
Group 6 (e.g., Der p 6)	39	25	Chymotrypsin
Group 7 (e.g., Der p 7)	38–53	26–31	Function unknown; belongs to the juvenile hormone binding family of proteins found in insects; may have lipid binding properties

TABLE 4-9 Physicochemical and Biochemical Characteristics of Arthropod-derived Indoor Allergens (Continued)

Allergen	Frequency of reactivity (%)	Mol. size (kDa)	Function
Group 8 (e.g., Der p 8)	40	27	Glutathione S-transferase
Group 9 (e.g., Der p 9)	>90	29	Collagenase-like serine protease
Group 10 (e.g., Der p 10)	81	36	Tropomyosin
Group 11 (e.g., Der f 11)	82	103	Paramyosin
Group 12 (e.g., Blo t 12)	50	16	May be a chitinase; shows homology with Der f 15 and 18 due to chitin-binding domain
Group 13 (e.g., Lep d 13)	11–23	15	Fatty acid-binding protein
Group 14 (e.g., Der f 14)	84	177	Vitellogenin or lipophorin
Group 15 (e.g., Der f 15)	95	98, 109*	Chitinase; shows homology with Blot 12 allergen
Group 16 (e.g., Der f 16)	50–62	53	Gelsolin
Group 17 (e.g., Der f 17)	35	30	Calcium-binding protein
Group 18 (e.g., Der f 18)	63	60	Chitinase
Group 19 (e.g., Blo t 19)	10	7	Antimicrobial peptide homology
Group 20 (e.g., Der p 20)	0–44	40	Arginine kinase
Group 21 (e.g., Der p 21)	26	15	Function unknown; shows homology with group 5 allergens
Group 22 (e.g., Der p 22)	?	?	Shows homology with group 2 mite allergen; belongs to MD-2-related lipid recognition (ML) domain family; implicated in lipid binding
Group 23 (e.g., Der p 23)	74	14	Unknown function; shows homology with peritrophin-A domain and contains a chitin-binding domain
Group 24 (e.g., Der f 24)	100?	13	Ubiquinol–cytochrome c reductase binding protein-like protein
Group 25 (e.g., Der f 25)	76	34	Triosephosphate isomerase
Group 26 (e.g., Der f 26)	?	18	Myosin alkali light chain
Group 27 (e.g., Der f 27)	?	48	Serpin (trypsin inhibitor)
Group 28 (e.g., Der f 28)	68	70	Heat shock protein
Group 29 (e.g., Der f 29)	70–86	16	Peptidyl-prolyl cis-trans isomerase (cyclophilin)
Group 30 (e.g. Der f 30)	63	16	Ferritin
Group 31 (e.g., Der f 30)		15	Colofin
Group 32 (e.g., Der f 32)		35	Secreted inorganic pyrophosphatase
Group 33 (e.g., Der f 33)		52	Alpha tubulin
Tyr p α-Tubulin	29	56	α-Tubulin found in *Tyrophagus putrescentiae*

*Glycosylated forms, DNA sequence indicates a non-glycosylated protein of 63 kDa. Frequency determined in dogs with atopic dermatitis.

HDM thrive in a warm, moist environment and, accordingly, mite abundance is seasonal (Fig. 4-8). The optimum growth temperature for mites is 18–27°C (65–80°F), and there is a requirement for atmospheric moisture (65–85% RH), which is absorbed through their leg joints or produced through metabolism because they are unable to drink. Domestic environments often show significant microclimatic variation such that when free air is relatively dry, mites are able to withdraw into the pockets of humidity within carpets, soft furnishings and clothing so that even with dehumidification (<50% RH) it may take months for mites to die, and longer for allergen levels to decline.

House-dust mites excrete digested food mixed with their digestive enzymes and other proteins as fecal pellets surrounded by a chitinous peritrophic membrane.[17] Although indoor allergens are carried on particles that are amorphous compared with pollen or fungal spores found outdoors, HDM fecal pellets are similar in diameter to pollen grains

TABLE 4-10   Physicochemical and Biochemical Characterization of Animal-derived Indoor Allergens

Allergen	Frequency of reactivity (%)	Mol. size (kDa)	Function
Cat (*Felix domesticus*)			
Fel d 1	95	33–39*	Tetramer of two heterodimers (chains 1 and 2), a possible ligand-binding molecule; chain 1 shows homology with 10-kDa secretory protein from human Clara cells, mouse salivary androgen-binding protein subunit, rabbit uteroglobin, and a Syrian hamster protein
Fel d 2	20–35	69	Serum albumin; food allergen, cross reacts with pork, beef albumin
Fel d 3	10	11	Cystatin
Fel d 4	60	20	Lipocalin
Fel d 5	38	400	Immunoglobulin A; food allergen, IgE is directed against the galactose β-1,3-galactose moiety, also found on the heavy chain of immunoglobulin M. Present in pork, beef, and lamb
Fel d 6	?	900	Immunoglobulin M
Fel d 7	38	18	Von Ebner gland protein, cysteine protease inhibitor
Fel d 8	19	24	Latherin, surfactant protein
Dog (*Canis familiaris*)			
Can f 1	50	19–25	Lipocalin; shows homology with Von Ebner gland protein, which has cysteine protease inhibitory activity
Can f 2	20–22	27	Lipocalin; shows homology with Can f 1 and Fel d 4, and with other lipocalin allergens
Can f 3	16–40	69	Serum albumin
Can f 4	35	23	Shows homology with bovine odorant-binding protein
Can f 5	70	28	Prostatic kallikrein; shows homology with human prostate-specific antigen (PSA), which is allergenic
Can f 6		20	Lipocalin
IgG	88	150	Immunoglobulin G
Horse (*Equus caballus*)			
Equ c 1	100	25	Lipocalin; shows homology with rodent urinary proteins
Equ c 2	100	17	Lipocalin; shows homology with rodent urinary proteins
Equ c 3	50	67	Serum albumin
Equ c 4	77	17, 20.5	Latherin, surfactant protein
Equ c 5	77–100	21	Function unknown
Cow (*Bos taurus*)			
Bos d 2	97	20	Lipocalin
Bos d 3	?	11	S100 calcium-binding protein
Bos d OSCP	31	21	Oligomycin sensitivity-conferring protein of the mitochondrial adenosine triphosphate synthase complex
BDA 11	?	12	Shows homology with human calcium-binding psoriasin protein
Guinea pig (*Cavia porcellus*)			
Cav p 1	70	20	Lipocalin; shows homology with Cav p 2
Cav p 2	65	17	Lipocalin; shows homology with Bos d 2
Cav p 3	54	19	Lipocalin
Mouse (*Mus musculus*)			
Mus m 1	>80	17	Major urinary protein; shows homology with lipocalins such as β-lactoglobulin, odorant-binding proteins, Rat n 2 Rat (*Rattus norvegicus*)

TABLE 4-10   Physicochemical and Biochemical Characterization of Animal-derived Indoor Allergens (Continued)

Allergen	Frequency of reactivity (%)	Mol. size (kDa)	Function
Rat (*Rattus norvegicus*)			
Rat n 1	>80	17	Lipocalin; shows homology with lipocalins such as β-lactoglobulin Bos d 5, odorant-binding proteins, Mus m 1
Albumin	24	69	Serum albumin
Rabbit (*Oryctolagus cuniculus*)			
Ory c 1	100	18	Lipocalin
Ory c 3	77 27/35	19–21	Lipophilin, glycosylated heterodimer and similar to Fel d 1
Ory c 4	?	25	Lipocalin
Ory c 6	9	69	Serum albumin

*Molecular size given represents dimer form, with two chains of approximately 18 kDa each. Note that for NAC (nascent polypeptide-associated complex alpha subunit) and keratin, deduced molecular masses are given.

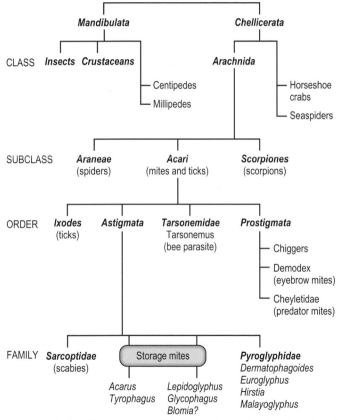

Figure 4-7 Phylogenetic relationships between different arthropods, showing the clinically important mite genera.

(10–35 μm) and contain a similar allergen load (~0.2 ng). Their contents are rapidly released (as with pollens) after impacting upon the hydrating environment of airway surface liquid, creating a high concentration of allergens at the site of deposition.

Mite Allergens

Mite species produce a number of allergens and the first mite allergens to be cloned were Der p 1, 2 and Der p 5 in the late 1980s. At least 34 groups of allergenic proteins have now been described, and the major allergens from different mite species include digestive enzymes (cysteine proteases, trypsins, chymotrypsins, amylases and chitinases),

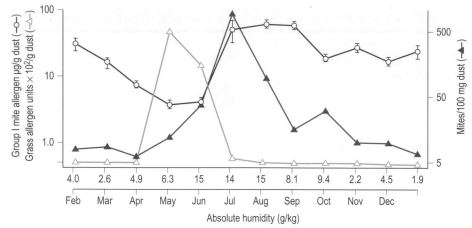

Figure 4-8 Seasonal variation in mites, mite allergen (group 1), and grass pollen allergen in a sofa followed over 1 year in central Virginia. A sharp rise in mite numbers (—▲—) follows the rise in outdoor absolute humidity. Mite allergen levels rise during the summer but remain high until after Christmas (—O—). Allergen from ryegrass pollen (—△—) was detected only in May, June, and July. *(Adapted from Platts-Mills TA, Hayden ML, Chapman MD, et al. Seasonal variation in dust mite and grass-pollen allergens in dust from the houses of patients with asthma. J Allergy Clin Immunol 1987; 79:781.)*

actin-associated proteins (tropomyosin, troponin C, and paramyosin,), ligand-binding proteins, or proteins of unknown function (Table 4-9). Traditionally, the clinically dominant mite allergens were considered to be the group 1 and 2 allergens, followed by the intermediate allergen groups 4, 5, and 6, and then a large group of minor allergens. However, recent data indicate that other allergens should now be considered to be major including the peritrophin-A related allergen involved in the formation of the chitin-containing peritrophic membrane (Fig. 4-9), and ubiquinol–cytochrome *c* reductase binding protein-like protein.[4]

Insecta

Insects such as cockroaches, moths, crickets, locusts, beetles, nimitti flies (midges), lake flies, houseflies, and lady beetles are established allergy triggers but of these, cockroaches form the most significant allergenic threat in the indoor environment, particularly in the inner city areas of the USA.[21,22,23] Sensitization is associated with *Blattella germanica*, *Periplaneta Americana* and *Periplaneta fuliginosa* (see Box 4-2), with the first of these common in urban settings where the climate is warm or domestic heating maintained. The allergenic components of cockroaches are associated with their feces, saliva, and the debris of dead insects, and substantial quantities of these aerodynamically large particulates can accumulate and persist even after the eradication of live insects. In contrast to HDMs, which predominate in the bedroom and living room, the greatest numbers of cockroaches are usually found in kitchens because of the proximity of food but cockroach allergen levels in bedrooms may correlate with the frequency of hospitalization.

Cockroach Allergens

Cockroaches produce a number of allergens and more than 10 groups have been delineated (Table 4-9). Unlike other sources, cockroach allergy is associated with several major allergens rather than with a single or small number of dominant ones, depending on the population studied. The first cockroach allergens to be cloned were shown to be a non-proteolytically active aspartate protease and a lipocalin.[24] Other allergens include the gut-associated group 1 allergens, which are thought to play a detoxifying function, digestive enzymes (amylase, trypsin), arginine kinases, and actin-associated proteins.

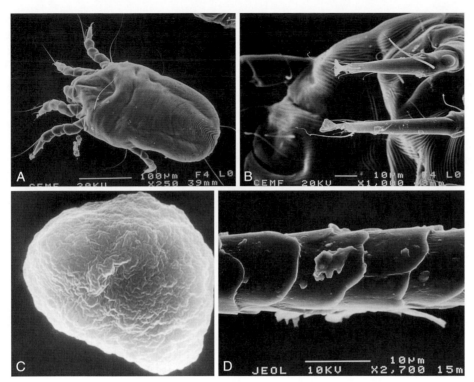

Figure 4-9 Photomicrographs of clinically important indoor allergen sources. **A.** *Dermatophagoides farinae*, showing legs and mouth parts. **B.** Details of the legs of a dust mite, showing the pads on their ends allowing them to hold on to surfaces. **C.** A mite fecal particle, with a chitinous, outer peritrophic membrane. **D.** Cat hair showing adherent particles of dander/skin scales that carry antigen. *(Scanning electron micrographs A–C, courtesy John Vaughan; D, courtesy Judith Woodfolk.)*

Indoor Allergen Sources – Mammalian

The clinically important animals in either domestic or occupational settings are cats, dogs, cows, rats, mice, horses, rabbits, mice, gerbils, and guinea pigs.[6] Their associated allergens are derived from dander, epithelium, fur, urine, or saliva and, in most of these species, the allergens fall into two major groupings, including the lipocalins (comprising >50% of all furry animal allergens thus far described) and the secretoglobins, and a diverse third minor group containing a small diversity of other proteins (Table 4-10).

Cats, Rabbits, and Dogs

Cat-allergic patients report symptoms on entering a house in which a cat is living, indicating that cat allergen can be airborne in undisturbed air. This is because 10–40% of cat allergens are carried on particles that are aerodynamically equivalent to 1- to 7-μm spheres that sediment only slowly, such that free undisturbed air concentrations of cat allergen may by 10 to 50 times higher than those of HDM allergens.[26] Modern housing is relatively airtight when windows are closed (0.2–0.5 air changes/hour),[27] so the beneficial effect of ventilation in removing small airborne particulates such as pet allergens is lost.

Compared with the mite allergen Der p 1, inhalational exposures to cat or dog allergens may be up to 100-fold (1 μg/day) greater in homes with pets. This situation results from the greater persistence of the pet allergens in air, and from the tendency of cat dander to be carried passively.[28] In a community where 20% or more of families have animals, these allergens will be measurable in dust from schools or in homes without a cat, and this can result in sensitization to animals occurring without direct exposure to the animals.[29,30,31]

Although inhalant exposure to cat allergens may be greater than for HDM allergens, this does not readily translate to individuals having a greater prevalence of cat sensitization or higher titer IgE antibodies against cat allergens. Indeed, there is clear evidence of greater sensitization to HDM, despite the imbalance in airborne concentrations. This paradox is complemented by studies reporting that living in a house with a cat is selectively protective against developing cat allergy[29–32] and that the dose–response relationship is bell-shaped rather than linear. Available evidence for exposure to dogs is less extensive, but data indicate they have an inhibitory effect on allergy in general.

These seemingly counterintuitive findings do not have proven explanations, but mechanisms have been proposed. In the case of cat allergens, which certainly do have the potential to evoke IgE-dependent sensitization and cause disease, the protection phenomenon may be a function of the dose, with high levels of allergens inducing tolerance, rather than sensitization, consistent with the apparently selective nature of the 'protection' and the ability of cat allergens to remain airborne for extended periods. The more general protective effect evoked by dogs may be related to increased LPS exposure.[33,34] Unlike dogs, having a cat in the home does not necessarily increase domestic LPS exposure.

Cat and Dog Allergens

The predominant allergens in cat and rabbit dander are secretoglobins (Table 4-10), which are common in other mammals.[25] They are small, protease-, heat- and pH-resistant proteins that form dimers before secretion from the skin and are thought to play a variety of biochemical roles including ligand transport, analogous to the lipocalins. They exist as tetramers comprising two heterodimers that form from two distinct disulfide-bonded peptides, designated chains 1 and 2. Their precise function is unclear but, like the lipocalin allergens, they may be immunomodulators because of their ability to bind lipid and activate TLR. There are no known cross-reactivities of this allergen, and secretoglobulins are thus a convenient marker to assess exposure. The other cat allergens are minor and include serum albumin, immunoglobulin, cystatin, lipocalin and latherin. The first two may be more important in relation to food allergy, since cross-reactivity with canine, porcine, and bovine albumins exists, giving rise to the so-called 'pork–cat' syndrome. However, the primary sensitization is environmental rather than dietary and the epitope recognized by IgE is the cross-reactive α-Gal epitope.

In addition to these groupings, mites also contain a number of diverse lipid-binding transport allergens including the groups 2/22, 5/21, 7, 13, and 14. For example, the group 2 allergens belong to the lipid-binding myeloid differentiation factor-2 (MD-2) family, members of which strongly bind the lipid-A moiety of LPS.[18,19] Similarly, the group 7 proteins belong to the juvenile hormone binding protein superfamily, some members of which bind LPS. However, the mite allergen does not bind LPS, but rather a gram-positive bacterial lipopeptide (polymyxin B).[20]

The size of any airborne particle determines its aerodynamic behavior and its distribution in the airways. Given the aerodynamic properties of HDM fecal pellets, it is unsurprising that airborne levels of HDM allergens decline after air disturbance ceases and little (<1 ng/m^3) is present in undisturbed air. This is in marked contrast to allergens from domestic pets, where the airborne persistence of respirable particles is a significant feature of their nuisance potential. Consequently, it is difficult to quantify the exact dose of HDM allergens to which the airways are exposed. It is estimated that because of the large sized particles and gentle mouth breathing, only low levels of natural exposure will result. However, people sleep with their heads next to materials that may be heavily infested with mites (pillows, blankets, duvets, mattresses), and atmospheric allergen levels are therefore probably poor estimates of true exposure.

In dogs, the major allergens are lipocalins, of which there are several and these belong to the calycine superfamily. They are produced in the liver or secretory glands, and members of this family play a role in the binding and transport of small hydrophobic molecules such as vitamins and steroids, because they possess a hydrophobic ligand-binding cavity. The identity of the ligands bound by them these allergens is unknown at present but, as with the cat allergen, they may possess immunomodulatory properties due to their interaction with LPS. The other dog allergens include serum albumin, immunoglobulins and kallikrein.

Rodent and Rodent Allergens

Rodents are not only a source of domestic indoor allergens but are also prominent sources in animal facilities, and are a well-recognized cause of occupational allergy. The National Cooperative Inner-City Asthma Study (NCICAS) showed the presence of mouse allergens in dust was correlated with IgE antibodies to these allergens and with asthma. Sensitization is common; in laboratory animal workers for example, allergy prevalence is in the order of about 40%, with most becoming sensitized within 3 years of exposure (~60%) and the remainder becoming sensitized within 5 to 20 years. The rat and mouse urinary lipocalin proteins (Table 4-10) induce IgE- and IgG-directed immune responses, with IgG and IgG$_4$ being seen in the absence of IgE in occupational cases. As with cat and dog allergens, rat and mouse allergens are formed on small particles and remain airborne for extended periods. When kept as pets, the quantity of allergen becoming and remaining airborne is dependent upon both disturbance and the condition of the animal litter; when dry, larger quantities will remain airborne longer.

ALLERGENS AND ALLERGENICITY

Why do some proteins trigger allergic responses? It is now apparent that there is no single mechanism that explains allergenicity, although the earliest attempts to grapple with this problem involved searches for such universal explanations. One early idea was that the amino acid sequence of an allergenic protein encoded a signal for allergenicity and that this signal was shared amongst all allergens. In essence, this concept is akin to there being a universal linear epitope for allergenicity. While linear epitopes are crucial immune recognition features, there is no evidence of a universal signature for allergenicity. Epitopes are also formed 3-dimensionally, so a further evolution of the coded message idea was the possible existence of a universal structural feature. Although not all allergen structures have been solved, it is clear that this idea does not explain allergenicity in a single mechanism, although it does highlight some similarities in structure between certain allergens and provides an explanation of the puzzle of cross-reactivity syndromes, e.g., pork–cat syndrome.

The molecular structure of allergens is of profound interest beyond the narrow confines of defining 3-dimensional epitopes. Molecular structure determines both protein function and molecular recognition on the broadest level. These key attributes are of relevance to allergenicity because they potentially provide some explanation of the bridge that needs to be made between innate and acquired immunity and the events that need to be activated in order to drive and maintain allergic sensitization. While there may be no specific universal mechanism, a general concept may apply. This concept has been dubbed the 'functionalist' view of allergenicity, in which understanding the IgE-independent bioactivity of an allergen helps to unlock some of the puzzles of allergenicity, such as why some allergens from the same source are clinically more important than others, and why some purified allergens are weak sensitizers alone but become strikingly allergenic when other allergens are present. Given the important link between innate and acquired immunity in the acquisition and maintenance of allergic sensitization, the functionalist view of allergenicity attempts to explain some of these phenomena in terms of the ability of different allergens to form an effective bridge between these arms of the immune system. The ability to form these bridges effectively actually resides in a small cadre.

Allergens that are proteolytically active and which are well represented in clinically important mites, fungi, and some occupational agents are pre-eminent members because they possess a bioactivity profile that fosters allergen delivery and the breaking of immune tolerance in a Th2-directed manner. Their ability to promote allergen delivery occurs by proteolysis of intercellular tight junctions in epithelial barriers[35] and their

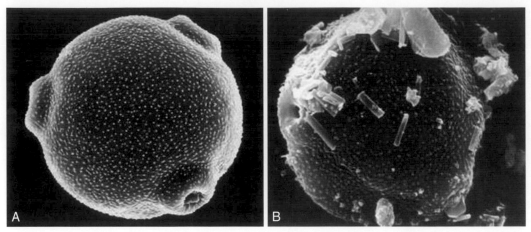

Figure 4-10 Pollen and particulate interactions. Scanning electron microscopy shows birch pollen grains before and after adsorption of particles collected over a highly polluted area. *(From Behrendt H, Friedrichs K, Kainka-Staenicke E, et al. Allergens and pollutants in the air—a complex interaction. In: Ring J, Przybilla B, editors. New trends in allergy, III. Berlin: Springer; 1991, p. 467–478.)*

ability to trigger the release of cytokines and chemokines that provide polarization to Th2 immune responses results from cleavage of protease activated receptors (PARs). Similarly, allergens with an ability to interact directly or indirectly with pattern recognition receptors (PRRs) and other cleavable targets, or to release damage associated molecular pattern molecules (DAMPs), display functional attributes that provide adjuvant-like activities, which drive the development of allergy.

Of those studied, PRRs of note include members of the Toll-like receptor family, C-type lectin receptors (CTLRs), which bind a variety of glycan moieties and PARs. DAMPs of note released by these allergens include ATP and the HMGB1 protein. In addition to these factors, pollens and some indoor allergens such as mites contain a variety of non-allergenic factors that may also contribute adjuvant-like properties to allergen sources. For example, pollen absorb bacteria and pollutants on to their surfaces (Fig. 4-10), and also carry pollen-derived biologically active lipid molecules, and mites possess endosymbiotic bacteria that possess significant amounts of both immunomodulatory LPS and peptidoglycan.

ENVIRONMENTAL MODIFIERS OF ALLERGIC SENSITIZATION AND DISEASE

In addition to genetic factors, environmental factors play a highly significant role in allergen aerobiology and allergic diseases and some have been alluded to in previous sections. In this section, the effects of climate and pollution on allergenicity and allergic diseases are discussed, as well as the impact of deliberate environmental intervention.

Avoidance Measures for Indoor Allergens

Reducing exposure to obvious trigger factors by modifying the patient's environment is a standard component of the management of allergic disease, and complete avoidance of allergens (sanatoria, clean rooms, and home modifications) can reduce the symptoms of asthma and bronchial hyperreactivity.[8] However, maintaining the strict regimens required for optimal results is onerous and the procedures achieve only a static improvement, which does not follow the daily perambulations of patients into allergen-laden environments. A further limitation is that many patients receive inadequate advice and fail to see the association between allergen exposure and disease. For allergen avoidance measures to produce clinical benefit, it is essential that the inciting trigger(s) be identified and the countermeasures adopted to achieve an effective reduction in allergen exposure. The former can be addressed by skin testing, which helps educate patients about exposure and disease, as well as confirming a diagnosis; the latter can be addressed by measuring specific allergens in the environment before and after instituting the avoidance measures.

House-dust Mites

Even with public awareness, it can be hard to convince patients of the association between HDM exposure and their allergic condition, as HDMs and their allergens cannot be perceived in the same way as some obvious outdoor pollutants. This failure to appreciate the association is one factor that can limit the acceptance of an allergen avoidance strategy. In addition, the perception of allergen avoidance has also been affected by a widely misunderstood meta-analysis of controlled trials of HDM allergen avoidance in homes, which concluded that it was not an effective treatment for asthma.[36] In fact, this meta-analysis was more a test of the achievability of allergen reduction under different regimens because the survey included trials that were of insufficient duration to achieve a reduction in HDM and their allergens.[37] In contrast, evidence from studies in sanatoria and in hospital clean rooms show that a reduction in HDM allergen levels is consistently effective in reducing symptoms and airway hyperreactivity, provided sufficient allergen reduction can be achieved. Controlled trials in homes, achieving a reduction for >6 months, have consistently reported a decrease in symptoms and/or bronchial hyperreactivity and, in atopic dermatitis, a highly significant improvement in symptoms and skin rash have been obtained.[38,39]

The necessary actions to reduce HDM exposure are divided into those for the bedroom and those for the remainder of the house (Box 4-3). In the bedroom, the most effective long-term measure is the removal of carpets but covering mattresses and pillows with impermeable covers, washing bedding at 55°C (130°F) weekly, are also effective. These should be supplemented with vacuum cleaning to eliminate dust where mites can grow but, elsewhere, the greatest problem comes from carpets and sofas. Carpets on unventilated damp floors are a particular problem (e.g., in basements and on ground floors of concrete slab construction) because water can accumulate by condensation on the cold surface of concrete, or because of leakage. Once the carpet is wet and the temperature rises, it provides an excellent growth environment for fungi and mites.

For mitigation, homes can be designed with uncarpeted floors and leather furniture to limit mite growth; ventilation and/or air conditioning can be used to control humidity and chemical treatments can be applied to carpets and furniture to control mite growth or denature allergens. While acaricides kill mites with varying efficacy, the challenge is to achieve a sufficient effect in a carpet but they do not tackle the reservoir of allergen already that is already dispersed in the carpet or furnishings. In contrast, 1–3% tannic acid may be used to inactivate allergens, but its effect is only temporary because it is not acaricidal.

Box 4-3   Avoidance Measures for Mite Allergens

BEDROOMS

- Cover mattresses and pillows with impermeable covers.*
- Wash bedding regularly at 55°C.
- Remove carpets, stuffed animals, and clutter from bedroom.
- Vacuum weekly (wearing a mask) using vacuum cleaner with a double-thickness bag or a high-efficiency particulate air (HEPA) filter.

REST OF HOUSE

- Minimize carpets[†] and upholstered furniture.
- Reduce humidity below 45% relative humidity (or 6 g H_2O/kg air).
- Treat carpets with benzyl benzoate or tannic acid.

*For pillow cases or duvets, covers should be 'fine woven'; for mattress covers, plastic or other impermeable fabrics can be used together with a mattress pad.[40]
†Carpets on unventilated floors (e.g., in basements) are difficult to keep dry.

Box 4-4   Avoidance Measures for Cat Allergens

- Removal of cat from the home.*
- Measures to reduce allergen with cat in situ:
  - Reduce reservoirs for cat allergen (e.g., carpets, sofas).
  - Use vacuum cleaners with effective filtration system.
  - Increase ventilation or use high-efficiency particulate air (HEPA) filters to remove small airborne particles.
  - Wash cat weekly, if possible.

---

*Reducing allergen levels requires about 12–16 weeks after cat is removed.

Domestic Animals

Avoiding allergens from domestic animals provides a special challenge and requires tact because many are considered full members of the family. As with HDM avoidance, the effects of removing a cat are progressive and >4 months may be required for levels to fall below 8 µg/g dust. This, and the airborne persistence of the allergens, explains why many patients with cat allergy find that they experience symptoms when they move into a home in which a cat has previously been present. Keeping a cat outdoors is only a partially successful measure because of the ease with which cat allergens are subject to passive transfer. Removal of carpets, air filtration, and regular washing of the cat (twice weekly) are additionally helpful (Box 4-4). Avoidance measures for dogs are similar.

Cockroaches and Other Allergens

In many inner cities of the USA, measures to avoid cockroaches are effective when part of an overall strategy, and include the use of poison bait, careful housekeeping to enclose all food sources, cleaning to remove and prevent allergen accumulation, and the sealing of access points. Insecticide sprays are generally ineffective, and the volatile organic vehicles in which their active ingredients are dissolved can be problematic for asthmatics. For wild rodents, the measures required are obvious, but it may be difficult to remove a domestic rodent pet. In urban areas of the midwestern and northeastern US, mice and rats are significant sources of allergens, and skin testing with rodent extracts should be routine in clinics that treat patients living in cities in these regions. Current recommendations for the avoidance of fungal allergens include controlling humidity, removing growth sites, cleaning with fungicides, and the avoidance of damp living environments. Closing of windows will reduce fungal entry from outside but, as this may also reduce ventilation, it could create conditions which allow other allergens to thrive or remain airborne.

Bacteria are generally discounted as a source of significant allergens, largely through a lack of evidence rather than evidence of absence. In contrast, data indicate that LPS from gram-negative bacteria significantly influence allergic disease. Exposure can both suppress and stimulate responses, suggesting that the operative mechanisms are complex and multifactorial. In farming villages, children who are exposed to cow barns in early life appear to be protected against sensitization and asthma. In homes generally, other data suggest that there is an inverse relationship between levels of LPS and the prevalence of allergic sensitization. Paradoxically, other data suggest that LPS exposure in the homes of mite-allergic children predicts the severity of asthma better than mite exposure.[41-43]

AIR POLLUTION, ALLERGIC SENSITIZATION, AND DISEASE

Interactions between genetic predispositions and allergen are crucial events in the development of allergic conditions but environmental factors are also relevant to disease pathogenesis (Box 4-5). For example, air pollution, a contamination of the indoor or outdoor atmosphere by chemical, physical or biologic agents, is one among many that might potentiate respiratory tract allergic conditions. Air pollution and poor air quality are global issues, which express themselves at macro (trans-boundary, outdoor

---

Box 4-5   Important Effects of Indoor and Outdoor Pollutants on Allergic Disease

- Air pollutants exacerbate asthma symptoms, and pollution may contribute to the development of asthma.
- Increasing global temperatures and rising carbon dioxide levels affect plant pollination potential and allergen potency.
- Ambient air pollutants can modify the allergen exposure of allergic persons.
- The WHO declared indoor air pollution one of the most preventable risk factors contributing to the global burden of disease.
- Indoor pollutants include biomass burning and tobacco smoke.
- Pollutant exposures can induce allergic and non-allergic inflammation in asthmatics.
- Genetic susceptibility to air pollution includes polymorphisms in oxidative stress response genes and in innate immunity genes.
- Public policy approaches to decrease ambient air pollutant levels have improved various parameters of public health outcomes, including asthma morbidity.

TABLE 4-11   Interactions between Pollutant and Allergen Exposures

Effect of airway pollutant challenge in allergic volunteers	Ozone	Diesel exhaust particles	Lipopolysaccharide
Response to recall eosinophilic response to nasal allergen challenge	Increased	Increased	Increased
Immediate phase response to inhaled allergen (PD_{20})	Increased	Unknown	Increased
Effect on development of IgE response to a neoantigen	Unknown	Increased	Unknown
Effect on local (airway) IgE levels	Unknown	Increased	Unknown

IgE, Immunoglobulin E; PD_{20}, provocative dose causing a 20% drop in forced expiratory volume in 1 second.
(From Peden DB. The epidemiology and genetics of asthma risk associated with air pollution. J Allergy Clin Immunol 2005; 115:213–220.)

---

atmospheric pollution) and micro (indoor air pollution) levels, although both are relevant to the health effects of indoor allergens.

Various mechanisms exist for an interaction between allergens and pollutants that might result in the exacerbation of allergic disease. While air pollution has the potential to affect all members of the population, some stratification exists through age (typically affecting the very young or the very old), the presence of pre-existing disease, genetic susceptibility, and socioeconomic factors. In some instances, the young, fit and active also form a vulnerable group because exposure of the respiratory tract to pollutants increases with physical activity. While air pollution has important associations with morbidities such as cardiovascular disease and cancer, there has, for obvious reasons, been considerable interest in understanding the primary medical effects of air pollution *per se* and addressing the issue of whether it has a significant role in the induction and/ or exacerbation of asthma and related conditions of the airways.

Sources of Air Pollution

The contaminants commonly responsible for poor air quality (both indoor and outdoor) are carbon monoxide, lead, sulphur dioxide, oxides of nitrogen, ozone, polyaromatic hydrocarbons, particulates, and miscellaneous biologics such as LPS. Permissible levels of pollutants are declared in air quality standards and air quality indices issued by a number of nation states and by the WHO (Tables 4-11, 4-12). Of the contaminants listed above, all except carbon monoxide and lead are potentially relevant to the pathogenesis and exacerbation of asthma through actions that directly affect airway tone or which promote inflammation directly or indirectly.

Regardless of whether the inciting pollutant is an oxidizing agent *per se*, oxidative stress is a component of the cellular mechanisms activated by these pollutants and responses will, therefore, be exaggerated in individuals with loss of function polymorphisms in antioxidant defense enzymes. Outdoor pollution ranges from discharges at

TABLE 4-12   National Ambient Air Quality Standards of the USA

Pollutant (final rule citation*)	Primary or secondary standards†	Average sampling time	Level	Limits
Carbon monoxide				
(76 FR 54294, Aug. 31, 2011)	Primary	8 h	9 ppm	Not to be exceeded more than once per year
		1 h	35 ppm	
Lead				
(73 FR 66964, Nov. 12, 2008)	Primary and secondary	Rolling 3 months average	0.15 µg/m³	Not to be exceeded
Nitrogen dioxide				
(75 FR 6474, Feb. 9, 2010)	Primary	1 h	10 ppb	98th percentile, averaged over 3 years
(61 FR 52852, Oct. 8, 1996)	Primary and secondary	1 year	53 ppb	Annual mean
Ozone				
(73 FR 16436, Mar. 27, 2008)	Primary and secondary	8 h	0.075 ppm	Annual fourth-highest daily maximum 8-h concentration, averaged over 3 years
Particle pollution				
(71 FR 61144, Oct. 17, 2006)	PM$_{2.5}$: secondary	1 year	15 µg/m³	Annual mean, averaged over 3 years
	PM$_{2.5}$: primary and secondary	24 h	35 µg/m³	98th percentile, averaged over 3 years
	PM$_{10}$: primary and secondary	24 h	150 µg/m³	Not to be exceeded more than once per year on average over 3 years
Sulfur dioxide				
(75 FR 35520, June 22, 2010)	Primary	1 h	76 ppb	99th percentile of 1-h daily maximum concentrations, averaged over 3 years
(38 FR 25678, Sept. 14, 1973)	Secondary	3 h	0.5 ppm	Not to be exceeded more than once per year

PM$_{10}$, particulate matter of ≤10 µm in diameter; PM$_{2.5}$, particulate matter of ≤2.5 µm in diameter.
*Citation of the final rule published in the Federal Register (FR) for the most recent update for each pollutant.
†Primary standards provide public health protection, including protecting the health of sensitive populations, such as asthmatics, children, and the elderly. Secondary standards provide public welfare protection, including protection against decreased visibility and damage to animals, crops, vegetation, and buildings.
(Modified from the U.S. Environmental Protection Agency (EPA), Air and Radiation, National Ambient Air Quality Standards (NAAQS). Available at: http://www.epa.gov/air/criteria.html (accessed February 7, 2013).)

point sources such as industrial plant and machinery to mobile sources such as motor vehicles, aircraft and marine craft, and the spectrum of outdoor pollutants is varied. The main sources of indoor air pollution, however, include biomass combustion (wood, crop, dung, grass and coal), nitrogen oxides (NO$_x$), tobacco smoke and LPS, and the WHO recognizes indoor air pollution as one of the top 10 preventable risk factors for global disease.

Biomass

Biomass combustion is used by 50% of the global population for cooking and/or heating. When this is conducted indoors on stoves lacking an effective flue, combustion is known to have a significant association with the development of chronic obstructive pulmonary disease (COPD) and is a risk factor for lung cancer due to deoxyribonucleic acid (DNA) damage. Women are at higher risk from biomass combustion because of their greater role in cooking and household management and their offspring have lower birth weight and are at risk of secondary impairment in lung function and/or lower respiratory tract infection. The adverse effects of biomass combustion are partly due to polyaromatic hydrocarbons that can be metabolized to oxidants, including quinones.[44]

Environmental Tobacco Smoke (ETS)

ETS is the major indoor source of pollutants of respirable size, and comprises both exhaled mainstream and sidestream smoke, from the burning end of cigarettes and related products. Both sources yield complex chemical mixtures rich in polyaromatic hydrocarbons and oxidants. ETS exacerbates illnesses that affect the airway lining and increases cancer risks through passive exposure. ETS is a major risk factor for asthma development; it is likely that multiple mechanisms, including long-term epigenetic changes, underlie this effect. Given the importance of ETS as a contributor to a range of diseases and the scale of tobacco usage, substantial effort has been directed towards understanding its mechanism of action. Evidence suggests that ETS enhances allergen-induced IgE and IgG_4 effects, and promotes a bias towards Th_2 (IL-4, -5 and -13-dependent) immune signaling at the expense of IFN-γ production (i.e. Th_1-mediated signaling).

Lipopolysaccharide (LPS)

LPS is a component of ambient air particulates, including ETS and, as alluded to earlier, its effects are complex.[45] Epidemiological studies have reported data, which support the hygiene hypothesis, namely that LPS exposure in early life is negatively linked to the development of allergy and asthma. However, it is clear that LPS also has exacerbating effects, a dichotomy illustrating the complexities of responses to inhaled agents. It is possible that this arises because the dose-response relationship for LPS may be bell-shaped. Inhaled LPS causes pathophysiological responses in both allergic and non-allergic airways, through activation of macrophages and neutrophils, but the airways of those with asthma are more sensitive. Although the mechanism is not conclusively established, monocyte and macrophage expression of CD14 (the LPS receptor) is upregulated in asthma and is correlated with neutrophil response to LPS. LPS may also prime the response to inhaled allergens through IgE-dependent mechanisms and also the presentation of antigen to mucosal T cells.[46]

TYPES OF POLLUTANT AND THEIR EFFECTS ON ALLERGENS, ALLERGIC SENSITIZATION, AND ASTHMA

Constituents of pollution may be categorized according to whether they are particulates or gases. Credible evidence reveals that atmospheric particulates lead to asthma exacerbations, but there is uncertainty whether they cause nascent asthma, but some evidence suggests it is possible. While for gaseous pollutants there is little doubt that they can trigger asthma exacerbations, only in the case of ozone are there currently grounds to think that gaseous pollution could be a cause of asthma *per se*. However, real-life exposures to pollutants will have both gaseous and particulate components in varying combinations, so the overall response to these pollutants depends upon the combination of materials and the forms in which they are presented to the airways. There is little mechanistic understanding of the consequences of exposure to 'real-life' mixtures of pollutants and whether these contribute to the etiology of asthma.

Particulates

Atmospheric particulate matter is heterogeneous in terms of its composition and physical behavior. Compelling evidence gathered across economically developed and less-developed countries, demonstrates that exposure to respirable particulates is associated with a range of major health conditions including asthma. In urban environments, vehicular traffic is an important source of these particulates and is associated with a risk of asthma exacerbations, and more recent data show an association between diesel exhaust particulates (DEPs) exposure, sensitization, and allergic rhinitis in young children.[47] This raises the question of whether this association can be accounted for by the effects of particulates modifying the responses to allergens, or modifying allergens themselves. In this regard, particulates and other environmental factors such as climate

TABLE 4-13   Environmental Modifiers of Allergens and Allergenicity of Outdoor Allergens

Pollutants*	Climate change†
Enhanced allergenicity due to adjuvant properties of particulates	Extended pollen seasons (earlier start, later finish)
Differential expression of allergens in pollen grains	Increased pollen production
Increased allergen content in pollen grains	Increased allergen expression in pollen grains
Increase in pollen protein expression with possibility of creating new allergens	Increased allergen content in pollen grains
Increased releasability of cytoplasmic allergens and allergen-laden granules from pollen grains	Increase in pollen protein expression with possibility of creating new allergens
Post-translational modification of pollen allergens	Change in distribution of pollen-producing plants
Enhanced antigen presentation	Induction of fungal sporulation
Alteration in pollen germination rate	

*Particulates, heavy metals, diesel exhaust particles (DEP), environmental tobacco smoke (ETS), NO_2, SO_2, O_3.
†Temperature, CO_2.
(Adapted from Stewart GA, Peden DP, Thompson PJ, Ludwig M. Allergens and air pollutants. In: Holgate ST, Church MK, Broide DH, Martinez FD, eds. Allergy. 4th edn. Edinburgh: Saunders; 2012. For a review, see Ziska, LH, Beggs PJ. Anthropogenic climate change and allergen exposure: The role of plant biology. J Allergy Clin Immunol 2012; 129:27–32.)

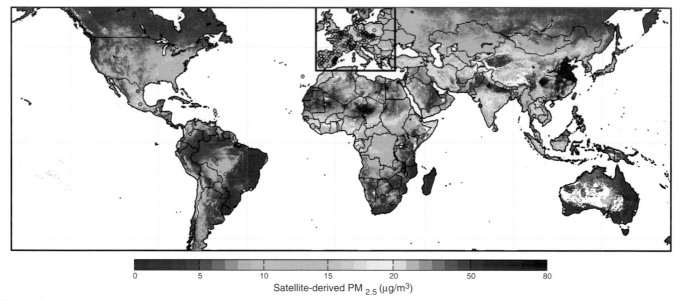

Satellite-derived PM$_{2.5}$ (µg/m³)

Figure 4-11 Global satellite-derived concentrations of particulate matter 2.5 µm or smaller in diameter (PM$_{2.5}$) were averaged from 2001 through 2006. White space indicates water or locations containing concentrations of <50 µg/m3. Circles correspond to values and locations of comparison sites outside Canada and the United States. The box outlines European sites. *(From van Donkelaar A, Martin RV, Brauer M, et al. Global estimates of ambient fine particulate matter concentrations from satellite-based aerosol optical depth: development and application. Environ Health Perspect 2010; 118:847–855.)*

change–associated temperatures and CO_2 concentrations, and gaseous pollutants such as NO_2 and O_3 have all been shown to influence allergenicity (Table 4-13).

The effects of particulates have been studied in detail (Fig. 4-11). Those with an aerodynamic diameter of 2.5 µm (PM$_{2.5}$) will gain entry to the whole respiratory tract and therefore potentially constitute a high health risk. Larger particulates (>2.5, <10 µm aerodynamic diameter) will impact in the larger airways, but not alveoli. However, there is no 'standard model' for the conduct of studies with respirable particulates, so approaches have ranged from the direct respiratory exposure to diluted diesel exhaust to the instillation of DEPs into the bronchial or nasal airways. Studies have also been conducted in-vitro. Collectively, available data suggest that DEPs cause airway inflammation in people regardless of whether they have asthma.

In asthma, responses mediated by IgE and IgG may be enhanced, but it is unclear whether this involves elevated IgE levels. Studies in humans and in experimental animal models suggest that DEPs also shift immune responses to a Th$_2$ phenotype. Challenge studies show that PM$_{2.5}$ particulates elicit a mild inflammatory response in the airways partly due to the presence of transition metals (e.g., Cu, Ni, Zn) within the particles. Particulate matter, especially DEPs, is also loaded with polyaromatic hydrocarbons, which can be converted to quinones and other oxidants. Studies in humans and experimental animal models confirm that the extent of hydrocarbon loading influences responses to particulates. However, particulates may be loaded with many substances, including fungal spores and pollens, which have a direct independent association with asthma. DEPs are also suggested to increase the susceptibility to viral infections and this may be of significance in asthma where interactions between allergens and respiratory viruses are central to the risk of asthma exacerbations. Evidence shows that pollutant exposure increases viral mRNA levels in allergic rhinitis, as well as promoting eosinophilic inflammation. Mechanistically, these responses to DEPs may be due to increased expression of TLR3.

Gaseous Pollutants

Exposure to pollutants sulfur dioxide (SO_2), nitrogen dioxide (NO_2) and ozone (O_3) may occur singly, but is more likely to occur in combination with each other and/or particulates. Gaseous pollutants, which exert effects on the integrity of the epithelial lining or which modify innate and/or acquired immune responses have a potential for interacting with inhaled allergens and thus an important question has been whether gaseous pollutants explain increases in the incidence of asthma. While current evidence indicates that pollution causes nascent asthma is weak, there are significantly stronger grounds to think that exposure to gaseous pollutants can exacerbate asthma when it is already established.

Sulfur Dioxide (SO_2)

Sulfur dioxide is a toxic gas with a pungent, rotten odor whose contribution to acid aerosol formation means that it is extensively studied.[48] Inhaling SO_2 is associated with shortness of breath, respiratory discomfort and premature death. Acutely, SO_2 exposure is linked with ER visits and hospital admissions. Chronically, it increases the likelihood of developing asthma or COPD and is correlated with the presence of current symptoms. The effects of SO_2 are rapid in onset (<2 min) resulting in a bronchospastic rather than inflammatory response, which involves wheezing, chest discomfort and dyspnea, but repeated exposure results in tachyphylaxis. Because the acute effects of inhaled SO_2 rely on absorption through the bronchial mucosa, they are exacerbated by exercise and are mitigated by nasal breathing, which redirects absorption via the nasal mucosa. However, this mitigation is reduced in asthma patients with nasal co-morbidities (e.g., rhinitis and sinusitis) where nasal airflow is decreased.

Nitrogen Dioxide (NO_2)

Epidemiologic surveys have consistently revealed a strong association between ambient NO_2 concentrations and both acute and chronic changes in lung function and the exacerbation of asthma. While the ability of NO_2 to enhance airway reactivity is equivocal at low exposure levels, at higher concentrations it has more notable effects on lung function in people with asthma in whom it augments the acute response to allergens.[49] The mechanism of NO_2 is an inflammatory neutrophilic infiltration. Studies in-vitro suggest that the airway epithelium has a significant role in orchestrating the inflammatory responses through cytokine production. Although definitive proof is awaited, there is an obvious potential for responses to NO_2 and allergens to interact at this level of inflammatory signaling and injury. Less clear is whether such an interaction promotes the nascent development of asthma.

Ozone (O_3)

Ozone is a pungent pale blue gas and its strongly oxidant action is damaging to mucous and respiratory tissues[50] and, therefore, has the potential to modify responses to inhaled allergens. Some data also suggest that it may be a cause of nascent asthma in addition to exacerbating established disease, for which stronger evidence exists. In the troposphere, ozone is formed by photochemical reaction between nitrogen oxides and volatile organic compounds from vehicle emissions and industrial discharges. This reaction is promoted by temperature and consequently the significance of ozone as a pollutant increases during warmer months, creating a photochemical smog. In the indoor environment, it may also be formed by electrical discharge in some types of electrical equipment. Ozone is an inherently unstable molecule whose breakdown generates reactive products, which themselves may be irritant and currently of unknown relevance to allergic disease.

O_3 is a well-recognized trigger for asthma exacerbations, even at low levels of exposure, and there is a significantly increased risk of death from respiratory causes at higher levels.[50] Controlled-exposure studies show that, acutely, O_3 induces a rapid decrease in FVC and FEV_1, a sensation of chest discomfort on deep breathing, and an increase in non-specific airway responsiveness mediated by sensory neural reflexes. These changes in lung function are accompanied by, but not correlated with, the onset of a moderately persistent (~24 h) neutrophilic inflammation. The increased susceptibility of people with asthma to O_3 is due to potentiation of allergic inflammation and innate immune responses. Mechanistic studies indicate that some responses are mediated by TLR4,[51] possibly activated by hyaluronic acid release, a known proinflammatory danger associated molecular pattern, from the airway epithelium. Levels of hyaluronic acid are increased in airway surface liquid in both non-asthmatics and asthmatics exposed to ozone. Other inflammatory events involve the release of cytokines, prostaglandins and leukotrienes. As with exposure to NO_2, physical activity (and thus raised respiratory rate) increases the effective lung dose of O_3, so it is recommended that persons at risk minimize exertion.

CONCLUSIONS

Our knowledge of allergens has grown enormously over the last three decades, and most, if not all of the major, clinically important allergens have been cloned. We know much about their functions in the original source, and we understand more about how they might interact with components of the innate immune system and modulate IgE responses. Detailed molecular knowledge of allergens is now being translated into the clinical sphere, particularly in the area of diagnostics where micro-arrayed recombinant indoor, outdoor and food allergens have become available. Whilst they are unlikely to replace skin-prick testing in the clinic or single source immunoassays, they are proving very useful in helping differentiate between primary sensitization and cross-reactivity in the diagnosis of food allergy, in rapidly determining whether patients are polysensitized, and in providing guidance in selecting patients for immunotherapy. Thus, a new lexicon has emerged with terms such as *molecular allergology*, *molecular-based allergy diagnostics* and *component resolved* diagnostics now being routinely used. In parallel, we are now acknowledging that patients do not just inhale benign proteins but rather collections of biologically active containers replete with both eukaryotic and prokaryotic components that contribute either to inflammation or its suppression in exposed individuals via our innate immune systems. Finally, it is clear that sensitization, disease manifestation and allergen production continues to be influenced by our internal and external environments, as it appears to have been since before the time Charles Blackley anecdotally described allergic diseases as being rare.

ACKNOWLEDGMENTS

The work of the authors described in this chapter was supported by Australia's National Health and Medical Research Council (NHMRC), The Asthma Foundation WA, Asthma UK, The Medical Research Council (UK), and The Wellcome Trust.

REFERENCES

1. Reese G, Ayuso R, Lehrer SB. Tropomyosin: an invertebrate pan-allergen. Int Arch Allergy Immunol 1999;119:247–58.
2. Radauer C, Bublin M, Wagner S, et al. Allergens are distributed into few protein families and possess a restricted number of biochemical functions. J Allergy Clin Immunol 2008;121:847–52.

3. Aalberse RC, Koshte V, Clemens JG. Immunoglobulin E antibodies that crossreact with vegetable foods, pollen, and Hymenoptera venom. J Allergy Clin Immunol 1981;68(5):356–64.

4. Platts-Mills TA, Schuyler AJ, Tripathi A, et al. Anaphylaxis to the carbohydrate side chain alpha-gal. Immunol Allergy Clin North Am 2015;35:247–60.

5. *Marsh DG, Goodfriend L, King TP, et al. Allergen nomenclature. Bull World Health Organ 1986;64:767–74.

6. *Radauer C, Breiteneder H. Pollen allergens are restricted to few protein families and show distinct patterns of species distribution. J Allergy Clin Immunol 2006;117:141–7.

7. Grote M, Valenta R, Reichelt R. Abortive pollen germination: a mechanism of allergen release in birch, alder, and hazel revealed by immunogold electron microscopy. J Allergy Clin Immunol 2003;111(5): 1017–23.

8. van Loon LC, Rep M, Pieterse CM. Significance of inducible defense-related proteins in infected plants. Annu Rev Phytopathol 2006;44:135–62.

9. *Vijay HM, Kurup VP. Fungal allergens. Clin Allergy Immunol 2008;21:141–60.

10. Pollart SM, Chapman MD, Flocco GP, et al. Epidemiology of acute asthma: IgE antibodies to common inhalant allergens as a risk factor for emergency room visits. J Allergy Clin Immunol 1989;83:875–82.

11. Sears MR, Herbison GP, Holdaway MD, et al. The relative risks of sensitivity to grass pollen, house dust mite and cat dander in the development of childhood asthma. Clin Exp Allergy 1989;19:419–24.

12. Sporik R, Holgate ST, Platts-Mills TA, et al. Exposure to house-dust mite allergen (Der p I) and the development of asthma in childhood. A prospective study. N Engl J Med 1990;323:502–7.

13. Gelber LE, Seltzer LH, Bouzoukis JK, et al. Sensitization and exposure to indoor allergens as risk factors for asthma among patients presenting to hospital. Am Rev Respir Dis 1993;147:573–8.

14. Illi S, Mutius E, Lau S, et al. for the Multicentre Allergy Study (MAS) group. Perennial allergen sensitisation early in life and chronic asthma in children: a birth cohort study. Lancet 2006;368:763–70.

15. Almqvist C, Larsson PH, Egmar AC, et al. School as a risk environment for children allergic to cats and a site for transfer of cat allergen to homes. J Allergy Clin Immunol 1999;103:1012–17.

16. Voorhorst R, Spieksma FT, Varekamp H, et al. The house-dust mite (*Dermatophagoides pteronyssinus*) and the allergens it produces. Identity with the house-dust allergen. J Allergy 1967;39:325–39.

17. Tovey ER, Chapman MD, Platts-Mills TA. Mite faeces are a major source of house dust allergens. Nature 1981;289:592–3.

18. Ichikawa S, Takai T, Yashiki T, et al. Lipopolysaccharide binding of the mite allergen Der f 2. Genes Cells 2009;14:1055–65.

19. Trompette A, Divanovic S, Visintin A, et al. Allergenicity resulting from functional mimicry of a Toll-like receptor complex protein. Nature 2009;457:585–8.

20. Mueller GA, Edwards LL, Aloor JJ, et al. The structure of the dust mite allergen Der p 7 reveals similarities to innate immune proteins. J Allergy Clin Immunol 2010;125:909–17.

21. Pollart SM, Smith TF, Morris EC, et al. Environmental exposure to cockroach allergens: analysis with monoclonal antibody-based enzyme immunoassays. J Allergy Clin Immunol 1991;87:505–10.

22. Kang BC, Wilson M, Price KH, et al. Cockroach allergen study: allergen patterns of three common cockroach species probed by allergic sera collected in two cities. J Allergy Clin Immunol 1991;87: 1073–80.

23. Rosenstreich DL, Eggleston P, Kattan M, et al. The role of cockroach allergy and exposure to cockroach allergen in causing morbidity among inner-city children with asthma. N Engl J Med 1997;336: 1356–63.

24. *Arruda LK, Vailes LD, Benjamin DC, et al. Molecular cloning of German cockroach (*Blattella germanica*) allergens. Int Arch Allergy Immunol 1995;107:295–7.

25. *Konradsen JR, Fujisawa T, van Hage M, et al. Allergy to furry animals: New insights, diagnostic approaches, and challenges. J Allergy Clin Immunol 2015;135:616–25.

26. Platts-Mills JA, Custis NJ, Woodfolk JA, et al. Airborne endotoxin in homes with domestic animals: implications for cat-specific tolerance. J Allergy Clin Immunol 2005;116:384–9.

27. Wright GR, Howieson S, McSharry C, et al. Effect of improved home ventilation on asthma control and house dust mite allergen levels. Allergy 2009;64:1671–80.

28. Munir AK, Einarsson R, Dreborg SK. Indirect contact with pets can confound the effect of cleaning procedures for reduction of animal allergen levels in house dust. Pediatr Allergy Immunol 1994;5:32–9.

29. Platts-Mills T, Vaughan J, Squillace S, et al. Sensitisation, asthma, and a modified Th2 response in children exposed to cat allergen: a population-based cross-sectional study. Lancet 2001;357:752–6.

30. Ownby DR, Johnson CC, Peterson EL. Exposure to dogs and cats in the first year of life and risk of allergic sensitization at 6 to 7 years of age. JAMA 2002;288:963–72.

31. Perzanowski MS, Rönmark E, Platts-Mills TA, et al. Effect of cat and dog ownership on sensitization and development of asthma among preteenage children. Am J Respir Crit Care Med 2002; 166:696–702.

32. Hesselmar B, Aberg N, Aberg B, et al. Does early exposure to cat or dog protect against later allergy development? Clin Exp Allergy 1999;29:611–17.

33. Ege MJ, Mayer M, Normand AC, et al. Exposure to environmental microorganisms and childhood asthma. N Engl J Med 2011;364:701–9.

34. Fujimura KE, Johnson CC, Ownby DR, et al. Man's best friend? The effect of pet ownership on house dust microbial communities. J Allergy Clin Immunol 2010;126:410–12, e3.

35. *Wan II, Winton HL, Soeller C, et al. Der p 1 facilitates transepithelial allergen delivery by disruption of tight junctions. J Clin Invest 1999;104:123–33.

36. Gotzsche PC, Johansen HK. House dust mite control measures for asthma: systematic review. Allergy 2008;63:646–59.

37. Platts-Mills TA. Allergen avoidance in the treatment of asthma: problems with the meta-analyses. J Allergy Clin Immunol 2008;122:694–6.

38. Piacentini GL, Martinati L, Mingoni S, et al. Influence of allergen avoidance on the eosinophil phase of airway inflammation in children with allergic asthma. J Allergy Clin Immunol 1996;97:1079–84.

39. Ehnert B, Lau-Schadendorf S, Weber A, et al. Reducing domestic exposure to dust mite allergen reduces bronchial hyperreactivity in sensitive children with asthma. J Allergy Clin Immunol 1992;90:135–8.
40. Platts-Mills TA, Vaughan JW, Carter MC, et al. The role of intervention in established allergy: avoidance of indoor allergens in the treatment of chronic allergic disease. J Allergy Clin Immunol 2000;106: 787–804.
41. Michel O, Ginanni R, Duchateau J, et al. Domestic endotoxin exposure and clinical severity of asthma. Clin Exp Allergy 1991;21:441–8.
42. Braun-Fahrländer C, Riedler J, Herz U, et al. Environmental exposure to endotoxin and its relation to asthma in school-age children. N Engl J Med 2002;347:869–77.
43. Ege MJ, Mayer M, Normand AC, et al. Exposure to environmental microorganisms and childhood asthma. N Engl J Med 2011;364:701–9.
44. Gilmour MI, Jaakkola MS, London SJ, et al. How exposure to environmental tobacco smoke, outdoor air pollutants, and increased pollen burdens influences the incidence of asthma. Environ Health Perspect 2006;114:627–33.
45. Alexis NE, Lay JC, Zeman K, et al. Biological material on inhaled coarse fraction particulate matter activates airway phagocytes in vivo in healthy volunteers. J Allergy Clin Immunol 2006;117:1396–403.
46. Peden DB. The role of oxidative stress and innate immunity in O_3 and endotoxin-induced human allergic airway disease. Immunol Rev 2011;242:91–105.
47. Codispoti CD, LeMasters GK, Levin L, et al. Traffic pollution is associated with early childhood aeroallergen sensitization. Ann Allergy Asthma Immunol 2015;114:126–33.
48. Bernstein JA, Alexis N, Barnes C, et al. Health effects of air pollution. J Allergy Clin Immunol 2004;114:1116–23.
49. Trasande L, Thurston GD. The role of air pollution in asthma and other pediatric morbidities. J Allergy Clin Immunol 2005;115:689–99.
50. Jerrett M, Burnett RT, Pope CA 3rd, et al. Long-term ozone exposure and mortality. N Engl J Med 2009;360:1085–95.
51. Bauer RN, Diaz-Sanchez D, Jaspers I. Effects of air pollutants on innate immunity: the role of Toll-like receptors and nucleotide-binding oligomerization domain-like receptors. J Allergy Clin Immunol 2012;129:14–24.

Key references are preceded by an asterisk.

CHAPTER 5

Principles of Allergy Diagnosis

Anca Mirela Chiriac, Jean Bousquet, and Pascal Demoly

CHAPTER OUTLINE

INTRODUCTION
HISTORICAL PERSPECTIVES
EPIDEMIOLOGY
PATHOGENESIS AND ETIOLOGY
CLINICAL FEATURES
THE ALLERGEN EXTRACTS
Skin Testing
  Skin Testing for a Specific Food
THE TECHNIQUE
Skin Tests Recommended in Clinical Practice
The Quantity of Allergen that Penetrates the Skin
Skin-prick and Intradermal Tests
Skin Reactivity
The Positivity of Skin Tests
Allergic Sensitization
Drug Interference with Skin Testing
  Antihistamines
  Imipramines, Phenothiazines, and Tranquilizers
  Corticosteroids

Other Immunomodulators
Other Drugs
THE PATIENT
Immediate-reading Skin Tests
Late Phase Reaction
Skin Test Risks
Skin Tests in Infancy
Regular Skin Testing
Anti-histaminic Treatment
Tested Allergens
Skin Test Areas
Allergic Profile
Systemic Allergic Reaction Follow-up
Immunotherapy Follow-up
Component Resolved Diagnosis
Skin Testing Reliability
REFERRAL
CONCLUSIONS

SUMMARY OF IMPORTANT CONCEPTS

- Immediate-reading allergy skin tests address type I hypersensitivity and can confirm sensitization to a specific allergen. They represent the primary diagnostic tool of immunoglobulin E (IgE)-mediated diseases.
- The value of skin tests relies on technically correct performance (i.e. technique, use of negative and positive controls, standardized allergen extracts whenever possible), reading (positivity criteria, timing), and on accurate interpretation in the context of the clinical history and physical examination findings, because sensitization is not always clinically relevant.
- Historically, skin tests have been improved in terms of the allergen extracts and devices used, but they have basically preserved their importance in allergy diagnosis for decades, alongside and despite new available and emerging technologies (particularly IgE molecular protein assessment).
- Performing skin tests enables the clinician to confirm or refute sensitization, which has important prognostic and therapeutic implications.
- In addition to their diagnostic value, skin tests are used in the standardization of allergen extracts and in pharmacologic, allergy immunotherapy, and epidemiologic studies.
- The clinical diagnosis benefits nowadays from input of the progress in biochemistry and molecular biology and the information obtained with conventional specific IgE antibody assays is enriched by the molecular allergy diagnosis, aiming to define allergic profiles, with therapeutic and prognostic implications.

INTRODUCTION

The cause–effect relationship between allergens and allergic disease was suspected (and investigated) long before the identification of immunoglobulin E (IgE) antibodies (the 'reagins'), half a century ago. Therefore, chronologically, skin testing took the lead on the detection and quantification of serum-specific IgE (sIgE).

Since the early recognition that allergic diseases (later described as IgE-mediated allergic diseases) are caused by exposure to allergens, it has been common practice to establish the presence or absence of sensitization by re-exposure of the individual to the allergen. This re-exposure should be progressive and it consists of tests that are performed either in vivo or in-vitro (Fig. 5-1). Skin tests have been the primary tool for investigation in allergy since their introduction in 1865 by Charles Harrison Blackley. The intracutaneous test proposed by Charles Mantoux in 1908 was rapidly applied to investigation of immediate hypersensitivity diseases. Some years later, Thomas Lewis and Ronald Thomson Grant described the skin-prick test. Without major modifications, these methods have been refined and further validated.

Skin tests can provide useful confirmatory evidence of sensitization to a specific allergen. The selection and number of allergens should be based on the history provided by the patient and his environment. Skin tests are simple, quick to perform, low cost, and highly sensitive, which explains their key position in allergy diagnosis. However, when improperly performed, skin tests can lead to false-positive or false-negative results. The main limitation of the skin test is that a positive reaction does not necessarily mean that patients will experience symptoms, because patients can have allergen sIgE without clinical symptoms. Skin tests are also used to help understand the pathophysiology of the allergic response, to evaluate the mechanisms of action of antiallergic treatments, to analyze general or specific population sensitization profiles in epidemiologic and pharmacologic studies, and to standardize allergen extracts.

HISTORICAL PERSPECTIVES

The first attempt to test an allergen on the skin is attributed to Blackley. It took place a century and a half ago, using raw pollen extract. The prick-puncture test was described

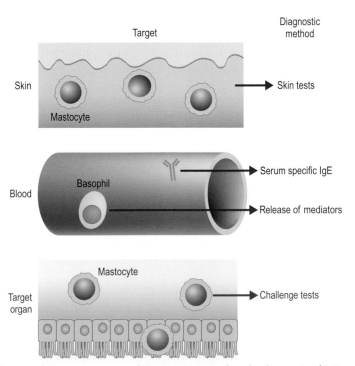

Figure 5-1 Differences between in-vivo and in-vitro tests used in the diagnosis of IgE-mediated allergic diseases.

later on, by Lewis and Grant (1924), and it became widespread in the 1970s after it was modified by Pepys. Today, prick-puncture tests are performed with different devices. Needles, as well as single or multi-headed devices have been proposed and used in order to decrease the variability of the prick-puncture procedure by different investigators, to increase acceptability (especially in children), to permit several tests to be performed with one application and thus minimize technician time and thereby increase efficiency.

Intradermal tests described by Charles Mantoux in 1908 are still used in clinical practice.

Regarding allergen extracts, probably the most significant novelty is the use of new technologies, such as recombinant allergens (rAllergens) for in-vivo diagnoses, so-called 'molecular allergology' and 'component resolved diagnosis' (CRD). However, they are not yet widely available in current allergy/clinical practices. These are available for in-vitro testing. These allergen protein components are the result of significant progress in biochemistry and molecular biology during the last two decades. In contrast to conventional sIgE antibody assays, CRD does not rely upon crude preparations obtained from natural allergen sources (generally poorly defined mixtures containing both allergenic and non-allergenic components) but on sIgE antibodies directed towards single components purified from natural sources or produced by recombinant techniques.[1]

EPIDEMIOLOGY

Skin tests and serum sIgE detection have been used in epidemiologic studies to assess the prevalence of sensitizations to common food and respiratory allergens in the general population[2] and how it compares with the prevalence and severity of symptomatic allergic or respiratory diseases, for long-term studies of the development of sensitization and natural desensitization and the factors that influence both. More recently, CRD has been used in epidemiological studies (serial cross-sectional and longitudinal cohorts) to study the changes in the allergy profile or the prediction of the occurrence of allergic disease over time.[3,4]

PATHOGENESIS AND ETIOLOGY

Skin tests aim to reproduce the IgE-dependent allergic reaction that occurs in the target organs. The IgE-mediated allergic response in the skin results in an immediate wheal and flare reaction that depends on proinflammatory and neurogenic mediators (i.e. immediate reaction). It is irregularly followed by a late phase reaction (LPR) starting 1 to 2 hours later, peaking at 6 to 12 hours, and resolving in approximately 24 to 48 hours. The LPR is represented by an erythematous inflammatory reaction.

The immediate reaction is essentially induced by mast cell degranulation after allergen challenge. Histamine and tryptase release begins about 5 min after allergen injection and peaks at 30 min. The injection of histamine into the skin by prick or intradermal techniques mimics the allergen-induced wheal and flare reaction. Histamine is the major, but not the sole, mediator of the wheal and flare reaction. The size of the wheal usually does not correlate with the concentration of histamine released.

Regarding detection and quantification of serum sIgE, the traditional radioallergosorbent test (RAST, which became commercially available shortly after the discovery of IgE) has been abandoned and replaced by a fluorescent immunoassay (FEIA).[1] The principle of detection and quantification of sIgE relies on the formation of an antigen-antibody immune complex between the protein extract (coupled on a solid phase or a polymer-coated slide) and the sIgE antibodies in the patients' serum recognizing the antigen. Subsequently, an antihuman-IgE antibody is added. In conventional FEIA, a substrate is then added and its metabolization by the enzyme-conjugated anti-IgE will result in a quantifiable fluorescence. In CRD, the anti-IgE may be fluorochrome labeled. The reaction is scanned in a laser scanner, and results are evaluated by image analysis software.[1]

CLINICAL FEATURES

The interpretation of skin tests depends on several variables. Amongst these, three are of major importance: the allergen extracts used, the technique, and the patient.

THE ALLERGEN EXTRACTS

Skin Testing

When non-commercialized and non-standardized allergens are tested, hygienic and non-irritant conditions should be observed. It is not acceptable to test with substances that may potentially contain infectious agents. Some substances (e.g., chemotherapy drugs such as vinorelbine) may elicit skin necrosis and their use should therefore be strictly avoided. Others should be diluted in order to respect the skin pH.

With respect to commercialized extracts, the quality of the allergen extract is of major importance. Some false-negative reactions are caused by the lack of sufficient allergens in non-standardized extracts. Although many years ago, skin test materials were often made directly in hospital laboratories or in physicians' offices by extracting allergenic raw materials, this practice is no longer recommended. Allergen extracts are marketed with documented potency (standardized using biologic methods and labeled in biologic units),[5] composition, and stability following regulatory agencies' guidelines. They are extracts from a single source material or mixtures of related, cross-reacting allergens, such as grass pollen, deciduous tree pollen, related ragweed pollen, and related mite allergen extracts. Mixtures of unrelated allergens are avoided because their use may result in false-negative responses due to over-diluted allergenic epitopes in some mixes[5] or enzymatic degradation by proteases.

Variations in the quality and potency of commercial extracts, which may be related or not to the differences between the US and the European standardization systems, are particularly found in extracts for mites, animal danders, molds, and pollens.[6] In addition to problems related to standardization, some extracts (e.g., *Hymenoptera* venoms) can induce false-positive reactions by non-immunologic mechanisms. Preservatives used in allergen extracts also may be irritants; thimerosal can elicit a wheal and flare reaction in non-sensitized subjects.

Because of the difficulties in preparing standardized extracts from natural raw material, new technologies have been tried. Starting from allergen-encoding cDNAs, large amounts of highly pure allergens with a high batch-to-batch consistency can be produced that satisfy the quality requirements of medicinal products manufactured by recombinant DNA technology (rAllergens). Recombinant allergens used for in-vivo diagnoses should have the same IgE binding activity as their natural counterparts. The rAllergens of various pollens, molds, mites, bee venom, latex, and celery have already been used for skin testing allergic and control individuals and skin-prick tests and intradermal tests with rAllergens have proved to be highly specific and safe. Although the diagnostic sensitivity of single rAllergens usually is lower than those obtained with allergen extracts, it can be increased by using rAllergen panels covering the most important allergenic structures in a given complex allergen extract. This type of approach with rAllergens may be of great importance for the diagnosis of allergy to unstable allergen extracts such as fruits and cross-reacting allergens.

Skin Testing for a Specific Food

The large spectrum of allergies makes it impossible to have commercialized and standardized extracts for all potential allergenic substances. When a suspicion of food allergy arises, it is common practice to perform prick tests with the culprit food itself. Thus, patients will be required to bring their own 'material' for skin testing, in accordance with the intake that elicited the reaction. However, fresh seasonal fruits, for instance, are not always available throughout the year, but allergists find a solution by using frozen aliquots of these fruits. The validity of this method has been confirmed, and skin testing with frozen fruits from different families (e.g., apple, peach) have proved to be a reliable alternative, with a performance similar to that of fresh fruits. This reasoning is generally extended to other foods, in daily activity, for practical purposes.

For skin testing with fresh foods, thermal denaturation of allergen structure by cooking has been well established. Therefore, the material used for skin testing should observe the same cooking conditions (raw or cooked food) as the culprit dish.

THE TECHNIQUE

Skin tests require skillful performance, reading, and interpretation. Although they are technically easy to perform, trained personnel are recommended in order to observe these three requirements.

Skin Tests Recommended in Clinical Practice

The skin-prick (prick-puncture) and intradermal tests are routinely used for skin testing. In the skin-prick method, antigen is placed on the skin and introduced into the epidermis with a variety of devices. In the intradermal method, the antigen is injected into the dermis using a hypodermic syringe and needle (Figs. 5-2, 5-3). Before initiating any skin test procedure, some precautions should be taken (Box 5-1). Common errors in skin testing are listed below (Boxes 5-2, 5-3).

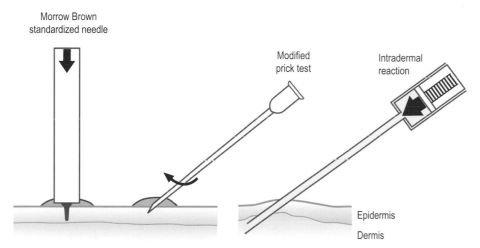

Figure 5-2 Common methods of skin testing.

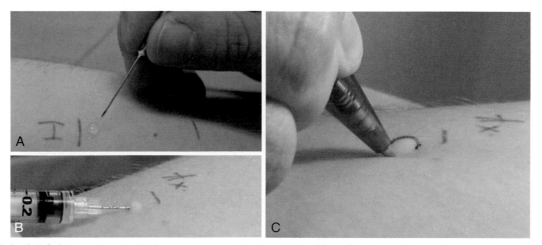

Figure 5-3 Methods of skin testing. **A.** Prick-puncture test. **B.** For the intradermal test, a volume of approximately 0.02–0.05 mL of allergen extract is injected intracutaneously to produce a small superficial bleb (2–4 mm in diameter). **C.** The size of skin tests may be outlined with a pen to obtain a permanent record.

Box 5-1   Skin Testing Precautions

1. Never perform skin tests unless a physician is immediately available to treat systemic reactions.
2. Have emergency equipment, including epinephrine, readily available.
3. Be careful with patients with current allergic symptoms.
4. Determine the potency and stability of the allergen extracts used.
5. Be certain that the test concentrations are appropriate.
6. Include a positive and a negative control solution.
7. Perform tests in normal skin.
8. Evaluate the patient for dermographism.
9. Determine and record medications taken by the patient and time of last dose.
10. Record the reactions at the proper time.

Box 5-2   Common Errors in Skin-prick Testing

1. Tests are placed too close together (<2 cm), and overlapping reactions cannot be separated visually.
2. Induction of bleeding can lead to false-positive results.
3. Insufficient penetration of skin by puncture instrument can lead to false-negative results; this occurs more frequently with plastic devices.
4. Allergen solutions can spread during the test or when the solution is wiped away.

Box 5-3   Common Errors in Intradermal Testing

1. Test sites are too close together, and false-positive results can be observed.
2. Volume injected is too large (>0.1 mL).
3. High concentration of allergen can lead to false-positive results.
4. Splash reaction is caused by air injection.
5. Subcutaneous injection leads to a false-negative test (i.e. no bleb formed).
6. Intracutaneous bleeding site is read as a positive test result.
7. Too many tests performed at the same time may induce systemic reactions.

The Quantity of Allergen that Penetrates the Skin

It has been shown that even when performed by a skilled operator and with standardized techniques, the skin-prick test shows great limits of reproducibility, at least as far as the size of the inoculum volume is concerned. The variability of the inoculum depends, in a statistically significant way, on the subject's individual characteristics and therefore can be reduced only within certain limits by the standardization and perfectibility of the technique. The average volume of the prick-test inoculum was equal to $0.016\,\mu L$, with a remarkable dispersion of the values around the mean. Regarding intradermal test, a volume of approximately 0.02–0.05 mL is injected into the dermis. The concentration of allergen extract required to elicit a positive reaction with intradermal testing is 1000–30 000 times smaller than that necessary for a positive prick-puncture test.

Skin-prick and Intradermal Tests

Out of safety concerns and in order to ensure the progressive increase in allergen input, intradermal tests should always be preceded by skin-prick tests. However, the latter are not always followed by intradermal tests. A comparison between prick-puncture and intradermal tests is shown in Table 5-1. The starting dose of solutions in patients with a preceding negative skin-prick test result should range between 100-fold and 1000-fold dilutions of the concentrated extract used for prick-puncture testing.

Skin Reactivity

Because of the variability in cutaneous reactivity, it is necessary to include negative and positive controls in every skin test evaluation. The negative control solutions are the diluents used to preserve the allergen extracts. All negative controls should be *totally* negative. The rare dermographic patient develops wheal and erythema reactions to the negative control. The negative control also detects traumatic reactivity induced by the skin test device (the wheal may approach a diameter of 3 mm with some devices)

TABLE 5-1 Relative Advantages of Skin-prick and Intradermal Tests

Advantages	Skin-prick test	Intradermal test
Simplicity	+++	++
Speed	++++	++
Interpretation of positive and negative reactions	++++	++
Discomfort	+	+++
False-positive reactions	Rare	Possible
False-negative reactions	Possible	Rare
Reproducibility	+++	++++
Sensitivity	+++	++++
Specificity	++++	+++
Detection of IgE antibodies	Yes	Yes
Safety	++++	++
Testing of infants	Yes	Difficult

+, Mild; ++, moderate; +++, high; ++++, very high.

or the technique of the tester.[5] Although any reaction at a negative control test site makes interpreting allergen sites more difficult, these responses are essential in accurately assessing the presence or absence of true allergic sensitization.[2]

Positive control solutions (histamine or mast cell secretagogues such as codeine phosphate) are used to detect suppression by medications or diseases and to detect exceptional patients who are poorly reactive to histamine. The mean wheal size for positive control solutions is 5 to 8 mm.

The Positivity of Skin Tests

Evaluation of the wheal or erythema is used to assess the positivity of skin tests. The positive control should optimally show a wheal diameter that is ≥3 mm.[6] Reactions to prick-puncture tests are regarded as positive and possibly indicative of clinical allergy if they are >3 mm in wheal diameter (i.e. wheal area of 7 mm^2) and >10 mm in flare diameter. Another criterion is the ratio of the size of the wheal induced by the allergen compared with the positive control. Any degree of positive response (i.e. small wheals of 1 to 2 mm with flare and itching) with appropriate positive and negative controls, indicates the presence of allergic sensitization to a particular allergen. Although significant in immunologic terms, small positive reactions do not necessarily indicate the presence of a clinically relevant allergy. Correlating skin test results with the clinical history is essential in interpreting the clinical significance of the testing procedure.

Allergic Sensitization

A positive skin test response confirms the presence of allergic sensitization but not the presence of allergic disease. Allergic sensitization with no correlative allergic disease is a common finding, occurring in 8–30% of the population when using a local standard panel of aeroallergens. However, positive skin test results for asymptomatic subjects may foreshadow the subsequent onset of allergic symptoms. Prospective studies have shown that 30–60% of sensitized-only individuals subsequently develop allergic symptoms that can be attributed to exposure to allergens that previously elicited positive skin test responses.[7]

With inhalant allergens, the skin-prick test is the cheapest and most effective method to diagnose respiratory allergies. Skin-prick tests give immediate information on sensitivity to individual allergens and should therefore be the primary method clinicians use to assess respiratory allergic diseases. Positive skin test results with a medical history that suggests clinical sensitivity strongly incriminate the allergen as a contributor to the disease process. Conversely, a negative skin test result with a negative history favors a non-allergic disorder. Interpretation of skin tests that do not correlate with the clinical history is difficult, and in these situations, measurements of allergen-specific IgE and provocative challenges are of interest.

Drug Interference with Skin Testing

Some drugs can interfere with the performance of skin tests and can modulate the wheal or the flare, complicating interpretation of skin tests. Other drugs used in allergic or asthmatic patients do not modify the cutaneous responsiveness, and they can be continued. Table 5-2 outlines the inhibitory effects of therapeutic drugs on skin tests and the delay of suppression of such treatments before performing skin tests.

TABLE 5-2   Inhibitory Effect of Drugs on IgE-mediated Skin Tests

Drugs	Degree	Suppression Duration (days)	Suppression Clinical significance*
H₁ antihistamines			
Azelastine	++++	3–10	Yes
Bilastine	++++	3–10	Yes
Cetirizine	++++	3–10	Yes
Chlorpheniramine	++	1–3	Yes
Clemastine	+++	1–10	Yes
Cyproheptadine	0 to +	1–8	Yes
Desloratadine	++++	3–10	Yes
Diphenhydramine	0 to +	1–3	Yes
Doxepin	++	3–11	Yes
Ebastine	++++	3–10	Yes
Hydroxyzine	+++	1–10	Yes
Ketotifen	++++	>5	Yes
Levocabastine	Possible		Yes
Levocetirizine	++++	3–10	Yes
Loratadine	++++	3–10	Yes
Mequitazine	++++	3–10	Yes
Mizolastine	++++	3–10	Yes
Promethazine	++	1–3	Yes
Tripelennamine	0 to +	1–3	Yes
H₂ antihistamines			
Cimetidine	0 to +		No
Ranitidine	+		No
Imipramines	++++	>10	Yes
Phenothiazines	++		Yes
Corticosteroids			
Systemic, short term	0		
Systemic, long term	Possible		Yes
Inhaled	0		
Topical skin	0 to ++		Yes
Theophylline	0 to +		No
Cromolyn	0		
β₂-Agonists			
Inhaled	0 to +		No
Oral, injection	0 to ++		No
Formoterol	Unknown		
Salmeterol	Unknown		
Dopamine	+		
Clonidine	++		
Montelukast	0		
Allergen immunotherapy	0 to ++		No

+, Mild; ++, moderate; +++, high; ++++, very high.
*Clinical significance for skin testing.

However, it is not reasonable to consider the suppression of antidepressant treatment in psychiatric disorders without consulting the prescribing doctor. In such a scenario, sIgE dosage could be the primary diagnostic tool, since it is not influenced by ongoing treatment.

Antihistamines

The H_1 antihistamines inhibit the wheal and flare response to histamine, allergen, and mast cell secretagogues. The duration of the inhibitory effect is linked to the pharmacokinetics of the drug and its active metabolites. First-generation H_1 antihistamines reduce skin reactivity for up to 24 hours or slightly longer (for >5 days for ketotifen). The second-generation H_1 antihistamines azelastine, bilastine, cetirizine, desloratadine, ebastine, fexofenadine, levocetirizine, loratadine, mizolastine, and rupatadine may suppress skin responses for 3 to 7 days. Some H_1 antihistamines, such as cetirizine, inhibit skin tests more than others, and this effect correlates with relief of allergic rhinitis symptoms. For other antihistamines, such as loratadine, blunting of skin-test reactivity to allergen or histamine is not necessarily predictive of the clinical efficacy of these drugs in seasonal allergic rhinitis treatment.

Topical H_1 antihistamines such as levocabastine or azelastine may suppress skin tests, especially if multiple doses are used, and these drugs should be discontinued for at least 48 hours before skin testing.

H_2 antihistamines used alone have a limited inhibitory effect on skin tests. Discontinuing H_2 antagonists on the day of testing is probably sufficient to prevent significant suppression of skin tests.

Imipramines, Phenothiazines, and Tranquilizers

Tricyclic antidepressants exert a potent and sustained reduction in skin responses to histamine. This effect may last for a few weeks. Tranquilizers and antiemetic agents of the phenothiazine class have H_1 antihistaminic activity and can abrogate skin test responses. Topical doxepin hydrochloride abolishes skin reactivity after 1 to 3 days of therapy and for up to 11 days after its discontinuation.

Corticosteroids

Short-term (<1 week) administration of corticosteroids used at therapeutic doses in asthmatic patients does not modify cutaneous reactivity to histamine or allergens. Long-term corticosteroid therapy does not alter histamine-induced vascular reactivity in skin but affects cutaneous mast cell responses and modifies the skin texture, which makes interpretation of immediate skin tests difficult in some cases. However, it has been shown that allergen-induced skin tests can be accurately performed in asthmatic patients receiving long-term oral corticosteroid treatment. The effects of inhaled corticosteroids have not been directly evaluated, but because therapeutic doses produce fewer systemic effects than oral steroids, their potential for interference is predictably insignificant. In contrast, the application of topical dermal corticosteroids for 1 week reduces the immediate and the late phase skin reaction induced by allergen.

Other Immunomodulators

Few data are available regarding the effect of other immunomodulating agents, including biologicals, on skin testing. During omalizumab treatment in asthmatic allergic patients, the size of allergen-induced early phase and late phase skin responses decreases.

Other Drugs

Theophylline slightly reduces skin tests, but its administration does not need to be stopped before skin testing.

Short-acting, inhaled β_2-agonists in doses approved for the treatment of asthma do not usually inhibit allergen-induced skin tests. Oral terbutaline can decrease the allergen-induced wheal, but this inhibitory effect has little significance in clinical practice. For long-acting, inhaled β_2-agonists, such as formoterol and salmeterol, definitive results are lacking. Conversely, β-blocking agents such as propranolol can significantly increase skin histamine reactivity.

Inhaled cromolyn and nedocromil do not alter the skin wheal response to skin tests with allergens or degranulating agents, and neither does cutaneously applied sodium cromoglycate. Dopamine and clonidine can decrease skin test reactivity, whereas this effect has not been observed with nifedipine and montelukast. Angiotensin-converting enzyme inhibitors moderately increase skin reactivity to allergen, histamine, codeine, and bradykinin. Topical pimecrolimus does not seem to modify skin reactivity.

THE PATIENT

Immediate-reading Skin Tests

Whatever method is used, the immediate skin test induces a wheal and flare response that reaches a peak in 8 to 10 min for histamine, 10 to 15 min for mast cell secretagogues, and 15 to 20 min for allergens. Globally, it takes 15 to 20 min for skin-prick tests and intradermal tests, respectively. Skin tests are read at the peak of their reaction and in a standard manner.[5,8] When the reactions are mature, the size of each reaction is measured with a millimeter rule. To obtain a permanent record, the size of the reaction is outlined with a pen, blotted onto cellophane tape, and stored on paper.

Late Phase Reaction

The immediate reaction resulting in a wheal and flare is irregularly followed by a LPR starting 1 to 2 hours later, peaking at 6 to 12 hours, and resolving in approximately 24 to 48 hours. The LPR is represented by an erythematous inflammatory reaction. Late phase reactions are not often recorded: not only are their mechanisms insufficiently characterized, but their exact clinical significance is unknown. Histamine accounts for only a limited portion of the LPR. Lymphocytes, predominantly CD4[+] T cells, play a key role in the generation and regulation of the LPR by the generation and release of cytokines. These findings are in contrast to delayed hypersensitivity, in which CD8[+] T cells are significant participants in the infiltrated erythema that characterizes a positive test. Interestingly, the same cellular pattern may be found after an immediate wheal and flare response that does not lead to a macroscopic LPR.

Skin Test Risks

Two iatrogenic risks have been evaluated: infectious and allergic. Skin tests with necrotizing drugs (e.g., vinorelbine) are not performed.

It could be argued that multiple-use vials of commercialized extracts may raise issues in terms of infectious risk. To date, no report regarding nosocomial infections resulting from skin-prick test procedures has been published. Nevertheless, even if no methicillin-resistant *Staphylococcus aureus* or vancomycin-resistant enterococci were observed in field samples, nosocomial infections may become a concern if skin tests are performed on subjects who are pathogen carriers. Skin bacteria such as *Staphylococcus epidermidis* can survive in allergen extracts for as long as 21 days. Simple prevention measures during pricking and storing of the vials are in place in all practices.

The risk to elicit a generalized reaction during skin-test performance is highest with intradermal tests and drugs than with prick-puncture tests and inhalant or food allergens. Of note, generalized reactions do not necessarily mean these are allergic reactions because vasovagal reactions are a frequent explanation.

The prick-puncture test appears to be safe. Systemic reactions after testing with inhalant allergens, although anecdotal, have been reported. The overall rate of generalized reactions is <0.5% in a large series (including thousands of pediatric and adult patients undergoing skin-prick tests for inhalant and food allergens).[9] Possible risk factors for adverse reactions during skin testing were suggested: low age and active eczema for generalized allergic reactions; female gender; and multiple skin-prick tests performed on a single patient for vasovagal reactions. No fatalities have been reported.

Intradermal tests on the other hand, bring an increase in the antigen load that the body is exposed to via the skin and therefore can provoke untoward, large local (immediate and late) and systemic reactions, with an incidence ranging from 0.02% to 1.4% of the tested patients. Some fatalities have been reported.[10] Therefore, several precautionary measures should be taken when using this technique:

- Intradermal tests may be performed by a nurse or a technician, but a physician should always be nearby.
- Performing prick-puncture tests before intradermal tests and using serial 10-fold dilutions of the usual test concentration, especially in patients with histories of anaphylaxis, are useful ways to minimize untoward adverse local and systemic reactions.
- A waiting period of 20 min in the office of the physician is recommended before the patient is released, and this period may be extended for high-risk patients (e.g., patients treated with β-blocking agents, which may increase the risk of fatal systemic reactions).

In case of a generalized anaphylactic reaction, a rubber tourniquet should be placed above the test site on the arm and a 1 : 1000 aqueous epinephrine (adrenaline) solution administered intramuscularly, preferably in the lateral thigh (i.e. vastus lateralis).

Skin Tests in Infancy

Skin test wheals increase in size from infancy to adulthood and then often decline after the age of 50. Using the prick-puncture test, it has been observed that a significant wheal is detectable after 3 months of age in most infants tested with histamine, codeine phosphate, or allergen extracts. Infants react predominantly with a large erythematous flare and a small wheal. It is therefore possible to perform skin tests to diagnose allergic disorders in infancy, but the size of the wheal is often reduced, and criteria of positivity should always compare the size of the wheal induced by allergen extracts with that elicited by positive control solutions.

Intradermal tests can elicit pain, and this may limit their use in very young children. The discomfort may be reduced by the use of a topical anesthetic cream such as the eutectic mixture of local anesthetics (e.g., EMLA), which reduces the flare but not the wheal responses.

Regular Skin Testing

In clinical practice, routine repeated skin testing and serum sIgE dosage is recommended for venom allergen immunotherapy, as an indirect measure of acquired tolerance.

Otherwise, it is not recommended. However, skin tests may be repeated for a variety of reasons,[5,6] including the age of the patient (i.e. allergic children have the tendency to acquire new sensitivities over time, beginning with foods and indoor allergens, and followed by pollens and outdoor molds); the patient's exposure to new allergens (e.g., acquisition of a new pet, geographic relocation, new job); or an increase and change in symptoms (raising the suspicion of new acquired sensitivities).

Anti-histaminic Treatment

Upon the allergist's decision, skin tests may be performed under anti-histaminic treatment (e.g., in patients with antidepressant treatment having antihistaminic properties, if the risk/benefit analysis is in favor of pursuing the treatment). However, in such circumstances, only positive results must be taken into account, and all negative results must be considered as potentially false-negatives. The allergy work-up can be supplemented in these cases with in-vitro allergen-specific IgE tests. Typically, skin tests are more sensitive than the latter, but using standardized extracts, the percentage agreement between in-vitro allergen-specific IgE tests and skin prick-puncture tests is between 85% and 95%, depending on the allergens being evaluated. Moreover, other in-vivo tests (e.g., bronchial, nasal, or oral challenges) can be considered, in an appropriate medical environment. For good clinical practice, H_1-antihistamines should be stopped 1 week before practicing immediate-reading skin tests.

Tested Allergens

The number of skin tests varies according to the age of the patient (i.e. fewer prick-puncture tests are needed in infants for food allergens, house-dust mites, indoor molds, indoor insects, and animal danders vs pollens; acceptability of skin tests in preschool children is essential and the number of skin tests should be reduced to a minimum based on the available evidence[5,6]); the geographic location of the patient; and the history of the allergic disease (e.g., persistent vs intermittent symptoms, clear causative factors).

The panel of tested allergens generally depends on the allergen exposure of the area but it should be kept in mind that allergic patients are travelling across countries and this demographic reality influences the patterns of sensitizations found in a certain area. In a large, multicenter European study involving more than 3000 subjects, sensitization rates were comparable for the most frequent inhalant allergens across Europe but depending on the country,[11] 2 to 9 allergens of 18 were sufficient to identify 95% of sensitized subjects, whereas 4 to 13 allergens were required to identify 100% of sensitized subjects. Similar surveys were undertaken in the USA. When testing certain allergens such as grass pollen, it should be kept in mind that the grass pollen mix selected should cover the regionally most dominant grasses, because non-cross-reactive species exist.

Detection of serum sIgE by qualitative tests to mixtures of common respiratory or food allergens is commercially available and could be an option when skin testing is not readily possible. However, their sensitivity is generally lower than that of skin testing, and a negative result cannot rule out allergic sensitization.

When using CRD, the number of tests necessary to enable a correct diagnosis increases significantly, thus increasing the costs, since more than one component needs to be included to allow identification of the exhaustive allergy profile for the sources of allergens of interest. The microarray technique for CRD enables sIgE antibody testing in a multiplex format and allows the simultaneous quantification of more than 100 sIgE antibodies. Sensitizations to respiratory and food allergenic components can be studied in parallel and cross-sensitizations with or without clinical impact can be identified. However, correct application and interpretation of multiplexed CRD requires training, since some of the information it provides may be clinically irrelevant. For example, it has repeatedly been shown that ubiquitous structures such as cross-reactive carbohydrate determinants (CCD) present on glycoproteins of plants and *Hymenoptera* venom, homologs of the major allergen Bet v 1 from birch pollen, profilins, and non-specific lipid transfer proteins can elicit a significant number of positive sIgE results without clinical significance.[1]

Skin Test Areas

Skin tests can be performed either on the back or on the forearm (or both, at the same time).

The back as a whole is more reactive than the forearm, and this differential effect is more pronounced for allergen extracts than for histamine solutions. Within these two areas, differences of reactivity have been shown: (1) the middle and upper back areas are more reactive than the lower back, and (2) the antecubital fossa is the most reactive portion of the arm, whereas the wrist is the least reactive (therefore, tests should not be placed in areas 5 cm from the wrist or 3 cm from the antecubital fossa). Apart from the practical aspect, performing skin tests on the forearm adds educational value to the test, because the patient can see the results for himself. Both forearms can be used. Whichever area is chosen, a safety distance of at least 2 cm between tests should be observed, in order to avoid cross-contamination.

Allergic Profile

With the growing knowledge in allergology, especially through the input of rAllergens, allergists now have the possibility to establish an allergic profile, that goes all the way down to the molecular level. Performing skin tests for inhalant allergens enables the allergist to search for atopic sensitization, as a screening test that may then be completed by in-vitro assessments of specific IgE. Cross-sensitizations between pollens and fruits/vegetables have been described and are known to lead to major clinical impact. Food allergies do not have the same clinical relevance, according to the geographical area where they are diagnosed (e.g., allergy to apple is generally less severe when sensitization to apple occurs via sensitization to birch pollen, as it is often the case in Northern Europe, as compared with Southern Europe, where primary sensitization responsible for apple allergy is to a different apple protein, known to elicit potentially life-threatening reactions).

Determining the allergen sensitization profiles is a major indication of CRD in food allergy.[1] Whether they are animal-derived (e.g., milk, egg, fish allergy), or plant-derived (by primary or secondary sensitization to the food itself), food allergies have largely benefited from the input of data obtained by CRD. In some allergies (e.g., peanut, hazelnut), CRD may discriminate between true allergy and merely sensitization, allowing an individual risk assessment of severity with impact upon dietary measures. Some secondary plant-derived food allergies are now well characterized: the oral allergy syndrome or 'birch-fruit-vegetable' syndrome, due to primary sensitization to the major birch pollen allergen Bet v 1 and its extensive cross-reactivity with its labile homologs in fruits, vegetables, and nuts; or the latex-fruit-vegetable syndrome, due to cross-sensitization between the allergenic components present in natural rubber and similar epitopes present in fruits such as kiwi or banana.[1]

Systemic Allergic Reaction Follow-up

After a systemic allergic reaction, a refractory period of up to 6 weeks has been described. This cutaneous anergy (or hypoergy) is attributed to the mediators' depletion after intense mast-cell degranulation. It was first described in systemic allergic reactions induced by *hymenoptera* sting and, in the absence of further studies, it has been applied to the exploration of other supposedly IgE-mediated reactions. Therefore, following a systemic reaction, an early evaluation might be performed, but only positive skin test results should be taken into account. If an early evaluation yields negative results, a re-test at 4 to 6 weeks is mandatory. Conversely, for certain allergens (e.g., drugs), skin-test reactivity may decrease in time and waiting too long a time (i.e. months to years) to perform skin tests after an allergic event is considered to be a potential source of false-negative results. Sensitization, as assessed by skin tests (and in-vitro IgE testing), may disappear after cessation of exposure, but there are few data on whether the loss of skin sensitization serves as a guarantee for systemic tolerance upon allergen challenge.

Immunotherapy Follow-up

Demonstrating allergen sensitization before starting allergen immunotherapy is mandatory. A decreased wheal and flare reaction has been observed in patients undergoing allergen immunotherapy (to inhalant or food allergens) as well as in patients who are spontaneously desensitized (e.g., professional beekeepers). However, with the exception of *Hymenoptera* venom immunotherapy, skin tests are not recommended in immunotherapy follow-up. They cannot be used to assess the efficacy of allergen immunotherapy in practice, nor should they be used to decide on the cessation of immunotherapy.

Component Resolved Diagnosis

Skin testing merely shows sensitization to the tested allergen sources, which are crude allergen extracts containing a mixture of both allergenic and non-allergenic components. In patients polysensitized to pollens, especially to pollens with overlapping pollination seasons, CRD allows the identification of the profile of sensitization[1] (i.e. to major or minor allergens), thus allowing targeting of patients who are sensitized to major allergens as candidates that would benefit most from allergen immunotherapy.[12,13] From these studies, it emerged that CRD results alter initial prescription of allergen immunotherapy in up to 50% of the patients, both children and adults.

Skin Testing Reliability

False-positive and false-negative skin test results may reflect improper technique or material. False-positive results may be provoked by impurities, contaminants, and non-specific mast cell secretagogues in the extract, as well as by dermatographism and non-specific enhancement from a nearby strong reaction. False-negative skin test results can be caused by extracts of poor initial potency or subsequent loss of potency; drugs modulating the allergic reaction; diseases attenuating the skin response; decreased reactivity of the skin in infants and elderly patients; improper technique (e.g., no or weak puncture); ultraviolet radiation exposure; a too-short or too-long time interval from the reaction; organ allergy; non-IgE-mediated mechanism; and infections, such as those by helminths. The use of positive and negative control solutions (or even the use of control subjects) may help to clarify some of the false-negative or false-positive results, because reactions are decreased or abolished in patients with weakly reactive skin, but are enhanced in those with dermographism or in cases where irritant extracts are used.

Learned societies across the world agree that when properly performed, prick-puncture tests are considered to be the most convenient and least expensive screening method for detecting respiratory and food allergic reactions in most patients. However, until the diagnostic efficacy of prick-puncture tests is fully established with standardized allergens and methods, negative prick-puncture results may be confirmed by more sensitive intradermal techniques, especially for drugs and stinging insect venoms. Even when false-positive and false-negative results have been eliminated, the proper interpretation of test results requires a thorough knowledge of the history and physical findings, because a positive skin test result alone does not confirm definite clinical sensitivity to an allergen.

REFERRAL

Allergies in general, and respiratory allergies in particular, are a growing primary care challenge because most patients consult primary care physicians when confronted with allergic symptoms. General practitioners play a major role in the management of allergic diseases, as they make the diagnosis, start the treatment, give relevant information, and monitor most of the patients. A structured allergy history appears to be insufficient when assessing patients with asthma and rhinitis in general practice. It has been demonstrated that performing skin tests can improve the positive predictive value of the clinical history alone, with up to 25% in respiratory allergies. For other allergies (*Hymenoptera* venom, food and drug allergies, anaphylaxis), there is no other solution than referral to the allergists. Indeed, strict avoidance without understanding better what is going on could be deleterious for the patient.

CONCLUSIONS

When properly performed, skin tests represent the major tool for the diagnosis of IgE-mediated diseases and are of particular importance in fields such as allergen standardization, pharmacology, and epidemiology. Although it is relatively easy to perform the tests, accurate interpretation requires investigators and clinician specialists to be experienced in the technical aspects and nuances of the testing procedures and in interpreting the observed findings in the context of the clinical history and physical examination findings. A major challenge of practitioners working in the allergy field is to create awareness, especially among primary care physicians, of the value of skin tests. Performing skin tests enables the clinician to confirm or refute sensitization and atopy, which has important prognostic implications for development of comorbid diseases such as asthma. The currently available technologies for detection and quantification of serum sIgE (and in particular CRD) have refined and increased the accuracy of allergy diagnosis, allowing identification of individual sensitization profiles that cannot be achieved by skin testing. After allergic sensitization and relevant diseases have been established, proper education regarding allergen avoidance and the prescribing of appropriate medical therapy (including allergen immunotherapy) can be safely and appropriately instituted.

REFERENCES

1. *Van Gasse AL, Mangodt EA, Faber M, et al. Molecular allergy diagnosis: Status anno 2015. Clin Chim Acta 2015;444C:54–61.
2. The International Study of Asthma and Allergies in Childhood Steering Committee. Worldwide variation in prevalence of symptoms of asthma, allergic rhinoconjunctivitis, and atopic eczema: ISAAC. Lancet 1998;351:1225–32.
3. Melioli G, Marcomini L, Agazzi A, et al. The IgE repertoire in children and adolescents resolved at component level: a cross-sectional study. Pediatr Allergy Immunol 2012;23(5):433–40.
4. *Westman M, Lupinek C, Bousquet J, et al., Mechanisms for the Development of Allergies (MeDALL) consortium. Early childhood IgE reactivity to pathogenesis-related class 10 proteins predicts allergic rhinitis in adolescence. J Allergy Clin Immunol 2015;135(5):1199–206.
5. Bernstein IL, Li JT, Bernstein DI, et al. American Academy of Allergy, Asthma and Immunology; American College of Allergy, Asthma and Immunology. Allergy diagnostic testing: an updated practice parameter. Ann Allergy Asthma Immunol 2008;100:S1–148.
6. *Bousquet J, Heinzerling L, Bachert C, et al. Practical guide to skin prick tests in allergy to aeroallergens. Allergy 2012;67:18–24.
7. Bodtger U, Poulsen LK, Malling HJ. Asymptomatic skin sensitization to birch predicts later development of birch pollen allergy in adults: a 3-year follow-up study. J Allergy Clin Immunol 2003;111:149–54.
8. The European Academy of Allergology and Clinical Immunology. Position paper: Allergen standardization and skin tests. Allergy 1993;48:48–82.
9. Liccardi G, D'Amato G, Canonica GW, et al. Systemic reactions from skin testing: literature review. J Investig Allergol Clin Immunol 2006;16:75–8.
10. *Lockey RF, Benedict LM, Turkeltaub PC, et al. Fatalities from immunotherapy (IT) and skin testing (ST). J Allergy Clin Immunol 1987;79:660–77.
11. Bousquet PJ, Burbach G, Heinzerling LM, et al. GA2LEN skin test study III: minimum battery of test inhalent allergens needed in epidemiological studies in patients. Allergy 2009;64:1656–62.
12. *Sastre J, Landivar ME, Ruiz-Garcia M, et al. How molecular diagnosis can change allergen-specific immunotherapy prescription in a complex pollen area. Allergy 2012;67:709–11.
13. *Moreno C, Justicia JL, Quiralte J, et al. Olive, grass or both? Molecular diagnosis for the allergen immunotherapy selection in polysensitized pollinic patients. Allergy 2014;69:1357–63.

Key references are preceded by an asterisk.

CHAPTER 6

Allergen-specific Immunotherapy

Anthony J. Frew and Helen E. Smith

CHAPTER OUTLINE

INTRODUCTION

HISTORICAL PERSPECTIVE

INDICATIONS FOR SPECIFIC ALLERGEN IMMUNOTHERAPY

CLINICAL EFFICACY WITH SPECIFIC ALLERGENS

Grass, Tree, and Weed Pollens

House-dust Mites

Domestic Pets

Fungi

Cockroach

Multiple Allergen Mixtures

SPECIFICITY OF ALLERGEN IMMUNOTHERAPY

EVIDENCE OF DISEASE MODIFICATION

Persistence of Clinical Improvement after Cessation of Immunotherapy

PHARMACOECONOMICS OF SIT

IMMUNOLOGIC RESPONSE TO INHALANT SIT

END-ORGAN CHANGES

OVERVIEW OF THE IMMUNE RESPONSE TO IMMUNOTHERAPY

INDICATIONS FOR SIT

Injection Schedules

Adverse Reactions to SIT

SIT in Pregnancy

Adherence to SIT

SUBLINGUAL IMMUNOTHERAPY

Mechanisms of SLIT

Side effects of SLIT

Efficacy of SLIT

SLIT for Asthma

Durability of Treatment

Effects of SLIT on the Natural History of Allergic Disease

Safety and Cost-effectiveness of SLIT

OTHER POTENTIAL MODES OF ADMINISTRATION

Intralymphatic Route

MODIFIED ALLERGEN EXTRACTS AND ADJUVANTS

Recombinant Allergen Vaccines

Unmodified Allergens

Peptides

Modified Allergens

THE FUTURE OF SLIT

CONCLUSIONS

SUMMARY OF IMPORTANT CONCEPTS

- Allergen immunotherapy is an effective treatment both for allergic rhinitis and for allergic asthma.
- Clinical effectiveness requires several years' treatment.
- Initially, SIT induces allergen-specific regulatory T cells that decrease T cell responses to allergens. Over time, there is immune deviation from a predominantly Th2 to a predominantly Th1 pattern of cytokine production.
- Immunotherapy modifies the course of allergic disease, as evidenced by reduction in rates of new allergic sensitizations, and prevention of progression from rhinitis to asthma.
- The clinical improvement achieved by SIT persists for years after it is discontinued.
- Several approaches have been tried to improve the safety and convenience of SIT. These include chemical modifications of allergen extracts and alternative routes of administration, with sublingual SIT appearing particularly promising.

INTRODUCTION

Allergic rhinitis is common and, in many cases, not very well controlled by standard drug therapy. Specific immunotherapy (SIT) offers a way to desensitize the patient, rendering them less sensitive to inhalation of seasonal or perennial allergens. This reduces their symptoms and improves quality of life, as well as reducing the need to use disease-suppressing medication such as antihistamines and nasal steroids. SIT can also help in selected patients with allergic asthma, who are especially affected by allergic triggers. SIT provides long-lasting benefits, beyond the period of treatment but SIT has to be given over several years to achieve maximal efficacy. Traditional SIT involves a course of injections, starting with a build-up phase of 7 to 12 weekly injections and followed by monthly maintenance injections for about 3 years. Current research focuses on ways to modify vaccines to improve efficacy with shorter courses and reduce the risk of side effects. Alternative routes of administration have also become fashionable, with sublingual immunotherapy showing comparable efficacy to injection SIT.

HISTORICAL PERSPECTIVE

Interest in the use of vaccination to treat allergy goes back to the late 19th century.[1] It had been well recognized that hay fever was a reaction against grass pollen, and that it involved immune recognition of pollen components so, although the exact mechanisms were unknown, different researchers attempted to immunize patients with pollen extracts. When early attempts led to anaphylaxis, progressive regimens were tried, starting with a very low dose and increasing gradually until a large dose could be given safely. In 1911, Noon and Freeman published the first paper on successful injection immunotherapy. Over the next decade, the practice of injection therapy for hay fever spread rapidly, especially in the US. The scope of immunotherapy was extended to treat perennial rhinitis and asthma, covering additional pollens and perennial allergens such as house dust and animal danders. SIT was one of the first treatments to be subjected to randomized controlled trials, with the trials taking place in the 1950s and 1960s.

For over 100 years, immunotherapy has been practiced by the same method as used by Noon, with injections at weekly intervals of progressively greater concentrations of extract, followed by a period of several years of maintenance injections. In the past 25 years, however, there has been increasing interest in administering immunotherapy by other routes, especially the sublingual, which is intended to reduce the risk of adverse reactions and increase convenience for patients. Other areas of research have focused on ways of modifying the vaccine so that only a small number of injections are required to achieve optimum desensitization.

INDICATIONS FOR SPECIFIC ALLERGEN IMMUNOTHERAPY

Specific immunotherapy (SIT) has three main indications: allergic rhinitis, allergic asthma, and anaphylaxis due to allergy to wasp and bee venom (Box 6-1). The efficacy of SIT in seasonal and perennial allergic rhinitis has been confirmed in many well designed clinical trials.[2]

SIT also works in asthma, although its relative role in treating asthma is less important than its role in treating allergic rhinitis. In placebo-controlled studies, SIT was shown to be effective in carefully selected patients with asthma caused by grass pollen, cats and house-dust mites (Fig. 6-1). The effect was most marked on allergen-specific

Box 6-1	Indications for SIT

- Allergic rhinitis
- Allergic asthma (if well controlled)
- Hymenoptera sensitivity

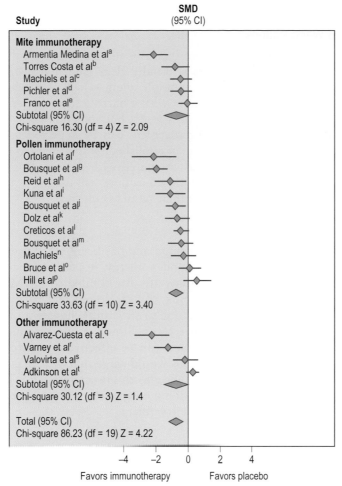

Figure 6-1 Odds ratios (SMD, standardized mean difference) and 95% confidence intervals (CIs) for clinical improvement, as evidenced by reduction in asthmatic symptoms after allergen immunotherapy in placebo-controlled studies. df, degrees of freedom. *(Modified from Abramson M, Puy R, Weiner J. Immunotherapy in asthma: an updated systematic review. Allergy 1999; 54:1022–1041. Referenced studies: a, Armentia Medina et al. Allergo Immunopathol (Madr) 1995; 23:211; b, Torres Costa et al. Allergy 1996; 51:238; c, Machiels et al. J Clin Invest 1990; 85:1024; d, Pichler et al. Allergy 1997; 52:274; e, Franco et al. Allergo Immunopathol (Madr) 1995; 23:58; f, Ortolani et al. J Allergy Clin Immunol 1984; 73:283; g, Bousquet et al. J Allergy Clin Immunol 1990; 85:490; h, Reid et al. J Allergy Clin Immunol 1986; 78:590; i, Kuna et al. J Allergy Clin Immunol 1989; 83:816; j, Bousquet et al. J Allergy Clin Immunol 1989; 84:546; k, Dolz et al. Allergy 1996; 51:489; l, Creticos et al. N Engl J Med 1996; 334:501; m, Bousquet et al. Clin Allergy 1985; 25:179; n, Machiels et al. Clin Exp Allergy 1990; 20; 653; o, Bruce et al. J Allergy Clin Immunol 1977; 59:449; p, Hill et al. BMJ 1982; 284:306; q, Alvarez-Cuesta et al. J Allergy Clin Immunol 1994; 93:556; r, Varney et al. Clin Exp Allergy 1997; 27:860; s, Valovirta et al. Ann Allergy 1986; 57:173; t, Adkinson et al. N Engl J Med 1997; 336:324.)*

bronchial hyperresponsiveness, but effects on lung function have been inconsistent. However, some carefully conducted studies of seasonal and/or perennial asthma have yielded only limited evidence of clinical improvement in patients with asthma. The critical issue is to be sure that the chosen allergen is responsible for causing symptoms in the individual patient, and that other factors have been addressed. Unstable asthma is a risk factor for adverse reactions to SIT, so patients must be carefully selected and the right allergens chosen if immunotherapy is to be of benefit for asthma.[3]

Systemic reactions to hymenoptera venom are relatively rare, but can be fatal. If there are no contraindications, SIT is the treatment of choice for this group of patients. The decision to treat is based on exposure risk and likely benefit, so these patients require specialist assessment and careful consideration of the risk to benefit ratio.

CLINICAL EFFICACY WITH SPECIFIC ALLERGENS

Grass, Tree, and Weed Pollens

Patients with seasonal allergic rhinitis are typically allergic to grass pollen, tree pollens or ragweed. The nature of the triggers is usually clear from the history, and can be confirmed by skin testing. Patients with multiple allergies will also benefit from pollen SIT, but the impact is most evident in those with a narrow range of sensitivities.[2] Typically, treatment is given pre-seasonally for 3 years, but sometimes SIT is given all year round, again for a total of 3 years. Improvement can be expected in about 80% of patients—symptoms are reduced rather than abolished, with a marked reduction in the number of days with very bad symptoms compared with untreated or placebo-treated controls. Patients who also have pollen-induced asthma will usually notice an improvement in their chest symptoms, as well as their nasal symptoms.

House-dust Mites

House-dust mite (HDM) sensitivity is common and has been implicated as a risk factor for developing asthma. However, unlike pollen allergy, it can be difficult to work out how much of a patient's rhinitis symptoms are attributable to HDM. This is partly because exposure to HDM allergens occurs all year round and partly because many patients with rhinitis also have symptoms due to structural changes and sinusitis that is independent of their mite allergy and therefore will not respond to mite-specific treatment. Nevertheless, SIT with HDM extracts can be effective in controlling symptoms of perennial allergic rhinitis. Most clinicians would agree that if there is no benefit after 6 months, the treatment is unlikely to become effective on continuing SIT. In some cases, an alternative allergen extract may be tried, but more often it is necessary to discontinue SIT and revert to standard pharmacologic treatment.

Domestic Pets

Sensitization to domestic pet allergens is associated with an increased risk of developing asthma. In theory, domestic pet allergen exposure is avoidable and, historically, SIT for pet allergy was only considered appropriate for people with occupational exposure (e.g., veterinarians, social workers, etc.). Clinical trials have shown reductions in asthma symptoms and medication usage, as well as improvements in non-specific bronchial hyperresponsiveness in cat-allergic patients who do not have cats at home, supporting the use of cat immunotherapy. Currently, there is no corresponding data for dog allergy.

Fungi

Airborne fungal spores are recognized causes of life-threatening episodes and epidemic outbreaks of asthma. Unfortunately, there is little accurate information on exposure patterns to most fungal species and, as there are thousands of different species of fungi, it is hard to know which fungi are relevant to any individual's allergic disease. Diagnosis is difficult because fungal extracts are of very variable quality, and there are no allergen extracts available for many genera of fungi, because they do not grow in artificial media. Some benefits on asthma and rhinitis symptoms have been reported in double-blind, controlled studies of SIT with extracts of *Cladosporium herbarum* and *Alternaria alternata*. With fungi, as with any allergen, the decision to use SIT is guided by the sensitivity and exposure of the patient, a pattern of symptoms consistent with the pattern of exposure, and the availability of an extract of sufficient quality to allow delivery of a therapeutically effective dose.

Cockroach

Cockroach sensitivity is now recognized as a major factor in the pathogenesis of inner city asthma, especially in warmer climates, but there have been no adequately controlled trials of cockroach SIT.

Multiple Allergen Mixtures

Most of the double-blind, placebo-controlled studies that confirmed the effectiveness of SIT in allergic rhinitis and bronchial asthma were performed with single allergen extracts. In contrast, a typical immunotherapy prescription in the United States contains multiple unrelated allergen extracts. Although current US guidance supports the use of allergen mixtures, it is recommended that patients should only be treated with relevant allergens and putting too many allergens into a maintenance injection may reduce the overall effectiveness.[4] Evidence supporting treatment with multiple allergens comes mainly from trials using mixtures of two allergens. Very few studies have examined true multi-allergen SIT mixes, and most of these were performed over 40 years ago, with different mixtures than those used today. However, clinical experience is that SIT with multiple allergen mixes can be effective, so long as the number of allergens used does not dilute out the individual constituents to ineffective concentrations.

SPECIFICITY OF ALLERGEN IMMUNOTHERAPY

Clinical improvement is only seen in the response to allergens contained within the treatment mixture. However, as some allergens have overlapping proteins, e.g., grasses, treatment with pollen from one grass species can reduce responses to pollens from other grasses, but there is no effect on unrelated allergens. For example, treating with grass pollen has no effect on sensitivity to ragweed and vice-versa. It follows that SIT is most effective where there is a limited range of allergic sensitivities and where there is clear evidence that those allergens are responsible for triggering symptoms. These conditions are best met for seasonal pollen allergens and for occupational exposure to domestic animals. It is more difficult to be sure that perennial allergens or people's own pets are truly responsible for ongoing symptoms. Where there is doubt about the role of allergens in causing symptoms or a large number of allergens are implicated, optimizing therapy with antihistamines and nasal steroids may be preferable to SIT.

EVIDENCE OF DISEASE MODIFICATION

Part of the argument in favor of SIT is that it may have long-term benefits by modifying the course of the disease, whereas drug therapies only suppress the symptoms for as long as they are taken (Box 6-2). Two outcomes are cited as evidence of disease modification – the prevention of asthma in patients treated for rhinitis and the prevention of new allergic sensitizations. A multicenter European study found that SIT with birch and/or timothy grass for 3 years reduced the risk of developing asthma by 2.5-fold in children who only had symptoms of rhinitis at the start of SIT.[5] This effect was still apparent 7 years after completing SIT. Three studies have reported reduced rates of development of new sensitivities after SIT, as indicated by newly positive skin-prick test results. In the two larger studies, the rate of new sensitization was reduced by 56–65% compared with the control group and this effect persisted for 3 years after 3 to 4 years of SIT. It seems unlikely that SIT with one allergen directly affects B cells that recognize unrelated allergens. However, SIT might reduce nasal inflammation and thereby alter the local environment to make it less likely that exposure to other allergens will lead to sensitization.

Persistence of Clinical Improvement after Cessation of Immunotherapy

Both open and blinded studies have shown a slow recurrence of grass pollen symptoms after completing 3 to 4 years of SIT, which reached 31% by the third year but with no

---

Box 6-2   Evidence of Disease Modification

- Prevention of asthma
- Prevention of new allergic sensitizations

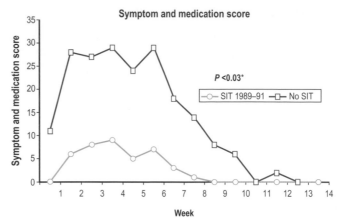

Figure 6-2 Persistence of effect of specific immunotherapy (SIT) 12 years after completing therapy. Graph shows symptoms scores during the pollen season in patients treated in childhood 12 years earlier (blue circles) compared with matched control group (red squares). *(From Eng et al. Allergy 2006; 61:198–201.)*

appreciable increase thereafter. This subjective benefit was supported by more objective measures, including conjunctival and skin sensitivity to grass pollen. The longest follow-up data has been reported in a 12-year open study of grass immunotherapy in children, in which the treated children still had decreased symptom and medication scores during the grass season and fewer new sensitizations compared with untreated controls (Fig. 6-2). Similar persistence of effect has been reported after immunotherapy with house-dust mite extract. Over a 3-year period after discontinuation, approximately half experienced a relapse in symptoms, but half remained symptom-free.

PHARMACOECONOMICS OF SIT

The fact that the benefits of SIT extend beyond the period of treatment is a key element of the economic argument for SIT. The possible cost benefits of SIT in children with newly diagnosed allergic rhinitis have been assessed in two US studies. Highly significant reductions were achieved in pharmacy claims, outpatient visits, and hospital admissions after SIT, compared with data for similar children not receiving SIT. The total medical costs were reduced by 25%, even when the cost of the immunotherapy was included. Another study compared 2771 children with newly diagnosed allergic rhinitis who received SIT and 11010 who did not. Healthcare utilization for the 18 months after starting SIT was US$3247 (including the cost of SIT), compared with US$4872 in the control group. Further studies of this type are needed with different extracts, in different healthcare systems, and in different age groups.

IMMUNOLOGIC RESPONSE TO INHALANT SIT

Much effort has gone into trying to understand the mechanisms of successful immunotherapy, partly to try to improve the efficacy and safety of SIT, and partly to try to find markers of treatment failure so that ineffective courses can be stopped early. Box 6-3 summarizes current understanding of the immunologic changes associated with successful immunotherapy for inhalant allergies.

END-ORGAN CHANGES

Since Noon's original report, it has been recognized that SIT induces increases in the conjunctival allergen threshold. SIT leads to a rapid reduction in the immediate skin reaction to allergen and within a few weeks there is a marked reduction in the late cutaneous reaction to allergen that develops 3 to 12 hours after intradermal injection of allergen. Nasal sensitivity to pollen is attenuated as are bronchial responses to inhaled

---

Box 6-3   The Immunologic Response to Immunotherapy

END-ORGAN RESPONSE

DECREASED EARLY AND LATE RESPONSES TO SPECIFIC ALLERGEN

- Conjunctiva
- Skin: early; late
- Nose
- Bronchi: early; late

DECREASED NON-SPECIFIC REACTION TO BRONCHIAL CHALLENGE

- Histamine
- Methacholine

DECREASED TISSUE INFLAMMATION

- Eosinophils
- Metachromatic cells

HUMERAL RESPONSE

IgE

- Early rise in specific IgE
- Suppression of seasonal rise in specific IgE
- Late decline in specific IgE

IgG

- Increase in specific IgG
- Early predominantly IgG$_1$
- Late predominantly IgG$_4$

CELLULAR RESPONSE

BASOPHILS

- Non-specific loss of responsiveness

LYMPHOCYTES AND PERIPHERAL BLOOD MONONUCLEAR CELLS

- Decreased serum IL-2R
- Decreased lymphocyte proliferation
- Generation of specific suppressor cells
- Regulatory T lymphocytes
  - Increased expression of Foxp3
  - Secreting IL-10
  - Secreting TGF-β

EVIDENCE OF IMMUNE DEVIATION

- Decreased stimulated release of Th2 cytokines
  - IL-4
  - IL-13
- Preferential deletion of Th2 T cells
- Increased stimulated release of Th1 cytokines
  - IFN-γ
- Increased stimulated mRNA for Th1 cytokines
  - IFN-γ
  - IL-12

OTHER IMMUNOLOGIC CHANGES

- Decrease in FcεRII/CD23 and B cell activation markers
- Decreased costimulatory molecules
- Decreased release of cytokines
  - IL-2
  - TNF
  - Histamine-releasing factors
  - Platelet-activating factor

IFN, interferon; *IgE, IgG*, immunoglobulins E and G; *IL*, interleukin; *IL-2R*, interleukin type 2 receptor; *mRNA*, messenger RNA; *TGF-β*, transforming growth factor-β; *TNF*, tumor necrosis factor.

allergen and non-specific agents (e.g., histamine or methacholine). Sensitivity to allergen on titrated skin prick testing, titrated conjunctival challenge, and titrated nasal challenge after SIT has been shown to correlate with symptoms of rhinitis during natural pollen exposure.

OVERVIEW OF THE IMMUNE RESPONSE TO IMMUNOTHERAPY

The effect of SIT on cellular inflammation has been studied exhaustively. In some ways, the immunologic responses to SIT may appear contradictory: some studies report induction of regulatory T cells that suppress both Th1 and Th2 cytokine responses to specific allergen stimulation, whereas other studies report an immune deviation from a Th2 to a Th1 response such that allergen stimulation of T cells results in increased synthesis of IL-12 and IFN-γ and decreased synthesis of IL-4. Current perspectives are that the regulatory T cell response occurs very early in the course of subcutaneous immunotherapy, but with time there is a more general suppression of T cell reactivity to the injected allergen.

A detailed discussion of the immunologic mechanisms of SIT is beyond the scope of this chapter. But the mechanisms involved can be summarized briefly as follows:

- Eosinophils, basophils and mast cells are thought to be the main effector cells of the allergic response.
- The increased levels of eosinophils seen during natural allergen exposure are reduced by SIT.
- Seasonal increases in nasal basophils and mast cells are also blunted.
- Allergen-specific IgE levels reduce slowly after SIT but the rate of change is much less than would be expected if this was an important mechanism.
- In contrast, allergen-specific IgG4 levels rise steeply after SIT. This is generally considered to be a direct consequence of the injection of foreign material rather

than the mechanism by which SIT works. The immediate cause of IgG4 production is likely to be induction of regulatory T cells producing IL-10.

Both during and after SIT, there is a general suppression of allergen-specific T cell responses, which is now thought to be due to induction of allergen-specific regulatory T cells, which produce two key cytokines: IL-10 and TGF-β (transforming growth factor-β). In parallel, there is suppression of allergen-specific lymphocyte proliferation and decreased production of interferon-γ (IFN-γ), IL-5, and IL-13. IL-10 is a general inhibitor of proliferative and cytokine responses in T cells, which inhibits IgE production and enhances IgG4 production. TGF-β induces an isotype switch towards IgA. At present, increased allergen-specific IL-10 production is considered a marker of successful SIT.

Two types of CD4+ helper T lymphocytes have been described: Th2 cells, which preferentially secrete IL-4, and Th1 cells, which preferentially secrete IFN-γ in response to allergen stimulation. Allergic individuals have increased numbers of allergen-specific Th2 cells in their peripheral circulation, but normal levels of antigen-specific Th1 and T regulatory cells. SIT leads to a decrease in allergen-specific Th2 cells, suggesting that SIT may work by deviating the immune response away from the Th2 pattern. This may be mediated through induction of cells producing IL-12. Increased numbers of cells expressing IL-12 mRNA have been noted in skin sites challenged with allergen after SIT. IL-12 promotes Th1 lymphocyte proliferation and suppresses Th2 cells, so the finding of increased IL-12-secreting cells is consistent with a shift from Th2 to Th1 allergen-specific responses after SIT.

INDICATIONS FOR SIT

In contrast to severe anaphylaxis to *Hymenoptera* venom, there are no absolute indications for SIT with inhalant allergens. Broadly speaking, SIT should be considered for patients who have troublesome symptoms of allergic rhinitis, rhinoconjunctivitis, or asthma after natural exposure to allergens and who demonstrate specific-IgE antibodies to relevant allergens. Other factors to consider are the severity and duration of symptoms, medication requirements, and patient preference. Because of the increased risk of side effects in patients with poorly controlled asthma, SIT should only be offered to patients with asthma if their asthma is under control and their forced expiratory volume in one second (FEV$_1$) is greater than the 70% predicted.

There is some evidence that SIT may have disease-modifying actions, preventing the onset of asthma in children with allergic rhinitis. If substantiated, this would mandate a more active approach to offering SIT to such children. Currently, we await further clinical trials, which are due to report in the next few years, before embarking on mass preventive programs in young children with allergic rhinitis.

Outside the US, most SIT injections involve single allergens, which are obtained commercially and used individually. However, within the US, it is common to use combinations of extracts and to mix the allergens in a single maintenance vial. Some caution is needed, however, because extracts from fungi and cockroaches contain proteases that can degrade the proteins in other extracts with which they may be mixed. Current best advice is not to mix cockroach or any fungal extract with extracts of pollens, mites, or danders, but other combinations are acceptable.

Effective SIT requires administration of sufficient allergenic protein. A variety of methods have been used to define the potency of allergen extracts. Experience gained over many years and many trials, has shown that a maintenance dose of approximately 6 to 20 μg of major allergen is needed to achieve clinical efficacy. The actual amount varies between manufacturers and allergens, and the lack of clarity on this point remains a matter of concern to practitioners and regulators alike.

Injection Schedules

An SIT schedule consists of two phases: the build-up phase going from very low dose to the full maintenance dose, and then a maintenance phase, in which the same dose is given at intervals over a number of years. Typically, the build-up phase is achieved by

Box 6-4   **Example of a Conventional US-Style Allergen Extract Treatment Schedule**

The following schedule should be used, with modification if necessary, as outlined in the accompanying instructions.

INSTRUCTIONS FOR THE INJECTION OF ALLERGENIC EXTRACTS

Begin with vial #**4** and progress to vial #**1**, which is the most concentrated or 'maintenance' solution. The injections should be given every **week**. Once maintenance is reached, the injection should be given every **3–4** weeks, with the following exceptions: **give weekly for first month and every 2 weeks for the second month**.

SCHEDULE

Vial #5	Vial #4	Vial #3	Vial #2	Vial #1
0.05 mL	0.05 mL	0.05 mL	0.05 mL	0.05 mL
0.10 mL	0.10 mL	0.10 mL	0.07 mL	0.07 mL
0.20 mL	0.20 mL	0.20 mL	0.10 mL	0.10 mL
0.40 mL	0.40 mL	0.40 mL	0.15 mL	0.15 mL
			0.25 mL	0.20 mL
			0.35 mL	0.30 mL
			0.50 mL	0.40 mL
				0.50 mL

The **bold-underlined** entries are representative instructions that would be placed in the blank spaces in the schedule.

TABLE 6-1   A European-style Injection Immunotherapy Schedule for Hay Fever, Giving Two Injections Each Week for 6 Weeks

Week no.	Injection no.	Allergen concentration	Volume (mL)	Amount of allergen (SQ-U)
1	1	1000	0.1	100
1	2	10000	0.1	1000
2	3	10000	0.2	2000
2	4	10000	0.4	4000
3	5	10000	0.6	6000
3	6	100000	0.1	10000
4	7	100000	0.1	10000
4	8	100000	0.2	20000
5	9	100000	0.3	30000
5	10	100000	0.3	30000
6	11	100000	0.5	50000
6	12	100000	0.5	50000

(Frew et al. 2006).

injections twice-weekly, weekly or alternate weeks (Box 6-4, Table 6-1). Various alternative schedules have been devised, with clusters of injections given at intervals or rush protocols, in which the full build-up phase is achieved in 1 to 2 days. Once patients reach the maintenance dose of their immunotherapy extract, injections are given at less frequent intervals, typically every 4 weeks. The basic treatment schedule may require modification, either because of missed visits or reactions to the previous injection. Reductions are not needed during a pollen season.

Adverse Reactions to SIT

Localized and systemic reactions may occur after SIT. Local reactions are more frequent during the build-up phase than during maintenance and, if large, may warrant adjustment to the schedule (e.g., repeating the last dose) or premedication with antihistamines.

The occurrence of local reactions after SIT does not predict subsequent occurrence of systemic reactions, so if the concern is solely about the possible occurrence of a systemic reaction, no dose adjustment is needed after a local reaction.

Systemic reactions are more serious and can occasionally prove fatal. The fatality rate in the US between 1985 and 2001 has been estimated to be about 1 per 2.5 million injections. In a national survey, three-quarters of systemic reactions were cutaneous or upper respiratory, while one-quarter was asthmatic; only 3% involved life-threatening respiratory compromise or hypotension. Although it used to be thought that patients are at increased risk for systemic reactions during their pollen seasons, no evidence of this has been found in large observational studies. Patients with asthma are at greater risk of adverse reactions, especially if their asthma is labile or symptomatic at the time of the injection, requires oral corticosteroid treatment, or has resulted in hospitalization or emergency room visits. This has led some authorities to say that SIT should not be given to anyone with asthma. However, with proper care and attention, it is reasonable to treat people whose asthma is mild and stable. Almost all severe reactions start within 20 min of the injection, and a minimum observation period of 30 min after injections is widely accepted as appropriate. Late-onset systemic reactions are relatively rare, but when they do occur, they are usually mild and subside spontaneously, without requiring epinephrine (adrenaline) or emergency department attendance.

SIT in Pregnancy

There are two specific concerns during pregnancy: the risk to the fetus of an anaphylactic reaction to SIT and potential effects on the development of the baby's immune system. Current advice is that SIT should not be started during pregnancy but maintenance treatment may be continued, provided there is no history of systemic reactions. There is no evidence of any increase in rates of prematurity, toxemia, abortion, neonatal death, or congenital malformations when SIT is continued in pregnancy. Whether maternal SIT has any beneficial effects on the unborn child in terms of preventing the development of allergic disease remains unanswered, and is unlikely ever to be studied formally.

Adherence to SIT

The long duration of allergen immunotherapy is an important factor in patients stopping prematurely. In different reports, 10–46% of patients do not complete their courses. These poor completion rates have led to an interest in developing more effective vaccines that can achieve the same benefits as conventional SIT, but in a shorter timeframe, and also in alternative routes of administration that may be easier for patients.

SUBLINGUAL IMMUNOTHERAPY

It has been known for many years that immunologic tolerance can be achieved by mucosal application of proteins. Sublingual immunotherapy (SLIT) exploits this by applying relatively large doses of allergen to the buccal mucosa. As this is safe and can be done at home, it is much more convenient for patients than standard injection immunotherapy. The immunologic mechanisms of successful SLIT are similar to those of injection allergen-specific immunotherapy, but dendritic cells in the buccal mucosa are thought to play a key role in inducing tolerance, most likely through regulatory T cells (Fig. 6-3). SLIT achieves most of the outcomes associated with successful injection SIT, with reduced symptoms and medication requirements, as well as disease modification. Economic considerations are crucial in deciding who should receive SLIT as the vaccine costs are relatively expensive compared with subcutaneous injection immunotherapy (SCIT).

Recent interest in SLIT has been driven by a perception that injection SIT is hazardous. When treating a relatively benign disease such as allergic rhinitis, the risk of serious adverse reactions weigh more heavily than when treating cancer or life-threatening autoimmune disease.

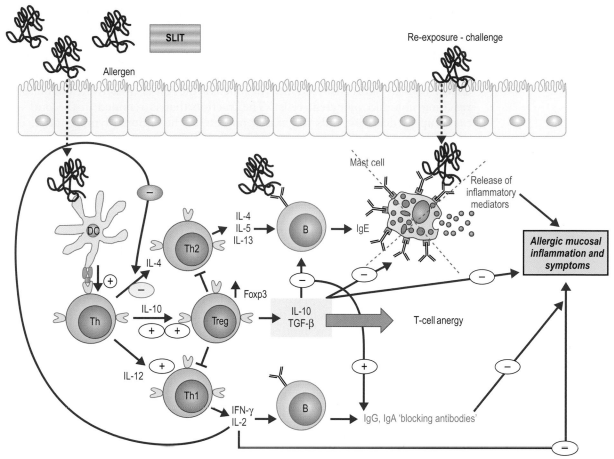

Figure 6-3 Immunologic mechanisms of specific sublingual immunotherapy (SLIT). Locally administered allergen using SLIT is taken up by mucosal dendritic cells (DCs) and then presented to T cells together with IL-12, biasing the response toward a Th1-like profile and away from the pro-IgE Th2 profile arbitrated by protolerogenic mechanisms mediated by the increased release of IL-10. There is enhanced secretion of interferon-γ (IFN-γ) and IL-2, which drive specific B cell production of non-pathogenic and protective IgG1 and IgG4 antibodies and decreased release of the Th2 pro-IgE cytokine IL-4. Oral mucosal DCs actively upregulate regulatory T cell (Treg) subtypes, including Forkhead box P3 protein (Foxp3)-expressing T cells, contributing to T cell anergy mediated by IL-10 and transforming growth factor-β (TGF-β). These interconnected pathways lead to reduction in allergic inflammation and symptoms.

Over the past 30 years, several different preparations of aqueous allergen extracts have been tried for sublingual use, including sprays, drops, and more recently, fast-dissolving tablets. Standardized extracts for SLIT are available for house-dust mite (*Dermatophagoides farinae* and *D. pteronyssinus*), cat dander, weeds (ragweed, *Parietaria*, mugwort), grasses, and tree pollens. To improve reliability of dosing and compliance, tablet formulations were developed with grass pollen SLIT tablets commercially available and approved for treating allergic rhinitis since 2009. The tablet formulation increases the stability of the product and improves standardization of doses. In pharmacologic terms, drops and tablets are equivalent: both deliver a sublingual solution of allergen extract. However, tablets simplify SLIT administration and minimize the potential risks of errors in dose administration.

Several large clinical trials have shown SLIT to be clinically effective, improving allergic rhinitis and asthma symptoms and reducing requirements for rescue medication. SLIT is now widely used in Europe, especially in France, Germany, and Italy. Different regimens have been employed: some include a rapid build-up phase, while others start directly at the maintenance dose. Depending on the manufacturer and preparation, SLIT doses are 50–110 times those used in SCIT. Local side effects are common, but serious side effects are very rare. In addition to its safer profile, SLIT is administered at home, an additional advantage over SCIT, which requires clinic visits.

Long-term data are lacking, but based on SCIT practice and limited evidence from clinical trials with seasonal allergens, 3 years or more of treatment is recommended.

Mechanisms of SLIT

When allergens are placed in contact with the oral mucosa, a small amount of the allergenic material is absorbed into the mucosa (the rest is swallowed and digested, never reaching immunocompetent cells). The fraction that is retained in the oral mucosa is taken up by dendritic cells (DCs) that migrate to the regional lymph nodes. Both standard allergens and chemically modified allergoids persist in the mouth for several hours, and small amounts can still be identified in the oral cavity up to 20 hours later. In theory, absorption from sites other than the oral mucosa might also contribute to the immunologic stimulus from SLIT, but there is minimal clinical benefit from allergens given orally and simply swallowed without a period of retention under the tongue.

The immunologic changes associated with successful SLIT are similar to those observed with SCIT (Fig. 6-3). These include enhanced suppressor activity of IL-10-secreting regulatory T cells (Tr cells), suppression of eosinophils, mast cells and basophils, and antibody isotype switching from IgE to IgG4. Current data suggest that IL-10-producing Tr cells are pivotal to the various changes induced by SIT. Once induced, chronic allergen exposure may favor expansion of Tr1 cells through IL-12 and IL-27 synthesis. Recruitment of these cells into areas of inflammation will lead to amplification of local cytokine responses, including IL-12, IL-10, and TGF-β1. The IL-12 will skew any Th2 and Th17 cells toward the Th1 phenotype, whereas IL-10 suppresses allergen-specific Th2 and Th17 responses, induces IgG4, and inhibits recruitment of mast cells, basophils, and eosinophils. Lastly, TGF-β1 blocks the Th2 response and decreases the activation of mast cells and eosinophils. Research in this area is now focused on identifying more efficient ways of inducing allergen-specific Tregs, including the use of appropriate immunologic adjuvants.

Most of these phenomena are also found after SLIT (Box 6-5), albeit with smaller changes in specific IgE, specific IgG, and cytokines compared with those identified in patients treated by injection SIT.[8] Induction of allergen-specific IgG4 is a consistent finding in most SLIT studies using large doses of allergen but some studies reporting good clinical responses to SLIT have not detected any change in allergen-specific IgE, IgG, or IgG4. This may partly reflect the timing of the immunologic analysis relative to administration of SLIT, but some doubts remain about the relationship between changes in these immunologic measures and the delivery of clinical benefit.[9]

Although there is considerable overlap in the immune responses found in individual studies of SCIT and SLIT, some differences have been found between injection and sublingual SIT. Because not all the phenomena reported after SCIT occur after SLIT, it is possible that different or additional mechanisms may occur in SLIT.

Side Effects of SLIT

SLIT has a much safer profile than SCIT, but local side effects are common, most frequently local irritation of the oral mucosa and sometimes local swelling. Systemic reactions are extremely rare, but caution is advised in patients who have experienced systemic side effects to other forms of SIT. Local side effects ease with repeated use, and rarely lead patients to discontinue therapy. To avoid unnecessary discontinuation,

---

Box 6-5   **Possible Mechanisms of Sublingual Immunotherapy**
• Induction of IgG (blocking) antibodies • Reduction in specific IgE (long term) • Reduced recruitment of effector cells • Altered helper T cell cytokine balance (shift to Th1 from Th2) • T cell anergy • B cell suppression • Increased regulatory T cell (Treg) function

patients should be supervised when they take their first doses. This allows any side effects to be explained and the natural history discussed.

Efficacy of SLIT

Several well-conducted clinical trials have shown 30–40% reductions in symptom score and rescue medication use in patients with seasonal allergic rhinitis after SLIT. In general, the trials show that clinically significant benefits are achieved in the first year of SLIT, but the magnitude of benefit does not increase much in the second and third years. However, it is likely that the second and third years of SLIT contribute to the overall durability of the response, which we know extends for at least 2 years after 3 years of therapy in double-blind, placebo-controlled trials (Fig. 6-4), supporting reports from open-label clinical practice that benefits are maintained for at least 7 years after ceasing SLIT. Lasting benefit seems to be more likely in those with more severe disease at enrolment.

SLIT with grass pollen tablets has also been studied in children and adolescents, in both Europe and North America. Grass pollen tablets were well tolerated and the levels of benefit achieved were comparable with those found in adults. These positive outcomes for grass pollen tablets contrast with earlier pediatric studies that found no benefit for grass pollen SLIT, given as liquid preparations (drops). It remains unclear whether these discordant results reflect the way the SLIT was given (drops vs tablets) or perhaps a less severely affected group of children (SLIT appears to have more impact in those with more prominent symptoms).

SLIT has been most extensively tested in grass pollen allergy, but tablet-based therapies are under development for tree pollen allergy, HDM allergy, and animal dander. Earlier forms of SLIT, in small studies using liquid preparations (drops), have shown some clinical benefit with immunologic effects similar to those in SCIT and grass pollen SLIT. House-dust mite allergy is a major focus for future development but thus far most relevant trials have been small, and need to be interpreted cautiously. However, it should be noted that HDM SLIT was ineffective in a study of Dutch children in primary care. It remains unclear whether this lack of effect is due to the type of preparation used for SLIT or to the relatively mild level of symptoms in this particular study population. Taking everything into consideration, it is clear that further large-scale placebo-controlled studies are needed in well-defined patient groups before SLIT can be recommended for HDM allergy.

SLIT for Asthma

Most clinical trials of SLIT have evaluated its efficacy in allergic rhinitis. Some of the trials included patients with asthma, and SLIT appears to reduce asthma symptoms and medication scores after 2 years of treatment. While this is promising, more robust data are needed from large studies with well-defined objective outcome measures for asthma. SLIT is currently recommended for patients with allergic rhinitis, with or without asthma, but is not currently recommended specifically for treatment of asthma.

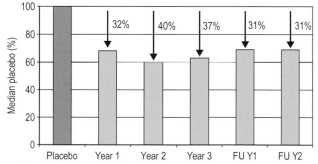

Figure 6-4 Efficacy of sublingual allergen tablets on rhinitis symptoms over 3 years treatment and 2 further years on placebo. *(Adapted from Durham SR et al. J Allergy Clin Immunol 2012; 129:717–725.)*

Durability of Treatment

A key question in deciding whether to use SLIT is how long the benefits of therapy extend beyond the period of treatment. Maintaining double-blind trials for years after completion of therapy is extremely difficult,[10] both for the investigators and for the control group participants who have to go without treatment for years to answer the question properly. Evidence from long-term follow-up of open-label therapy has shown that the longer the course of treatment, the longer the benefit persists. Five years of SLIT gave benefits for at least 7 years, whereas the benefit of 3 to 4 years of SLIT seemed to wear off more quickly. The recent double-blind, placebo-controlled studies continued for 2 years after completing therapy, demonstrating a durable response, but longer-term follow-up seems unlikely. Unfortunately, accurate cost–benefit analysis requires an estimate of the durability of therapeutic effect, so the lack of long-term data remains a problem for policymakers and manufacturers alike.

Effects of SLIT on the Natural History of Allergic Disease

As discussed above, there is considerable interest in the possibility that SIT may modify the course of allergic disease. If proved, this effect would dramatically alter the economic argument in favor of SIT because one could discount the costs of treatment against the costs of the future condition that has been avoided. Data have been presented in two areas: prevention of new sensitizations and prevention of asthma. As with SCIT, atopic children treated with SLIT acquire fewer new sensitivities over 3 years, compared with untreated children. SLIT also seems capable of preventing children with rhinitis from progressing to develop asthma. In a 3-year study, 18 of 44 control children developed asthma versus only 8 of 45 SLIT-treated children (Fig. 6-5). A more formal trial of this concept is under way and will report in a few years.

Thus, both SCIT and SLIT appear to modify the course of allergic disease, by reducing the incidence of new sensitizations, preventing the development of clinical asthma and/or speeding up its resolution. The mechanism remains unclear but probably involves a combination of immunologic effects and downstream changes to the structure and function of the small airways. Better data are needed, but if confirmed, these disease-modifying and preventive effects of SIT would have a major impact on any cost–benefit analysis.

Safety and Cost-Effectiveness of SLIT

One of the main drivers behind the development of SLIT was awareness of risks associated with SCIT. Although SIT is usually quite safe in patients who do not have asthma, occasional serious adverse events do happen, but these are rarely fatal. In most reports, the rate of serious systemic reactions in patients with rhinitis is about 1 in 500

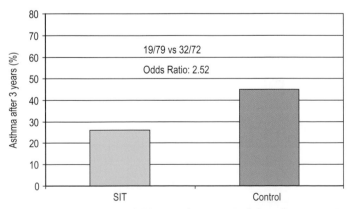

Figure 6-5 Pollen SIT reduces asthma in children with seasonal allergic rhinitis. *(Adapted from Möller et al. J Allergy Clin Immunol 2002; 109:251–256.)*

injections. Most clinical trials of SLIT report local side effects, particularly itching of the mouth and palate, but there were few serious systemic side effects. Since SLIT preparations became available commercially, a small number of serious adverse events have been reported, mainly in patients who had already experienced problems with conventional SCIT. These episodes were not witnessed by medical personnel, so some doubt remains about their precise nature, but clearly some caution is required if SLIT is given to such patients. The first dose of SLIT should normally be taken in the physician's office, particularly in patients who previously experienced problems with SCIT. In some series, up to 11.6% of patients had experienced wheezing or worsening of nasal symptoms on one or more occasions after a SLIT dose, although the overall frequency of systemic adverse reactions was only 1 in 3000 doses.

No discussion of new therapeutic options is complete without consideration of the economic aspects. Rhinoconjunctivitis is a common condition, and standard therapies such as antihistamines and even nasal corticosteroids are relatively inexpensive compared with forms of SIT. SLIT offers improvements that cannot be achieved by standard pharmacotherapy, but it is relatively expensive compared with antihistamine therapy, which is adjusted according to symptoms. Cost-effectiveness analysis requires assumptions on the likely durability of benefits and the period over which they impact relevant financial outcomes. Some evidence of cost-effectiveness has been presented, indicating a cost of 13 000–18 000 euros (US$17 000–25 000) per quality-adjusted life year (QALY) gained. The benefit consisted of reductions in rescue medication and fewer hours lost from work (production loss). The analysis used a horizon of 9 years and assumed that the clinical benefit achieved in the first years of therapy would be sustained throughout. On this basis, tablet-based SLIT could be considered as cost-effective at current prices compared with standard thresholds applied by national regulatory bodies.[6,7]

In summary, favorable cost–benefit analysis has been presented, although not all healthcare systems have been convinced. SLIT vaccines are relatively expensive, especially compared with standard drug treatment for allergic rhinitis, and therefore SLIT needs to be targeted to patients with significant disease.

OTHER POTENTIAL MODES OF ADMINISTRATION

Intralymphatic Route

Given that SIT is thought to work through an effect on T cells, it seemed logical to try delivering the allergen direct to the lymph nodes. The clinical and immunologic response to three injections of grass pollen extract into an inguinal lymph node has been compared with SCIT using the same extract for a period of 3 years in 112 subjects sensitive to grass. The total dose by the intralymphatic route was less than one-thousandth of that given by subcutaneous injection. Systemic reactions were fewer and less severe with intralymphatic injection. A more rapid increase in tolerance to intranasal challenge with grass pollen extract was observed in the intralymphatic group, and after 3 years, the clinical and immunologic outcomes were identical in the two groups. Confirmatory studies are needed, but intralymphatic immunotherapy has several attractive features: it uses currently approved extracts, multiple allergen mixes can be administered, and it would not require an expensive development program to gain approval.

MODIFIED ALLERGEN EXTRACTS AND ADJUVANTS (BOX 6-6)

A major disadvantage of conventional SIT is the considerable investment in time and money required on the part of the patient to achieve and maintain effective doses of allergen extract. To address this, allergists began experimenting over 60 years ago with ways of slowing the absorption of allergen from the injection site in order to decrease the number of injections required and/or improve safety. Various depot preparations have been tried: alum precipitation reduces the risk of systemic side effects but all trials

> **Box 6-6   Modifications to Allergen Extracts and Routes of Administration***
>
> - Depot preparations
>   - Aluminum adsorption
>   - Tyrosine adsorption
>   - Liposome-encapsulated
> - Allergoids
> - Recombinant technology
>   - Unmodified major allergens
>   - Mutated or deleted major allergens
>   - T cell epitope peptides
> - Toll-like receptor stimulation
>   - 3-Deacylated monophosphoryl lipid A
>   - CpG (type A and type B): combined with allergen or administered without allergen
> - Intralymphatic
> - Transcutaneous
> - Transmucosal
>   - Oral
>   - Intranasal
>   - Sublingual

*In clinical use or under investigation.

with modified vaccines have shown that 3 years of treatment is required for maximum efficacy.

Various adjuvants have been tried in order to increase the immunologic effect of a given amount of allergen. Two of these involved stimulation of Toll-like receptors (TLRs), which are cell surface receptors that recognize molecular patterns commonly found in bacteria and viruses. When allergens are given together with TLR stimulation, the immunologic effect is altered, biasing the response towards a Th1 pattern. Unmethylated CpG DNA motifs stimulate TLR9, and lipopolysaccharides and a derivative, monophosphoryl lipid A (MPL) stimulate TLR4. SIT studies using MPL as an adjuvant have shown clinical efficacy after only four injections, but further data on durability is needed before this can be adopted into routine use. Immunostimulation with CpG-containing DNA sequences has been tested for ragweed and house-dust mite allergy. Initial trials were promising, although later ragweed studies have proved less effective.

Allergenic proteins can be cross-linked with formaldehyde or glutaraldehyde to produce larger molecules, which are less able to react with IgE antibodies. Such allergen extracts are called 'allergoids' and have proved effective in clinical trials, although their clinical use has been limited in the US. In contrast, allergoids have proved more popular in Europe, allowing rapid build-up regimens and delivery of large amounts of allergen in fewer injections. Encapsulation of unmodified house-dust mite allergen extracts in liposomes has also been investigated. Liposomes are lipid vesicles formed by one or more phospholipid bilayers that entrap the water-soluble extract in their internal aqueous compartment. They are biodegradable and stable and prolong the half-life of the encapsulated drug, while acting as an adjuvant, inducing a Th1 response. To date, the clinical effectiveness of this approach has not been confirmed.

Recombinant Allergen Vaccines

In theory, recombinant technology offers the possibility of improving the standardization and safety of allergen SIT. Most of the key components of inhaled allergens have been identified, cloned, sequenced, and expressed in various systems. This allows production of virtually unlimited quantities of allergenic proteins, mutated proteins, or fragments of allergenic proteins.

Unmodified Allergens

There have been several trials of SIT with unmodified purified major allergens. To date, the trials have shown efficacy but no real superiority to standard SIT. In theory, SIT vaccines could be personalized to the individual's serologic pattern of reaction, but this approach raises awkward regulatory questions, which remain unanswered.

Peptides

Because we know that the clinical response to allergen immunotherapy seems to involve the induction of non-responsiveness in T lymphocytes, it should be possible to treat patients with allergen-derived peptides (T cell–activating epitopes), which do not react with IgE antibodies and therefore will not cause systemic side effects. Clinical trials of peptide vaccines for ragweed and cat allergy have shown some reduction in symptoms compared with placebo, and there are ongoing trials for grass and tree pollen allergy, but this development is ongoing and unlikely to hit the market within the next 5 years.

Modified Allergens

Genetic modification can produce hypoallergenic variants of allergenic proteins, which may reduce the risk of IgE-mediated side effects, while allowing T cell effects to continue. This approach has mainly been studied for birch pollen. Other genetically modified allergens reported in papers include hybrid molecules derived from house-dust mite, timothy grass and cat dander.

THE FUTURE OF SLIT

Future developments in SLIT may take several forms, including mucoadhesives, allergoids, adjuvants, and new allergens (latex, foods). The delivery of allergen to the mucosa may be improved by creating formulations that adhere better to the mucosa and deliver the necessary amount of allergen more efficiently. Such mucoadhesives could allow smaller amounts of allergen to be given, thereby reducing the risk of local side effects and adverse reactions. The efficiency of SLIT might also be improved by more persistent presence of the allergen. Experimental data from mouse models are promising, but this approach has yet to be tested in humans.

As with SCIT, it may be possible to use modified allergens. For example, allergoids, which retain the ability to stimulate T cells while having reduced binding to IgE. This should reduce side effects and has been tested in patients with grass pollen allergy, in whom it appears effective, both when given all-year-round and when used pre-seasonally. Adjuvants that selectively induce IL-10 could also enhance the efficacy of SLIT vaccines. A combination of dexamethasone and 1,25-dihydroxyvitamin D_3 has been tested in models and induces IL-10 production by human and murine DCs, leading to differentiation of $CD4^+$ naive T cells toward a Tr profile. Another adjuvant, *Lactobacillus plantarum*, deviates T cells toward a mixed Th1/Tr pattern. Both these adjuvants have enhanced the efficacy of SLIT in a mouse model of asthma.

CONCLUSIONS

Allergen immunotherapy has been practiced with only relatively modest changes for more than 100 years. The clinical effectiveness of adequate doses in appropriate patients for both allergic rhinitis and bronchial asthma has been repeatedly confirmed. Treatment by the sublingual route is becoming increasingly popular. SLIT appears to be as effective as SCIT for allergic rhinitis and is certainly more convenient for patients. The precise mechanisms of SIT action remain uncertain. Both SCIT and SLIT are associated with induction of regulatory T cells, expression of IL-10 and TGF-β1, and secretion of allergen-specific IgG4. The major threat to future use of SCIT and SLIT is the lack of comprehensive cost-effectiveness data, which is increasingly required by healthcare commissioners when deciding which treatments to fund. Future developments will include a wider range of allergens, adaptations with mucoadhesives and adjuvants to refine the immunologic response, and research into the durability of responses to determine cost-effectiveness.

As well as confirming primary efficacy, clinical trials of SCIT and SLIT have confirmed a persisting beneficial effect after immunotherapy is discontinued. These findings suggest that immunotherapy has the potential to be used more widely. Increased utilization would be facilitated by alternative extracts and better methods of administration making SIT safer and more convenient for the patient.

REFERENCES

1. Frew AJ. Hundred years of immunotherapy. Clin Exp Allergy 2011;41:1221–5.
2. Frew AJ, Powell RJ, Corrigan CJ, et al. Clinical efficacy and safety of specific allergy vaccination with Alutard Grass in seasonal allergic rhinoconjunctivitis: a large-scale randomised double-blind placebo-controlled multi-centre study (UKIS – The UK Immunotherapy Study). J Allergy Clin Immunol 2006;117:319–25.
3. Abramson MJ, Puy RM, Weiner JM. Injection allergen immunotherapy for asthma. Cochrane Database Syst Rev 2010;(8):CD001186.
4. Cox L, Nelson H, Lockey R. Allergen immunotherapy: a practice parameter third update. J Allergy Clin Immunol 2011;127:S1–55.
5. Jacobsen L, Niggemann B, Dreborg S, et al. Specific immunotherapy has long-term preventive effect on seasonal and perennial asthma: 10-year follow-up on the PAT study. Allergy 2007;62:943–8.
6. Hankin CS, Cox L, Lang D, et al. Allergen immunotherapy and health care cost benefits for children with allergic rhinitis: a large-scale, retrospective, matched cohort study. Ann Allergy Asthma Immunol 2010;104:79–85.
7. Bachert C, Vestenbaek U, Christensen J, et al. Cost-effectiveness of grass allergen tablet (Grazax) for the prevention of seasonal grass pollen induced rhinoconjunctivitis: a Northern European perspective. Clin Exp Allergy 2007;37:772–9.
8. Bohle B, Kinaciyan T, Gerstmayr M, et al. Sublingual immunotherapy induces IL-10-producing T regulatory cells, allergen-specific T-cell tolerance, and immune deviation. J Allergy Clin Immunol 2007;120:707–13.
9. Novak N, Bieber T, Allam JP. Immunologic mechanisms of sublingual allergen-specific immunotherapy. Allergy 2011;66:733–9.
10. Durham SR, Emminger W, Kapp A, et al. SQ-standardized sublingual grass immuno-therapy: confirmation of disease modification 2 years after 3 years of treatment in a randomized trial. J Allergy Clin Immunol 2012;129:717–25.

CHAPTER 7

Asthma

Stephen T. Holgate and Mike Thomas

CHAPTER OUTLINE

INTRODUCTION AND OVERVIEW
Background
Diagnosis
Airway Inflammation and Remodeling
Treatment
Prevalence and Impact of Asthma
HISTORICAL PERSPECTIVE
EPIDEMIOLOGY
Incidence
Prevalence
Changing Trends
PATHOGENESIS AND ETIOLOGY
Inflammatory Changes
Structural Changes and Airway Remodeling
Immunologic Factors
Genetics and Epigenetics
CLINICAL FEATURES AND PHENOTYPES OF ASTHMA
Phenotypes of Adult Asthma
Phenotypes in Children
EVALUATION AND DIAGNOSIS
Diagnosis in Adults
    Risk Factors
    History and Examination
    Lung Function
    Bronchial Hyperreactivity (BHR)
    Determination of the Allergic Status
    Assessment of Airway Inflammation
    Imaging
Asthma Diagnosis in Specific Settings
    Occupational Asthma
    Asthma in the Elderly
    Asthma in the Athlete
    Conditions that May Mimic Asthma
Diagnosis in Children
    History and Examination
    Radiographic Studies
    Pulmonary Function Tests
    Laboratory Evaluation
Monitoring Asthma
    Severity
    Symptom Control
    Exacerbations

Asthma-related Quality of Life
Lung Function
Rescue Medication Use
Adherence with Regular Medication and Inhaler Technique
Personal Asthma Action Plan
ASTHMA MANAGEMENT
Long-term Management in Adults
    Control of Environmental Factors
    Comorbidity
Pharmacologic Treatment in Adults
    Quick-relief Medications
    Long-term Control Medications
Step Care Approach to Asthma Management
    Intermittent Asthma
    Persistent Asthma
Asthma Management in Infants and Children
Non-pharmacologic Management in Children
    Environmental Control
    Psychosocial Factors
Asthma Education
    Pharmacologic Therapy in Children
ACUTE ASTHMA AND REFERRAL FOR HOSPITAL CARE
Introduction
Evaluation
Treatment
    Adults: Home Management of Asthma Exacerbation
    Adults: Hospital and Emergency Department Care
Care after Hospitalization and ED Visits
Managing Exacerbations in Children
Home Management
Office or Emergency Department Management in Children
Hospital Management in Children
Post-hospital Care
CONCLUSIONS
Asthma Diagnosis and Monitoring
Asthma Treatment
    Better Use of Current Treatments
    New Treatments
Prevention

SUMMARY OF IMPORTANT CONCEPTS

- Asthma is a common but complex clinical syndrome affecting people of all ages, characterized by variable airflow obstruction, bronchial hyperresponsiveness and airway inflammation, and manifesting as differing phenotypes.
- The symptoms of asthma are non-specific, and diagnosis may not be straightforward in community settings. Spirometry is used to demonstrate the airflow obstruction, and patient-held peak expiratory flow (PEF) meters to show variable airflow obstruction.
- Symptoms and airflow limitation vary between individuals and over time, either spontaneously, in response to triggers (such as allergens and viral infection), or as a result of treatment.
- Step-wise treatment is advocated, with step-up if control is inadequate and step-down when stable. Regular inhaled corticosteroids (ICS) are the primary treatment of persistent asthma, with inhaled bronchodilators used as rescue medication.
- Most patients have inadequate asthma control for a variety of reasons, which include severe disease, inadequate or ineffective treatment, non-adherence to treatment, and the effects of comorbidities.

INTRODUCTION AND OVERVIEW

Background

Asthma is a complex clinical syndrome characterized by variable airflow obstruction, bronchial hyperresponsiveness (BHR), and cellular inflammation. Asthma is defined by the Global Initiative in Asthma (GINA)[1] as *"a heterogeneous disease, usually characterized by airway inflammation. It is defined by the presence of respiratory symptoms such as wheeze, shortness of breath, chest tightness and cough that vary over time and in intensity, together with variable expiratory airflow limitation."*

Asthma is a common and potentially serious condition affecting an estimated 300 million individuals of all ages worldwide, comprising 1–18% of the population in different countries; highest in economically developed countries but rising over time in low- and middle-income countries.[2,3] It poses a major burden on patients, their families and communities, and on health economies.[4]

Asthma results in variable respiratory symptoms and variable airflow limitation, leading to activity and quality of life impairment and sometimes in episodic flare-ups ('asthma attacks' or exacerbations) that may result in emergency healthcare utilization, hospitalization and in rare cases, even death. Classic asthma symptoms include breathlessness, wheezing, chest tightness, phlegm production, and cough, particularly at night or early morning. Asthma may manifest only as a chronic cough (cough-variant asthma) or as exercise intolerance.

Symptoms and airflow limitation vary between individuals and over time, either spontaneously, in response to triggers, or as a result of treatment. Although treatable with effective inhaled, oral and parental therapies, there is no cure. Asthma therefore imposes a major burden on health systems, on societies through costs of treatment and lost productivity, and on personal and family life. As it is such a common condition, the bulk of diagnosis and management occurs in primary care in most economically developed countries, with specialist care generally reserved for those with severe disease, poor control, or diagnostic uncertainty.

The airways in people with asthma usually show persistent but therapeutically modifiable inflammation and demonstrate bronchial (airway) hyperresponsiveness (BHR, i.e. increased sensitivity to bronchoconstrictor stimuli). BHR is found in almost all symptomatic asthmatic patients,[5] can increase after sensitizing exposures, and can decrease after anti-inflammatory treatment. Provocation of asthma can occur through interaction with a variety of trigger factors, including allergens, airborne irritants, viral respiratory infections, and occupational exposure, each of which likely acts through different pathways to produce the same end result: multicellular inflammation, BHR, and airflow obstruction. Exposure to triggers can result in bronchospasm, respiratory symptoms, and asthma attacks, particularly in those with uncontrolled or under-treated asthma.

Diagnosis

The symptoms of asthma are non-specific and shared with other respiratory and non-respiratory conditions, and diagnosis may not be straightforward. Airway inflammation and BHR are fundamental to the definition of asthma, but are currently rarely measured in primary care. Spirometry is used to demonstrate the presence and reversibility of airflow obstruction, and patient-held peak expiratory flow (PEF) meters can be used to show variable airflow obstruction over a period of time (e.g., 2–4 weeks). Variable and reversible airway obstruction is specific but insensitive in the diagnosis of asthma, as airway physiology may be normal in the absence of asthma triggers.[6] Although there is evidence of 'under-diagnosis,' based on the presence of suggestive symptoms and findings in population-based surveys in people without a diagnosis of asthma,[7] there is also growing evidence that a considerable minority of patients diagnosed and treated for asthma in the community lack objective evidence of the disease.[8,9] Lung function testing with spirometry and PEF monitoring is possible in primary care settings, but needs to be of a high standard. Lung function can be difficult to measure in younger children. The criteria for the diagnosis of asthma should be (but are often not) recorded in the medical record.

Airway Inflammation and Remodeling

Airway inflammation is the principal mechanism of asthma, and the main treatment target. Typical features of airway inflammation are increased eosinophils, mast cells, and lymphocytes and a predominance of type 2 helper T lymphocytes (Th2 cells), which produce mediators such as interleukin-3 (IL-3), IL-4, IL-5, IL-13, and granulocyte-macrophage colony-stimulating factor (GM-CSF). However, some patients exhibit different patterns of inflammation, including neutrophilic bronchitis or, less frequently, few inflammatory cells (pauci granulocytic phenotype).[10]

Asthma is characterized by structural changes in the airway that may precede the development of asthma, including epithelial damage, subepithelial fibrosis, increased airway vasculature, and increased smooth muscle mass.[11] Mucous hypersecretion is associated with an increase in the number of secretory glands and goblet cells.

Treatment

A step-wise approach to treatment is generally applied and is advocated in guidelines,[12,13] based on the effectiveness, safety, cost, and availability of medication. Treatment step is increased in those not achieving control and reduced after a period (e.g., 3–6 months) of full control. Regular 'controller' therapy with inhaled corticosteroids (ICS) is advocated for most, for symptom control and risk reduction. Inhaled short-acting inhaled bronchodilators are provided as 'rescue' medication to temporarily reverse bronchospasm, usually in the form of short-acting inhaled β_2-agonists. In those uncontrolled on standard doses of ICS, long-acting bronchodilators (usually as long-acting β_2-agonists, LABA) may be added to ICS, often in the form of a fixed dose ICS-LABA combination inhaler. Other add-on treatments may be used in those not achieving control, including leukotriene receptor antagonists (LTRA), theophyllines, and inhaled long-acting anti-muscarinic cholinergic antagonists (LAMA). Newer treatments for specific groups of patients with difficult-to-control asthma include parenteral monoclonal antibodies targeted at different parts of the complex inflammatory pathway (e.g., anti-IgE).

Prevalence and Impact of Asthma

Asthma prevalence has ranged from 3% to 5% in developing countries to >20% in developed countries, affecting people of all ages. The disability-adjusted life years lost due to asthma is estimated at 15 million per year, which equates to 1% of total global health impairment and is similar to the impact of diabetes, cirrhosis of the liver and schizophrenia. Although some countries have reported a reduction in hospitalization and deaths in recent years, for many economically developed countries, the improvements seen over the last decades of the last century have plateaued in the new millennium. The prevalence of asthma is increasing in many developing countries. In clinical trials, most (but not all) patients are able to achieve high levels of control,[14] yet surveys repeatedly show that in 'real life,' most patients continue to suffer significant levels of symptoms and many have asthma attacks.[15] This is sometimes related to biologically severe, therapy-resistant disease, but more often to avoidable behavioral factors such as poor adherence to treatment, poor inhaler technique, or to unaddressed comorbidities. A recent UK national review of asthma deaths[16] reported preventable factors in most.

HISTORICAL PERSPECTIVE

While originally considered a disease of bronchospasm treated purely with bronchodilators, overuse of inhaled β-agonist bronchodilators in the 1970s and 1980s and an associated increase in mortality led to a re-evaluation of the disease as one of airway inflammation in genetically susceptible individuals driven by environmental exposures mostly to inhaled allergens and viral infections. It is the variable characteristics of asthma that has given rise to the concept of differing subtypes (phenotypes) with differing natural histories over the life course and differing responses to therapeutic interventions. Allergic-type asthma is frequently accompanied by other manifestations of allergy such as allergic rhinitis and atopic dermatitis (AD).

EPIDEMIOLOGY

Asthma (Fig. 7-1) usually begins in early childhood, although it may later remit (sometimes recurring in adult life). Of asthma sufferers, 95% have their first episode of wheezing before the age of 6 years. Adult-onset asthma occurs more rarely, and should raise consideration of occupational asthma (see below). Adult-onset asthma is more common in women and is associated with more persistent airflow obstruction, a lack of association with atopy, and a worse prognosis.[17]

Early-life wheezing often remits, but asthma lasting into adult life is likely to be persistent. Asthma is more common in boys than girls, but more common in women than men, the gender switch occurring in adolescence. Asthma has become more common in all ages in recent decades, paralleled by similar increases in sensitization and allergic diseases such as atopic dermatitis and allergic rhinitis. It is associated with Western lifestyles and prevalence increases as populations adopt such lifestyles and become urbanized. In total, 250 000 people die from asthma each year, accounting for 1 in every 250 deaths worldwide.

Incidence

Currently, there are no international measures of asthma incidence, or the risk of developing asthma within a specified time. A US study found the incidence of asthma in the first year of life was 3%, dropping to 0.9% and then to 0.1% in the age group 1 to 4 years and after the age of 15 years, respectively. A New Zealand cohort study reported that at age 9 years, 27% of all children had a history of at least one episode of wheezing, and 4.2% were receiving asthma therapy. These figures are similar in US and Australian cohort studies[18,19]; in all, the age of first reported wheeze was greatest in the first year and levelled off in the teenage years.

Adult onset asthma is unusual, with an estimated incidence of 4.6 cases per 1000 person-years in females and 3.6 in males.

Prevalence

Due to the intermittent nature of asthma, wheezing at any time in the previous 12 months is often used to define asthma. The recognition of differing wheezing

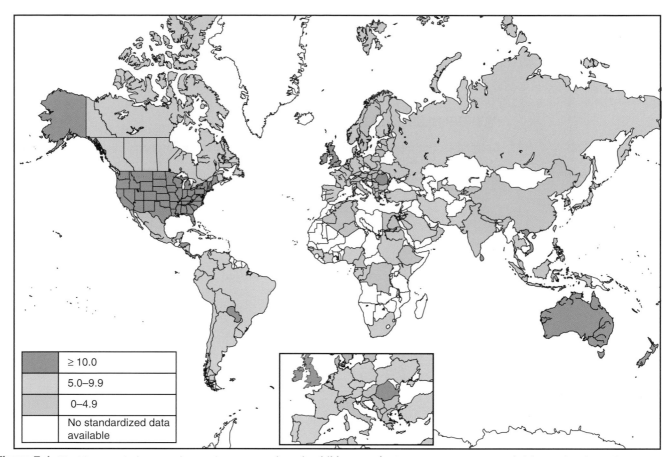

Figure 7-1 World map of the prevalence of current asthma in children aged 13–14 years. Map provided by Richard Beasley. Data are based on ISAAC III.[3] The prevalence of current asthma in the 13–14 year age group is estimated as 50% of the prevalence of self-reported wheezing in the previous 12 months. *(From Global Initiative For Asthma®, Online Appendix, Global Strategy For Asthma Management and Prevention, Revised 2014.)*

phenotypes, particularly in younger children, hampers the definitive labeling of asthma. The International Study of Asthma and Allergies in Childhood (ISAAC) reported the 12-month prevalence of symptoms ranged from 3% to 5% in countries that included Indonesia, China, and Greece, to >20% in Canada, Australia, New Zealand, and the UK.[20] The prevalence of childhood asthma in Western countries either remained steady or decreased somewhat in the 7 years between the ISAAC surveys, but increased in many low-prevalence non-Western countries. The plateau in Western countries may represent the population having achieved its genetic potential: all children predisposed to develop asthma now do so. The increase in low-prevalence countries appears as the economy develops and the countries become more 'Westernized.' Research is needed to understand the mechanisms underlying changes in prevalence, such as alteration in the microbial colonization in the lung and gastrointestinal tract, differing exposures to environmental chemicals and pollutants and differing diets that accompany Western-type lifestyles. In developed countries, a close association exists between early life allergic sensitization and childhood asthma,[18] but not in many developing countries, where non-atopic asthma may predominate.[21]

Changing Trends

Asthma in many countries is increasing in prevalence. The proportion of US children up to 17 years with asthma over a 12-month period increased from 3.6% in 1980, to 7.5% in 1995. US asthma prevalence has risen from 8.7% in 2001 to 9.6% in 2009. Boys experience an elevated prevalence rate until 17 years, from when prevalence in girls is higher. Children of American Indian or Alaska Native descent have asthma prevalence rates 25% higher than black and 60% higher than white children. Puerto Rican children have the highest prevalence of all groups, 140% higher than non-Hispanic white children, whereas Mexican and Asian children have low reported rates. The increases in asthma prevalence in Africa, Latin America, and Asia result in a growing global burden of asthma.

PATHOGENESIS AND ETIOLOGY

Asthma is a complex syndrome manifesting through an interaction of genetic and environmental factors. Persistent airway inflammation is a key feature, accompanied by airway wall remodeling. Structural changes occur primarily in the major bronchi but as asthma becomes severe, it also involves smaller bronchi and bronchioles.[22] Alveolar inflammation can occasionally occur.[23] Chronic inflammation is accompanied by structural changes referred to as *remodeling*. At least two thirds have features of allergy, constituting *allergic* or *extrinsic asthma*, usually accompanied by elevated levels of circulating immunoglobulin E (IgE), and usually beginning in childhood. In contrast, *nonallergic* or *intrinsic* asthma is not associated with atopy, and often begins later in life.

Inflammatory Changes

Airway inflammation is the dominant abnormality, occurring even in the earliest stages. Airway mucosa inflammatory cells include lymphocytes, plasma cells, mast cells, and macrophages, typically associated with eosinophils (Fig. 7-2).[24] Neutrophils are found in some patients, particularly smokers.[25] In allergic asthma, most cells exhibit a helper T cell type 2 (Th2) profile of cytokine secretion, characterized by production of interleukin-4 (IL-4), IL-5, IL-9, granulocyte-macrophage colony-stimulating factor, and IL-1.[26]

However, some patients do not show eosinophilic inflammation and or Th2 cytokine responses. These respond less well to inhaled corticosteroids[27] and other interventions targeting Th2 cytokines. They have a predominantly mononuclear inflammatory cell airway response, with T lymphocytes and activated macrophages. Neutrophils may be prominent in some.

Structural Changes and Airway Remodeling

Structural alterations of the lung are termed *airway remodeling* (see Ch. 1).[28] Airway wall thickening in large and small airways is characteristic, involving all airway wall components. The epithelium is hyperplastic and injured (Fig. 7-3), and autopsies in fatal asthma show epithelial sloughing. Epithelial cells lie on a basement membrane thickened

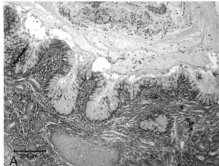
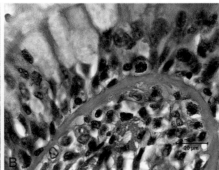
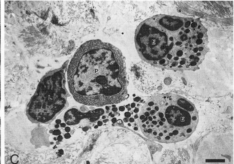

Figure 7-2 A. A low-magnification light micrograph of the bronchial wall in a person with moderate asthma shows mucosal inflammation, increased airway smooth muscle and bronchial gland mass, mucous cell hyperplasia in the surface epithelium, and a prominent mucus plug in the lumen. **B.** Higher magnification of a region of epithelium shown in A demonstrates eosinophils in the epithelial layer and lamina propria, with thickening of the reticular basement membrane. **C.** Transmission electron micrograph of cells in the mucosa from a patient with mild asthma shows a lymphocyte (L), plasma cell (P), and adjacent eosinophils (E) (bar = 2 μm).

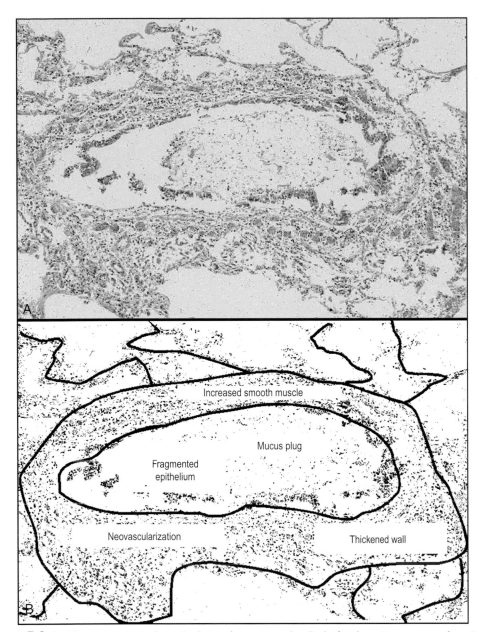

Figure 7-3 **A.** Airway specimen from the lung of a patient who died of asthma (i.e. status asthmaticus) shows profound structural changes (i.e. remodeling). **B.** The airway wall is thickened by cellular infiltration, extracellular matrix deposition, and expansion of smooth muscle, and there is pronounced neovascularization. The epithelium is friable and disintegrating, and a mucus plug occupies the airway lumen (hematoxylin-eosin stain, ×100).

by subepithelial fibrosis, with hyperplasia and hypertrophy of mucus-secreting cells. The airway walls have increased vascularity and smooth muscle hypertrophy or hyperplasia. Stiffness and loss of elasticity of the parenchyma occurs, contributing to air trapping and hyperinflation. The normal parenchyma is linked to the airway by alveolar septa, which apply traction to the airway (Fig. 7-4), but their effectiveness is affected by subepithelial fibrosis and inflammation.

Immunologic Factors

Immunologic and early life immune development factors play a crucial role in the development of asthma and other allergic diseases, which frequently become evident in infancy and early childhood. Early events and exposures affect the developing immune system, with the 'hygiene hypothesis' positing that a lack of exposure to microbial

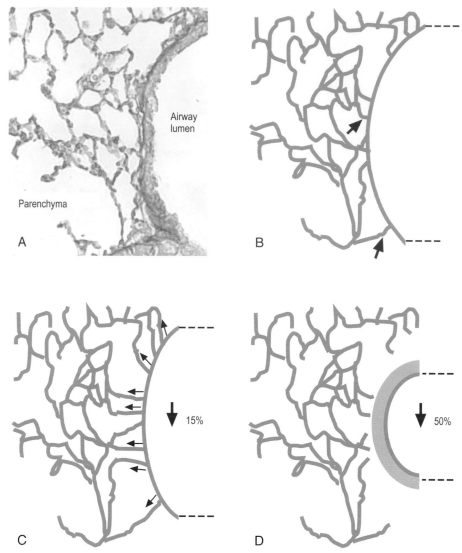

Figure 7-4 Parenchyma-airway interdependence. **A.** The airway and parenchyma are apparent in the stained histologic section of a lung. **B.** The alveolar septa attach to the outer portion of the airway wall (arrows). **C.** The attachments function as tethers that apply outward tension (small arrows) when a normal (unremodeled) airway constricts. **D.** When an airway is remodeled (shaded area), the tethers are effectively broken, allowing the airway to constrict more than occurs in an unremodeled airway.

antigens in early life leads to allergy.[29] Allergic children show differences in both innate and adaptive immune responses that contribute to the production of allergen-specific IgE and so to allergy and asthma. A range of factors (microbial contact, diet, cigarette smoke, other airborne pollutants) increase the risk of allergic disease (Figs. 7-5, 7-6).

Genetics and Epigenetics

Susceptibility to asthma and allergy results from many genetic factors. Multiple genes, each with a modest effect, combine with environmental factors to produce the phenotypes of asthma. Genome-wide association studies (GWAS) have provided insights into pathogenesis, but these have so far failed to translate into novel therapeutic or preventative interventions. Increasing numbers of genes have been identified as asthma-susceptibility genes by the use of GWAS (Table 7-1).[30–45] Gene–environment interaction studies have demonstrated the importance of environmental triggers for initiation, exacerbation, and persistence of asthma. Candidate gene association studies evaluate

Text continued on p. 164

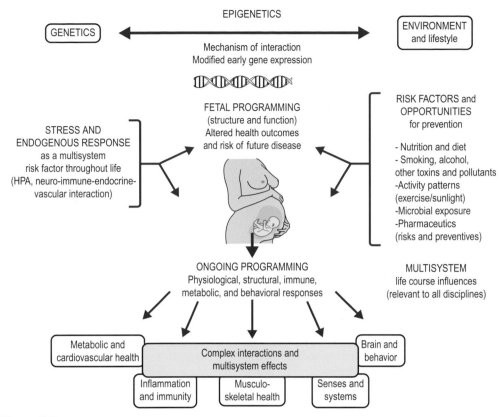

Figure 7-5 Importance of early life events in the programming of structural and functional development. Physiologic, immune, metabolic, and behavioral patterns of response are determined early in development and may be modified by events and exposures early in life. Epigenetic effects provide a mechanism for gene–environment interactions, which may alter future disease risk with potentially greater effects in early life, when systems are developing. The same developmental plasticity provides opportunities early in life for disease prevention. HPA, hypothalamic–pituitary axis. *(Adapted from the University of Western Australia Developmental Origins of Health and Disease [DOHaD] Consortium, Perth, Australia, 2012.)*

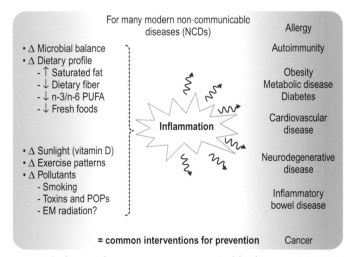

Figure 7-6 Common risk factors for many non-communicable diseases (NCDs); inflammation is a common element. Lifestyle changes are associated with an increase in inflammatory diseases, suggesting common risk factors and a central role for the immune system. Many risk factors for allergic disease are also implicated in many other NCDs, highlighting the need for a multidisciplinary approach to disease prevention. EM, Electromagnetic; POPs, persistent organic pollutants; PUFA, polyunsaturated fatty acid.

TABLE 7-1 Genome-wide Association Studies for Asthma and Allergic Disease

Study	Discovery population	Study size	Phenotype analyzed	Genes or loci*	Gene product and functional role
Moffatt et al. (2007)[30]	UK (Caucasian), German	994 asthmatics and 1243 controls; replicated in 2320 (German) and 3301 (UK) individuals	Childhood-onset asthma	ORMDL3, GSDMA or GSDMB	Orosomucoid 1–like 3: transmembrane protein anchored in the endoplasmic reticulum but function unknown gasdermin A and B: expressed in epithelium and gut but function unknown; locus also associated with Crohn's disease and ulcerative colitis
Weidinger et al. (2008)[31]	European	1530 individuals, replication in four independent samples ($n = 9769$)	IgE levels, allergic sensitization	FCER1A	Fc fragment of IgE high-affinity receptor 1, alpha polypeptide: IgE receptor α unit initiates inflammation and hypersensitivity responses to allergens
				RAD50	RAD50 homolog (S. cerevisiae): important for DNA double-strand break repair, cell cycle checkpoint activation, telomere maintenance, and meiotic recombination; adjacent to the IL-4, IL-13 cytokine locus
Gudbjartsson et al. (2009)[32]	Icelandic, European, East Asians, 10 different populations	9392 (Icelandic); 12 118 (European); 5212 (East Asian); 7996 cases and 44 890 controls (10 populations)	Blood eosinophil counts	IL1RL1	IL-1 receptor–like 1: murine studies suggest receptor is induced by proinflammatory stimuli and may be involved in helper T cell function
				WDR36, TSLP	WD repeat domain 36: may facilitate formation of heterotrimeric or multiprotein complexes; family members involved in many cellular processes, including cell cycle progression, signal transduction, apoptosis, and gene regulation; gene adjacent to TSLP. Thymic stromal lymphopoietin: epithelial cell–derived cytokine with a key role in induction of allergic inflammation
				RAD50 MYB	See earlier. Myeloblastosis viral oncogene homolog: nuclear transcription factor implicated in proliferation, survival, and differentiation of hematopoietic stem and progenitor cells
				IL33	IL-33: epithelial cell–derived IL-1–like cytokine ligand for the IL-1 receptor–related protein ST2; activates mast cells and Th2 lymphocytes
Kim et al. (2009)[33]	Korean	84 TDI asthma cases and 263 unexposed, healthy controls	TDI asthma	CTNNA3	Catenin (cadherin-associated protein), alpha 3: key molecule in the E-cadherin–mediated cell–cell adhesion complex; α-catenin suppresses invasion and tumor growth and inhibits RAS-MAPK activation; genetic polymorphisms may disturb defense systems of the airway epithelium, increasing airway hyperresponsiveness to environmental toxins such as TD

TABLE 7-1 Genome-wide Association Studies for Asthma and Allergic Disease (Continued)

Study	Discovery population	Study size	Phenotype analyzed	Genes or loci*	Gene product and functional role
Moffatt et al. (2010)[34]	European	10 365 persons with physician-diagnosed asthma and 16 110 unaffected persons	Asthma	IL18R1	IL-18 receptor 1: member of the IL-1 receptor family; DC-derived IL-18 drives Treg differentiation and plays a role in airway inflammation in murine asthma models; IL-18 expression increased in asthma; adjacent to IL1RL1 (see earlier)
				HLA-DQ	MHC class II, DQ members: due to extensive linkage disequilibrium across the HLA region, difficult to identify specific genes that underlie association signals in this locus; extended haplotypes across the HLA region have been studied in relation to specific allergen sensitization and production of TNF-α, which is encoded in the HLA class III region
				IL33	See earlier
				SMAD3	SMAD family member 3: transcription modulator activated by TGF-β, a cytokine that controls proliferation, differentiation, and other functions in many cell types, including Tregs; Smad3-deficient mice have increased levels of proinflammatory cytokines in lungs; potential role in airway remodeling
				IL2RB	IL-2 receptor, beta: IL-2 controls survival and proliferation of Tregs; implicated in differentiation and homeostasis of effector T cell subgroups, including Th1, Th2, Th17, and memory CD8+ T cells
				IL13	IL-13: Th2 cytokine that drives IgE production by B cells and goblet cell differentiation and mucus production by airway epithelial cells
				RORA	RAR-related orphan receptor A: encodes member of NR1 subfamily of nuclear hormone receptors; expressed at high levels in keratinocytes with cluster of proteins that form the structural and innate immune defenses of the epithelial barrier
				SLC22A5	Solute carrier family 22 (organic cation transporter), member 5: encodes a carnitine transporter
			IgE levels	IL13	See earlier
				HLA locus	See earlier
				STAT6	Signal transducer and activator of transcription 6: transcription factor critical to IL-4 and IL-13 intracellular signaling regulating IgE and Th2 cytokine production

Continued on following page

TABLE 7-1   Genome-wide Association Studies for Asthma and Allergic Disease (Continued)

Study	Discovery population	Study size	Phenotype analyzed	Genes or loci*	Gene product and functional role
				IL4R, IL21R	IL-4 receptor: a subunit of the IL-4/IL-13 receptor IL-21 receptor: IL-21 and its receptor (IL-21R) are upregulated in skin lesions of patients with active atopic dermatitis and in murine models; they play a critical role in sensitization and allergic inflammation in skin
Sleiman et al. (2010)[35]	US	793 asthmatic children and 1988 matched controls of European ancestry (discovery set); 917 asthmatics and 1546 matched controls of European ancestry (replication 1); 1667 North American children of African ancestry who had asthma and 2045 ancestrally matched controls (replication 2)	Asthma	DENND1B	DENN/MADD domain–containing 1B: gene is expressed by NK cells and DCs; DENND1B protein predicted to interact with the TNF-α receptor
Li X et al. (2010)[36]	US (Caucasian)	473 severe asthmatics and 1892 general population controls	Severe or difficult-to-treat asthma	RAD50-IL13 and HLA-DR and -DQ regions	See earlier
Ferreira et al. (2011)[37]	Australian (Caucasian)	2669 physician-diagnosed asthmatics and 4528 controls from Australia, combined with data from Moffatt et al. (2010) ($n = 26\,475$); further replication in additional 25\,358 independent samples	Asthma	IL6R	IL-6 receptor: increased sIL-6R level in serum and airways of asthma patients; correlates with Th2 cytokine production in the lung; selective blockade of sIL-6R in mice suppresses IL-4, IL-5, and IL-13 production and decreases eosinophil numbers in the lung
				11q13.5 near C11orf30, LRRC32	Leucine-rich repeat containing 32: this locus is also associated with atopic dermatitis (see later) and Crohn disease
Hirota T et al. (2011)[38]	Japanese	7171 cases, 27\,912 controls	Adult asthma	USP38 and GAB1	Ubiquitin-specific peptidase 38: function is unclear GRB2-associated binding protein 1: scaffolding adopter protein that plays an important role in the signaling pathway activated by cytokine receptors for IL-3, IL-6, IFN-αI, IFN-γ, and B cell and T cell receptors
				A locus on chromosome 10p14	Region contains no reported genes but is located 1 Mb downstream of GATA3, a master regulator of Th2 cell differentiation
				A gene-rich region on chromosome 12q13	Associated with type 1 diabetes and alopecia areata; strongest associated SNP is located 2 kb upstream from IKZF4 (i.e. EOS), which is involved in differentiation of regulatory T cells

TABLE 7-1   Genome-wide Association Studies for Asthma and Allergic Disease (Continued)

Study	Discovery population	Study size	Phenotype analyzed	Genes or loci*	Gene product and functional role
Torgerson et al. (2011)[39]	European-American, African-American or African-Caribbean, and Latino ancestry	3246 cases with asthma, 3385 non-asthmatic controls, 1702 asthma case-parent trios, and 355 family-based cases and 468 family-based controls	Asthma	*PYHIN1*	Pyrin and HIN domain family member 1: asthma susceptibility specific to persons of African descent
Tantisira et al. (2011)[40]	US (Caucasian)	Four independent populations totaling 935 persons	Improvement in lung function in response to glucocorticoid therapy for asthma	*GLCCI1*	Glucocorticoid-induced transcript 1: expressed in lung and immune cells; expression is significantly enhanced by glucocorticoids in asthma-like conditions
Du et al. (2012)[41]	US (Caucasian)	403 subjects and trios; replication in 584 children from a Costa Rican cohort	Gene–vitamin D interaction in asthma exacerbations	*CRTAM*	Cytotoxic and regulatory T cell molecule: this class I MHC-restricted T cell–associated molecule is highly expressed in activated human CD8+ and NK T cells, both implicated in asthma pathogenesis
Esparza-Gordillo et al. (2009)[42]	European	939 cases, 975 controls. 270 complete nuclear families with two affected siblings	Atopic dermatitis	C11orf30 locus	See earlier
Paternoster et al. (2011)[43]	European	5606 cases and 20 565 controls from 16 population-based cohorts; replication in 5419 cases and 19 833 controls from 14 studies	Atopic dermatitis	*OVOL1* Locus near *ADAMTS10* and *ACTL9* *KIF3A*	Ovo-like 1: belongs to highly conserved family of genes that regulate development and differentiation of epithelial tissues and germ cells; regulates epidermal proliferation and differentiation ADAM metallopeptidase with thrombospondin type 1 motif and actin-like 9: most strongly associated SNP is upstream of ADAMTS10 and downstream of ACTL9 (encoding a hypothetical protein); ADAMTS proteins are complex, secreted, zinc-dependent metalloproteinases that bind to and cleave extracellular matrix components and are involved in connective tissue remodeling and extracellular matrix turnover Kinesin family member 3A: located within the Th2 cytokine cluster at 5q31.1
Sun et al. (2011)[44]	Chinese Han	1012 cases and 1362 controls; replication in 3624 cases and 12 197 controls	Atopic dermatitis	*TMEM232* and *SLC25A46*	Transmembrane protein 232: encodes a protein belonging to the functional class of tetraspan transmembrane proteins. Solute carrier family 25, member 46: this family encodes mitochondrial carrier proteins, which may shuttle metabolites across the inner mitochondrial membrane

Continued on following page

TABLE 7-1   Genome-wide Association Studies for Asthma and Allergic Disease (Continued)

Study	Discovery population	Study size	Phenotype analyzed	Genes or loci*	Gene product and functional role
				TNFRSF6B and ZGPAT	Tumor necrosis factor receptor superfamily, member 6B decoy: important role in adaptive immune responses Zinc finger, CCCH type with G patch domain: located at 20q13.3; limited analysis of variants found no significant association
Ramasamy et al. (2012)[45]	European	3933 self-reported cases and 8965 controls	Allergic rhinitis	HLA-DRB4 C11orf30 locus TMEM232 and SLC25A46	HLA locus (see earlier) See earlier See earlier

*Genes or loci identified in addition to those previously identified in genome-wide association studies.
DC, Dendritic cell; HLA, human leukocyte antigen; IFN-γ, interferon-γ; IgE, immunoglobulin E; IL, interleukin; MAPK, mitogen-activated protein kinase; MHC, major histocompatibility complex; NK, natural killer; sIL-6R, soluble IL-6 receptor; SMAD, derived from *Drosophila* mothers against decapentaplegic (Mad) and *C. elegans Sma* genes; SNP, single-nucleotide polymorphism; TDI, toluene diisocyanate induced; TGF-β, transforming growth factor-β; Th1, helper T cell type 1; Th2, helper T cell type 2; Th17, helper T cell type 17; TNF-α, tumor necrosis factor-α; Treg, regulatory T cell; US, United States.

genetic variation in genes involved in disease pathogenesis (e.g., genes encoding cytokines, chemokines, and receptors). For example, *ADAM33* was identified as an asthma-susceptibility gene, with a polymorphism associated with early-life measures of lung function.[46]

Pharmacogenetics refers to the relationship between genetic variation and drug response, with research focused on the β2-adrenoceptor encoded by the gene ADRB2. Specific alleles for this gene predict response to short-acting β-agonists. Responses to ICS and leukotriene antagonists vary between individuals, and polymorphisms in steroid-signaling and other pathways may be important. In the future, systems incorporating genetic predictors of response may enable targeted treatment.

Epigenetic processes result from modifications of DNA structure without a change in the sequence in response to environmental exposures, and may be passed between generations. Epigenetic factors are a particular focus of interest in current research, are important modifiers of susceptibility, and may contribute to heritability.

CLINICAL FEATURES AND PHENOTYPES OF ASTHMA

Phenotypes of Adult Asthma

Asthma is not a single disease but a group of clinical entities that share common features. The term *phenotype* refers to the observable characteristics of an individual or group resulting from interaction of its genotype with its environment. Phenotypes reflect the heterogeneity of asthma. Asthma develops from complex interactions of environmental exposures and underlying genetic predispositions, resulting in heterogeneity.[47,48] Phenotypes are defined by clinical features, pattern of inflammation, pulmonary function, triggers or on comorbidity (Box 7-1). Variability is noted in age of onset, allergy versus no allergy, inflammatory patterns, and response to treatment. Cluster analyses have identified clinically distinct phenotypes in adults.[49] An *endotype* is a subtype defined by distinct functional or pathophysiologic mechanisms, and addresses etiology and pathophysiology.[50] Assessment of phenotypes potentially allows effective targeting of therapy, but is still at an early stage in routine clinical care. Asthma is often associated with comorbidities such as rhinitis, sinusitis, gastroesophageal reflux disease (GERD), obstructive sleep apnea (OSA), hormonal disorders, and psychological disturbances (Table 7-2).[51]

TABLE 7-2 Tests for Asthma-related Comorbidities

Comorbidity	Potentially useful tests

Rhinitis
  Allergic
 	
  Non-allergic
  Associated with nasal polyps
  CRS and sinusitis
	
	Allergy skin-prick test
	Serum-specific IgE
	ENT examination
	Sinus radiography/CT scan

GERD	Proton-pump inhibitor treatment trial 24-h esophageal pH measurement Imaging techniques
Obesity	BMI and other obesity measures Detection of metabolic syndrome
OSA	Sleep studies: polysomnography
Psychopathologies	Psychological evaluation
Dysfunctional breathing	Nijmegen questionnaire[30]
VCD	Flow-volume loop Visualization of the pharynx: laryngoscopy
Hormonal and metabolic disorders	Hormone measurements
COPD and smoking	Pulmonary function tests Chest radiography/CT scan Biomarkers

Infections
  Viral
  Bacterial
  Fungal
	
	Specific serologies
	Various identification measures
	Precipitins for *Aspergillus*/fungal cultures/*Aspergillus* serology

BMI, Body mass index; COPD, chronic obstructive pulmonary disease; CRS, chronic rhinosinusitis; CT, computed tomography; ENT, ear, nose, and throat; GERD, gastroesophageal reflux disease; IgE, immuno globulin E; OSA, obstructive sleep apnea; VCD, vocal cord dysfunction.
(Adapted from Boulet LP, Boulay MÈ. Asthma-related comorbidities. Expert Rev Respir Med 2011; 5:377–393.)

Box 7-1 Phenotypes of Asthma

BASED ON AIRWAY INFLAMMATION

- Eosinophilic
- Neutrophilic
- Pauci-granulocytic

BASED ON CLINICAL FEATURES

- Mild, moderate, or severe asthma
- Exacerbation-prone
- Treatment-resistant
- Early-onset or late-onset asthma
- Asthma in the elderly

BASED ON PULMONARY FUNCTION

- With a component of fixed airway obstruction
- With marked/rapid fluctuations of airway caliber
- With marked hyperinflation

BASED ON TRIGGERS

- Allergic or non-allergic asthma
- Aspirin or non-steroidal anti-inflammatory drugs

- Occupational allergens or irritants
- Hormones: premenstrual and menopausal asthma
- Exercise- or cold air–induced asthma
- Asthma in the high-level athlete
- Asthma in the smoker

BASED ON ASSOCIATED COMORBID CONDITIONS

- Rhinitis/rhinosinusitis, nasal polyps, and aspirin intolerance
- Psychological disturbances (e.g., depression, anxiety disorders)
- With dysfunctional breathing (hyperventilation syndrome, vocal cord dysfunction)
- With associated chronic obstructive pulmonary disease
- Asthma in the obese

Phenotypes in Children

Symptoms and clinical features are broadly similar in children, but childhood phenotypes of wheezing illnesses are complex, particularly in younger children. The Tucson Children's Respiratory Study (TCRS) identified four wheezing phenotypes: (1) never (51%); (2) transient early (20%), with onset of wheezing before age 3 years and wheezing resolved by age 6; (3) persistent (14%), with onset of wheezing before age 3 years with continued wheezing at age 6; and (4) late onset (15%), with onset of wheezing between 3 and 6 years of age, and differences in risk factors and persistence between atopic and non-atopic wheezers. Early transient wheezing is the most prevalent phenotype, characterized by recurrent episodes in the first year. Of children who wheeze in the first 3 years, 60% have resolution of their symptoms by 6 years of age. Transient wheezing has no significant relationship to atopy, but is associated with maternal smoking during pregnancy (odds ratio [OR], 2.2; 95% confidence interval [CI], 1.3–3.7). Transient wheezing is associated with lower levels of lung function. Less than one quarter of transient wheezers continue to wheeze during adolescence. Children with transient wheezing do not have increased methacholine reactivity or PEF variability at age 11 years.

Non-atopic persistent wheezing is associated with the first episode of wheezing occurring before the age of 1 year, representing 20% of wheezy children under 3 years of age. Episodes become less frequent by teenage years. Children have a lower level of prebronchodilator lung function and enhanced airway reactivity. IgE-associated atopic persistent wheezing is found in 20% of children who wheeze during the first 3 years, with symptoms first presenting after age 1 year and an association with early sensitization to food or aeroallergens. Risk factors include male gender, parental asthma, atopic dermatitis, eosinophilia at 9 months, and history of wheezing with infections. Children have normal lung function in infancy but reduced lung function at age 6 years. BHR is often observed.

Persistent wheezers continue to have symptoms and lower airflow as they reach teenage years, but no progressive deficits in lung function. Other longitudinal birth cohort studies have reported similar results, although these have suggested additional phenotypes. The European Respiratory Society has defined symptom-based phenotypes: 'episodic' (or 'viral') and 'multi-trigger' wheeze.[52] Children with episodic (viral) wheeze have discrete symptomatic periods. Children with multi-trigger wheeze have wheezing both during exacerbations and between episodes in response to various triggers, including viruses, allergens, exercise, and cigarette smoke, and also have lower airway function.[53]

EVALUATION AND DIAGNOSIS

The lack of a simple gold standard diagnostic test and limited availability of diagnostic tests may lead to difficulties in primary care, and there is evidence of both over- and under-diagnosis.[9]

Diagnosis in Adults

Risk Factors

Potential risk factors for the development of asthma should be ascertained and documented. These include a personal or family history of asthma and allergy; exposure to airborne allergens, tobacco smoke, or other pollutants; and past respiratory infections (Box 7-2).[54]

History and Examination

Asthma is a symptomatic condition. Symptom pattern and triggers should be documented. However, symptoms do not accurately predict pulmonary function and are not reliable to establish a diagnosis in isolation.[8,55] Physical examination is often normal unless the disease is severe or the examination is performed during an exacerbation or exposure to triggers, when wheezes can be heard on auscultation, with prolonged expiratory time.

Lung Function

Pulmonary function tests should always be performed in the diagnosis of asthma (Box 7-3). Spirometry is the preferred method to measure airway obstruction.[13] A ratio of

---

Box 7-2   Suggested Items for Medical History*

A detailed medical history of the new patient who is known, or thought, to have asthma should address the following items:

1. Symptoms
   - Cough
   - Wheezing
   - Shortness of breath
   - Chest tightness
   - Sputum production
2. Pattern of symptoms
   - Perennial, seasonal, or both
   - Continual, episodic, or both
   - Onset, duration, frequency (number of days or nights, per week or month)
   - Diurnal variations, especially nocturnal and on awakening in early morning
3. Precipitating and/or aggravating factors
   - Viral respiratory infections
   - Environmental allergens, indoor (e.g., mold, house-dust mite, cockroach, animal dander or secretory products) and outdoor (e.g., pollen)
   - Characteristics of home, including: age, location, cooling and heating system, wood-burning stove, humidifier, carpeting over concrete, presence of molds or mildew, characteristics of rooms where patient spends time (e.g., bedroom and living room with attention to bedding, floor covering, stuffed furniture)
   - Smoking (patient and others in home or day-care)
   - Exercise
   - Occupational chemicals or allergens
   - Environmental change (e.g., moving to new home; going on vacation; alterations in workplace, work processes, or materials used)
   - Irritants (e.g., tobacco smoke, strong odors, air pollutants, occupational chemicals, dusts and particulates, vapors, gases, aerosols)
   - Emotions (e.g., fear, anger, frustration, hard crying or laughing)
   - Stress (e.g., fear, anger, frustration)
   - Drugs (e.g., aspirin and other non-steroidal anti-inflammatory drugs, β-blockers including eye drops, others)
   - Food, food additives, and preservatives (e.g., sulfites)
   - Changes in weather, exposure to cold air
   - Endocrine factors (e.g., menses, pregnancy, thyroid disease)
   - Comorbid conditions (e.g., sinusitis, rhinitis, GERD)
4. Development of disease and treatment
   - Age of onset and diagnosis
   - History of early-life injury to airways (e.g., bronchopulmonary dysplasia, pneumonia, parental smoking)

- Progression of disease (better or worse)
- Present management and response, including plans for managing exacerbations
- Frequency of using SABA
- Need for oral corticosteroids and frequency of use
5. Family history
   - History of asthma, allergy, sinusitis, rhinitis, eczema, or nasal polyps in close relatives
6. Social history
   - Day-care, workplace, and school characteristics that may interfere with adherence
   - Social factors that interfere with adherence, such as substance abuse
   - Social support/social networks
   - Level of education completed
   - Employment
7. History of exacerbations
   - Usual prodromal signs and symptoms
   - Rapidity of onset
   - Duration
   - Frequency
   - Severity (need for urgent care, hospitalization, ICU admission)
   - Life-threatening exacerbations (e.g., intubation, ICU admission)
   - Number and severity of exacerbations in the past year
   - Usual patterns and management (what works?)
8. Impact of asthma on patient and family
   - Episodes of unscheduled care (ED, urgent care, hospitalization)
   - Number of days missed from school/work
   - Limitation of activity, especially sports and strenuous work
   - History of nocturnal awakening
   - Effect on growth, development behavior, school or work performance, and lifestyle
   - Impact on family routines, activities, or dynamics
   - Economic impact
9. Assessment of patient's and family's perceptions of disease
   - Patient's, parents', and spouse's or partner's knowledge of asthma and in the chronicity of asthma and in the efficacy of treatment
   - Patient's perception and beliefs regarding use and long-term effects of medications
   - Ability of patient and parents, spouse, or partner to cope with disease
   - Level of family support and patient's and parents', spouse's, or partner's capacity to recognize severity of an exacerbation
   - Economic resources
   - Sociocultural beliefs

*This list does not represent a standardized assessment or diagnostic instrument. The validity and reliability of this list has not been assessed.
ED, Emergency department; GERD, gastroesophageal reflux disease; ICU, intensive care unit; SABA, short-acting β-agonists.
(From National Heart, Lung, and Blood Institute. Expert Panel Report 3 (EPR-3): Guidelines for the Diagnosis and Management of Asthma: Full Report 2007. Available at: <http://www.nhlbi.nih.gov/files/docs/guidelines/asthgdln.pdf>; [accessed July 7, 2015.])

---

forced expiratory volume in 1 second (FEV_1) to forced vital capacity (FVC) of <0.7 generally defines obstruction. FEV_1 is an absolute measure of the volume of air exhaled in the first second of forced expiration, and normative tables are available for groups, stratified by ages and sex, allowing the determination of the percent predicted FEV_1. A reduced percent predicted FEV_1 with a low FEV_1/FVC ratio indicates the presence of airway obstruction. Significant reversibility (usually defined as an increase in FEV_1 of 12% or more with at least a 200 mL change) after a bronchodilator or following 4 weeks of anti-inflammatory treatment with ICS suggests asthma. Spirometry is reliable and reproducible when performed correctly,[56] and is entirely possible to perform in primary care settings. However, staff require training, quality assurance is needed, and equipment requires maintenance and calibration. Ideally, spirometers should produce a visible or hard-copy 'flow-volume' or 'volume-time' trace to allow inspection of the adequacy of the test. It has been recommended to use the 5th percentile as the 'lower limit of normal' because these values are not always proportional to the percent of

---

Box 7-3   Diagnosis of Asthma in Adults

Symptoms of episodic breathlessness, wheezing, cough, chest tightness, phlegm production (one or more)
 *PLUS**
 Increase in FEV_1 after a bronchodilator or after a course of controller therapy ≥12% (and a minimum ≥200 mL)
 OR
 Increase in PEF after a bronchodilator or after a course of controller therapy of 60 L/min (minimum ≥20%) or an increase ≥20%, based on multiple daily readings
 OR
 Methacholine PC_{20} <4 mg/mL (4–16 mg/mL is borderline)
 OR
 Decrease in FEV_1 after exercise challenge ≥10–15%[†]

---

*Ideally with an FEV_1/FVC less than the lower limit of normal value (<0.075–0.8).
[†]If exercise-induced asthma is suspected, eucapnic voluntary hyperpnea or mannitol/hyperosmolar challenges may be used if available.
FEV_1, Forced expiratory volume in 1 second; FVC, forced vital capacity; PC_{20}, provocative concentration that induces a 20% fall in FEV_1; PEF, peak expiratory flow.
(Adapted from Global Initiative for Asthma (GINA) 2011. Available at: <http://www.ginasthma.org/guidelines-gina-report-global-strategy-for-asthma.html>; and Lougheed MD, Lemiere C, Ducharme FM, et al.; Canadian Thoracic Society Asthma Clinical Assembly. Canadian Thoracic Society 2012 guideline update: diagnosis and management of asthma in preschoolers, children and adults. Can Respir J 2012; 19:127–64.)

predicted value. However, fixed-ratio lower limit of normal for FEV_1/FVC (70%) and percent of predicted FEV_1 are still most commonly used.

PEF measurements with a portable peak flow meter may be used, although are more dependent on patient effort. Domiciliary morning and night monitoring of PEF (usually as the best of three tests) can be used to demonstrate peak flow variability over a period of time (e.g., 2 weeks) to support the diagnosis of asthma. PEF should be compared with the patient's best value, as normative values are unreliable. Characteristically monitoring in untreated patients produces a 'saw-tooth' pattern, with significant diurnal variability (lower values on morning readings). Diurnal PEF variability is calculated as the highest PEF of the day minus the lowest PEF reading divided by the mean of the day's highest and lowest readings, and averaged over a 1- to 2-week period. Average diurnal variability is >10%, and the greater the variation, the greater is the support for the diagnosis.

Bronchial Hyperreactivity (BHR)

Bronchial provocation tests provide an objective test of the constriction thresholds or 'twitchiness' of the airways. In these tests, patients inhale (usually via a nebulizer) increasing concentrations or cumulative doses of a bronchoconstrictor, and spirometry is repeated until a 20% reduction in baseline FEV_1 is observed. In patients with normal pulmonary function or non-significant reversibility of airway obstruction, a broncho-provocation test can be performed to confirm BHR. Direct challenges involve the inhalation of a bronchoconstrictor; the lower the concentration or dose required, the more hyperreactive are the airways. Direct bronchial challenge tests are highly sensitive judged against a gold standard of a subsequent diagnostic review made by an experienced clinician with the aid of all diagnostic tests and response to treatment over a period of time of some months, and negative tests help exclude asthma. The commonest test used is the methacholine inhalation test, measuring the provocative concentration of methacholine inducing a 20% fall in FEV_1 (PC_{20}). The test is sensitive but not specific, and may be positive in conditions such as rhinitis or chronic obstructive pulmonary disease (COPD). Regular use of ICS may normalize the test.

Indirect bronchial stimuli such as exercise, hypertonic aerosols such as saline or mannitol, adenosine monophosphate, and eucapnic voluntary hyperpnea (EVH) have also been used, and correlate better with airway inflammation.

Determination of the Allergic Status

Asthma is often allergic, and allergy skin-prick tests help identify allergens. The temporal relationship of symptoms with allergen exposure should be documented, but subclinical inflammation after allergen exposure may be insufficient to induce acute symptoms. Measurement of specific immunoglobulin E (IgE) in the serum (e.g., by a radioallergosorbent test [RAST] or ImmunoCAP®) can also identify sensitization to a particular allergen. Although total IgE levels suggest an atopic status, they do not help to establish a diagnosis of asthma and are of limited clinical value.

Assessment of Airway Inflammation

Non-invasive assessments of airway inflammation are helpful in cases of diagnostic difficulty, including induced sputum analysis and measurement of fractional nitric oxide concentration in exhaled breath (FeNO). In general, they are underused.[57] Nebulized hypertonic saline is used to induce sputum, from which inflammatory cell numbers and types are recorded, generally reserved for patients with severe asthma in research and hospital settings. Levels of FeNO are increased in asthma and correlate with the presence of eosinophilic airway inflammation. Production of nitric oxide (NO) by airway epithelial cells is driven by inducible NO synthase (iNOS) and is upregulated in asthmatic inflammation, while the expression of iNOS is decreased by corticosteroid therapy. A recent clinical guideline stated that FeNO may help to detect eosinophilic inflammation, assess the likelihood of corticosteroid responsiveness, contribute to the monitoring of corticosteroid needs, and detect non-adherence.[58] This test is simple to perform, relatively inexpensive and can potentially be performed in primary care settings,[59] although the precise role in diagnosis and monitoring is still being defined.

The usefulness of substances in exhaled breath condensate and of volatile organic compounds (olfactometry) in asthma care remains to be established.

Imaging

Imaging studies are not useful in the diagnosis or follow-up of asthma, but can be used to investigate diagnostic difficulties when they arise such as allergic bronchopulmonary aspergillosis, COPD (emphysema), and interstitial diseases. Lung hyperinflation, a mosaic perfusion pattern at full inspiration (reflecting ventilation-perfusion inequalities), and increased airway wall thickness are more prevalent on high-resolution chest computed tomography in severe asthma.

Asthma Diagnosis in Specific Settings

Occupational Asthma

There is growing recognition that work-related asthma is a major public health concern, and is frequently unrecognized. *Work-related asthma* is a broad term indicating asthma worsened by the workplace,[60] encompassing *occupational asthma* (OA), which is caused by a specific workplace agent, and *work-exacerbated asthma* (WEA), which is asthma worsened by stimuli at the workplace (Fig. 7-7).[61] A widely cited definition emphasizes the causal relationship between asthma and the workplace: '*Occupational asthma is characterized by airway inflammation, variable airflow limitation, and airway hyper-responsiveness due to causes and conditions attributable to a particular occupational environment and not to stimuli encountered outside the workplace.*'[62]

A pooled analysis of studies published up to 2007 indicated that 17.6% of all cases of adult-onset asthma are attributable to workplace exposures.[63] Cohort studies reported incidence rates of 2.7 to 3.5 cases of OA per 100 person-years amongst workers exposed to laboratory animals;[64] 4.1 per 100 person-years amongst those exposed to wheat flour;[65] and 1.8 per 100 person-years amongst dental health apprentices exposed to latex gloves.[66] The pathophysiology in most cases is an immunoglobulin E (IgE)-dependent mechanism. The agents and occupations most commonly implicated are listed in Table 7-3.

The diagnosis is difficult, and requires specialist referral. It is important, as early removal of the sensitizing factor may allow full resolution. Occupational asthma may be suspected from the temporal relationship between asthma symptoms and exposure to workplace sensitizers. To confirm the diagnosis, serial measures of airway responsiveness and PEF can be used, or specific bronchoprovocation tests performed.[67]

TABLE 7-3   Principal Agents Causing Immunologic Occupational Asthma

Agent		Workers/occupations at risk
High-molecular-weight agents		
Cereals (flour)	Wheat, rye, barley, buckwheat	Millers, bakers, pastry makers
Latex	Gloves	Healthcare workers, laboratory technicians
Animals	Mice, rats, cows, seafood	Laboratory workers, farmers, seafood processors
Enzymes	α-Amylase, maxatase, alcalase, papain, bromelain, pancreatin	Baking products manufacture, bakers, detergent production, pharmaceutical industry, food industry
Low-molecular-weight agents		
Isocyanates	Toluene diisocyanate (TDI), methylene diphenyl-diisocyanate (MDI), hexamethylene diisocyanate (HDI)	Polyurethane production, plastic industry, molding, spray painters, insulation installers
Metals	Chromium, nickel, cobalt, platinum	Metal refinery, metal alloy production, electroplaters, welders
Biocides	Aldehydes, quaternary ammonium compounds	Healthcare workers, cleaners
Persulfate salts	Hair bleach	Hairdressers
Acid anhydrides	Phthalic, trimellitic, maleic, tetrachlorophthalic acids	Epoxy resin workers
Reactive dyes	Reactive black 5, pyrazolone derivatives, vinyl sulfones, carmine	Textile workers, food industry workers
Acrylates	Cyanoacrylates, methacrylates, di- and triacrylates	Manufacture of adhesives, dental and orthopedic materials, sculptured fingernails, printing inks, paints and coatings
Wood dusts	Red cedar, iroko, obeche, oak	Sawmill workers, carpenters, cabinet and furniture makers

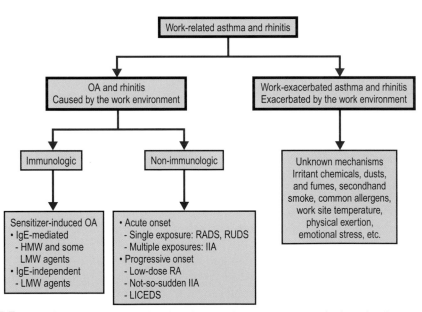

Figure 7-7 Classification of work-related asthma and rhinitis. HMW, high-molecular-weight; IgE, immunoglobulin E; IIA, irritant-induced asthma; LICEDS, low-intensity chronic exposure dysfunction syndrome; LMW, low-molecular-weight; OA, occupational asthma; RADS, reactive airways dysfunction syndrome; RUDS, reactive upper airways dysfunction syndrome.

Asthma in the Elderly

Elderly patients may have difficulty in performing pulmonary function tests and may show a different pattern of asthma, mostly a combined neutrophilic and eosinophilic inflammatory pattern with more severe airway obstruction and physiologic features related to the aging of the lung.[68] COPD is often misdiagnosed in this population.

Box 7-4	Differential Diagnosis of Asthma

- Bronchiolitis
- Cardiac condition (e.g., heart failure)
- Chronic obstructive pulmonary disease
- Cystic fibrosis
- Deconditioning
- Dysfunctional breathing (e.g., hyperventilation syndrome)
- Foreign body aspiration
- Laryngotracheomalacia, tracheal stenosis
- Obstructive sleep apnea
- Other causes of cough (e.g., chronic eosinophilic bronchitis, GERD, ACE-inhibitor)
- Pulmonary embolism
- Pulmonary infiltrate with eosinophilia (PIE syndrome)
- Tracheobronchial tumor
- Upper airways diseases (e.g., upper airway cough syndrome)
- Vocal cord dysfunction

ACE, Angiotensin-converting enzyme; GERD, gastroesophageal reflux disease.

Asthma in the Athlete

Athletes may present with asymptomatic BHR or asthma that is less responsive to therapy.[69] Because symptoms are unreliable and expiratory flows are often normal, bronchoprovocation tests are often needed.

Conditions that May Mimic Asthma

Many conditions may be confused or associated with asthma, and can influence its manifestations (Box 7-4). These conditions include dysfunctional breathing syndromes such as vocal cord dysfunction and hyperventilation syndrome,[70,71] upper airways diseases, deconditioning, obesity-related symptoms, pulmonary embolism, obstructive sleep apnea (OSA), and airway neoplasms. Smoking-induced COPD and cardiac insufficiency may manifest with asthma-like symptoms in elderly patients. Less common masqueraders include bronchiectasis, vasculitis (e.g., Churg–Strauss syndrome), cystic fibrosis, and mastocytosis.

Diagnosis in Children

The natural history of pediatric wheezing is complex. The evaluation is made more complicated by difficulty in obtaining objective lung function measurements and the complexity of wheezing phenotypes.

History and Examination

The presence of multiple key indicators increases the probability that a child has asthma (Box 7-5). Documenting risk factors, symptoms, triggers, and reversible airflow obstruction where possible are needed, as with adults.

Risk factors include a personal or family history of atopic disease. Age of onset, timing and pattern of wheezing, relationship of episodes to viral illness and feeding, comorbidities, response to previous treatments, and socioenvironmental factors contributing to morbidity should be documented (Box 7-2).

Atypical features suggesting an alternative diagnosis include symptoms starting at birth, continuous wheezing, failure to thrive, failure to respond to medications, and no association with typical triggers such as viral upper respiratory infections or exposure to allergens after sensitization. Box 7-6 lists the differential diagnosis of asthma and comorbid diseases, and Table 7-4 shows their relative frequency by age. Physical examination may be normal; findings that increase the probability are: chest hyperinflation, use of accessory muscles, hunched shoulders, barrel chest, wheezing during normal breathing or forced expiration, rhinitis, and dermatitis. Unilateral wheezing may indicate foreign body aspiration.

Box 7-5   Key Symptom Indicators for Considering a Diagnosis of Asthma

1. Wheezing—high-pitched wheezing sounds when breathing out (normal chest exam without wheezing does not exclude asthma)
2. History of any of the following:
   - Cough (worse particularly at night)
   - Recurrent wheeze
   - Recurrent difficulty breathing
   - Recurrent chest tightness
3. Symptoms occur or worsen in the presence of:
   - Exercise
   - Viral Infection
   - Inhalant allergens (e.g., animals with fur or hair, house-dust mites, mold, pollen)
   - Irritants (tobacco or wood smoke, airborne chemicals)
   - Changes in weather
   - Strong emotional expression (laughing or crying hard)
   - Stress
   - Menses
4. Symptoms occur or worsen at night, waking the patient

(Modified from National Heart, Lung, and Blood Institute. Expert Panel Report 3 (EPR-3): Guidelines for the Diagnosis and Management of Asthma: Full Report 2007. Available at: <http://www.nhlbi.nih.gov/files/docs/guidelines/asthgdln.pdf>; [accessed July 7, 2015.])

Box 7-6   Differential Diagnosis for Asthma in Infants and Children

UPPER AIRWAY DISEASES

- Allergic rhinitis and sinusitis

OBSTRUCTIONS INVOLVING LARGE AIRWAYS

- Foreign body in the trachea or bronchus
- Vocal cord dysfunction
- Vascular rings or laryngeal webs
- Laryngotracheomalacia, tracheal stenosis, or bronchostenosis
- Enlarged lymph nodes or tumor

OBSTRUCTIONS INVOLVING SMALL AIRWAYS

- Viral bronchiolitis or obliterative bronchiolitis
- Cystic fibrosis
- Bronchopulmonary dysplasia (chronic lung disease of prematurity)
- Heart disease

OTHER

- Recurrent cough not caused by asthma (infection, habit cough, postnasal drip)
- Aspiration from swallowing mechanism dysfunction or gastroesophageal reflux disease

---

(Modified from National Heart, Lung, and Blood Institute. Expert Panel Report 3 (EPR-3): Guidelines for the Diagnosis and Management of Asthma: Full Report 2007. Available at: <http://www.nhlbi.nih.gov/files/docs/guidelines/asthgdln.pdf>; [accessed July 7, 2015.])

Radiographic Studies

Radiographic studies are not required in routine diagnosis, although may be useful in cases of diagnostic uncertainty.

Pulmonary Function Tests

Pulmonary function testing with spirometry should be possible in primary care in the majority of children over the age of 6 years. PEF is well suited for monitoring trends in asthma control over time in children age 4 years and older, but less useful in diagnosing asthma or classifying severity. FEV_1 is generally normal in children with asthma, but FEV_1/FVC decreases as asthma severity increases. Pre- and post-bronchodilator determinations can be obtained with improvements of 12% or greater for FEV_1 clinically significant, although many will not reach this degree of reversibility.[72] Specialized PFTs include body plethysmography, impulse oscillometry, and infant testing and are available in most pediatric medical centers, but not in primary care. Plethysmography allows the measurement of lung volumes and airway mechanics (resistance, conductance, specific conductance). Impulse oscillometry (IOS) measurements are based on respiratory system resistance and reactance produced by a loudspeaker on the child's respiratory system during quiet tidal breathing. A lung function test using rapid thoracoabdominal compression has similar results in infants as produced by voluntary maneuvers performed by adults. These tests require sedation but are well tolerated. If the diagnosis is not clear bronchial provocation testing may be useful.

TABLE 7-4   Age-related Differential Diagnosis for Wheezing

Condition	Relative frequency of occurrence		
	Infancy	Childhood	Adolescence
Asthma	+	+++	+++
Airway malacia	++	+	−
Cystic fibrosis	+++	+	±
Foreign body	++	+++	±
Airway infection	+++	++	+
Bronchopulmonary dysplasia	+++	+	−
Primary ciliary dyskinesia	+	++	+
Bronchiectasis	+	+	+
Congenital anomalies (vascular ring)	+++	+	−
Vocal cord dysfunction	−	±	++
Tumors	±	±	±
Aspiration syndromes	+	±	±
Pulmonary edema	+	+	+

−, Unlikely to present in this age group; +, likely to present in this age group; ± may present in this age group.
(Modified from Bierman CW, Pearlman DS, eds. Allergic diseases from infancy to adulthood. 2nd edn. Philadelphia: Saunders; 1988.)

Laboratory Evaluation

These are not generally needed in the diagnosis of childhood asthma. The presence of eosinophilia or an elevated total serum IgE level is supportive but not necessarily diagnostic of asthma. Evaluation of immune competence might disclose an immune deficiency. Sweat chloride testing, a biopsy to evaluate ciliary structure, and bronchoscopy are important in diagnosing other diseases. Allergen-specific IgE to mites, tree pollen, grass pollen, or animal dander is uncommon during the first year of life but increases during the preschool years. A total of 60% of children at high risk for development of asthma were sensitized to aeroallergen and/or food allergen by ages 2 and 3 years. The presence of allergen-specific IgE is determined using the radioallergosorbent test (RAST or ImmunoCAP®) or skin-prick testing.

Monitoring Asthma

Asthma is a variable condition, and monitoring is required to ensure both current control and reduction in future risk. According to GINA, asthma is controlled if there are no daytime symptoms, no limitations of activities, no nocturnal symptoms or awakenings, no need for reliever medication, normal or near-normal pulmonary function, and no exacerbations (Table 7-5). The goal of therapy is to maintain control with the least amount of medication. Assessment of control is based on the patient's response to treatment (Table 7-6); categories are *well-controlled*, *not well-controlled*, and *very poorly controlled*. Although high levels of control are possible for most patients with mild to moderate asthma in clinical trials, in 'real-world' asthma care, poor control is not uncommon and often not volunteered by patients or fully appreciated by clinicians. Structured proactive care by primary care clinicians, with at least an annual assessment of control and including instruction in self-management, improves asthma outcomes.[73,74]

Since asthma is primarily an inflammatory disorder of the airways, disease activity can be monitored by using inflammatory biomarkers such as sputum eosinophils and FeNO. While the former is more difficult to perform in primary care, FeNO is now feasible using the modern smaller measurement devices.[57]

TABLE 7-5   Levels of Asthma Control

A. Assessment of current clinical control (preferably over 4 weeks)

Characteristic	Controlled (all of the following)	Partially controlled (any measure present)	Uncontrolled
Daytime symptoms	None (twice or less/week)	More than twice/week	Three or more features of partially controlled asthma*,†
Limitation of activities	None	Any	
Nocturnal symptoms/awakening	None	Any	
Need for reliever/rescue treatment	None (twice or less/week)	More than twice/week	
Lung function (PEF or FEV₁)‡	Normal	<80% predicted or personal best (if known)	

B. Assessment of future risk (risk of exacerbations, instability, rapid decline in lung function, side-effects)

Features that are associated with increased risk of adverse events in the future include poor clinical control, frequent exacerbations in past year,* ever admission to critical care for asthma, low FEV₁, exposure to cigarette smoke, high-dose medications.

*Any exacerbations should prompt review of maintenance treatment to ensure that it is adequate.
†By definition, an exacerbation in any week makes that an uncontrolled asthma week.
‡Without administration of bronchodilator. Lung function is not a reliable test for children 5 years and younger.
(From Global Initiative for Asthma (GINA), 2012. Available at: <http://www.ginasthma.org/guidelines-gina-report-global-strategy-for-asthma.html>.)

TABLE 7-6   Assessment of Asthma Control in Patients 12 Years of Age and Older

Control category/component	Asthma control classification: frequency/nature of component		
	Well-controlled	Not well-controlled	Very poorly controlled
IMPAIRMENT			
Symptoms	≤2 day/week	>2 day/week but not daily	Throughout the day
Nighttime awakenings	≤2×/month	3–4×/month	7×/week
Interference with normal activity	None	Minor limitation	Extremely limited
SABA use for symptom control	≤2 day/week	>2 day/week	Several times a day
FEV₁ or peak flow	>80% predicted or personal best	60–80% predicted or personal best	<60% predicted or personal best

Validated questionnaire scores
   ATAQ
   ACQ
   ACT
	0
	≤0.75
	≥20
		1–2
		≥1.5
		16–19
			1–2
			N/A
			≤15

RISK			
Exacerbations requiring oral systemic corticosteroids	0–1/year	≥2/years	
	Consider severity and interval since last exacerbation.		
Progressive loss of function	Evaluation requires long-term follow-up care.		
Treatment-related adverse effects	Medication side effects can range in intensity from none to very troublesome and worrisome. The level of intensity does not correlate with specific levels of control but should be considered in the overall assessment of risk.		
Recommended action for treatment	Maintain current level of step care. Regular follow-up every 1–6 months to maintain control. Consider step-down if asthma is well controlled for at least 3 months.	Step-up 1 step and re-evaluate in 2–6 weeks. For side effects, consider alternative treatment options.	Consider short course of oral systemic corticosteroids. Step-up 1–2 steps and reevaluate in 2 weeks. For side effects, consider alternative treatment options.

ACQ, Asthma Control Questionnaire; ACT, Asthma Control Test; ATAQ, Asthma Treatment Assessment Questionnaire; FEV₁, forced expiratory volume in 1 second; FVC, forced vital capacity; N/A, not applicable; SABA, short-acting β₂-agonist.
(From National Heart, Lung, and Blood Institute. Expert Panel Report 3 (EPR-3): Guidelines for the Diagnosis and Management of Asthma: Full Report 2007. Available at: <http://www.nhlbi.nih.gov/files/docs/guidelines/asthgdln.pdf>; [accessed July 7, 2015.])

Box 7-7   Domains of Outcomes Used in the Assessment of Asthma Severity and Disease Control

IMPAIRMENT

- Symptoms
- Nighttime awakenings
- Use of short-acting β_2-agonists for symptom control
- Interference with normal activity
- Lung function

RISK

- Exacerbations
- Progressive loss of lung function
- Side effects from medications

(From National Heart, Lung, and Blood Institute. Expert Panel Report 3 (EPR-3): Guidelines for the Diagnosis and Management of Asthma: Full Report 2007. Available at: <http://www.nhlbi.nih.gov/files/docs/guidelines/asthgdln.pdf>; [accessed July 7, 2015.])

Severity

Asthma severity reflects underlying disease activity, and definition is based on intensity and frequency of symptoms and degree of impairment of pulmonary function.[75] Severity is assessed prior to commencing therapy or by the level of medication needed to achieve asthma control. Severity can vary over time, reflecting changes in response to treatment or in the intrinsic nature of the disease.

Mild or intermittent asthma is characterized by minimal symptoms and near-optimal pulmonary function, usually requiring no more than infrequent use of a SABA. Mild persistent asthma is defined as requiring a low dose of ICS to achieve control, moderate asthma as requiring a higher dose of ICS or additional medication, and severe asthma as requiring high ICS doses plus add-on medication with or without oral corticosteroids. Within the scope of asthma severity and control are two major domains: impairment and risk (Box 7-7). *Impairment* refers to the frequency and intensity of current symptoms, based on five factors: daytime symptoms, nighttime awakenings, SABA use for symptom control, interference with activity, and lung function. *Risk* focuses on three elements: exacerbations; progressive loss of lung function; and side effects from medications.

Symptom Control

Validated questionnaires (such as the Asthma Control Questionnaire, ACQ; the Asthma Control Scoring System, ACSS; the Asthma Control Test, ACT; and pediatric equivalents, such as the Pediatric Asthma Control Test) have been standardized to quantify asthma control. These are preferable to single questions, because they assess overall control of the disease. Cut-off threshold for 'controlled,' 'partially controlled,' and 'not-controlled' asthma are available for most questionnaires. Uncontrolled patients require an assessment of adherence, inhaler technique and self-management behavior, but escalation of treatment may be needed. By contrast, for well-controlled patients, it may be possible to reduce the level of treatment.

Exacerbations

Exacerbations are defined by the need for short courses of oral corticosteroids and/or for emergency care. Frequency of oral corticosteroid use, emergency department visits, hospital admissions, and unscheduled healthcare use should all be recorded. Whenever possible, the frequency, severity, and causes of asthma exacerbations should be documented. Exacerbation occurring in the recent past is a strong predictor of future exacerbations.[76] All patients who have experienced an exacerbation need to have their disease self-management behavior investigated and an updated written self-management plan provided. Poor adherence with ICS medication, overuse of SABA medication, at-risk behaviors such as smoking, and poor inhaler technique may be important and potentially reversible factors increasing exacerbation risk.

Asthma-related Quality of Life

Quality of life (QoL) is a patient-centered dimension of asthma that may not correlate well with current control, pulmonary function or biomarkers, but reflects how the patient experiences asthma in their life. Quality of life and symptoms are overlapping but discrete domains of asthma control; for instance, it is possible to have low symptoms but impaired QoL, for example in the case of a patient who avoids physical exercise or sport to prevent exercise-induced asthma symptoms. Validated QoL questionnaires, either 'generic,' measuring overall health status (e.g., SF36, EQ5D), or 'disease-specific,' measuring the specific impact of asthma (e.g., Asthma QoL Questionnaire) may help to predict healthcare use and future exacerbations and to characterize the impact of disease on the individual. These questionnaires are commonly used in research settings, but their place in the routine clinical monitoring of asthma is less well established.

Lung Function

Measures of PEF should be used for monitoring control. PEF should ideally be compared with the patient's best value, and can be used for domiciliary monitoring. It is most useful in labile, severe asthma or when patients have difficulties in interpreting their respiratory symptoms (so-called 'under-perceivers,' who may only become aware of bronchoconstriction when it is advanced). It is also helpful in documenting the effects of therapy or environmental triggers, particularly in the workplace. Such patients can benefit from an asthma action plan based on PEF in addition to or instead of symptoms. Repeated spirometry (e.g., on an annual basis) can demonstrate the development of fixed or deteriorating lung function, which may indicate an asthma-COPD overlap syndrome (ACOS) in smokers or the development of airway remodeling and the possible need for more intensive treatment.

Rescue Medication Use

When asthma is well-controlled, use of short-acting rescue bronchodilators should be occasional or absent. The requirement for rescue medication use on more than 2 days a week is indicative of suboptimal control and the need for a review of maintenance therapy. If available, the frequency of ordering of refill prescriptions for SAB medication is a useful guide to SAB use, which is frequently under-reported by patients. Overuse of SABA medication is associated with increased risk of exacerbation, hospitalization, and mortality.

Adherence with Regular Medication and Inhaler Technique

An important and often neglected aspect of monitoring asthma is an assessment of whether the prescribed medication is being used correctly. Underuse of regular medication, particular with ICS preparations, is very common and is associated with poor control.[77] The reasons for non-adherence are complex, and may be broadly categorized as 'non-intentional' and 'intentional' non-adherence.[78] In non-intentional non-adherence, the patient forgets to take the medication, is unable to obtain medication, or has poor inhalational technique, resulting in lung low deposition of medication. 'Intentional non-adherence' occurs when a patient makes a decision not to use the medication as prescribed, usually affecting ICS medication. This is often due to an under-appreciation of the effectiveness of ICS and an over-perception of side-effect risks, and points to the need for improved self-management education. Detection of ICS non-adherence through refill prescription monitoring or other methods, and a following discussion with the patient, has been shown to improve adherence and asthma outcomes.[79]

Personal Asthma Action Plan

A key factor in successful asthma care is effective self-management, and all patients should have asthma education and the provision of a written personal asthma action plan.[80] This should be reviewed and reinforced annually and after any episode of loss of control. The action plan should include instructions on daily management, as well as specific strategies to deal with worsening of asthma symptoms and loss of disease control. A written action plan should be provided (Fig. 7-8). Traditionally, the action plan includes three levels: '*I feel good*' (green zone); '*I do not feel good*' (yellow zone); and '*I feel awful*' (red zone). An action plan includes symptoms and may include lung function, usually with a peak flow meter. It is critical to provide understandable and acceptable instructions on actions to take in the face of a loss of control.

ASTHMA MANAGEMENT

Long-term Management in Adults

As a long-term variable condition, a key factor is establishing a successful partnership between patient and clinician, involving education in self-management. This includes: identification of the characteristics of the patient's asthma; education of what constitutes control; review of medications, including their actions and use; and development of an action plan.

Control of Environmental Factors

It is important to identify environmental factors that may affect asthma control. Allergens can be identified by means of skin or serologic testing, and by correlation of exposure to symptoms. Although allergen avoidance has limitations, efforts should be made to reduce exposure where possible. Active and passive cigarette smoke exposure should be minimized, as smoking increases asthma severity and reduces response to ICS.[81]

Comorbidity

Treatment of coexisting conditions, such as chronic rhinosinusitis, gastroesophageal reflux disease, obesity, and psychosocial issues, should be addressed. Obesity with increases in body mass index (BMI) have become a significant public health problem and may compromise pulmonary physiology. An increase in BMI is associated with greater asthma morbidity and the need for multiple medications.[49] Psychological problems are up to six times more common in people with asthma than in the general population, and outcomes of all varieties are associated with poor asthma control. The mechanisms underlying this relationship and the effectiveness of psychological interventions are poorly understood. Psychological factors may affect immunologic pathways, perception of symptoms, and behavior.[82] Breathing control exercises, encouraging slow steady nasal diaphragmatic breathing, and discouraging hyperventilation, may be helpful as adjuvant treatment in patients with symptoms and quality of life impairment, despite standard pharmacotherapy.[83]

Pharmacologic Treatment in Adults

Medications used in asthma treatment are categorized as: *quick-relief* and *long-term control* (Box 7-8). Quick-relief drugs (e.g., SABAs) act to rapidly reduce airflow obstruction, and long-term control medications (e.g., corticosteroids) regulate airway inflammation and its consequences.

Quick-relief Medications

Short-acting β_2-Agonists. The SABAs, albuterol (salbutamol), levalbuterol, and pirbuterol, are effective inhaled bronchodilators and the agents of choice for the acute relief of symptoms.

Anticholinergics. Ipratropium bromide is a muscarinic cholinergic antagonist and is used in asthma, primarily in patients who either are intolerant of β_2-agonists or are experiencing limited benefit from SABA use.[84] Tiotropium is a long-acting anticholinergic agent used in COPD, but data are emerging for its use in asthma.[85]

My Asthma Action Plan

Patient name: _____

Medical record #: _____

Physician's name: _____   DOB: _____

Physician's phone #: _____   Completed by: _____   Date: _____

Long-Term-Control Medicines	How Much To Take	How Often	Other Instructions
		_____ times per day EVERY DAY!	
		_____ times per day EVERY DAY!	
		_____ times per day EVERY DAY!	
		_____ times per day EVERY DAY!	

Quick-Relief Medicines	How Much To Take	How Often	Other Instructions
		Take ONLY as needed	NOTE: If this medicine is needed frequently, call physician to consider increasing controller medications.

Special instructions when I feel ●*good*, ○*not good*, and ●*awful*.

GREEN ZONE

I feel *good*.
(My **peak flow** is in the **GREEN** zone.)

Peak Flow
My Personal Best

Prevent asthma symptoms every day:
☐ Take my long-term-control medicines (above) every day.
☐ Before exercise, take _____ puffs of
_____
☐ Avoid things that make my asthma worse like: _____
_____

YELLOW ZONE

I do *not* feel *good*.
(My **peak flow** is in the **YELLOW** zone.)
My symptoms may include one or more
of the following:

• Wheeze
• Tight chest
• Cough
• Shortness of breath
• Waking up at night with asthma symptoms
• Decreased ability to do usual activities
• _____
• _____

80% Personal Best

CAUTION: I should continue taking my long-term-control asthma medicines every day AND:

☐ Take _____
_____

If I still do not feel good, or my peak flow is not in the *Green Zone* within 1 hour, then I should:

☐ Increase _____
☐ Add _____
☐ Call _____

RED ZONE

I feel *awful* :
(My **peak flow** is in the **RED** zone.)
Warning signs may include one or more
of the following:

• It's getting harder and harder to breathe.
• Unable to sleep or do usual activities because of trouble breathing.

50% Personal Best

Liters/Min.
Peak Flow Meter

MEDICAL ALERT! Get help!

☐ Take _____
until I get help immediately!
☐ Take _____
☐ Call _____

DANGER!
Get help immediately!

Call 9-1-1 if you have trouble walking or talking due to shortness of breath or lips or fingernails are gray or blue.

Source: Adapted and reprinted with permission from the Regional Asthma Management and Prevention (RAMP) initiative, a program of the Public Health Institute. http://www.calasthma.org/uploads/resources/actionplanpdf.pdf. San Francisco Bay Area Regional Asthma Management Plan.

Figure 7-8 Sample asthma action plan—adult, as presented in the Expert Panel Report 3 (EPR-3). *(From National Heart, Lung, and Blood Institute. Expert Panel Report 3 (EPR-3): Guidelines for the Diagnosis and Management of Asthma: Full Report 2007. Available at: <http://www.nhlbi.nih.gov/files/docs/guidelines/asthgdln.pdf>; [accessed July 7, 2015.])*

Box 7-8   **Classification of Asthma Treatment Medications**

QUICK-RELIEF MEDICATIONS

- Short-acting β_2-agonists
- Anticholinergics
- Systemic corticosteroids

LONG-TERM CONTROLLERS

- Corticosteroids—inhaled and systemic
- Long-acting β_2-agonists
- Leukotriene receptor antagonists
- Methylxanthines
- Cromolyn/nedocromil
- Anticholinergics
- Omalizumab

TABLE 7-7   Estimated Comparative Daily Dosages for Inhaled Corticosteroids for Older Children* and Adults with Asthma

Drug	Low daily dose, adult	Medium daily dose, adult	High daily dose, adult
Beclomethasone HFA 40 or 80 µg/puff	80–240 µg	241–480 µg	>480 µg
Ciclesonide MDI 80 µg/puff, 160 µg/puff	80–240 µg	241–320 µg	>320 µg
Budesonide DPI 90, 180, or 200 µg/inhalation	180–600 µg	601–1200 µg	>1200 µg
Flunisolide 250 µg/puff	500–1000 µg	1001–2000 µg	>2000 µg
Flunisolide HFA 80 µg/puff	320 µg	321–640 µg	>640 µg
Fluticasone HFA/MDI: 44, 110, or 220 µg/puff	88–264 µg	265–440 µg	>440 µg
DPI: 50, 100, or 250 µg/inhalation	100–300 µg	301–500 µg	>500 µg
Mometasone DPI 200 µg/inhalation	200 µg	400 µg	>400 µg
Triamcinolone acetonide 75 µg/puff	300–750 µg	751–1000 µg	>1500 µg

*12 years of age and older.
DPI, Dry powder inhaler; HFA, hydrofluoroalkane; MDI, metered-dose inhaler.
(From National Heart, Lung, and Blood Institute. Expert Panel Report 3 (EPR-3): Guidelines for the Diagnosis and Management of Asthma: Full Report 2007. Available at: <http://www.nhlbi.nih.gov/files/docs/guidelines/asthgdln.pdf>; [accessed July 7, 2015.])

Long-term Control Medications

Medications for long-term control are used on a daily basis to regulate airway inflammation.

Corticosteroids. Corticosteroids are the primary anti-inflammatory medication used in long-term control of asthma. They improve both impairment and risk but do not have disease-modifying activities, and effects recede once discontinued.[86] Their anti-inflammatory actions are broad-based and affect lymphocyte function, principally helper T cell type 2 (Th2) generation, and inflammatory cell migration and activation.

Inhaled corticosteroids (ICS) have minimal long-term side effects in low to moderate doses. Multiple formulations are available; these may be used in low, medium, or high doses, depending on underlying severity (Table 7-7). Oral corticosteroids are used in short-term bursts for acute exacerbations, and regular use limited by associated side-effects.

Leukotriene Modifiers. Leukotriene modifiers interfere with the leukotriene pathway, and included LTRAs montelukast and zafirlukast and also zileuton, which inhibits the 5-lipoxygenase pathway. Leukotriene modifiers, such as montelukast, are alternative choices for mild persistent asthma,[87] and may be used in combination with ICS in more severe asthma.

Long-acting β₂-Agonists. LABAs—salmeterol and formoterol (Table 7-8)—are inhaled bronchodilators that improve airflow for at least 12 hours. They are not used alone in asthma for safety reasons, but given in combination with an ICS (e.g., fluticasone-salmeterol [Advair]; budesonide-formoterol [Symbicort]; and mometasone-formoterol [Dulera]) (Table 7-9). Combination ICS-LABA medications are available in low, medium, and high doses, based on ICS dose and lead to greater control of impairment and exacerbations.[88] Indacaterol is an LABA with 24-hour duration of bronchodilation, but its use in asthma is not yet approved by the US Food and Drug Administration (FDA).

Immunomodulation. At present, omalizumab (Xolair®), or anti-IgE, is the only approved immunomodulator and is given as an injectable monoclonal antibody to bind to IgE, preventing receptor binding and as a consequence, leads to loss of IgE receptors. Omalizumab is recommended for patients with severe asthma in the US Guidelines for the Diagnosis and Management of Asthma (EPR-3) at Steps 5 and 6, in those with poor control, raised IgE, and evidence of allergen-specific IgE. It improves control and reduces

TABLE 7-8 Usual Dosages of Long-acting β₂-Agonists (LABAs) for Older Children* and Adults with Asthma

Medication	Formulation	Dose	Comments
			Inhaled LABAs should not be used alone for symptom relief or exacerbations. Use with ICS.
Salmeterol	DPI 50 µg/blister	1 blister q12h	Decreased duration of protection against EIB may occur with regular use.
Formoterol	DPI 12 µg/single-use capsule	1 capsule q12h	Each capsule is for single use only; additional doses should not be administered for at least 12 h. Capsules should be used only with the Aerolizer inhaler and should not be taken orally.

*12 years of age and older.
DPI, Dry powder inhaler; EIB, exercise-induced bronchospasm; ICS, inhaled corticosteroid.
(Modified from National Heart, Lung, and Blood Institute. Expert Panel Report 3 (EPR-3): Guidelines for the Diagnosis and Management of Asthma: Full Report 2007. Available at: <http://www.nhlbi.nih.gov/files/docs/guidelines/asthgdln.pdf>; [accessed July 7, 2015.])

TABLE 7-9 Usual Dosages for Combination Inhaled Corticosteroid and Long-acting β₂-Agonist (ICS-LABA) Treatment for Older Children* and Adults with Asthma

Combination agent	Formulation	Dose	Comments
Fluticasone-salmeterol (Advair)	DPI 100 µg/50 µg, 250 µg/50 µg, or 500 µg/50 µg HFA 45 µg/21 µg, 115 µg/21 µg, or 230 µg/21 µg	1 inhalation BID; dose depends on severity of asthma	*100/50 DPI or 45/21 HFA*: for patient whose asthma is not controlled on low- to medium-dose ICS *250/50 DPI or 115/21 HFA*: for patients whose asthma is not controlled on medium- to high-dose ICS
Budesonide-formoterol (Symbicort)	HFA, MDI 80 µg/4.5 µg, 160 µg/4.5 µg	2 inhalations BID; dose depends on severity of asthma	*80/4.5*: for patients whose asthma is not controlled on low- to medium-dose ICS *160/4.5*: for patients whose asthma is not controlled on medium- to high-dose ICS
Mometasone-formoterol (Dulera)	HFA, MDI 50 µg/5 µg, 100 µg/5 µg, or 200 µg/5 µg,	2 inhalations BID; dose depends on the severity of asthma	*50/5*: for patients whose asthma is not controlled on low-dose ICS *100/5*: for patients whose asthma is not controlled on medium-dose ICS *200/5*: for patients whose asthma is not controlled on high-dose ICS

*12 years of age and older.
DPI, Dry powder inhaler; HFA, hydrofluoroalkane; MDI, metered-dose inhaler.
(From National Heart, Lung, and Blood Institute. Expert Panel Report 3 (EPR-3): Guidelines for the Diagnosis and Management of Asthma – Full Report 2007. Available at: <http://www.nhlbi.nih.gov/files/docs/guidelines/asthgdln.pdf>; [accessed July 7, 2015.])

asthma exacerbations. Other immunomodulators: methotrexate, cyclosporine, and intravenous immunoglobulin, have been evaluated in asthma, with inconsistent effects.

Methylxanthines. Sustained-release theophylline has modest bronchodilator activity, and its use in asthma is limited by toxicity and modest efficacy and the need for monitoring of serum theophylline levels.

Cromolyn Sodium and Nedocromil Sodium. Cromolyn sodium and nedocromil sodium interfere with mast cell activation mechanisms to reduce inflammatory mediator release. Although these compounds are extremely safe, their use in patients older than 12 years of age is limited, and in some countries availability is now limited.

Step Care Approach to Asthma Management

Guidelines recommend that therapy be tailored to needs, circumstances, and responsiveness of the individual patient. The step care approach to asthma (Fig. 7-9) is based on the premise that increasing severity is most effectively controlled by greater amounts of medication, particularly of anti-inflammatory agents.

Intermittent Asthma

Step 1 Care. Intermittent asthma characterized by: symptoms on less than 3 days per week; nighttime awakenings less than twice per month; use of SABA no more than 2 days per week; normal activity; normal lung function; exacerbation frequency of 0 to 1 per year (Table 7-10).

SABAs are effective in relieving symptoms and normalizing pulmonary function. Short-acting anticholinergic agents, are not generally recommended owing to a slower

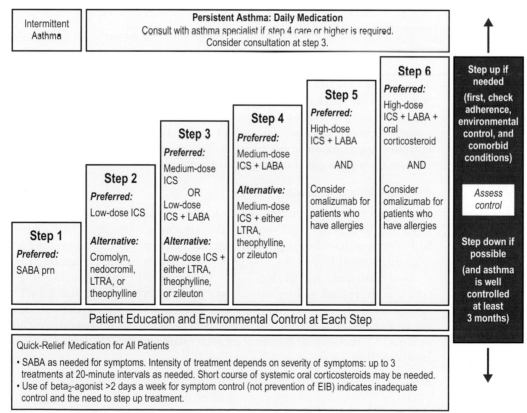

Figure 7-9 Step-care approach to asthma treatment according to disease severity, as presented in the Expert Panel Report 3 (EPR-3). EIB, exercise-induced bronchospasm; ICS, inhaled corticosteroid; LABA, long-acting β-agonist; LTRA, leukotriene receptor antagonist; SABA, short-acting β₂-agonist. *(From National Heart, Lung, and Blood Institute. Expert Panel Report 3 (EPR-3): Guidelines for the Diagnosis and Management of Asthma: Full Report 2007. Available at: <http://www.nhlbi.nih.gov/files/docs/guidelines/asthgdln.pdf>; [accessed July 7, 2015.])*

TABLE 7-10   Assessment of Asthma Severity in Patients 12 Years of Age and Older

| Severity category/component | Asthma severity classification: frequency/nature of component | | | |
| | Intermittent | Persistent | | |
		MILD	MODERATE	SEVERE
Impairment				
Symptoms	≤2 day/week	>2 day/week but not daily	Daily	Throughout the day
Nighttime awakenings	≤2×/month	3–4×/month	>1×/week but not nightly	7×/week
SABA use for symptom control	≤2 day/week	>2 day/week but not >1×/day	daily	Several times a day
Interference with normal activity	None	Minor limitation	Some limitation	Extremely limited
Lung function *Normal FEV₁/FVC:* 8–19 years: 85% 20–39 years: 80% 40–59 years: 75% 60–80 years: 70%	Normal FEV_1 between exacerbations FEV_1 >80% predicted FEV_1/FVC normal	FEV_1 ≥80% predicted FEV_1/FVC normal	FEV_1 >60% but <80% predicted FEV_1/FVC reduced 5%	FEV_1 <60% predicted FEV_1/FVC reduced >5%
Risk				
Exacerbations requiring oral systemic corticosteroids	0–1/year	≥2/years		
	Consider severity and interval since last exacerbation. Frequency and severity may fluctuate over time for patients in any severity category. Relative annual risk of exacerbations may be related to FEV_1			
Recommended step for initiating treatment	STEP 1	STEP 2	STEP 3	STEP 4 or 5 Consider short course of oral corticosteroids.
	In 2–6 weeks, evaluate level of control that is achieved and adjust therapy accordingly.			

FEV₁, Forced expiratory volume in 1 second; *FVC*, forced vital capacity; *SABA*, short-acting β₂-agonist.
(From National Heart, Lung, and Blood Institute. Expert Panel Report 3 (EPR-3): Guidelines for the Diagnosis and Management of Asthma – Full Report 2007. Available at: <http://www.nhlbi.nih.gov/files/docs/guidelines/asthgdln.pdf>; [accessed July 7, 2015.])

onset of action and less bronchodilation. SABAs can be used every 4 to 6 hours for 24 hours if needed (e.g., during a viral infection). If regular use for more than 24 hours is needed, additional treatment, such as a short course of oral corticosteroids, may be needed. If episodes requiring more frequent SABAs occur more often than every 6 weeks, consideration should be given to step-up treatment.

Persistent Asthma (Fig. 7-9)

Step 2 Care: Mild Persistent Asthma. Mild persistent asthma characterized by: symptoms less than 3 days per week; nighttime awakenings 3 to 4 times per month; use of SABA on less than 3 days per week; no activity limitation; normal lung function between exacerbations (FEV_1 of 80%; 0 to 1 exacerbation in the preceding year (Table 7-10).

Low-dose daily ICS (Table 7-7) is the preferred treatment, resulting in fewer symptoms, a decreased exacerbation risk, and improved lung function.[89] LTRAs relieve symptoms and improve lung function, but are less effective than ICSs,[90] although may be an option in non-adherent patients,[91] or those with concomitant exercise induced asthma.[92] Theophylline has limited anti-inflammatory effects and a narrow therapeutic profile (Table 7-6).

Step 3 Care: Moderate Persistent Asthma. Moderate persistent asthma is characterized by: daily symptoms; nighttime awakening more than once per week; need for daily SABA use; limitation in daily activity; and compromises in lung function (FEV_1 >60% but <80%); an average of two exacerbations in the previous year (Table 7-10).

EPR-3 has two preferred recommendations for Step 3: medium dose of ICS (Table 7-7) or combination therapy with low-dose ICS and an LABA (Table 7-9). The observation[93] that the addition of LABA to low-dose ICS had greater efficacy than doubling the dose of ICS has been substantiated by many subsequent studies. Effects include improvement in lung function, symptoms, exacerbations, and a lessened need for SABA. Evidence also supports increasing the dose of ICS to achieve improved lung function, symptoms and exacerbations. In GINA, Step 3 recommends low-dose ICS plus LABA as the preferred treatment. Both options improve control, but the addition of LABA has been consistently found to be superior. In observational data,[94] LABA addition was superior in symptom control, but an increase in ICS dose more effective in reducing exacerbations, plausibly explained by improved inflammation control translating to fewer exacerbations.

There have been concerns over life-threatening events, including death, associated with LABA use following the Salmeterol Multicenter Asthma Research Trial (SMART) study, a randomized controlled trial involving 26 355 asthma subjects randomized to receive salmeterol alone or albuterol, along with ICS; among patients in the salmeterol treatment group, an increased incidence in life-threatening events and respiratory-related or asthma-related deaths was noted.[95] A meta-analysis performed by the US FDA also found an added risk with LABA use.[96] As a result, the FDA issued an advisory statement and a 'black box' warning label to all LABA inhalers, advising that LABAs should not be used as monotherapy. The FDA further recommended that once control is achieved, step-down should be considered, with discontinuation of LABA therapy if possible.[97] However, the increased risks were largely seen with LABAs used as monotherapy.

GINA also recommends that the combination therapy of budesonide and formoterol can be used for both maintenance and rescue treatment in a 'single maintenance and reliever therapy' (SMART) regimen. This involves regular once or twice daily combination inhaler use, with additional inhalations for relief of symptoms. Although not approved by the US FDA, the SMART regimen has been shown to reduce exacerbations, and is used in other parts of the world.

Acceptable, non-preferred alternatives for add-on therapy include LTRAs and theophylline. In one study, the addition of LTRA to ICS was found to be equivalent to doubling ICS[98]; however, a systematic review of studies comparing the add-on of LABA with ICS and of LTRA with ICS found superiority with the LABA-ICS combination.[99]

Theophylline remains an alternative, especially when cost is an issue and when adherence with or use of inhaled medication is problematic.[100]

Steps 4 to 6 Care: Severe Persistent Asthma. Patients at Steps 4 to 6 care have severe persistent asthma (Fig. 7-9). Their impairment includes symptoms throughout the day; sleep disturbance; need for frequent daily SABA; activity limitations; and compromise in lung function (FEV$_1$ <60% predicted). These patients also have frequent exacerbations.

The evidence base for treatments is less defined. The US EPR-3 guideline recommends medium-dose ICS in combination with LABA, especially in those with exacerbations, emergency department (ED) visits, or hospitalizations. Non-preferred options include add-on therapy with LTRA, zileuton (a leukotriene synthesis inhibitor), or theophylline. Control achieved in patients at Steps 4 to 6 care is often worse than in milder disease. At high ICS doses, adrenal function may be suppressed and cataracts or osteoporosis may develop in some patients, although risks are far less than associated with systemic corticosteroids.

Steps 5 and 6 Care in Severe Persistent Asthma. For patients at Steps 5 and 6, it is recommended to advance the ICS dose to higher doses (Table 7-9), although evidence for added effectiveness is limited.[101]

The addition of omalizumab can be considered. A systematic review[102] of omalizumab supported decreases in exacerbations, hospitalizations, reduction in inhaled and oral corticosteroids without loss of control, and patients' significant improvement in quality of life, although not lung function.

Step 6 includes consideration of oral corticosteroids (OCS) at the lowest possible dose, with monitoring for adverse effects, while attempting to reduce dose once control is achieved.

In 2010, bronchial thermoplasty was approved. The procedure involves using a bronchoscopy to deliver radiofrequency energy to the airways, transiently heating the airway to 65°C on three separate occasions a month apart, to reduce airway smooth muscle. Experience with thermoplasty still remains limited.

Step-up and Step-down Considerations. After initiation or adjustment, follow-up evaluation should occur in 2 to 6 weeks. If asthma remains uncontrolled, advancement to the next step is indicated—or a course of oral corticosteroids initiated to achieve control. If controlled for 3 months, a step-down in therapy may be considered. Close monitoring is essential. Approaches for step-down are not well established.[103] Before any step-up in treatment is considered, it is important to assess that the patient is adherent to treatment recommendations and that the recommended inhalation technique for the device used, is being used (see above).

Immunotherapy. In selected patients, the US EPR-3 guideline recommends consideration of allergen-specific immunotherapy for patients at Steps 2 to 4,[104] derived from studies with subcutaneous immunotherapy (SCIT), rather than sublingual immunotherapy (SLIT). However, many studies were conducted with a single allergen, whereas patients often have multiple sensitivities. It is unclear which asthma outcome is most appropriate to use—symptoms, lung function, or exacerbations. Finally, patients are often on maximal therapy. Consensus from meta-analyses favors immunotherapy, which may have disease-modifying effects through enhancement of regulatory T cell activity, the production of blocking antibodies, or upregulation of regulatory T cells.

Vaccination. It is advised that people with moderate or severe asthma should receive an annual influenza vaccine. Inactivated influenza vaccines are associated with fewer side effects and are safer to administer to adults and to children over the age of 3 years, including those with 'difficult to control' asthma.[1] People with asthma should receive other vaccinations according to the local schedules and recommendations unless there are specific contraindications.

Food Allergy and Anaphylaxis. Food allergy is uncommon as an exacerbating factor in asthma, and occurs primarily in young children.[1] Food avoidance should not be recommended until allergy has been demonstrated, usually by an oral challenge, and suspected food allergy should trigger a referral to an allergy specialist. Food additives and preservatives (such as sulfites, tartrazine, and monosodium glutamate) may occasionally cause worsening of asthma, but confirmation requires referral and blinded oral challenges.[1]

Anaphylaxis is a potentially life-threatening condition that can both mimic and complicate severe asthma, and can occur in any situation in which medication or biological substances are given, particularly by injection. Airway anaphylaxis can cause sudden onset asthma attacks in people with severe asthma.[105] The symptoms include flushing, pruritus, urticaria, angioedema, dyspnea, stridor, wheezing, gastrointestinal symptoms, and hypotension. Prompt treatment is vital, and includes epinephrine followed by systemic corticosteroids, with bronchodilators and circulatory support if required. Everyone experiencing anaphylaxis should undergo a full specialist assessment to identify triggers and instigate avoidance measures and training in self-administration of emergency treatment with preloaded epinephrine syringes.[106]

Asthma Management in Infants and Children

As with adults, attaining and sustaining asthma control in children and infants requires four components: (1) assessment and monitoring; (2) education; (3) control of triggers (environmental factors and comorbid conditions); (4) pharmacologic therapy. As with adults, EPR-3 designates four categories of severity: intermittent, mild persistent, moderate persistent, and severe persistent. Control level is used to adjust therapy by category: well-controlled, not well-controlled, and poorly controlled. Severity and control are evaluated as *impairment* (current asthma symptoms and pulmonary function) and *risk* (exacerbations and side to effects).

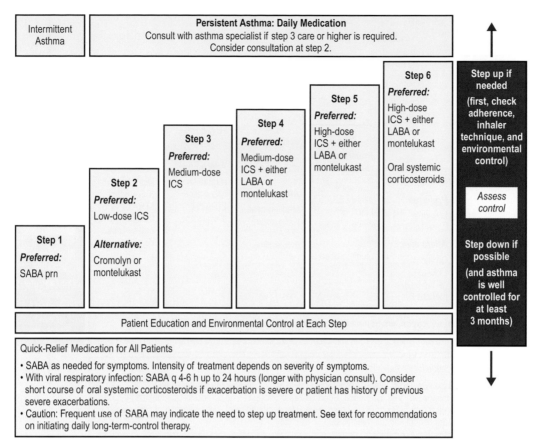

Figure 7-10 Step-wise approach to therapy in children 0–4 years of age, as presented in the Expert Panel Report 3 (EPR-3). ICS, Inhaled corticosteroid; LABA, long-acting β₂-agonist; SABA, short-acting β-agonist. *(From National Heart, Lung, and Blood Institute. Expert Panel Report 3 (EPR-3): Guidelines for the Diagnosis and Management of Asthma: Full Report 2007. Available at: <http://www.nhlbi.nih.gov/files/docs/guidelines/asthgdln.pdf>; [accessed July 7, 2015.])*

EPR-3 describes a step-wise approach in three age ranges: 0 to 4 years (infants and young children), 5 to 11 years, and 12 years of age and older (Figs. 7-10–7-12, respectively).

As with adults, *long-term control medications* are taken daily to achieve and maintain control, and *quick-relief, rescue* or *reliever medications* produce rapid reversal of acute airflow obstruction. Therapy should be maintained for 3 to 6 months if stable, after which 'step-down' is considered. Unfortunately, data to help guide step-down are lacking. Giving daily long-term controller therapy only during specific exposures or seasons can also be considered. For example, in children who experience episodes related to viral infections, stepping up therapy at high-risk times of the year (school attendance) or social situations (day-care settings) may be appropriate. Patient education and environmental control should be discussed at every step.

Non-pharmacologic Management in Children

Environmental Control

Aeroallergen sensitization is associated with risk of developing asthma.[107] Dust mite exposure in older children correlates with wheezing and BHR. Pet dander exposure can occur without the presence of an animal in the home and may trigger worsening asthma in sensitized children.[108] Reduction of house-dust mite exposure may decrease symptoms and bronchial hyperresponsiveness in sensitized children, although can be hard to achieve in practice.[109] EPR-3 recommends that children with persistent asthma be evaluated by history for seasonal fluctuations with substantiation by skin testing or specific IgE antibodies.

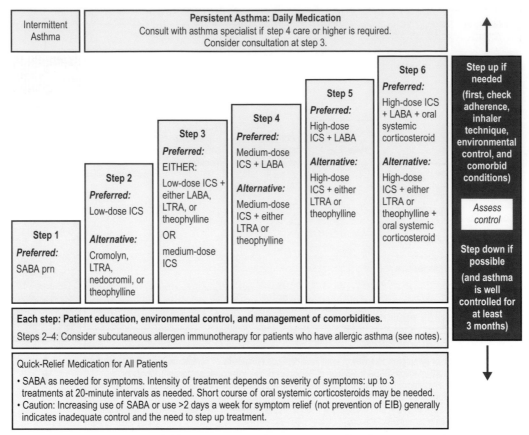

Figure 7-11 Step-wise approach to therapy in children 5–11 years of age, as presented in the Expert Panel Report 3 (EPR-3). EIB, exercise-induced bronchospasm; ICS, inhaled corticosteroid; LABA, long-acting β-agonist; LTRA, leukotriene receptor antagonist; SABA, short-acting β₂-agonist. *(From National Heart, Lung, and Blood Institute. Expert Panel Report 3 (EPR-3): Guidelines for the Diagnosis and Management of Asthma: Full Report 2007. Available at: <http://www.nhlbi.nih.gov/files/docs/guidelines/asthgdln.pdf>; [accessed July 7, 2015.])*

Passive smoke exposure adversely influences asthma incidence, BHR, symptoms, exacerbations, and overall lung function, yet many parents and caregivers continue to smoke.

Psychosocial Factors

Observational studies have identified an association between stress and depression and poorly-controlled asthma. Stress is associated with an increased prevalence[110] and risk of exacerbations in children with negative life events.[111] Emotions can influence airway function, interpretation of symptoms, and the ability to react appropriately to them. Conversely, asthma may influence psychosocial adaptations in the home and at school. Asthmatic children have significantly more anxiety disorders, lower self-esteem, greater functional impairment, greater school problems, psychiatric illnesses, and intrafamily stress. Psychosocial factors such as conflict between family and the medical staff, inappropriate self-care, depressive symptoms, behavioral problems, and disregard of symptoms may occur.[112] Parental mental status is a predictor of asthma morbidity, hospitalization, and poor adherence to therapy.

Asthma Education

Education of children with asthma and their caregivers on skills of self-assessment, use of medications, and actions to prevent or control exacerbations is associated with reduction in urgent care visits and hospitalizations, reduction in school absences, and improvement in health status (Fig. 7-13).

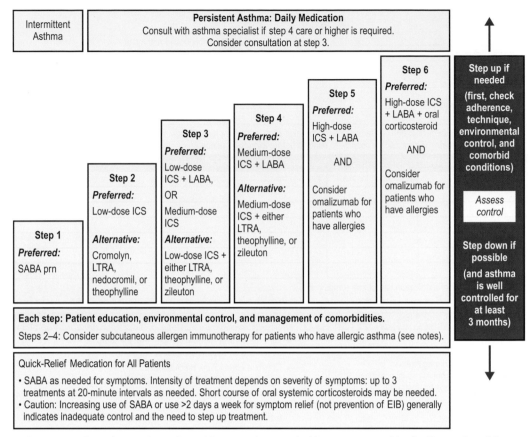

Figure 7-12 Step-wise approach to therapy in patients 12 years of age and older, as presented in the Expert Panel Report 3 (EPR-3). *EIB, Exercise-induced bronchospasm; ICS, inhaled corticosteroid; LABA, long-acting β₂-agonist; LTRA, leukotriene receptor antagonist; SABA, short-acting β₂-agonist. (From National Heart, Lung, and Blood Institute. Expert Panel Report 3 (EPR-3): Guidelines for the Diagnosis and Management of Asthma: Full Report 2007. Available at: <http://www.nhlbi.nih.gov/files/docs/guidelines/asthgdln.pdf>; [accessed July 7, 2015.])*

Pharmacologic Therapy in Children

Across all ages, therapy of *intermittent* asthma involves the use of β-agonists on an as-needed basis. Inhalation remains the preferred route of administration.

For persistent disease, options for step-up and step-down are more variable. Features relevant include age, dosing, delivery system, the risk–benefit ratio, and cost-effectiveness of each medication by itself and in combination.

Inhaled Corticosteroids. ICSs are the first-line prophylactic therapy in all pediatric age groups.[113-115] ICS decrease BHR, inflammation, attenuate late phase allergen reaction, lessen symptoms, and exacerbations risk,[1] but are not disease modifying.[116] Effectiveness must be weighed against toxicity, particularly regarding growth. Although numerous studies have established the safety of ICS in children, potential to decrease growth rate exists,[117] influenced by: dose and potency of specific ICS; delivery device; age, gender, weight; individual susceptibility. The small risk of side effects must be balanced against the ability of ICSs to improve impairment and risk with long-term use. Systemic bioavailability results from the oral (swallowed fraction) and lung components. A balanced approach between the extremes of refusing to prescribe ICS because of steroid phobia and insistence that all need to be on these is advised, and approaches must reflect the observation in adults that the regular use of low-dose ICS decreases mortality.[77]

Long-acting Bronchodilators (LABAs). Salmeterol and formoterol that have been evaluated in children. In the USA, salmeterol delivered by metered-dose inhaler (MDI) has been approved for children aged 12 and older; and by dry powder inhaler (DPI) for those 4 years and older; and formoterol has been approved for 5 years and older.

Asthma Action Plan

Name: _____

Date of birth: _____

My best peak-flow is: _____

Quick Relief Medication: _____

Controlled Asthma Is:
1. No cough or wheeze during day or night.
2. Sleep through the night.
3. No missed school/work/play.
4. No emergency visits for asthma.

Rescue or quick-relief medication is used as needed for relief of asthma symptoms (cough, wheezing, chest tightness or shortness of breath). It may also be used 5–15 minutes before exercise if needed.

Green Zone: Doing Well		Use these controller medications everyday	
Medicine	How much to take	When to take it	Special Instructions

→ Take quick-relief medication for asthma symptoms

Peak Flow: from _____ to _____

Yellow Zone: Asthma Getting Worse	Begin yellow zone medications at first signs of a cold or asthma symptoms
Asthma Symptoms • Cough, wheezing • Starting to cough during sleep • Can do some, but not all, usual activities • Decreased response to albuterol Peak Flow: from _____ to _____	→ Take quick-relief medication up to every 4 hours as needed for asthma symptoms → Continue Green Zone medication ☐ → Add/Change to the following medication(s): _____ _____ (use for 5–7 days or until 2 days of being symptom free or back in green zone)

Red Zone: Severe Asthma Signs	Take quick-relief medication and CALL YOUR DOCTOR NOW
• Yellow Zone medications are not helping • Constant cough and/or wheezing • Coughs during sleep most nights • Fast breathing and shortness of breath • Poor response to albuterol Peak Flow: less than _____	→ Take quick-relief medication for asthma symptoms (repeat in 15 minutes if needed) Continue quick-relief medication every 2–4 hours as needed → Continue Green Zone medication ☐ → Add the following medication: _____ _____

If you see any of the following call 911 or go to the EMERGENCY ROOM now:
• Pulling in neck or chest muscles to breathe   • Not able to speak or talk because of asthma • No response to albuterol (rescue medication)   • Lips or fingernails look blue or gray

Provider/Doctor's Name _____   Clinic's Phone Number _____

Return to Clinic _____   Hospital/Emergency Room _____

Signature: _____   Date: _____   Time: _____

Figure 7-13 Sample asthma action plan for home management of asthma, as presented in the Expert Panel Report 3 (EPR-3). *(From National Heart, Lung, and Blood Institute. Expert Panel Report 3 (EPR-3): Guidelines for the Diagnosis and Management of Asthma: Full Report 2007. Available at: <http://www.nhlbi.nih.gov/files/docs/guidelines/asthgdln.pdf>; [accessed July 7, 2015.])*

Salmeterol has a delayed (10–15 min) onset of action but the duration of 12–18 hours vs 3–6 hours for albuterol. Formoterol has a similar onset of action to short-acting bronchodilators. Meta-analyses of trials in patients 12 years and older report greater benefit in improving symptoms, exacerbations and lung function with addition of LABA than with ICS dose.[118,119] The bronchodilating effect of LABAs, however, may diminish with time.[120] Use of LABAs as monotherapy is contraindicated.

In patients 12 years of age and older, the ICS-LABA combination therapy may permit reductions in ICS without worsening of control. LABAs should therefore be used as adjunctive therapy in patients older than 5 years not controlled on low-dose ICS. In EPR-3, equal consideration can be given to increasing ICS dose to the addition of a LABA or LTRA to ICS.

Leukotriene Modifiers. Only two leukotriene modifiers are approved for use in children younger than 12 years of age, in the USA: montelukast (in those at least 1 year of age) and zafirlukast (in those at 7 years of age and older). Both improve lung function and response to allergen and exercise challenge in children. However, the overall efficacy of LTRA in comparison with low-dose ICS is lower, with most outcome measures (symptoms, exacerbations, and lung function) significantly favoring ICS.

Use of LTRA as add-on therapy to low-dose inhaled steroids has not been studied satisfactorily in children 5 to 11 years of age and has not been examined at all in younger children. Adverse events in clinical trials have been mild. EPR-3 recommends that LTRAs be used as an alternative, not a preferred, treatment option for mild persistent asthma, and as alternative, not preferred, adjunctive treatment with ICS in moderate or severe asthma.

Cromolyn Sodium and Nedocromil Sodium. Cromolyn sodium is available only in nebulized form and is approved for use in children older than 2 years of age. Nedocromil sodium is no longer available in the US, but may be available in other countries. Clinical studies evaluating the efficacy of cromolyn sodium and nedocromil sodium in children and adolescents have demonstrated some efficacy. EPR-3 suggests use as an alternative but not a preferred medication for patients with mild persistent asthma.

Theophylline. Theophylline is effective as monotherapy for persistent asthma and has a steroid-sparing effect in children with moderate to severe persistent asthma,[121] although the efficacy of theophylline is less than that of ICS in controlling persistent asthma. As an adjunctive therapy to ICS, theophylline produces a small improvement in lung function similar to that obtained with doubling the dose of ICS. EPR-3 recommends that sustained-release theophylline be used as an alternative, not a preferred, adjunctive agent with ICS. When prescribed, monitoring of serum theophylline levels is needed (target level of 5–15 µg/mL).

Immunomodifiers. Studies of omalizumab in children have demonstrated efficacy in those 5 to 18 years of age.[122] As an add-on to ICS or an ICS-LABA combination, omalizumab leads to improvement in symptoms but has greatest benefit in the prevention of exacerbations. Despite studies demonstrating efficacy, omalizumab is not FDA-approved for use in children younger than 12 years of age. EPR-3 suggests that omalizumab be considered for adjunctive therapy in persons 12 years of age and older who have severe asthma (Step 5 or 6; Fig. 7-12).

Immunotherapy. Subcutaneous allergen immunotherapy (SCIT) is the only childhood treatment shown to potentially modify allergic sensitization and reduce allergic asthma in regard to specific exposures.[123] A meta-analysis has confirmed the effectiveness of immunotherapy in asthma, with reductions in symptoms, medication use and bronchial hyperreactivity.[124] Nevertheless, a large placebo-controlled clinical trial evaluating the efficacy of multiallergen immunotherapy in children was not able to demonstrate a significant effect. Allergen immunotherapy has been recommended in patients with stable asthma sensitized to that particular allergen if clear association between symptoms and allergen exposure can be established.

ACUTE ASTHMA AND REFERRAL FOR HOSPITAL CARE

Introduction

Severe episodes are described as *asthma attacks* or *exacerbations*, with a distinction between an acute flare-up and the day-to-day fluctuations. In the US, 12.8 million have an asthma attack each year.[125] The highest attack prevalence is among children 5 to 17 years of age.

Box 7-9   Risk Factors for Death from Asthma

ASTHMA HISTORY

- Previous severe exacerbation (e.g., intubation or ICU admission for asthma)
- Two or more hospitalizations for asthma in the past year
- Three or more ED visits for asthma in the past year
- Hospitalization or ED visit for asthma in the past month
- Using more than two canisters of SABA a month
- Difficulty perceiving asthma symptoms or severity of exacerbations
- Other risk factors: lack of a written asthma action plan, sensitivity to *Alternaria*

SOCIAL HISTORY

- Low socioeconomic status or inner-city residence
- Illicit drug use
- Major psychosocial problems

COMORBID CONDITIONS

- Cardiovascular disease
- Other chronic lung disease
- Chronic psychiatric disease

ED, Emergency department; ICU, intensive care unit; SABA, short-acting β_2-agonist.

Data sources (see National Heart, Lung, and Blood Institute. Expert Panel Report 3): Abramson et al., 2001; Greenberger et al., 1993; Hardie et al., 2002; Kallenbach et al., 1993; Kikuchi et al., 1994; O'Hollaren et al., 1991; Rodrigo and Rodrigo, 1993; Strunk and Mrazek, 1986; Suissa et al., 1994.

(From National Heart, Lung, and Blood Institute. Expert Panel Report 3 (EPR-3): Guidelines for the Diagnosis and Management of Asthma: Full Report 2007. Available at: <http://www.nhlbi.nih.gov/files/docs/guidelines/asthgdln.pdf>; [accessed July 7, 2015.])

Although most exacerbations are mild and can be managed at home, severe exacerbations prompt emergency department (ED) visits and occasionally hospitalization. ED visits and hospitalizations together account for approximately 15–50% of the billions of US dollars spent on asthma each year.[126] Indirect costs (e.g., lost productivity) add additional billions. In the US, acute asthma accounts for approximately 1.7 million ED visits and 444 000 hospitalizations annually. Acute presentations are precipitated by many factors, commonly upper respiratory tract infections and environmental allergies.

Exacerbations are important events for patients and their families, associated with morbidity, disruption and, occasionally, mortality. Exacerbations persist for many days, and patients remain at risk for subsequent relapses for weeks after.[127] Frequently, ED visits are followed by inadequate subsequent care; in an observational study, 50% of patients seen in Canadian EDs had not had a follow-up examination within 3 weeks.[128]

EPR-3 provides general strategies to manage an exacerbation (Box 7-9).

Evaluation

Key elements in the history include details of the current exacerbation (e.g., time of onset, potential causes), severity of symptoms (especially compared with previous exacerbations), response to treatment, current medications, asthma history (i.e. number of previous unscheduled office visits, ED visits, and hospitalizations), and other comorbid conditions (e.g., other pulmonary or cardiac diseases).

Key elements of the initial physical examination are assessment of overall status (e.g., alertness, fluid status, respiratory distress); vital signs (including pulse oximetry); and chest findings (e.g., use of accessory muscles, wheezing). Examination should also focus on identification of complications (e.g., pneumonia, pneumothorax). In children, the examination should also rule out upper airway obstruction (e.g., foreign bodies). Most patients do not require any laboratory studies, although pulse oximetry can be useful in determining hypoxia.

Pulmonary function should be measured. Although FEV_1 is preferred, serial PEF measurements can provide an estimate of severity and can be used to guide emergency management. Pulmonary function testing is not necessary for patients in extreme respiratory distress. The percentage of predicted FEV_1 or PEF cut-offs for asthma exacerbation severity are 40% for severe and 70% for mild episodes.

Treatment

Table 7-11 summarizes essential information for the major therapeutic options: inhaled, short-acting β_2-agonists (SABAs); systemic (injected) β_2-agonists; anticholinergics; and systemic corticosteroids.

Adults: Home Management of Asthma Exacerbation

Home management (Fig. 7-14) includes an assessment of severity (Fig. 7-15). Initial treatment begins with an increase in frequency of SABA use, usually 2 to 6 puffs, 20 min

TABLE 7-11   Dosages of Drugs for Asthma Exacerbations

Medications	Dosages Children*	Dosages Adults	Comments
Inhaled short-acting β_2-agonists			
Albuterol			
Nebulizer solution (0.63 mg/3 mL, 1.25 mg/3 mL, 2.5 mg/3 mL, 5.0 mg/mL)	0.15 mg/kg (minimum dose, 2.5 mg) every 20 min for 3 doses, then 0.15–0.3 mg/kg up to 10 mg every 1–4 h as needed, or 0.5 mg/kg per h by continuous nebulization	2.5–5 mg every 20 min for 3 doses, then 2.5–10 mg every 1–4 h as needed, or 10–15 mg/h continuously	Only selective β_2-agonists are recommended. For optimal delivery, dilute aerosols to minimum of 3 mL at gas flow of 6–8 L/min. Use large-volume nebulizers for continuous administration; may mix with ipratropium nebulizer solution
MDI (90 µg/puff)	4–8 puffs every 20 min for 3 doses, then every 1–4 h inhalation maneuver as needed; use VHC; add mask for children <4 years	4–8 puffs every 20 min up to 4 h, then every 1–4 h as needed	In mild-to-moderate exacerbations, MDI plus VHC is as effective as nebulized therapy with appropriate administration technique and coaching by trained personnel
Bitolterol			
Nebulizer solution (2 mg/mL)	See albuterol dose; thought to be half as potent as albuterol on mg basis	See albuterol dose	Has not been studied in severe asthma exacerbations; do not mix with other drugs
MDI (370 µg/puff)	See albuterol MDI dose	See albuterol MDI dose	Has not been studied in severe asthma exacerbations
Levalbuterol (R-albuterol)			
Nebulizer solution (0.63 mg/3 mL, 1.25 mg/0.5 mL, 1.25 mg/3 mL)	0.075 mg/kg (minimum dose, 1.25 mg) every 20 min for 3 doses, then 0.075–0.15 mg/kg up to 5 mg every 1–4 h as needed	1.25–2.5 mg every 20 min for 3 doses, then 1.25–5 mg every 1–4 h as needed	Levalbuterol administered in one half (mg) of the albuterol dose provides comparable efficacy and safety; has not been evaluated by continuous nebulization
MDI (45 µg/puff)	See albuterol MDI dose	See albuterol MDI dose	
Pirbuterol			
MDI (200 µg/puff)	See albuterol MDI dose; thought to be one half as potent as albuterol on a milligram basis	See albuterol MDI dose	Has not been studied in severe asthma exacerbations
Systemic (injected) β_2-agonsts			
Epinephrine 1:1000 (1 mg/mL)	0.01 mg/kg up to 0.3–0.5 mg every 20 min for 3 doses SQ	0.3–0.5 mg every 20 min for 3 doses SQ	No proven advantage of systemic therapy over aerosol
Terbutaline (1 mg/mL)	0.01 mg/kg every 20 min for 3 doses SQ, then every 2–6 h as needed	0.25 mg every 20 min for 3 doses SQ	No proven advantage of systemic therapy over aerosol

Continued on following page

TABLE 7-11   Dosages of Drugs for Asthma Exacerbations (Continued)

Medications	Dosages		Comments
	Children*	Adults	
Anticholinergics			
Ipratropium bromide			
Nebulizer solution (0.25 mg/mL)	0.25–0.5 mg every 20 min for 3 doses, then as needed	0.5 mg every 20 min for 3 doses, then as needed	May mix in same nebulizer with albuterol; should not be used as first-line therapy; should be added to SABA therapy for severe exacerbations; addition of ipratropium not shown to provide further benefit after patient is hospitalized
MDI (18 μg/puff)	4–8 puffs every 20 min as needed up to 3 h	8 puffs every 20 min as needed up to 3 h	Should use with VHC and face mask for children <4 years; studies have examined ipratropium bromide MDI for up to 3 h
Ipratropium with albuterol			
Nebulizer solution (each 3 mL vial contains 0.5 mg ipratropium bromide and 2.5 mg albuterol)	1.5 mL every 20 min for 3 doses, then as needed	3 mL every 20 min for 3 doses, then as needed	May be used for up to 3 h in initial management of severe exacerbations; addition of ipratropium to albuterol not shown to provide further benefit after patient is hospitalized
MDI (each puff contains 18 μg ipratropium bromide and 90 μg of albuterol)	4–8 puffs every 20 min as needed up to 3 h	8 puffs every 20 min as needed up to 3 h	Should use with VHC and face mask for children <4 years
Systemic corticosteroids†			
Prednisone Methylprednisolone Prednisolone	1 mg/kg in 2 divided doses (maximum, 60 mg/day) until PEF is 70% of predicted or personal best	40–80 mg/day in 1 or 2 divided doses until PEF reaches 70% of predicted or personal best	For outpatient burst, use 40–60 mg in single dose or 2 divided doses for total of 5–10 days in adults (children: 1–2 mg/kg per day maximum, 60 mg/day for 3–10 days)

*Children ≤12 years of age.
†Dosages and comments apply to all three corticosteroids. There is no known advantage for higher doses of corticosteroids in severe asthma exacerbations, nor is there any advantage for intravenous administration over oral therapy if gastrointestinal transit time or absorption is not impaired. The total course of systemic corticosteroids for an asthma exacerbation requiring an ED visit or hospitalization may be 3–10 days. For corticosteroid courses of less than 1 week, there is no need to taper the dose. For slightly longer courses (e.g., up to 10 days), there probably is no need to taper, especially if patients are concurrently taking ICs. The ICs can be started at any point in the treatment of an asthma exacerbation.
ED, Emergency department; ICs, inhaled corticosteroids; MDI, metered-dose inhaler; PEF, peak expiratory flow; SABA, short-acting β₂-agonists; VHC, valved holding chamber.
(From National Heart, Lung, and Blood Institute. Expert Panel Report 3 (EPR-3): Guidelines for the Diagnosis and Management of Asthma: Full Report 2007. Available at: <http://www.nhlbi.nih.gov/files/docs/guidelines/asthgdln.pdf>; [accessed July 7, 2015.])

apart. Initiation of an oral corticosteroid course can reduce duration of the exacerbation, prevent hospitalizations, and reduce relapse rates. Some patients may be provided with self-held oral corticosteroid courses as part of an action plan. Response to initial treatment is graded as good, incomplete, or poor, based on a reassessment of symptoms and airflow obstruction. With a good response, SABA can be used frequently over the next 24 to 48 hours, along with a short course of prednisone if appropriate. The most effective dosing schedule and duration for systemic corticosteroids are unclear, but a commonly suggested regimen is 0.5 to 1.0 mg of prednisone/kg of body weight for 3 to 7 days. Depending on the individual patient, prednisone can be stopped or rapidly tapered once control has been re-established.

For patients experiencing an incomplete response, the approach is continued SABA use and initiation of a course of prednisone, and the clinician should be involved in supervision of treatment. In patients with a poor response to inhaled SABAs, oral corticosteroids should be started, and transfer to a medical facility is indicated.

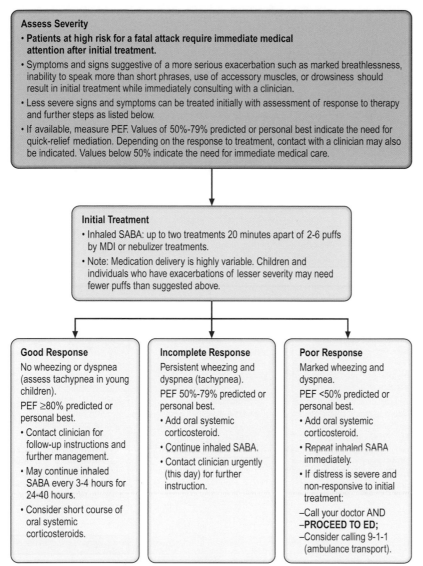

Assess Severity
- **Patients at high risk for a fatal attack require immediate medical attention after initial treatment.**
- Symptoms and signs suggestive of a more serious exacerbation such as marked breathlessness, inability to speak more than short phrases, use of accessory muscles, or drowsiness should result in initial treatment while immediately consulting with a clinician.
- Less severe signs and symptoms can be treated initially with assessment of response to therapy and further steps as listed below.
- If available, measure PEF. Values of 50%-79% predicted or personal best indicate the need for quick-relief mediation. Depending on the response to treatment, contact with a clinician may also be indicated. Values below 50% indicate the need for immediate medical care.

Initial Treatment
- Inhaled SABA: up to two treatments 20 minutes apart of 2-6 puffs by MDI or nebulizer treatments.
- Note: Medication delivery is highly variable. Children and individuals who have exacerbations of lesser severity may need fewer puffs than suggested above.

Good Response

No wheezing or dyspnea (assess tachypnea in young children).

PEF ≥80% predicted or personal best.
- Contact clinician for follow-up instructions and further management.
- May continue inhaled SABA every 3-4 hours for 24-40 hours.
- Consider short course of oral systemic corticosteroids.

Incomplete Response

Persistent wheezing and dyspnea (tachypnea).

PEF 50%-79% predicted or personal best.
- Add oral systemic corticosteroid.
- Continue inhaled SABA.
- Contact clinician urgently (this day) for further instruction.

Poor Response

Marked wheezing and dyspnea.

PEF <50% predicted or personal best.
- Add oral systemic corticosteroid.
- Repeat inhaled SABA immediately.
- If distress is severe and non-responsive to initial treatment:
  –Call your doctor AND
  –**PROCEED TO ED;**
  –Consider calling 9-1-1 (ambulance transport).

Figure 7-14 Management of asthma exacerbations: Home treatment. ED, Emergency department; MDI, metered-dose inhaler; PEF, peak expiratory flow; SABA, short-acting β2-agonist (quick-relief inhaler). *(From National Asthma Education and Prevention Program. Expert Panel Report 3: guidelines for the Diagnosis and Management of Asthma. Full report 2007. Washington DC: US Government Printing Office; 2007.)*

Although commonly recommended, doubling the dose of ICS is not beneficial, although some data suggest a four-fold increase in ICS may be beneficial.[129]

Adults: Hospital and Emergency Department Care

For patients with severe potentially life-threatening asthma exacerbations, assessment and treatment in hospital settings is needed. The goal of emergency care is to ensure adequate oxygenation, to reverse the obstruction, and to initiate anti-inflammatory therapy. Laboratory studies (e.g., arterial blood gas testing) are used for detection of actual or impending respiratory failure and to detect conditions complicating emergency management (e.g., electrocardiogram to rule out cardiac ischemia, chest radiograph to rule out pneumonia).

Oxygen. Supplemental oxygen is recommended for initial ED or inpatient treatment, administered by nasal cannula or mask, to maintain an arterial oxygen saturation (SaO_2) of ≥90% or ≥95% in pregnant women and those with cardiac disease.

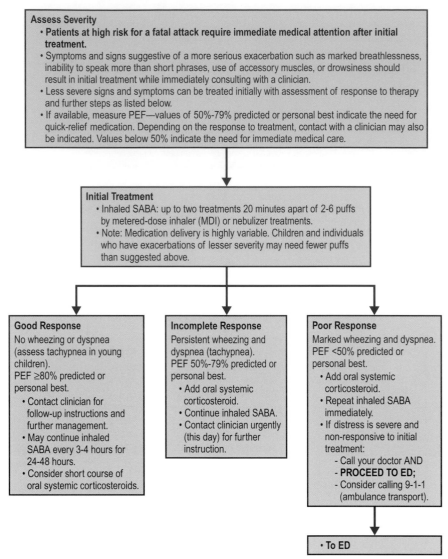

Assess Severity
- **Patients at high risk for a fatal attack require immediate medical attention after initial treatment.**
- Symptoms and signs suggestive of a more serious exacerbation such as marked breathlessness, inability to speak more than short phrases, use of accessory muscles, or drowsiness should result in initial treatment while immediately consulting with a clinician.
- Less severe signs and symptoms can be treated initially with assessment of response to therapy and further steps as listed below.
- If available, measure PEF—values of 50%-79% predicted or personal best indicate the need for quick-relief medication. Depending on the response to treatment, contact with a clinician may also be indicated. Values below 50% indicate the need for immediate medical care.

Initial Treatment
- Inhaled SABA: up to two treatments 20 minutes apart of 2-6 puffs by metered-dose inhaler (MDI) or nebulizer treatments.
- Note: Medication delivery is highly variable. Children and individuals who have exacerbations of lesser severity may need fewer puffs than suggested above.

Good Response
No wheezing or dyspnea (assess tachypnea in young children).
PEF ≥80% predicted or personal best.
- Contact clinician for follow-up instructions and further management.
- May continue inhaled SABA every 3-4 hours for 24-48 hours.
- Consider short course of oral systemic corticosteroids.

Incomplete Response
Persistent wheezing and dyspnea (tachypnea).
PEF 50%-79% predicted or personal best.
- Add oral systemic corticosteroid.
- Continue inhaled SABA.
- Contact clinician urgently (this day) for further instruction.

Poor Response
Marked wheezing and dyspnea.
PEF <50% predicted or personal best.
- Add oral systemic corticosteroid.
- Repeat inhaled SABA immediately.
- If distress is severe and non-responsive to initial treatment:
  - Call your doctor AND
  - **PROCEED TO ED;**
  - Consider calling 9-1-1 (ambulance transport).

- **To ED**

Figure 7-15 Management of asthma exacerbations in adolescents and adults: home treatment. (Figure numbers refer to those in cited source.) ED, emergency department; PEF, peak expiratory flow; SABA, short-acting β₂-agonist [quick-relief medication]. *(Modified from National Heart, Lung, and Blood Institute. Expert Panel Report 3 (EPR-3): Guidelines for the Diagnosis and Management of Asthma: Full Report 2007. Available at: <http://www.nhlbi.nih.gov/files/docs/guidelines/asthgdln.pdf>; [accessed July 7, 2015.])*

Inhaled, Short-acting β₂-Agonists. Early treatment is with inhaled selective SABAs (i.e. albuterol [salbutamol], levalbuterol, pirbuterol) because of the rapid effect on bronchospasm. Whether the drug is most effective delivered through a nebulizer or through a metered-dose inhaler (MDI) with a holding chamber or spacer remains an area of research. A Cochrane systematic review[130] found that either delivery method produced similar outcomes. In children, but not adults, MDI with holding chamber or spacer appeared to offer advantages in terms of ED length of stay and adverse effects (e.g., tachycardia). Nebulizer therapy may still be preferred, however, for patients who are unable to cooperative effectively in using an MDI because of their age, agitation, or severity of acute asthma. For patients with life-threatening exacerbations, continuous nebulization[131] may be considered. EPR3 recommendations are summarized in Figures 7-14 and 7-16 and in Table 7-11.

Inhaled Anticholinergic Agents. There is support, particularly in children, for adding the anticholinergic agent ipratropium bromide to β₂-agonist therapy in severe asthma

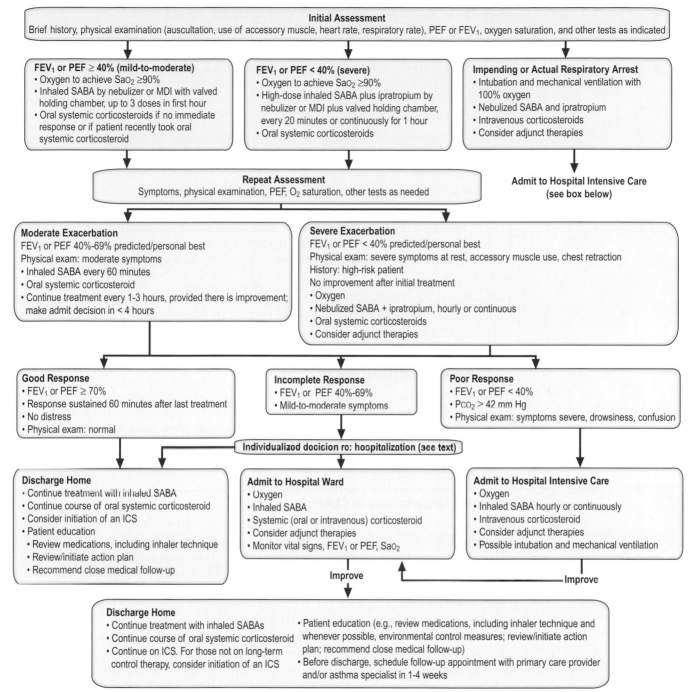

Figure 7-16 Management of asthma exacerbations: Emergency department and hospital-based care. FEV₁, Forced expiratory volume in 1 second; ICs, inhaled corticosteroids; MDI, metered-dose inhaler; PCO₂, partial pressure of carbon dioxide; PEF, peak expiratory flow; SABA, short-acting β₂-agonist(quick-relief inhaler); SaO₂, arterial oxygen saturation. *(From National Heart, Lung, and Blood Institute. Expert Panel Report 3 (EPR-3): Guidelines for the Diagnosis and Management of Asthma – Full Report 2007. Available at: <http:// www.nhlbi.nih.gov/files/docs/guidelines/asthgdln.pdf>; [accessed July 7, 2015.])*

exacerbations.[132] Multiple doses of ipratropium bromide result in a clinically significant improvement in FEV₁ and reduced the risk of hospitalization by 25%.

Systemic Corticosteroids. Early use of systemic corticosteroids (i.e. within 1 hour of the presentation) delivered by oral or intravenous routes continues to be the principal treatment choice. Early use of corticosteroids in the ED reduces admission rates (OR = 0.40), with a number needed to treat (NNT) of 8, particularly for those not already receiving systemic corticosteroids. Intravenous corticosteroids should be reserved for those who are too breathless to swallow, obtunded or intubated, or unable to tolerate oral medications.

Magnesium Sulfate. Magnesium sulfate ($MgSO_4$) is used in unresponsive acute asthma, with immediate bronchodilator and mild anti-inflammatory effects.[133] Although uncertainties remain, EPR3 recommend consideration of intravenous $MgSO_4$ in patients with life-threatening exacerbations.

Heliox. Another controversial area is the role of heliox, a helium-oxygen mixture, which has been used sporadically since the 1930s. A 2006 Cochrane review yielded a borderline-significant group difference. EPR3 guidelines recommend consideration of heliox in patients who have life-threatening exacerbations.

Leukotriene Modifiers. Intravenous montelukast may be beneficial in cases of moderate to severe exacerbations, with significant improvement in FEV_1 within 10 min of administration.[134] For rapid bronchodilation, the intravenous route is required because an oral formulation of montelukast does not provide benefit until approximately 90 min after administration.

Other Therapies. The benefits of agents such as aminophylline[135] are limited. Antibiotics should not be used routinely for acute asthma.[136] Despite this, many clinicians continue to prescribe antibiotics for the viral upper respiratory tract infections triggering asthma, a focus for future quality improvements to decrease inappropriate antibiotic use.

Care after Hospitalization and ED Visits

Approximately 10–20% of ED patients treated for acute asthma and sent home will relapse within 2 weeks of discharge.[90] The use of oral corticosteroids for a short period (e.g., 5–7 days) is appropriate for patients discharged after an acute asthma episode, with a medical review arranged prior to discontinuation. All should also receive ICS if they were not already receiving them. However, in the US, only 11% of discharged patients were prescribed ICS.[137]

Managing Exacerbations in Children

In the Childhood Asthma Management Program study of school-aged children with asthma, 40% of the children in the ICS treatment group experienced exacerbation, compared with 75% in those receiving placebo.[113] Many can be managed at home, but as with adults, more severe exacerbations require ED and hospital care.

Home Management

Inhaled SABAs can be delivered by MDI with or without a spacer device, as dry powder formulations, or by handheld nebulizer. Children younger than 5 years of age require the use of a mask with nebulizer treatments or with an MDI and valved spacer system for effective delivery of medication into the airways. Some patients and families prefer nebulizer treatments, which require only slow tidal breathing. Both high-dose MDI and nebulized delivery, however, have been shown to be equally efficacious. If the attack is severe and unresponsive to therapy, the family caregiver and/or the patient should be instructed to contact a healthcare provider. Home therapy may involve the introduction of short course oral corticosteroids, which reduce the duration and severity of the exacerbation and prevent hospitalization.[138] Quadrupling but not doubling the dose of ICS at the first sign of worsening symptoms in patients already receiving ICS may prevent exacerbations requiring oral corticosteroids.[139] The increased SABA use during an exacerbation should continue until the level of asthma symptom control and PEF values return to the patient's baseline.

Office or Emergency Department Management in Children

If early intervention at home fails, the family should be instructed to take the child to an urgent care center, or hospital ED for further management. The initial assessment should include a brief history, physical examination focused on the work of breathing,

PEF determination or spirometry, and measurement of oxygen saturation. Blood gas analysis is not routinely indicated. Routine chest radiographs are not necessary.

In a mild to moderate exacerbation (FEV_1 or PEF of $\geq 40\%$), initial therapy includes oxygen to keep oxygen saturations higher than 90% and up to three doses in the first hour of inhaled SABA delivered by either nebulizer or MDI with spacer, and oral corticosteroids if no immediate response to bronchodilators is obtained. In severe exacerbations (FEV_1 or PEF $<40\%$), therapy should include prompt administration of oxygen, high-dose inhaled SABA plus ipratropium every 20 min or continuously for the first hour, and oral corticosteroids. Severe exacerbations are potentially life-threatening, so transfer to an ED is required in most cases to permit close observation for deterioration, repeated assessments, and frequent administration of indicated treatments. Most studies evaluating the use of intravenous theophylline in the treatment of acute exacerbations have been unable to demonstrate any additional benefit.

Hospital Management in Children

An incomplete response in symptoms or lung function (FEV_1 or PEF of 40–69%) despite aggressive treatment, warrants hospitalization for continued inhaled SABA, systemic corticosteroids, oxygen (if needed), and close monitoring. Hospitalization should be considered for infants with oxygen saturation <92% on room air.[140]

Post-Hospital Care

In addition to acute management, a most important aspect should be preventing recurrence. Asthma education is appropriate in the clinic, ED, and hospital settings, and communication with primary care health providers is crucial.

CONCLUSIONS

Asthma care has seen remarkable developments over the last 30 years, with greater understanding of the diverse factors comprising the asthma syndrome leading to therapeutic advances and to improved outcomes. However, asthma remains common, incurable, the global prevalence continues to increase, and the improvements in outcomes seen over the last decades of the last century have stalled in most economically developed countries. Although we have superior insights into the biologic basis of asthma, the complex genetic and environmental factors interacting to manifest as asthma in susceptible individuals, and greater understanding of the immunologic pathways underpinning asthma, translating this knowledge into patient benefit, has lagged. The complexity of asthma is now appreciated, with the various phenotypes and endotypes comprising the asthma syndrome progressively becoming clearer. Asthma guidelines are based on group mean data from clinical trials, and use a stepped approach for all, based on severity and control, yet the heterogeneity of individual responses to different interventions is increasingly apparent. Future developments in asthma care, as with other long-term conditions, are likely to involve 'stratified' or 'personalized' approaches to asthma care. Since the final manifestation of the various pathologic processes involved in the asthma syndrome can be very similar, yet the drivers be diverse, it is likely that further improvements in asthma outcomes will rely on targeting interventions onto appropriately identified individuals with specific characteristics. This will involve better characterization at an individual patient level and an approach that encompasses this diversity by detecting poor control, assessing the reasons for it and directing the most appropriate treatments to improve it. Such a 'stratified' approach is starting to occur in severe asthma, where the development of expensive new biological treatments that are very effective for appropriately characterized patients (accompanied by biomarkers to characterize responders) is being driven by economic considerations. However, it is possible that similar stratified approaches can be applied in community practice.

Asthma Diagnosis and Monitoring

There is concern that the diagnosis of asthma is sometimes inappropriately applied, and that asthma is inadequately monitored. The symptoms of asthma are non-specific, and supporting objective criteria (such as reversible variable airflow obstruction, bronchial hyperresponsiveness or airway inflammation) are often not measured or recorded. General practitioners and community-based non-specialists frequently lack access to the more sophisticated diagnostic tests needed to confirm or refute the diagnosis in the (frequent) cases of diagnostic uncertainty. This may result in patients with non-specific respiratory symptoms being labeled as having asthma and commenced on anti-asthma medication (commonly anti-inflammatory treatment with ICS) without evidence of a corticosteroid-responsive disease. Lack of response often leads to escalation of treatment rather than a review of the diagnosis. Asthma is defined as an inflammatory disease of the airways characterized by BHR, yet inflammation and hyperreactivity are commonly not assessed outside of research or specialist settings. Recent advances in technology potentially allow greater use of objective testing in routine community settings (including blood biomarkers, exhaled biomarkers such as FeNO and even bronchial challenge tests such as with inhaled mannitol), which may have significant implications for the diagnosis, monitoring and therapeutic decision making in asthma care.

Poor control is frequently not detected by clinicians and not volunteered by patients, who have come to accept the status quo as a fact of life. More objective assessments of control are possible with currently available tools (both patient-reported and using biomarkers).

Asthma Treatment

Improvements in asthma therapeutics are likely to involve both more effective use of currently available therapies, and the development of new treatments for the small but important subgroup with genuine therapy resistant disease.

Better Use of Current Treatments

The most common reasons for suboptimal outcomes in asthma relate to poor adherence and poor inhaler technique. Greater awareness of these important factors and greater partnership with patients (including wider use of self-management education) is a challenge for primary care asthma providers. Improved patient characterization is likely to assist in the better targeting of current therapies. For instance, in the case of a patient receiving low-dose ICS who remains uncontrolled, current guidelines suggest that addition of a LABA is the preferred option. However, the ability to measure airway inflammation could guide the decision-making process; evidence of ongoing inflammation could point to inadequate delivery of ICS (e.g., non-adherence or poor inhaler technique) or to the need for increased doses or potency of anti-inflammatory medication, whereas normal inflammatory indices would support the use of a bronchodilator or other approaches to achieve control.

Considerable interest exists in the use of combination ICS-fast acting bronchodilator inhalers as rescue medication, in theory allowing increased delivery of anti-inflammatory medication as symptoms (and inflammation) worsen; the 'single maintenance and reliever' inhaler approach is now possible with more than one product, and as required use at 'Step 1' under investigation. The effectiveness and positioning of these strategies will become clearer in coming years

Current trends in chronic disease management of involving patients (where possible) in decision making and sharing uncertainty is likely if applied effectively to improve adherence, patient outcomes, expectations, and satisfaction.

New Treatments

There continues to be new products (Fig. 7-17) for treating asthma reaching the market, although most consist of new versions of existing therapy classes. The availability of more potent and longer-acting molecules within currently available drug classes (e.g., once daily ICS and LABAs) potentially have limited incremental benefits that may be helpful to some patients. New inhaler devices and delivery systems that are easier for patients to use and for professionals to teach, may again benefit some patients and allow existing classes of medications to be used more effectively.

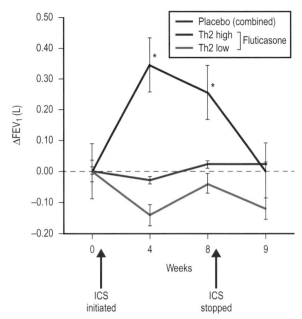

Figure 7-17 Responsiveness of 'Th2 high' asthma to inhaled corticosteroids (ICS) and placebo in a randomized controlled trial. FEV$_1$ measured at baseline (week 0), after 4 and 8 weeks on daily fluticasone (500 μg twice a day), and 1 week after the cessation of fluticasone (week 9). No significant change in FEV$_1$ in response to placebo is seen at any time point in either group, Th2 low, and placebo. *(From Woodruff PG, Modrek B, Choy DF, et al. T-helper type 2-driven inflammation defines major subphenotypes of asthma. Am J Respir Crit Care Med 2009;180:388–95.)*

Although the majority of patients could be well controlled on existing therapy classes, there are some (estimated to be 5–10% of the total asthma population) with more severe, therapy-resistant, 'difficult to control' disease who currently have poor outcomes and high associated healthcare use and cost. The greater understanding of the various biologic and immunologic abnormalities present in these patients has led to the development of a number of new treatments, currently undergoing clinical trials. Most of these treatments involve synthesized human monoclonal antibodies targeted upon Th2 cytokines such as Il-4, -5, and -13, and several are currently in clinical trials, with the promise of effective new therapeutic options targeted at specific asthma endotypes.[141] Some asthmatics show abnormalities in innate immunity leading to viral triggered asthma, and again novel interventions such as inhaled interferon-β are undergoing trials and hold promise for selected patients.[142] A minority of patients with asthma do not show Th2 driven inflammation, with neutrophilic or pauci-granulocytic disease observed; this challenging group of patients show poor responsiveness to corticosteroids, and new approaches are under investigation. Macrolide antibiotics hold some promise for this subgroup of patients, with trials currently under way.

Prevention

The causes of the increasing global prevalence of asthma remain incompletely understood, with a number of large birth cohort studies ongoing in different parts of the world. These have provided important information on factors associated with asthma (e.g., early life microbial exposure; family size and birth rank; early contact with animals) but have not yet provided public health strategies for prevention. The complexity and interdependence of factors promoting or protecting against asthma is slowly being unraveled. Interventions studied have included environmental (e.g., intensive aeroallergen avoidance measures in the home), vaccination, and diet, with generally disappointing results. Advances in computing techniques in large databases are allowing databases to be combined and it is likely that important new information will become available in the coming years.

REFERENCES

1. *Global Initiative for Asthma. Global strategy for asthma management and prevention 2014. Online. Available: <www.ginasthma.org>.
2. *The International Study of Asthma and Allergies in Childhood (ISAAC) Steering Committee. Worldwide variation in prevalence of symptoms of asthma, allergic rhinoconjunctivitis, and atopic eczema: ISAAC. Lancet 1998;351:1225–32.
3. *Asher MI, Montefort S, Björkstén B, et al. Worldwide time trends in the prevalence of symptoms of asthma, allergic rhinoconjunctivitis, and eczema in childhood: ISAAC Phases one and three repeat multicountry cross-sectional surveys. Lancet 2006;368:733–43.
4. *Masoli M, Fabian D, Holt S, et al. The global burden of asthma: executive summary of the GINA Dissemination Committee report. Allergy 2004;59:469–78.
5. Cockcroft DW. Bronchoprovocation methods: direct challenges. Clin Rev Allergy Immunol 2003;24:19–26.
6. Shaw D, Green R, Berry M, et al. A cross-sectional study of patterns of airway dysfunction, symptoms and morbidity in primary care asthma. Prim Care Respir J 2012;21(3):283–7.
7. *To T, Stanojevic S, Moores G, et al. Global asthma prevalence in adults: findings from the cross-sectional world health survey. BMC Public Health 2012;12:204.
8. Thomas M, Wilkinson T. Asthma diagnosis in the community: time for a change? Clin Exp Allergy 2014;44(10):1206–9.
9. Aaron SD, Vandemheen KL, Boulet LP, et al. Overdiagnosis of asthma in obese and non-obese adults. CMAJ 2008;179:1121–31.
10. Wenzel SE. Phenotypes in asthma: useful guides for therapy, distinct biological processes, or both? Am J Respir Crit Care Med 2004;170:579–80.
11. Bergeron C, Boulet LP. Structural changes in airway diseases: characteristics, mechanisms, consequences, and pharmacologic modulation. Chest 2006;129:1068–87.
12. *British Thoracic Society, Scottish Intercollegiate Guideline Network. British Guideline on the Management of Asthma. A national clinical guideline. Revised 2014. Online. Available: <https://www.brit-thoracic.org.uk/document-library/clinical-information/asthma/btssign-asthma-guideline-2014/>.
13. *National Asthma Education and Prevention Program (NAEPP). Expert Panel Report 3 (EPR-3): Guidelines for the diagnosis and management of asthma. NIH Publication No. 07-4051. Bethesda, MD: US Department of Health and Human Services, National Institutes of Health; 2007.
14. *Bateman ED, Boushey HA, Bousquet J, et al. Can guideline-defined asthma control be achieved? The Gaining Optimal Asthma Control study. Am J Respir Crit Care Med 2004;170(8):836–44.
15. *Demoly P, Gueron B, Annunziata K, et al. Update on asthma control in five European countries: results of a 2008 survey. Eur Respir Rev 2010;19(116):150–7.
16. *Levy M, Andrews R, Buckingham R, et al. Why asthma still kills: the National Review of Asthma Deaths (NRAD) Confidential Enquiry report. London: RCP; 2014 Online. Available: <https://www.rcplondon.ac.uk/sites/default/files/why-asthma-still-kills-full-report.pdf>.
17. de Nijs SB1, Venekamp LN, Bel EH. Adult-onset asthma: is it really different? Eur Respir Rev 2013;22(127):44–52.
18. *Martinez FD, Wright AL, Taussig LM, et al. Asthma and wheezing in the first six years of life. The Group Health Medical Associates. N Engl J Med 1995;332:133–8.
19. Guilbert T, Moss MH, Lemanske RF Jr, et al. Approach to infants and children with asthma. In: Adkinson NF, Busse WW, Bochner BS, editors. Middleton's allergy: principles and practice. 7th ed. St Louis: Mosby; 2009. p. 1319–43.
20. Pearce N, Ait-Khaled N, Beasley R, et al. Worldwide trends in the prevalence of asthma symptoms: Phase III of the International Study of Asthma and Allergies in Childhood (ISAAC). Thorax 2007; 62:758–66.
21. Pereira MU, Sly PD, Pitrez PM, et al. Non-atopic asthma is associated with helminth infections and bronchiolitis in poor children. Eur Resp J 2007;29:1154–60.
22. James AL. Localization of pathology in asthma. Clin Exp Allergy 2009;39:1450–2.
23. Kraft M, Djukanovic R, Wilson S, et al. Alveolar tissue inflammation in asthma. Am J Respir Crit Care Med 1996;154:1505–10.
24. Shaver JR, Zangrilli JG, Cho SK, et al. Kinetics of the development and recovery of the lung from IgE-mediated inflammation: dissociation of pulmonary eosinophilia, lung injury, and eosinophil-active cytokines. Am J Respir Crit Care Med 1997;155:442–8.
25. Bessa V, Tseliou E, Bakakos P, et al. Non-invasive evaluation of airway inflammation in asthmatic patients who smoke: implications for application in clinical practice. Ann Allergy Asthma Immunol 2008;101:226–32, quiz 32–34, 78.
26. Hamid Q, Azzawi M, Ying S, et al. Expression of mRNA for interleukin-5 in mucosal bronchial biopsies from asthma. J Clin Invest 1991;87:1541–6.
27. Woodruff PG, Modrek B, Choy DF, et al. T-helper type 2-driven inflammation defines major subphenotypes of asthma. Am J Respir Crit Care Med 2009;180:388–95.
28. Bosse Y, Reisenfeld EP, Pare PD, et al. It's not all smooth muscle: non-smooth-muscle elements in control of resistance airflow. Annu Rev Physiol 2010;72:937–62.
29. Strachan DP. Hay fever, hygiene, and household size. BMJ 1989;299:1259–60.
30. Moffatt MF, Kabesch M, Liang L, et al. Genetic variants regulating ORMDL3 expression contribute to the risk of childhood asthma. Nature 2007;448:470–3.
31. Weidinger S, Geiger C, Rodriguez E, et al. Genome-wide scan on total serum IgE levels identifies FCER1A as novel susceptibility locus. PLoS Genet 2008;4:e1000166.
32. Gudbjartsson DF, Bjornsdottir US, Halapi E, et al. Sequence variants affecting eosinophil numbers associate with asthma and myocardial infarction. Nat Genet 2009;41:342–7.

33. Kim SH, Cho BY, Park CS, et al. Alpha-T catenin (CTNNA3) gene was identified as a risk variant for toluene diisocyanate-induced asthma by genome-wide association analysis. Clin Exp Allergy 2009;39:203–12.
34. Moffatt MF, Gut IG, Demenais F, et al. A largescale, consortium-based genomewide association study of asthma. N Engl J Med 2010;363:1211–21.
35. Sleiman PM, Flory J, Imielinski M, et al. Variants of DENND1B associated with asthma in children. N Engl J Med 2010;362:36–44.
36. Li X, Howard TD, Zheng SL, et al. Genome-wide association study of asthma identifies RAD50-IL13 and HLA-DR/DQ regions. J Allergy Clin Immunol 2010;125:328–35.
37. Ferreira MA, Matheson MC, Dufy DL, et al. Identification of IL6R and chromosome 11q13.5 as risk loci for asthma. Lancet 2011;378:1006–14.
38. Hirota T, Takahashi A, Kubo M, et al. Genomewide association study identifies three new susceptibility loci for adult asthma in the Japanese population. Nat Genet 2011;43:893–6.
39. Torgerson DG, Ampleford EJ, Chiu GY, et al. Meta-analysis of genome-wide association studies of asthma in ethnically diverse North American populations. Nat Genet 2011;43:887–92.
40. Tantisira KG, Lasky-Su J, Harada M, et al. Genomewide association between GLCCI1 and response to glucocorticoid therapy in asthma. N Engl J Med 2011;365:1173–83.
41. Du R, Litonjua AA, Tantisira KG, et al. Genome-wide association study reveals class I MHC-restricted T cell-associated molecule gene (CRTAM) variants interact with vitamin D levels to affect asthma exacerbations. J Allergy Clin Immunol 2012;129:368–73.
42. Esparza-Gordillo J, Weidinger S, Fölster-Holst R, et al. A common variant on chromosome 11q13 is associated with atopic dermatitis. Nat Genet 2009;41:596–601.
43. Paternoster L, Standl M, Chen CM, et al. Metaanalysis of genome-wide association studies identifies three new risk loci for atopic dermatitis. Nat Genet 2012;44:187–92.
44. Sun LD, Xiao FL, Zhou WM, et al. Genomewide association study identifies two new susceptibility loci for atopic dermatitis in the Chinese Han population. Nat Genet 2011;43:690–4.
45. Ramasamy A, Kuokkanen M, Vedantam S, et al. Genome-wide association studies of asthma in population-based cohorts confirm known and suggested loci and identify an additional association near HLA. PLoS ONE 2012;7(9):e44008.
46. Simpson A, Maniatis N, Jury F. Polymorphisms in a disintegrin and metalloprotease 33 (ADAM33) predict impaired early-life lung function. Am J Respir Crit Care Med 2005;172:55–60.
47. Haldar P, Pavord I, Shaw D, et al. Cluster analysis and clinical asthma phenotypes. Am J Respir Crit Care Med 2008;178(3):218–24.
48. Anderson GP. Endotyping asthma: new insights into key pathogenic mechanisms in a complex, heterogeneous disease. Lancet 2008;372(9643):1107–19.
49. Moore WC, Meyers DA, Wenzel SE, National Heart, Lung, and Blood Institute's Severe Asthma Research Program, et al. Identification of asthma phenotypes using cluster analysis in the Severe Asthma Research Program. Am J Respir Crit Care Med 2010;181:315–23.
50. Lotvall J, Akdis CA, Bacharier LB, et al. Asthma endotypes: a new approach to classification of disease entities within the asthma syndrome. J Allergy Clin Immunol 2011;127:354–60.
51. Boulet LP. Influence of comorbid conditions on asthma. Eur Respir J 2009;33:897–906.
52. Brand PL, Baraldi E, Bisgaard H, et al. Definition, assessment and treatment of wheezing disorders in preschool children: an evidence-based approach. Eur Respir J 2008;32:1096–110.
53. Sonnappa S, Bastardo CM, Wade A, et al. Symptom-pattern phenotype and pulmonary function in preschool wheezers. J Allergy Clin Immunol 2010;126:519–26.
54. Morgan WJ, Martinez FD. Risk factors for developing wheezing and asthma in childhood. Pediatr Clin North Am 1992;39:1185–203.
55. Thomas M. Asthma diagnosis: not always simple or straightforward ... J Thorac Dis 2014;6(5):409–10.
56. Miller MR, Hankinson J, Brusasco V, et al. Standardisation of spirometry. Eur Respir J 2005;26:319–38.
57. Pavord ID, Bush A, Holgate S. Asthma diagnosis: addressing the challenges. Lancet Respir Med 2015;3(5):339–41.
58. Dweik RA, Boggs PB, Erzurum SC, et al. An official ATS clinical practice guideline: interpretation of exhaled nitric oxide levels (FeNO) for clinical applications. Am J Respir Crit Care Med 2011;184:602–15.
59. Gruffydd-Jones K, Ward S, Stonham C, et al. The use of exhaled nitric oxide monitoring in primary care asthma clinics: a pilot study. Prim Care Respir J 2007;16:349–56.
60. Malo JL, Vandenplas O. Definitions and classification of work-related asthma. Immunol Allergy Clin North Am 2011;31:645–62.
61. Henneberger PK, Redlich CA, Callahan DB, et al. An official American Thoracic Society statement: work-exacerbated asthma. Am J Respir Crit Care Med 2011;184:368–78.
62. Bernstein I, Chan-Yeung M, Malo J, et al. Definition and classification of asthma in the workplace. In: Bernstein IL, Chan-Yeung M, Malo JL, editors. Asthma in the workplace. 3rd ed. New York: Francis & Taylor. 2006. p. 1–8.
63. Torén K, Blanc PD. Asthma caused by occupational exposures is common – a systematic analysis of estimates of the population-attributable fraction. BMC Pulm Med 2009;9:7.
64. Cullinan P, Cook A, Gordon S, et al. Allergen exposure, atopy and smoking as determinants of allergy to rats in a cohort of laboratory employees. Eur Respir J 1999;13:1139–43.
65. Cullinan P, Cook A, Nieuwenhuijsen M, et al. Allergen and dust exposure as determinants of work-related symptoms and sensitization in a cohort of flour-exposed workers; a case-control analysis. Ann Occup Hyg 2001;45:97–103.

66. Archambault S, Malo J, Infante-Rivard C, et al. Incidence of sensitization, symptoms and probable occupational rhinoconjunctivitis and asthma in apprentices starting exposure to latex. J Allergy Clin Immunol 2001;107:921–3.

67. Lemière C, Chaboilliez S, Trudeau C, et al. Characterization of airway inflammation after repeated exposures to occupational agents. J Allergy Clin Immunol 2000;106:1163–70.

68. Gibson PG, McDonald VM, Marks GB. Asthma in older adults. Lancet 2010;376(9743): 803–13.

69. Fitch KD, Sue-Chu M, Anderson SD, et al. Asthma and the elite athlete: summary of the International Olympic Committee's consensus conference, Lausanne, Switzerland, January 22–24, 2008. J Allergy Clin Immunol 2008;122:254–60.

70. Ibrahim WH, Gheriani HA, Almohamed AA, et al. Paradoxical vocal cord motion disorder: past, present and future. Postgrad Med J 2007;83:164–72.

71. Thomas M, McKinley RK, Freeman E, et al. Prevalence of dysfunctional breathing in patients treated for asthma in primary care: cross sectional survey. BMJ 2001;322:1098–100.

72. Galant SP, Morphew T, Amaro S, et al. Value of the bronchodilator response in assessing controller naive asthmatic children. J Pediatr 2007;151:457–62.

73. Baishnab E, Karner C. Primary care based clinics for asthma. Cochrane Database Syst Rev 2012;(4):CD003533.

74. Pinnock H, Thomas M. Does self-management prevent severe exacerbations? Curr Opin Pulm Med 2015;21(1):95–102.

75. Cockcroft DW, Swystun VA. Asthma control versus asthma severity. J Allergy Clin Immunol 1996;98(6 Pt 1):1016–18.

76. Adams RJ, Smith BJ, Ruffin RE. Factors associated with hospital admissions and repeat emergency department visits for adults with asthma. Thorax 2000;55:566–73.

77. *Suissa S, Ernst P, Benayoun S, et al. Low-dose inhaled corticosteroids and the prevention of death from asthma. N Engl J Med 2000;343(5):332–6.

78. Horne R. Compliance, adherence, and concordance: implications for asthma treatment. Chest 2006;130(1 Suppl.):65S–72S. PMID: 16840369.

79. Gamble J, Stevenson M, Heaney LG. A study of a multi-level intervention to improve non-adherence in difficult to control asthma. Respir Med 2011;105(9):1308–15. doi:10.1016/j.rmed.2011.03.019; PMID: 21511454.

80. Gibson PG, Coughlan J, Wilson AJ, et al. Self-management education and regular practitioner review for adults with asthma. The Cochrane Library 2003;(1):CD001117.

81. Bel EH. Smoking: a neglected cause of glucocorticoid resistance in asthma. Am J Respir Crit Care Med 2003;168:1265–6.

82. Thomas M, Bruton A, Moffat M, et al. Asthma and psychological dysfunction. Prim Care Respir J 2011;20(3):250–6.

83. Thomas M, McKinley RK, Mellor S, et al. Breathing exercises for asthma: a randomised controlled trial. Thorax 2009;64:55–61.

84. Westby M, Benson M, Gibson P. Anticholinergic agents for chronic asthma in adults. Cochrane Database Syst Rev 2004;(3):CD003269.

85. Kerstjens HA, Engel M, Dahl R, et al. Tiotropium in asthma poorly controlled with standard combination therapy. N Engl J Med 2012;67:1198–207.

86. Adams N, Bestall J, Jones PW. Budesonide for chronic asthma in children and adults. Cochrane Database Syst Rev 2001;(1):CD003274.

87. Malmstrom K, Rodriguez-Gomez G, Guerra J, et al. Oral montelukast, inhaled beclomethasone, and placebo for chronic asthma. A randomized, controlled trial. Montelukast/Beclomethasone Study Group. Ann Intern Med 1999;130:487–95.

88. Nelson HS, Busse WW, Kerwin E, et al. Fluticasone propionate/salmeterol combination provides more effective asthma control than low-dose inhaled corticosteroid plus montelukast. J Allergy Clin Immunol 2000;106:1088–95.

89. Pauwels RA, Pedersen S, Busse WW, et al. Early intervention with budesonide in mild persistent asthma: a randomised, double-blind trial. Lancet 2003;361:1071–6.

90. Emerman CL, Woodruff PG, Cydulka RK, et al. Prospective multicenter study of relapse following treatment for acute asthma among adults presenting to the emergency department. Chest 1999;115:919–27.

91. Price D, Musgrave SD, Shepstone L, et al. Leukotriene antagonists as first-line or add-on asthma-controller therapy. N Engl J Med 2011;364:1695–707.

92. Edelman JM, Turpin JA, Bronsky EA, et al. Oral montelukast compared with inhaled salmeterol to prevent exercise-induced bronchoconstriction. Ann Intern Med 2000;132:97–104.

93. Greening AP, Ind PW, Northfield M, et al. Added salmeterol versus higher-dose corticosteroid in asthma patients with symptoms on existing inhaled corticosteroid. Allen & Hanburys Limited UK Study Group. Lancet 1994;344:219–24.

94. Thomas M, von Ziegenweidt J, Lee AJ, et al. High-dose inhaled corticosteroids versus add-on long-acting beta-agonists in asthma: an observational study. J Allergy Clin Immunol 2009;123:116–21.

95. Nelson HS, Weiss ST, Bleecker ER, SMART Study Group, et al. The Salmeterol Multicenter Asthma Research Trial: a comparison of usual pharmacotherapy for asthma or usual pharmacotherapy plus salmeterol. Chest 2006;129:15–26.

96. McMahon AW, Levenson MS, McEvoy BW, et al. Age and risks of FDA-approved long-acting beta(2)-adrenergic receptor agonists. Pediatrics 2011;128:e1147–54.

97. Chowdhury BA, Dal Pan G. The FDA and safe use of long-acting beta-agonists in the treatment of asthma. N Engl J Med 2010;362:1169–71.

98. Price DB, Hernandez D, Magyar P, et al. Randomised controlled trial of montelukast plus inhaled budesonide versus double dose inhaled budesonide in adult patients with asthma. Thorax 2003;58:211–16.

99. Ram FS, Cates CJ, Ducharme FM. Long-acting beta2-agonists versus anti-leukotrienes as add-on therapy to inhaled corticosteroids for chronic asthma. Cochrane Database Syst Rev 2005;(1):CD003137.

100. Kidney J, Dominguez M, Taylor PM, et al. Immunomodulation by theophylline in asthma. Demonstration by withdrawal of therapy. Am J Respir Crit Care Med 1995;151:1907–14.

101. Faurschou P, Steffensen I, Jacques L. Effect of addition of inhaled salmeterol to the treatment of moderate-to-severe asthmatics uncontrolled on high-dose inhaled steroids. European Respiratory Study Group. Eur Respir J 1996;9:1885–90.

102. Rodrigo GJ, Neffen H, Castro-Rodriguez JA. Efficacy and safety of subcutaneous omalizumab vs placebo as add-on therapy to corticosteroids for children and adults with asthma: a systematic review. Chest 2011;139:28–35.

103. Thomas A, Lemanske RF Jr, Jackson DJ. Approaches to stepping up and stepping down care in asthmatic patients. J Allergy Clin Immunol 2011;128:915–24.

104. Viswanathan RK, Busse WW. Allergen immunotherapy in allergic respiratory diseases: from mechanisms to meta-analyses. Chest 2012;141:1303–14.

105. Ayres JG, Jyothish D, Ninan T. Brittle asthma. Paed Respir Review 2004;5(1):40–4.

106. Joint task force on Practice Parameters, American Academy of Allergy, Asthma and Immunology, et al. The diagnosis and management of anaphylaxis. J Allergy Clin Immunol 1998;101(6 Pt 2): S465–528.

107. Möller C, Dreborg S, Ferdousi HA, et al. Pollen immunotherapy reduces the development of asthma in children with seasonal rhinoconjunctivitis (the PAT-Study). J Allergy Clin Immunol 2002;109:251–6.

108. Moss MH, Gern JE, Lemanske RF Jr, et al. Asthma in infancy and childhood. In: Adkinson NF Jr, Yunginger JW, Busse WW, editors. Middleton's allergy principles and practice. 6th ed. Philadelphia: Mosby; 2003. p. 1225–55.

109. Morgan WJ, Crain EF, Gruchalla RS, et al. Inner-City Asthma Study Group. Results of a home-based environmental intervention among urban children with asthma. N Engl J Med 2004;351:1068–80.

110. Wright RJ, Cohen S, Carey V, et al. Parental stress as a predictor of wheezing in infancy: a prospective birth-cohort study. Am J Respir Crit Care Med 2002;165:358–65.

111. Sandberg S, Paton JY, Ahola S, et al. The role of acute and chronic stress in asthma attacks in children. Lancet 2000;356:982–7.

112. Strunk RC. Death due to asthma. New insights into sudden unexpected deaths, but the focus remains on prevention. Am Rev Respir Dis 1993;148:550–2.

113. The Childhood Asthma Management Program Research Group. Long-term effects of budesonide or nedocromil in children with asthma. N Engl J Med 2000;343:1054–63.

114. Guilbert TW, Morgan WJ, Zeiger RS, et al. Long-term inhaled corticosteroids in preschool children at high risk for asthma. N Engl J Med 2006;354:1985–97.

115. Sorkness CA, Lemanske RF Jr, Mauger DT, Childhood Asthma Research and Education Network of the National Heart, Lung, and Blood Institute, et al. Long-term comparison of 3 controller regimens for mild-moderate persistent childhood asthma: the Pediatric Asthma Controller Trial. J Allergy Clin Immunol 2007;119:64–72.

116. Murray CS, Woodcock A, Langley SJ, et al. Secondary prevention of asthma by the use of Inhaled Fluticasone propionate in Wheezy INfants (IFWIN): double-blind, randomised, controlled study. Lancet 2006;368:754–62.

117. Guilbert TW, Mauger DT, Allen DB, et al. Childhood Asthma Research and Education Network of the National Heart, Lung, and Blood Institute. Growth of preschool children at high risk for asthma 2 years after discontinuation of fluticasone. J Allergy Clin Immunol 2011;128:956–63, e1–e7.

118. *Ni CM, Greenstone IR, Ducharme FM. Addition of inhaled long-acting beta2-agonists to inhaled steroids as first line therapy for persistent asthma in steroid-naive adults. Cochrane Database Syst Rev 2005;(2):CD005307.

119. Masoli M, Weatherall M, Holt S, et al. Moderate dose inhaled corticosteroids plus salmeterol versus higher doses of inhaled corticosteroids in symptomatic asthma. Thorax 2005;60:730–4.

120. Simons FE. A comparison of beclomethasone, salmeterol, and placebo in children with asthma. Canadian Beclomethasone Dipropionate-Salmeterol Xinafoate Study Group. N Engl J Med 1997;337:1659–65.

121. Nassif EG, Weinberger M, Thompson R, et al. The value of maintenance theophylline in steroid-dependent asthma. N Engl J Med 1981;304:71–5.

122. Busse WW, Morgan WJ, Gergen PJ, et al. Randomized trial of omalizumab (anti-IgE) for asthma in inner-city children. N Engl J Med 2011;364:1005–15.

123. Joint Task Force on Practice Parameters. Allergen immunotherapy: a practice parameter. American Academy of Allergy, Asthma and Immunology. American College of Allergy, Asthma and Immunology. Ann Allergy Asthma Immunol 2003;90(1 Suppl. 1):1–40.

124. Abramson MJ, Puy RM, Weiner JM. Allergen immunotherapy for asthma. Cochrane Database Syst Rev 2003;(4):CD001186.

125. American Lung Association. Trends in asthma morbidity and mortality. September 2012. Online. Available: <http://www.lungusa.org/finding-cures/our-research/trend-reports/asthma-trend-report.pdf>; [accessed December 10, 2012].

126. Barnett SB, Nurmagambetov TA. Costs of asthma in the United States: 2002–2007. J Allergy Clin Immunol 2011;127:145–52.

127. Emerman CE, Cydulka RK, Crain EF, et al. Prospective multicenter study of relapse following treatment for acute asthma among children presenting to the emergency department. J Pediatr 2001;138: 318–24.

128. Rowe BH, Voaklander DC, Wang D, et al. Asthma presentations by adults to emergency departments in Alberta, Canada: a large population-based study. Chest 2009;135:57–65.

129. Brenner BE, Chavda KK, Camargo CA Jr. Randomized trial of inhaled flunisolide versus placebo among asthmatics discharged from the emergency department. Ann Emerg Med 2000;36:417–26.

130. Cates CJ, Crilly JA, Rowe BH. Holding chambers (spacers) versus nebulisers for beta-agonist treatment of acute asthma. Cochrane Database Syst Rev 2006;(2):CD000052.

131. Camargo CA Jr, Spooner CH, Rowe BH. Continuous versus intermittent beta-agonists for acute asthma. Cochrane Database Syst Rev 2003;(4):CD001115.
132. Plotnick LH, Ducharme FM. Combined inhaled anticholinergic agents and beta-2-agonists for initial treatment of acute asthma in children. Cochrane Database Syst Rev 2000;(2):CD000060.
133. Rowe BH, Bretzlaff JA, Bourdon C, et al. Magnesium sulfate for treating exacerbations of acute asthma in the emergency department. Cochrane Database Syst Rev 2000;(1):CD001490.
134. Camargo CA Jr, Gurner DM, Smithline HA, et al. A randomized placebo-controlled study of intravenous montelukast for the treatment of acute asthma. J Allergy Clin Immunol 2010;125:374–80.
135. Parameswaran K, Belda J, Rowe BH. Addition of intravenous aminophylline to beta2-agonists in adults with acute asthma. Cochrane Database Syst Rev 2000;(4):CD002742.
136. Graham V, Lasserson T, Rowe BH. Antibiotics for acute asthma. Cochrane Database Syst Rev 2001;(3):CD002741.
137. Rowe BH, Bota GW, Clark S, et al. Comparison of Canadian versus American emergency department visits for acute asthma. Can Respir J 2007;14:331–7.
138. Rachelefsky G. Treating exacerbations of asthma in children: the role of systemic corticosteroids. Pediatrics 2003;112:382–97.
139. Foresi A, Morelli MC, Catena E. Low-dose budesonide with the addition of an increased dose during exacerbations is effective in long-term asthma control. On behalf of the Italian Study Group. Chest 2000;117:440–6.
140. Solé D, Komatsu MK, Carvalho KV, et al. Pulse oximetry in the evaluation of the severity of acute asthma and/or wheezing in children. J Asthma 1999;36:327–33.
141. Holgate ST. Stratified approaches to the treatment of asthma. Br J Clin Pharmacol 2013;76(2):277–91.
142. Djukanović R, Harrison T, Johnston SL, INTERCIA Study Group, et al. The effect of inhaled IFN-(on worsening of asthma symptoms caused by viral infections. A randomized trial. Am J Respir Crit Care Med 2014;190(2):145–54.

Key references are preceded by an asterisk.

CHAPTER 8

Allergic Rhinitis and Conjunctivitis

CHAPTER OUTLINE

INTRODUCTION
HISTORIC PERSPECTIVE
EPIDEMIOLOGY
Incidence and Prevalence
Quality of Life and Economic Impact
Associated Diseases
PATHOGENESIS AND ETIOLOGY
Clinical Features
Patient Evaluation, Diagnosis, and Differential
    Diagnosis
    Physical Examination
    Fiberoptic Rhinoscopy
Laboratory Testing
    Testing for Specific Immunoglobulin E
    Blood Eosinophils and Total Serum
        Immunoglobulin E
    Radiographic Imaging
    Other Tests
Differential Diagnosis of Allergic Rhinitis
    Work-related Rhinitis
    Chronic Rhinosinusitis with and without Nasal
        Polyps
    Non-allergic Rhinitis
    Nasal and Pharyngeal Structural Abnormalities
Differential Diagnosis of Allergic Conjunctivitis
    Other Allergy-associated Forms of Conjunctivitis
    Infectious Conjunctivitis
    Dry Eye Syndrome

Blepharitis
Toxic Conjunctivitis
Ocular Rosacea
Keratitis
Angle Closure Glaucoma
TREATMENT
Allergen Avoidance
Pharmacotherapy
    Antihistamines
    Decongestants
    Intranasal Corticosteroids
    Systemic Corticosteroids
    Leukotriene Inhibitors
    Cromolyn Sodium
    Anticholinergics
    Medications for Ocular Symptoms
    Combinations of Medications
Allergen Immunotherapy
Surgery
Overall Approach to Treatment
    Allergic Rhinitis
    Non-allergic Rhinitis
Treatment Considerations in Select Populations
    Pregnancy
    Elderly
INDICATIONS FOR REFERRAL
CONCLUSIONS

SUMMARY OF IMPORTANT CONCEPTS

- The incidence of chronic rhinitis has increased significantly during the last two decades, particularly in Western countries.
- Moderate to severe rhinitis has been shown to adversely affect performance at work and school, thereby contributing significantly to the indirect economic costs of this disease.
- Approximately 50–60% of patients with allergic rhinitis have associated symptoms of allergic conjunctivitis.
- The presence of rhinitis has significant effects on the development and severity of other disorders, including bronchial asthma, sinusitis, middle ear disease, and dental malocclusion.
- The two most common rhinitis syndromes are allergic rhinitis and idiopathic rhinitis, and differentiation of these two disorders requires an assessment of specific immunoglobulin E (IgE).

- A small subset of patients with rhinitis may have symptoms caused by strictly localized allergic mechanisms with no systemic evidence of specific IgE.
- Although rhinitis can be treated effectively with a number of medications, both over-the-counter and prescription products, allergen immunotherapy remains the only disease-modifying treatment capable of causing long-term improvement with respect to nasal symptoms and reduction in incident cases of asthma.

INTRODUCTION

Chronic rhinitis is an increasingly common condition that is now recognized to have a major impact on human health. Persistent nasal dysfunction may have significant effects on physical and emotional functioning, which result in absences from school and work, reduced worker productivity, and impaired school performance. In addition, chronic nasal inflammation may aggravate or lead to the development of other significant disorders, including asthma, rhinosinusitis, and middle ear disease. Recent improvements in current understanding of the pathologic mechanisms of rhinitis are providing key insights into the development of new treatments, including novel immunologic therapies. This chapter presents an overview of the epidemiology, diagnosis, pathophysiology, and treatment of allergic and non-allergic rhinitis and conjunctivitis.

HISTORIC PERSPECTIVE

John Bostock was an English physician who personally suffered from symptoms of 'summer catarrh' every June, since childhood. The symptoms of this newly described malady included nasal congestion, sneezing, and tiredness, which he believed were brought on by the exhausting heat of summer. In 1859, Charles Blackley, who also suffered from this recurrent ailment, became convinced that pollen was linked to these summer nasal symptoms, and that a toxin was the most likely culprit. In his 1873 volume *Experimental Researches on the Cause and Nature of Catarrhus Aestivus*, he reported the results of the first intranasal challenge with rye grass pollen and noted the immediate occurrence of profuse coryza followed 30 min later by nasal blockage.[1] He then attempted the first effort at pollen immunotherapy by repeatedly applying pollen grains to his abraded skin, which was not effective. In 1911, Noon published the first seminal trial of immunotherapy with a grass pollen extract.[2] Following this study, injections of grass pollen extracts became accepted as an important treatment for seasonal rhinitis, and, in 1954, Augustin presented the first double-blind, placebo-controlled trial of pollen extract injection to demonstrate efficacy.[3]

EPIDEMIOLOGY

Incidence and Prevalence

The increase in the prevalence of allergic diseases began to garner attention from epidemiologists in the late 1980s. The International Study of Asthma and Allergies in Childhood (ISAAC) was initiated to establish the prevalence of allergic diseases in 257 800 schoolchildren aged 6 to 7 years and in 463 801 children aged 13 to 14 years, using standardized, validated questionnaires.[4] The prevalence rates for rhinitis collected across all centers ranged from 0.8% to 14.9% (median, 6.9%) in the 6- to 7-year-olds and from 1.4% to 39.7% (median, 13.6%) in the 13- to 14-year-olds.[4] The highest prevalence rates for rhinitis were observed in parts of Western Europe, North America, and Australia, whereas the lowest rates were found in parts of Eastern Europe and south and central Asia. Select analyses revealed that the prevalence rates had increased, with 12-month prevalence rates of 1.8–24.2% in children aged 6 to 7 years (median, 8.5%) and 1.0–45% (median, 14.6%) in 13- to 14-year-olds[5]; these findings strongly indicated that the prevalence of rhinitis had increased over a relatively short period of time, mostly in Westernized countries with a higher standard of living. In a subgroup analysis of

Box 8-1   **Factors that Influence the Development of Allergic Rhinitis**

INCREASED RISK
- Female gender
- Particulate air pollution
- Maternal smoking

DECREASED RISK
- Increased number of siblings
- Grass pollen exposure
- Farm environment
- Mediterranean diet

2810 German children followed from age 9 to 11 years until age 15 to 18 years,[6] the incidence of allergic rhinitis increased from an initial rate of 7% to 14%. These longitudinal data offer compelling evidence that the incidence of allergic rhinitis increases significantly as children grow from childhood into adolescence. A number of exposures in early childhood may act to increase the risk of developing rhinitis (Box 8-1).

Historically, the available data regarding the epidemiology of chronic rhinitis in adults are much more limited. Based on data for 15 394 adults of 20 to 44 years of age, in the European Community Respiratory Health Survey I (ECRHS I), the prevalence of allergic rhinitis ranged from 4.6% in Oviedo, Spain, to 31.8% in Melbourne, Australia.[7] In the most recent (US) National Health and Nutrition Examination Survey (NHANES), conducted in 2005–2006, the 12-month prevalence of rhinitis for the entire cohort was 23.5%, with a peak of 31.3% in patients 40 to 49 years of age.[8] For the group as a whole, 24% had seasonal rhinitis and 10% had perennial rhinitis.

Quality of Life and Economic Impact

Large, population-based studies have revealed that chronic rhinitis significantly impairs health-related quality of life. Questionnaires that focus on general quality of life (as used in the SF 36 Health Survey) have demonstrated significant decreases in physical functioning, energy, general health perception, social functioning, emotions, mental health, and pain, in patients with moderate to severe perennial allergic rhinitis compared with control subjects.[9] Sleep loss may play a key role in determining quality of life, in that it may lead to daytime fatigue and poor concentration in school, resulting in learning impairment.[10]

Quality of life questionnaires have shown that chronic rhinitis may also influence mood and cognitive function. Studies conducted during and after the allergy season reveal that subjects with seasonal allergic rhinitis had significant decreases in verbal learning, decision-making speed, psychomotor speed, reaction time tests, and positive affect scores, as well as workplace productivity compared with those reported for non-allergic control subjects.[11]

Associated Diseases

Approximately 40% of patients with chronic rhinitis have asthma, and 80% of patients with asthma suffer with persistent nasal symptoms.[12] Allergic rhinitis, particularly perennial disease, is a significant independent risk factor for the development of asthma.[13] Nasal disease is also an important risk factor for worsening asthma in patients who have both rhinitis and asthma; the frequency of both emergency department visits and hospitalizations is greater in patients with moderate to severe rhinitis than in patients who have mild or no rhinitis.[14]

Rhinosinusitis is commonly identified in patients with allergic rhinitis. As many as 30% of patients with acute sinusitis, 67% with unilateral chronic sinusitis, and 80% with bilateral chronic sinusitis, have allergic rhinitis.[15] Nasal allergy most likely precipitates acute sinusitis by inducing sinus ostial edema, resulting in impairment of sinus drainage, a shift to anaerobic conditions inside of the sinus cavity, and finally bacterial proliferation. The relationship between allergy and chronic sinus disease is more complex and involves anti-staphylococcal IgE antibodies in some patients.[16]

A considerable proportion of patients with allergic rhinitis his concomitant otitis media with effusion (OME).[17] Pollen exposure has been shown to cause eustachian tube dysfunction, which induces negative pressure in the middle ear space, followed by transudation of fluid.[18]

Adults and children with allergic rhinitis frequently have poor-quality sleep, including difficulty getting to sleep, waking up during the night, and lack of a 'good night's sleep.'[19] Nasal obstruction associated with allergic rhinitis has been shown to be a risk factor for a variety of problems during sleep, including microarousals, hypopneas, and apnea. Persistent, severe rhinitis in children may also cause chronic mouth breathing, particularly at night, which has been linked to alterations in the palatal anatomy and dental malocclusion.[20]

PATHOGENESIS AND ETIOLOGY

Sensitization of the nasal mucosa to certain airborne allergens entails multiple interactions between antigen presenting cells (i.e. dendritic cells), CD4 Th2 lymphocytes, and B cells that lead to the production of antigen-specific IgE antibodies, which then bind to mast cells and basophils.[21] Subsequent allergen exposure leads to cross-linking of specific IgE molecules on mast cells and their resultant degranulation, with the release of preformed mediators (e.g., histamine) and synthesis of newly generated mediators (e.g., leukotriene C4, prostaglandin D2). Other proinflammatory substances are also generated after allergen exposure, including toxic eosinophil products (e.g., eosinophil cationic protein) and cytokines (e.g., IL-4, -5, and -13). Cytokines are thought to be generated by both Th2 lymphocytes and by mast cells. Cytokines upregulate adhesion molecules on the vascular endothelium, and possibly on marginating leukocytes, and lead to the migration of these inflammatory cells, including lymphocytes, eosinophils, and basophils, into the site of tissue inflammation. Various cytokines will also promote the chemotaxis and survival of these recruited inflammatory cells and lead to a secondary immune response by virtue of their capability to promote IgE synthesis by B cells. The nervous system also plays an important role by amplifying and perpetuating allergic reactions. These inflammatory changes lower the threshold of mucosal responsiveness to various specific and non-specific stimuli, making allergic patients more responsive to stimuli to which they are exposed every day (Fig. 8-1).

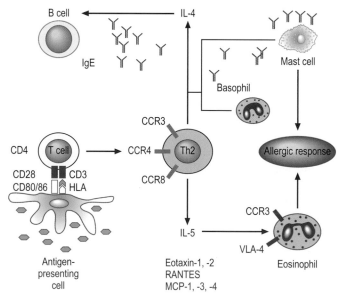

Figure 8-1 Overview of pathophysiology of allergic rhinitis. CCR, Chemokine (C-C motif) receptor; HLA, human leukocyte antigen; IgE, immunoglobulin E; IL, interleukin; MCP, monocyte chemoattractant protein; RANTES, regulated on activation, normal T expressed and secreted; Th2, helper T cell type 2; VLA-4, very late antigen 4.

Clinical Features

Typical signs and symptoms of allergic rhinitis with or without conjunctivitis include some combination of congestion, sneezing, rhinorrhea (anterior and/or posterior), and pruritus of the nose, eyes, oral mucosa, or face and watering and redness of the eyes. Nasal congestion frequently alternates between both sides of the nose as a function of the physiologic nasal cycle.[22] In addition, during sleep, the dependent side of the nose may become preferentially obstructed. Persistent unilateral obstruction strongly suggests the possibility of an anatomic defect (e.g., nasal septal deviation, concha bullosa of the middle turbinate), inflammatory mass (e.g., nasal polyp), or tumor. Sneezing may be extremely variable but in allergic disease often marked by explosive paroxysms of 5 to 10 sneezes or more. In allergic rhinitis, rhinorrhea most often is clear to white in color, and the presence of purulent secretions strongly indicates the possibility of chronic sinusitis or atrophic rhinitis. Ocular signs and symptoms, including redness, itching, and watering, constitute a major cause of suffering in at least half of the patients with allergic rhinitis,[23] the presence of which will dramatically alter which therapy is selected. Other signs and symptoms, such as headache, a feeling of facial fullness, reduction in or loss of sense of smell, cough, and halitosis, should be noted because presence of any of these will affect both the diagnosis and choice of treatment. When anosmia is the most prominent symptom and nasal or ocular symptoms are minimal or absent, primary central nervous system lesions should be considered.[24]

Once the spectrum of symptoms has been established, the presence of temporal patterns and specific triggers should be sought. Symptoms of allergic rhinitis often are most intense during the early morning hours as a consequence of circadian variations in inflammation.[25] Aggravation of symptoms while indoors and after exposure to house dust, furry pets, mildew, or cockroaches suggests the presence of IgE-mediated allergy to those specific allergens. Conversely, clear-cut worsening of symptoms in outside environments indicates the probability of allergy to an outdoor allergen such as pollen or mold. Occurrence of symptoms during well demarcated seasons, as documented in the medical history, usually is diagnostic of allergic rhinitis that is due to an outdoor allergen. Symptoms that occur during the spring usually are ascribed to tree pollen exposure, in summer to grass and outdoor molds, and in fall to weeds and outdoor molds; precise start and stop dates of specific pollination seasons varies geographically.

A large number of triggers may act as irritants rather than as allergens, including volatile organic compounds (e.g., perfumes, paints, cleaning fluids)[26] and particulates (e.g., certain types of outdoor air pollution, construction dust). These substances may be important in provoking nasal symptoms in both allergic and non-allergic rhinitis patients (see below). Changes in climatic factors, such as temperature, humidity, and barometric pressure, are most important in patients with non-allergic rhinitis.[27]

Patient Evaluation, Diagnosis, and Differential Diagnosis

Physical Examination

The routine physical examination provides important information regarding both the cause and severity of rhinitis, as well as potential comorbid conditions, such as conjunctivitis, otitis media, and asthma. Additionally, in young children, the examination may suggest the presence of dental malocclusion and/or facial deformities (e.g., retracted mandible, high-arched palate) that may result from chronic, severe nasal obstruction.[28]

The nose should first be examined for outward signs of prior bony fractures (seen as deformities of the nasal bridge), asymmetry of the nostrils, and in children, a transverse crease over the lower portion of the nose caused by repetitive pushing of the nose upward in response to nasal itching or discharge. The interior of each nostril should be carefully examined using either a handheld otoscope or nasal speculum and headlamp. In patients with moderate to severe mucosal swelling of the inferior or middle turbinates, the examination also should be conducted after the instillation of a topical decongestant such as oxymetazoline. The nasal airway should be examined systematically, to look for and establish the degree of swelling and color of the mucosa; the presence, color, and consistency of secretions; alterations in internal structures (e.g., septal deviation or perforation); and the presence of any abnormal mass lesions (e.g., nasal polyp) or foreign body. The mucosa in patients with symptomatic allergic rhinitis most often is swollen and pale in color, whereas patients with idiopathic rhinitis more typically have pink or erythematous mucous membranes. Great variability in appearance of the nasal airway is the rule, however, and these characteristics are not reliable for establishing a diagnosis. In patients with allergic rhinitis, the discharge is clear to white in color; the presence of discolored secretions suggests chronic rhinosinusitis. Crusting, particularly with dried blood, should alert the physician to the possibility of atrophic rhinitis. An anterior nasal septal deviation may be easily visible, whereas more posterior abnormalities may be detected only with flexible rhinoscopy or computed tomography (CT) imaging. Nasal polyps most commonly are seen coming from the superior portion of the airway and are not difficult to distinguish from turbinates by virtue of their gray, glistening, 'grape-like' appearance.

Examination of the eyes reveals conjunctival injection in approximately half of patients with allergic rhinitis, which may be associated with erythema and bogginess of the upper and lower eyelids brought on by frequent rubbing. Cyanosis of the infraorbital tissues ('allergic shiners') is thought to be caused by venous stasis and may be seen with any chronic nasal or sinus disorder and is not pathognomonic of allergy.[29]

Fiberoptic Rhinoscopy

Visualization of the nasal airway with a rhinoscope may serve as a very useful adjunct to the routine examination.[30] Flexible rhinoscopes are employed regularly by otorhinolaryngologists, as well as some allergists and primary care physicians, and provide an enhanced view of structures in the superior and posterior regions of the nose. These normally unseen regions include the posterior nasal septum, superior nasal turbinates, middle meatus, adenoid gland, and eustachian tube orifices. Flexible rhinoscopy should therefore be considered in cases of rhinitis in which nasal obstruction is unilateral or refractory to therapy in the absence of any discernible anatomic cause on routine examination. Rigid rhinoscopes are used nearly exclusively by otorhinolaryngologists for visualizing the ostiomeatal complexes of the paranasal sinuses as well as performing nasal or sinus surgery.

Laboratory Testing

Testing for Specific Immunoglobulin E

Assessments of allergen-specific IgE are necessary to distinguish allergic rhinitis from non-allergic rhinitis. Allergy skin testing using the prick-puncture method is considered to provide the best combination of sensitivity and specificity, although in-vitro testing has demonstrated comparable performance characteristics for some but not all allergens[31] (see Ch. 5 for a complete discussion of skin and in-vitro testing). Although IgE most commonly is distributed systemically and can be identified by allergy skin testing or blood assays, in a subset of patients with allergic rhinitis, specific IgE can be identified only in the nose. This finding, referred to as *local allergic rhinitis*, or entopy, has been suspected for several decades but has only recently undergone rigorous investigation.[32] Nasal allergen challenge is required to clinically confirm this diagnosis, which is performed primarily in research settings. In the near future, this procedure may become part of the clinically accepted evaluation for patients with suspected local allergic rhinitis.

Blood Eosinophils and Total Serum Immunoglobulin E

Large, population-based studies reveal that mean concentrations of total serum IgE and circulating blood eosinophils are increased in allergic rhinitis. Although recent analyses have demonstrated utility using a combination of threshold values for total IgE and blood eosinophils,[33] a great deal of overlap with values in asymptomatic persons is typical, thereby limiting the diagnostic value of these markers.

Radiographic Imaging

The most accurate test for evaluating possible inflammation of the paranasal sinuses is computed tomography.[34] Frequently, mild mucoperiosteal thickening can be seen in patients with uncomplicated allergic rhinitis and non-allergic rhinitis.[35] Radiographic studies should be considered in patients with symptoms that are not typical of rhinitis and are unresponsive to medical therapy, such as chronic purulent rhinorrhea, alterations in sense of smell, or headaches.

While both plain sinus films and ultrasonography of the maxillary sinuses have been shown to accurately predict acute maxillary sinusitis, neither method is useful for chronic disease.[36]

Other Tests

Histologic analyses of blown nasal secretions or scrapings taken from the inferior turbinates have been used historically but are no longer employed routinely in clinical practice. Similarly, tests of nasal patency, such as rhinomanometry or nasal peak flow, are not utilized frequently in clinical practice and are relegated primarily to research studies.

Differential Diagnosis of Allergic Rhinitis

For the classification of chronic rhinitis, see Box 8-2.

Work-Related Rhinitis

Rhinitis related to the workplace is characterized by intermittent or persistent nasal symptoms attributable to exposures incurred in a particular work environment.[41] Work-related rhinitis may be due to immunologic hypersensitivity, including the presence of IgE, or may be non-allergic in etiology. Occupations that carry a high risk for development of work-related rhinitis include laboratory workers, furriers, and bakers (Table 8-1). Diagnosis of work-related rhinitis relies heavily on a history of symptomatic worsening during the work week, with improvement over the weekend and during vacations, when the putative trigger is absent. Eventually, symptoms may persist during periods away from work as mucosal inflammation becomes more established. In situations in which the workplace exposure is a protein, skin or blood testing for specific IgE may be very helpful (see Ch. 14 for detailed commentary).

Chronic Rhinosinusitis with and Without Nasal Polyps

Chronic rhinosinusitis (CRS) is an inflammatory disease of the paranasal sinuses that has been present for 12 weeks or longer.[37] The four cardinal symptoms of CRS are mucopurulent drainage, nasal obstruction, facial discomfort, and decreased sense of smell; two of these must be present, along with CT or endoscopic evidence of sinus mucosal inflammation in order to establish this diagnosis. Up to one third of patients with CRS present with nasal polyps, which are likely to cause anosmia.[38]

Box 8-2 Differential Diagnosis of Chronic Rhinitis

ALLERGIC
- Systemic
- Local (entopy)

WORK-RELATED
- Irritant
- Corrosive
- Immunologic

INFECTIOUS (RHINOSINUSITIS)
- Allergic
- Non-allergic

NON-ALLERGIC
- Idiopathic (vasomotor)
- Non-allergic with eosinophilia
- Atrophic
    - Primary
    - Secondary
- Medication-related
- Topical vasoconstrictors (rhinitis medicamentosa)
    - Oral medications
- Exercise-induced
- Cold air–induced
- Gustatory
- Hormonal
- Aging
- Systemic diseases

TABLE 8-1   Occupations with Increased Prevalence of Work-related Rhinitis

Category	Occupation	Likely Trigger
Irritant	Drywall installer	Gypsum dust
	Makeup artist	Cosmetic power, perfume
Corrosive	Janitor	Ammonia
	Chemistry technician	Hydrochloric acid
Immunologic		
Immunoglobulin E	Baker	Grain flour
	Furrier	Animal dander
	Livestock breeder	Animal dander
	Veterinarian	Animal dander
	Food processing worker	Foodstuffs
	Pharmacist	Medication powders
Low-molecular-weight substances	Boat builder	Anhydrides

Non-allergic Rhinitis

Idiopathic Non-allergic Rhinitis (Vasomotor Rhinitis). Idiopathic non-allergic rhinitis, also referred to as vasomotor rhinitis, manifests with chronic or intermittent symptoms of nasal congestion and/or watery rhinorrhea that worsen acutely in response to non-specific provocateurs, including cold air, exercise, pungent odors, smoke, alcohol, and specific physiologic states, such as sexual arousal and emotional upset.[39] One trigger, which deserves special mention, is eating, which most often causes isolated watery discharge and has been referred to as gustatory rhinitis. Patients with idiopathic rhinitis have negative responses on skin or blood tests for specific IgE, including to potential food allergens, although occasionally patients may exhibit a small number of positive reactions that do not correlate with the clinical pattern of symptoms and are considered clinically irrelevant.

Non-allergic Rhinitis with Eosinophilia. Studies of nasal histopathology reveal that one third of patients with non-allergic rhinitis have an increased percentage of eosinophils, a condition that has previously been referred to as 'non-allergic rhinitis with eosinophilia' or 'eosinophilic non-allergic rhinitis.'[40] Nasal congestion and discharge are the most frequently reported symptoms, and these patients develop nasal polyps more frequently than other groups of rhinitis patients. It has been speculated, that at least in some cases, non-allergic rhinitis with eosinophilia may represent local allergic rhinitis with local IgE to an unknown allergen. As cytologic analyses of nasal mucus or epithelium are not performed routinely in clinical practice, this subtype of non-allergic rhinitis is not usually identified by physicians.

Atrophic Rhinitis. Atrophic rhinitis is a chronic condition characterized by symptoms of nasal crusting, purulent discharge, nasal obstruction, and halitosis.[42] Primary atrophic rhinitis is most prevalent in areas with prolonged warm seasons, including south Asia and the Middle East and is more common in women. Although primary atrophic rhinitis has no known specific cause, many patients are found to have chronic bacterial infection of the nose and sinuses due to any of a large number of organisms, the most common of which is *Klebsiella ozaenae*. Secondary atrophic rhinitis presents with symptoms similar to those noted above and is the more common form of this disease in the developed world. It is most likely to occur in older patients who have undergone multiple or aggressive nasal surgeries,[42] nasal trauma, or nasal irradiation; in the case of nasal surgery, it has been referred to as the 'empty nose syndrome.'

Rhinitis Associated with Drugs. Repetitive use of topical α-adrenergic decongestant nasal sprays (e.g., oxymetazoline, phenylephrine) for more than a few days may result in rebound nasal congestion,[43] most likely secondary to downregulation of the α-agonist receptor. With long-term use of these agents, patients may develop a chronic form of rhinitis referred to as *rhinitis medicamentosa*. This disorder most often manifests with severe nasal congestion without other significant symptoms. Cocaine use also has been implicated in causing rhinitis medicamentosa but usually results in significantly more

TABLE 8-2   Medications Associated with Chronic Nasal Symptoms

Category	Example(s)
Antihypertensives	Angiotensin-converting enzyme inhibitors β-Adrenergic blockers Amiloride Prazosin Hydralazine
Psychotropics	Risperidone Chlorpromazine Amitriptyline
Phosphodiesterase-5 inhibitors	Sildenafil Tadalafil Vardenafil
Non-steroidal anti-inflammatory drugs	Ibuprofen
Others	Gabapentin

crusting, bleeding, and ultimately septal perforation than topical decongestant drugs. Physical examination in patients with rhinitis medicamentosa often reveals swollen, red nasal mucous membranes with minimal discharge.[43]

A number of systemic medications have been shown to be associated with increased nasal symptoms, particularly congestion and rhinorrhea.[44] General classes of medications that have been implicated in causing rhinitis symptoms include antihypertensives, drugs for erectile dysfunction, psychiatric drugs, and non-steroidal anti-inflammatory drugs (Table 8-2).

Hormonal Rhinitis. Approximately 20–30% of pregnant women will develop rhinitis of pregnancy, defined as new-onset nasal symptoms (usually congestion and/or rhinorrhea) in the absence of another known cause that lasts ≥6 weeks and resolves within 2 weeks after delivery.[45] Uncontrolled rhinitis during pregnancy may be a cause of severe snoring, which has been associated with an increased risk of gestational hypertension, preeclampsia, and intrauterine growth retardation.[46] Although abundant data are available to link pregnancy to nasal symptoms, much less is known regarding the relationship between the menstrual cycle or use of exogenous ovarian hormones (i.e. oral contraceptives, hormone replacement therapy) and rhinitis.

The relationship between rhinitis and hypothyroidism and other abnormal hormonal states has not been substantiated by research.

Rhinitis Related to Systemic Disease. A number of systemic diseases may be occasionally associated with symptoms of rhinitis. These include granulomatous diseases (e.g., granulomatosis with polyangiitis, sarcoidosis, midline granuloma), cystic fibrosis, ciliary dyskinesia syndromes, and immunodeficiencies. In most of these conditions, both the nose and sinus cavities are affected. In these disorders, patients often present with multisystem involvement, particularly the lungs and associated constitutional complaints, such as fatigue and poor appetite.

Nasal and Pharyngeal Structural Abnormalities

A number of anatomic abnormalities in the nose and pharynx can cause chronic partial or complete nasal blockage without other significant symptoms (Box 8-3). Concha bullosa (aeration of the middle turbinate bones with expansion of the turbinates) has been shown to be present in varying degrees in approximately two thirds of the general population; in a small number of affected persons, however, the condition is extensive enough to result in unilateral or bilateral nasal obstruction.[47] Nasal septal deviation can be identified in nearly 20% of people but only a small fraction of that group will have significant symptoms.[47] Adenoidal enlargement may cause some degree of nasal obstruction in approximately 50% of children; the majority of these will resolve spontaneously without the need for surgical intervention.[48] Children presenting with chronic unilateral

Box 8-3   **Anatomic Abnormalities Causing Nasal Obstruction**
• Concha bullosa • Nasal septal deviation • Adenoidal enlargement • Nasal polyps • Nasal cancer • Nasal foreign body

nasal obstruction should be evaluated for a possible foreign body in the nose, with the most common examples including peanuts, beads, and buttons. Nasal cancers are very rare with a prevalence of 0.001%.[49] Nasal cancer should be suspected in older persons with unilateral nasal obstruction and bleeding of gradual onset.

Differential Diagnosis of Allergic Conjunctivitis

Other Allergy-Associated Forms of Conjunctivitis

Three allergy-associated forms of conjunctivitis may occasionally be difficult to differentiate from typical allergic conjunctivitis. Vernal keratoconjunctivitis is usually a more severe conjunctival disorder that most often affects young males living in warm climates.[50] Symptoms include ocular itching, mucus discharge, and cobblestoning of the eye which may vary in severity according to the seasons. Giant papillary conjunctivitis represents a hypersensitivity reaction to medical appliances placed on or into the eyes, including contact lenses and ocular implants. The most common symptoms include itching and a gritty sensation.[51] Atopic keratoconjunctivitis can affect the conjunctiva, cornea and eyelid, and is most commonly diagnosed in middle-aged adults (30–50 years of age) with atopic dermatitis.[52] Patients usually complain of severe itching of the eyes with associated thickening and lichenification of the eyelids.

Infectious Conjunctivitis

Viral infections may be either unilateral or bilateral, while bacterial conjunctivitis usually affects one eye.[53] Most types of bacterial and viral conjunctivitis are self-limited and do not have significant pruritus. In most cases, bacterial infections are associated with purulent discharge, while viral conjunctivitis is characterized by a clear, watery discharge and may be occasionally difficult to distinguish from acute allergic conjunctivitis.

Dry Eye Syndrome

Dry eye syndrome, or xerophthalmia, may present as an isolated finding or may present as part of a systemic disease, such as Sjögren syndrome or sarcoidosis.[54] Dry eyes are capable of minimal tear production, creating a sensation of grittiness and discomfort. Medications, particularly those with anticholinergic side effects, are a frequent cause of dry eye syndrome and patients should undergo a trial of discontinuation before embarking on an in-depth evaluation. A Schirmer test is a convenient and inexpensive method for documenting dry eyes.

Blepharitis

Anterior blepharitis occurs at the front edge of the eyelid where the eyelashes are attached, while posterior blepharitis affects the inner edge of the eyelid that comes in contact with the eyeball.[55] Individuals with blepharitis experience a gritty or burning sensation in their eyes, excessive tearing, itching and swelling of the eyelids, or crusting of the eyelids. The prominent inflammation of the lids and lesser degree of eye involvement help distinguish blepharitis from allergic conjunctivitis.

Toxic Conjunctivitis

Toxic conjunctivitis is an irritant reaction to ocular medications which usually occurs after long periods of use.[56] The most commonly implicated agents are preservatives in eye medications, contact lens solutions, and artificial tears. The findings are non-specific and consist of conjunctival erythema, mucus discharge, and itching. The eyelids can eventually become swollen, thickened, and excoriated, findings which are uncommon in allergic conjunctivitis.

Ocular Rosacea

Ocular rosacea commonly presents with burning, itching, sensation of a foreign body, dryness, tearing, or photophobia and may occasionally occur in the absence of rosacea elsewhere on the face.[57] Physical findings include conjunctival erythema, blepharitis, and lid margin telangiectasias.

Keratitis

Keratitis, defined as inflammation of the cornea, most often occurs in response to contact lens use but may also be associated with *Herpes simplex* infections.[58] This condition typically presents with unilateral findings, often consisting of intense erythema and pain, and may be associated with vision loss. The presence of corneal infiltrates distinguishes this condition from allergic conjunctivitis.

Angle Closure Glaucoma

Angle closure glaucoma may present with injection of the affected eye, but is most always associated with severe unilateral eye pain and vision loss due to corneal edema.[59]

TREATMENT

Allergen Avoidance

Multiple measures for allergen avoidance have been advocated and are most commonly directed at house-dust mites, animal danders, and molds. All environmental control recommendations should be predicated upon a positive finding to an allergy skin test or in-vitro test.

House-dust mites (*Dermatophagoides farinae* and *pteronyssinus*) are found in most places with relative indoor humidity levels higher than 45%. These microscopic arachnids are found in highest concentrations in carpeting, pillows, mattresses (including foam mattresses), and upholstered furniture. As mite allergen proteins are quite large and heavy, they are unlikely to become airborne for any significant lengths of time. Recent studies have demonstrated that single measures, such as pillow encasings, are not effective in reducing symptoms in patients with allergic rhinitis.[60] However, the simultaneous combination of multiple interventions, including pillow and mattress encasings, acaricidal sprays and powders for carpeting, and frequent washing of bed linens in hot water are beneficial in reducing rhinitis symptoms due to dust mites.[61] High-efficiency particulate air (HEPA) filters have never been shown to be helpful in dust mite-induced rhinitis.

Nearly 50% of American households own at least one cat, and 25% of allergic rhinitis sufferers are allergic to cats. One study of cat allergen avoidance measures demonstrated that a combination of carpet removal, frequent washing of bedding, and washing the cat resulted in large reductions of levels of major cat allergen with an attendant reduction of rhinitis symptoms.[62] HEPA filters used as a solitary measure, however, have not been found to be effective.[63] Overall, the most practical and effective approach to reduction of indoor cat allergen is removal of the cat from the indoor environment. Even this measure, however, may not be immediately effective because residual allergen may remain at relatively high levels in the carpeting and upholstered furniture for several months or longer.[63] After removal of the cat, therefore, all carpeting should be removed and upholstered furniture cleaned.

Indoor mold growth usually results from water intrusion into the living space. Air sampling can accurately identify relevant species and numbers of spores in water-damaged buildings. When mold growth affects large areas of the indoor environment, abatement of damaged areas and corrective measures to prevent future water leakage are often beneficial in reducing rhinitis symptoms in mold-allergic individuals.

Exposure to outdoor allergens, such as grass, tree and weed pollens, and outdoor mold spores, is very difficult to control. Avoidance of outdoor activity during peak pollen hours (usually between 11:00 hours and 15:00 hours) may be helpful in some patients. In general, however, allergy to these ubiquitous triggers is therefore best addressed with pharmacotherapy and/or immunotherapy.

Pharmacotherapy

Antihistamines

H_1-antihistamines block histamine at the H_1 receptor and are commonly used in the treatment of allergic rhinitis and conjunctivitis. Oral H_1-antihistamines have been shown to reduce histamine-mediated symptoms and signs such as sneezing, itching, rhinorrhea, and eye symptoms but are not as effective in alleviating nasal congestion.[64] They are rapidly absorbed after oral administration and usually begin to provide relief within 1 to 2 hours. Oral H_1-antihistamines also have been shown to be safe and effective in children, and many are available in liquid form.[65] The side effects of first-generation antihistamines (e.g., diphenhydramine) can be bothersome and include sedation and anticholinergic effects, such as constipation, dry mouth and eyes, and urinary outlet obstruction. Newer antihistamines have a low reported incidence of sedation as well as minimal or no anticholinergic effects. H_1-antihistamines also are available for intranasal administration. Azelastine hydrochloride and olopatadine hydrochloride both have a more rapid onset of action than oral antihistamines, usually within 15 to 30 min, and result in significant reduction of nasal congestion as well as itching, sneezing, and runny nose. These medications may cause alteration of taste sensation and occasionally somnolence.[66,67]

Decongestants

Decongestants reduce nasal congestion but have no other significant effects on the symptoms of rhinitis. Both topical and systemic decongestants act by α-adrenergic stimulation, which results in vascular constriction and a reduction of nasal blood supply to the sinusoids. Topical decongestants can be either catecholamines (such as phenylephrine) or imidazoline derivatives (such as xylometazoline or oxymetazoline) and have a more rapid onset of action and stronger effect than systemic decongestants. Topical decongestants do not have systemic side effects; however, in children there have been rare case reports of seizures. When these agents are used for longer than 5 days, rebound nasal congestion may develop in some patients. Therefore, topical decongestants should be used primarily to reduce nasal congestion in patients with acutely severe rhinitis in order to facilitate the penetration of intranasal corticosteroids.

Oral decongestants do not cause rebound congestion but are not as effective as topical formulations. Agents that combine an oral decongestant, usually pseudoephedrine, with an antihistamine are frequently used for the treatment of acute and chronic rhinitis due to a variety of causes. The most common side effects of oral decongestants are insomnia and irritability, which can occur in as many as 25% of patients taking these medications. At normal doses, aggravation of hypertension and cardiac arrhythmias may occur. Taken in overdose, these agents may result in renal failure, psychosis, strokes, and seizures. They should therefore be largely avoided in patients with hypertension, heart disease, seizure disorders, hyperthyroidism, and prostatic hypertrophy and in those taking monoamine oxidase inhibitors.

Intranasal Corticosteroids

Intranasal corticosteroids are the most potent drugs available for the management of allergic rhinitis, and have been shown to significantly reduce all nasal symptoms of allergic rhinitis. In comparative studies in allergic rhinitis, intranasal steroids (INSs) have been shown to be superior in efficacy to both H_1-antihistamines[68] and leukotriene receptor antagonists.[69] An unexpected benefit of use of INSs in patients with allergic rhinitis is a significant reduction in concomitant allergic ocular symptoms[70] (see Medications for Ocular Symptoms, below). INSs begin to have effects within 7 to 8 hours of dosing, although some reports demonstrate an effect within 2 hours.[71] Although continuous use is usually recommended, some studies have demonstrated that as-needed use of intranasal fluticasone propionate is superior to placebo.[72] The main side effects of INSs include local nasal irritation (in 5–10% of patients) and epistaxis (4–8%). In patients with perennial rhinitis treated with fluticasone propionate or mometasone furoate continuously for 1 year, nasal mucosal biopsy specimens showed no evidence of atrophy and normalization of the epithelium.[73] Rarely, septal perforations and *Candida* overgrowth have been reported. With regard to potential systemic effects, INSs that have been subjected to rigorous study have not been shown to affect parameters such as growth in children.[74] Despite these reassuring findings, it is recommended that pediatric patients receiving INSs be evaluated every 6 months using a stadiometer to monitor growth.

INSs also have been shown to be effective in the treatment of non-allergic rhinitis. Among the available preparations, fluticasone propionate and fluticasone furoate are approved by the FDA for the treatment of non-allergic rhinitis in addition to allergic rhinitis.

Systemic Corticosteroids

The role of systemic steroids in the treatment of rhinitis is limited because of their adverse effects and the limited morbidity of the disease. They are best reserved for patients with any type of rhinitis who present initially with severe nasal obstruction. A short course of oral prednisone, 30 mg daily for 3 to 5 days, usually will significantly decrease nasal edema and allow for enhanced penetration of INS.

Intramuscular injections of corticosteroids have been a popular therapy, dating back many years. Data demonstrating efficacy are limited, however. Use of intramuscular injections of depot steroids generally should be avoided for the treatment of seasonal allergic rhinitis because of the risk of rare but potentially catastrophic side effects, particularly aseptic necrosis of the femoral head. In addition, as seasonal rhinitis is usually a life-long disease, patients who request and receive this treatment multiple times per year for many years may be at increased risk for long-term effects of systemic corticosteroids, such as cataracts and osteoporosis.

Leukotriene Inhibitors

Montelukast has comparable efficacy with oral antihistamines for the relief of all ocular and nasal symptoms of allergic rhinitis, including congestion, rhinorrhea, and sneezing.[75] As montelukast is also approved for the treatment of asthma, it may be an effective first-line treatment in patients with both allergic rhinitis and asthma.

Cromolyn Sodium

Intranasal cromolyn sodium 4% solution is available over-the-counter and has been shown to be clinically effective in the treatment of allergic rhinitis. As with antihistamines, it is more helpful for sneezing, itching, and rhinorrhea and less effective in relieving nasal congestion. Treatment is most effective when dosing is started before the onset of symptoms. The recommended dosage frequency is four times daily, leading to compliance problems, but the drug is very safe, especially in children and pregnant women.

Anticholinergics

Anticholinergic drugs are useful in the treatment of those patients in whom rhinorrhea is the predominant complaint. Ipratropium bromide has little or no systemic effect when administered intranasally and has been shown to be effective in controlling watery nasal discharge in perennial allergic rhinitis.[76] It has no effect, however, on sneezing, itching, or nasal congestion. Ipratropium can be used in conjunction with drugs of other classes, such as antihistamines or INSs, for the treatment of rhinorrhea in patients with allergic rhinitis.

Ipratropium bromide also is useful for the treatment of watery discharge that occurs in patients with perennial non-allergic rhinitis.[77] In addition, ipratropium has been found to effectively reduce rhinorrhea associated with gustatory rhinitis and rhinorrhea induced by exposure to cold, dry air.[78]

Medications for Ocular Symptoms

Oral H_1-antihistamines and leukotriene receptor antagonists have demonstrated efficacy in reducing ocular redness, tearing, and itch. Topical ocular antihistamines frequently are prescribed as adjunctive agents for patients with rhinoconjunctivitis and as the primary medication for patients with isolated allergic conjunctivitis.[79] As would be expected with topical therapy, these drugs begin to work within a few minutes and have a 12- to 24-hour duration of action. The various agents are available as both over-the-counter and prescription products.

INSs also have been shown to have significant effects in reducing allergic eye symptoms. In a meta-analysis comparing oral H_1-antihistamines and INSs for the control of ocular symptoms, no difference was found in the efficacy of these two classes.[80] The mechanism of this favorable effect of INSs is speculated to be reduced intranasal inflammation, which in turn inhibits the nasal ocular reflex initiated by allergen contact to the nasal mucosa.

Combinations of Medications

Often, a single pharmacologic agent does not effectively reduce symptoms of rhinitis. As noted above, oral antihistamines are frequently combined with oral decongestants to treat allergic rhinitis. The combination of an INS plus an intranasal antihistamine, including both azelastine and olopatadine, has been shown to be more effective than either agent given alone.[81] Recently, a combination spray composed of fluticasone propionate and azelastine hydrochloride was made commercially available. In clinical practice, oral antihistamines frequently are combined with INSs in patients who do not respond to antihistamines alone. Nevertheless, studies of INS given together with oral H_1-antihistamines, including loratadine and cetirizine, have not shown that the combination is significantly better than INS given alone.[82]

With respect to combination treatment of eye symptoms, intranasal fluticasone propionate plus intraocular olopatadine was significantly more effective than the combination of fluticasone and fexofenadine, tested using an ocular challenge model.[83]

Allergen Immunotherapy

Specific allergen immunotherapy has been shown to be effective in seasonal and perennial allergic rhinitis.[84] The principal advantages of immunotherapy over pharmacotherapy are that it generally is more efficacious and that two consecutive years of treatment results in persistent tolerance.[85] Immunotherapy should be considered in a number of clinical scenarios, including severe allergic rhinitis unresponsive to usual pharmacotherapy and allergen avoidance measures; allergic rhinitis complicated by other disorders, particularly new-onset or worsening asthma; and occurrence of significant adverse effects from medications for rhinitis. In addition, in patients who desire a more lasting improvement in their allergic rhinitis, a strong case can be made that immunotherapy is a cost-effective alternative to pharmacotherapy.[86] Subcutaneous immunotherapy is the predominant route of administration employed in the US, although sublingual immunotherapy is now commercially available with both ragweed and northern pasture grasses. Experimental comparisons between these two modes of delivery, as well as studies of which allergens provide optimal efficacy, are ongoing and conceivably will resolve many of the controversies that currently exist (see Ch. 6 for detailed commentary).

Surgery

Individuals with a significant anatomic nasal defect (e.g., nasal septal deviation) may require surgery if nasal obstruction is of a degree that adversely affects quality of life. In patients with chronic rhinitis, in the absence of a structural abnormality, surgery is rarely indicated. Turbinate reduction surgery should be used in patients with refractory mucosal edema only if pharmacotherapy and immunotherapy have been tried and failed.

Overall Approach to Treatment

Allergic Rhinitis

The following approach to treatment is based on recent national and global recommendations (Fig. 8-2).[84] In patients with *mild, intermittent* symptoms of allergic rhinitis who complain primarily of rhinorrhea or sneezing, an oral or topical intranasal antihistamine, taken as needed, often is very effective. In patients with intermittent symptoms of nasal congestion, an intranasal antihistamine or an antihistamine-decongestant combination pill, taken as needed, may be helpful. If persistent symptoms are present, particularly nasal congestion, an INS given regularly is usually most effective.

Patients with *moderate* to *severe* symptoms should be re-evaluated after 2 to 4 weeks to assess their response to therapy. With an excellent response, anticipated exposures should be considered and the patient treated accordingly. With a partial response, residual complaints should be identified and targeted with specific medications. For significant eye symptoms, an intraocular antihistamine can be taken as needed. If significant redness of the eye persists, referral to an ophthalmologist should be considered. For residual nasal congestion, the addition of an intranasal antihistamine may be the most useful of all options. If rhinorrhea persists as a primary problem, ipratropium bromide may provide additional benefit. If the patient does not improve after maximal medical therapy, the diagnosis should be reconsidered, along with the need for additional diagnostic testing (e.g., CT of the sinuses or nasal endoscopy). For refractory allergic rhinitis that fails to respond to the foregoing treatments, in the absence of obvious complicating factors, consideration for allergen immunotherapy is in order. A stepped-care approach to the treatment of allergic rhinitis is shown in Figure 8-2.

Non-allergic Rhinitis

In patients with persistent anterior or posterior discharge associated with any of the forms of non-allergic rhinitis, particularly when it is thick in consistency, nasal irrigation

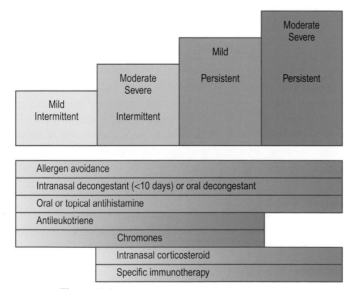

Figure 8-2 Stepped therapy for allergic rhinitis.

with saline may be very helpful. Nasal saline washes are also extremely important in the management of nasal crusting, as seen in atrophic rhinitis. Nasal saline may have no effect on nasal congestion, however, and other medications will be important in alleviating this symptom.

In patients with chronic congestion, an INS or intranasal azelastine should be administered as a first-line pharmacologic agent, used on an intermittent basis. As in allergic rhinitis, if either agent alone is not completely effective, the addition of the other drug may be useful.

In patients with intermittent acute, watery rhinorrhea caused by irritant or cold air exposure, exercise, or food, ipratropium bromide used before symptoms occur can be very effective.

For patients using medications for systemic diseases, such as antihypertensives, a change in therapy should be considered. If, however, a particular medication is deemed necessary and irreplaceable, the nasal side effects may need to be medicated. This is best accomplished with topical therapy in order to avoid drug interactions and/or additional systemic adverse effects.

Treatment Considerations in Select Populations

Pregnancy

In pregnant women with rhinitis, non-drug therapies should be tried first. Nasal rinsing with normal saline helps to remove thick nasal secretions and over-the-counter mechanical nasal dilators[87] may improve nasal congestion and snoring at night in some women. In many women, medications will still be required. Nasal cromolyn, one spray four times daily, should be tried next, because of its excellent safety profile and FDA pregnancy category B rating.[88] If a 2-week course of cromolyn is not helpful, particularly if nasal congestion is present, a trial of an INS is indicated. Although most INS are given an FDA pregnancy category C rating (with the exception of budesonide, in category B), gestational risk has not been confirmed in observational human data, and the reported safety data on all of the available compounds are reassuring. When INS therapy is started during pregnancy, budesonide frequently is the drug of choice because of the category B rating.[89] Oral antihistamines may be worth considering if primary complaints include rhinorrhea, sneezing, and pruritus and the patient prefers oral therapy. If use of an oral antihistamine is appropriate, both diphenhydramine and chlorpheniramine have a very long record of use in pregnancy and frequently are the drugs of choice for obstetric patients.[90] In a significant subset of women, however, the central nervous system and anticholinergic effects of these agents will prove difficult to tolerate. Loratadine and cetirizine have been extensively studied during pregnancy, and both belong to pregnancy category B. Topical antihistamines, including olopatadine and azelastine, do not have a long history of use in pregnancy and belong to FDA category C. For these reasons, the other medications listed here would be considered more appropriate choices in pregnancy. Oral decongestants should be avoided, if possible, during the first trimester because of conflicting reports of an association of phenylephrine and pseudoephedrine with congenital malformations such as gastroschisis and small intestinal atresia. Specific allergen immunotherapy for allergic rhinitis may be continued during pregnancy if it is providing significant benefit and has not caused systemic reactions. Allergen extract doses should be maintained and not increased until the completion of the pregnancy. For these same reasons, immunotherapy should not be started during pregnancy.

Elderly

Two of the most important aspects of treating rhinitis in older patients are improving intranasal moisture content and removing dried secretions.[91] Nasal irrigation using buffered saline or a saline nasal spray should be used by most elderly people with chronic rhinitis, particularly those with non-allergic rhinitis. INS, although generally safe, may cause more bleeding than is usually seen in younger patients, owing to the increased fragility of the nasal mucous membranes in this population. In general, older-generation

---

Box 8-4 **Indications for Referral**

TO ALLERGIST/IMMUNOLOGIST

1. Poor response to multiple medications for rhinitis
2. Significant drug-related side effects
3. Secondary complications of rhinitis, including:
   a. Chronic sinusitis/nasal polyposis
   b. Persistent middle ear disease
   c. Poorly-controlled asthma
4. Consideration of allergen immunotherapy or complex allergen avoidance measures

TO OTOLARYNGOLOGIST

Consideration of surgical treatment for chronic sinusitis/nasal polyposis, adenoidal enlargement, or other anatomic obstructions

---

oral antihistamines should be avoided because of their potential to sedate or cause anticholinergic effects. Oral decongestants should be similarly avoided owing to possible adverse effects on blood pressure (hypertension), cardiac rhythm (extrasystoles, arrhythmias), central nervous system (insomnia, agitation), and urinary tract (obstruction).

INDICATIONS FOR REFERRAL

A number of different patient profiles should be considered for referral to an allergist: (1) patients whose rhinitis symptoms have not responded adequately to combination pharmacotherapy; (2) patients with significant adverse side effects due to pharmacotherapy; (3) patients with secondary complications from their rhinitis, including recurrent or chronic sinusitis, nasal polyposis, recurrent or persistent middle ear disease, and poorly controlled asthma; and (4) patients with positive in-vitro or skin tests to a perennial allergen in order to consider and implement a program of allergen avoidance. In addition, because of the significant cost savings associated with allergen immunotherapy for allergic rhinitis, any patient requiring year-around, long-term treatment with combination therapy should also be considered for referral to an allergist. Referral to an otolaryngologist is most important when surgical treatment for nasal polyposis, chronic sinusitis, significant adenoidal enlargement, or anatomic obstructions is being considered (Box 8-4).

CONCLUSIONS

During the past 10 to 15 years, prospective studies of large populations have significantly improved our understanding of the epidemiology of chronic rhinitis in both children and adults. Simultaneously, advances in the basic science of allergic mechanisms have provided new and important insights into the pathophysiology of rhinitis. An integrated approach to therapy, including environmental control measures, pharmacotherapy, and allergen immunotherapy, will provide significant relief of symptoms and improvements in quality of life in the vast majority of patients with allergic rhinitis.

REFERENCES

1. Blackley CH. Experimental researches on the cause and nature of Catarrhus Aestivus. Oxford: Oxford Historical Books; 1988.
2. Noon L. Prophylactic inoculation against hay fever. Lancet 1911;1:1572–3.
3. Frankland AW, Augustin R. Prophylaxis of summer hayfever and asthma: controlled trial comparing crude grass pollen extracts with isolated main protein component. Lancet 1954;4:1055.
4. *Strachan D, Sibbald B, Weiland S, et al. Worldwide variations in prevalence of symptoms of allergic rhinoconjunctivitis in children: the International Study of Asthma and Allergies in Childhood (ISAAC). Pediatr Allergy Immunol 1997;8:161–76.
5. Bjorksten B, Clayton T, Ellwodd P, et al. ISAAC Phase III Study Group. Worldwide time trends for symptoms of rhinitis and conjunctivitis: phase III of the International Study of Asthma and Allergies in Childhood. Pediatr Allergy Immunol 2008;19:110–24.
6. Kellberger J, Dressel H, Vogelberg C, et al. Prediction of the incidence and persistence of allergic rhinitis in adolescence: a prospective cohort study. J Allergy Clin Immunol 2012;129:397–402.

7. Bousquet PJ, Leynaert B, Neukirch F, et al. Geographical distribution of atopic rhinitis in the European Community Respiratory Health Survey I. Allergy 2008;63:1301–9.
8. Salo PM, Calatroni A, Gergen PJ, et al. Allergy-related outcomes in relation to serum IgE: results from the National Health and Nutrition Examination Survey 2005–2006. J Allergy Clin Immunol 2011;127:1226–35.
9. *Bousquet J, Bullinger M, Fayol C, et al. Assessment of quality of life in patients with perennial allergic rhinitis with the French version of the SF-36 Health Status Questionnaire. J Allergy Clin Immunol 1994;94(2 Pt 1):182–8.
10. Simons FE. Learning impairment and allergic rhinitis. Allergy Asthma Proc 1996;17:185–9.
11. Marshall PS, Colon EA. Effects of allergy season on mood and cognitive function. Ann Allergy 1993; 71:251–8.
12. Bousquet J, Van Cauwenberge P, Khaltaev N. Allergic rhinitis and its impact on asthma. J Allergy Clin Immunol 2001;108(5 Suppl.):S147–334.
13. Laynaert B, Neukirch C, Kony S, et al. Association between asthma and rhinitis according to atopic sensitization in a population-based study. J Allergy Clin Immunol 2004;113:86–93.
14. Bousquet J, Gaugris S, Kocevar VS, et al. Increased risk of asthma attacks and emergency visits among asthma patients with allergic rhinitis: a subgroup analysis of the investigation of montelukast as a partner agent for complementary therapy [corrected]. Clin Exp Allergy 2005;35:723–7.
15. Fokkens W, Lund V, Mullol J. European Position Paper on Rhinosinusitis and Nasal Polyps group. European position paper on rhinosinusitis and nasal polyps 2007. Rhinol Suppl 2007;20:1–136.
16. Van Crombruggen K, Zhang N, Gevaert P, et al. Pathogenesis of chronic rhinosinusitis: inflammation. J Allergy Clin Immunol 2011;128:728–32.
17. Tewfik TL, Mazer B. The links between allergy and otitis media with effusion. Curr Opin Otolaryngol Head Neck Surg 2006;14:187–90.
18. Hurst DS. The role of allergy in otitis media with effusion. Otolaryngol Clin North Am 2011; 44:637–54.
19. Lund M, Craig T. Rhinitis and sleep. Sleep Med Rev 2011;15:293–9.
20. Hannuksela A, Väänänen A. Predisposing factors for malocclusion in 7-year-old children with special reference to atopic diseases. Am J Orthod Dentofacial Orthop 1987;92:299–303.
21. *Sin B, Togias A. Pathophysiology of allergic and non-allergic rhinitis. Proc Am Thorac Soc 2011;8:106–14.
22. Eccles R. A role for the nasal cycle in respiratory defence. Eur Respir J 1996;9:371–6.
23. Singh K, Axelrod S, Bielory L. The epidemiology of ocular and nasal allergy in the United States, 1988–1994. J Allergy Clin Immunol 2010;126:778–83.
24. Pinto JM. Olfaction. Proc Am Thorac Soc 2011;8:46–52.
25. Smolensky MH, Lemmer B, Reinberg AE. Chronobiology and chronotherapy of allergic rhinitis and bronchial asthma. Adv Drug Deliv Rev 2007;59:852–82.
26. Billionnet C, Gay E, Kirchner S, et al. Quantitative assessments of indoor air pollution and respiratory health in a population-based sample of French dwellings. Environ Res 2011;111:425–34.
27. Jacobs R, Lieberman P, Kent E, et al. Weather/temperature-sensitive vasomotor rhinitis may be refractory to intranasal corticosteroid treatment. Allergy Asthma Proc 2009;30:120–7.
28. Weider DJ, Baker GL, Salvatoriello FW. Dental malocclusion and upper airway obstruction, an otolaryngologist's perspective. Int J Pediatr Otorhinolaryngol 2003;67:323–31.
29. Marks MB. Allergic shiners: dark circles under the eyes in children. Clin Pediatr 1966;5:655–8.
30. Castellanos J, Axelrod D. Flexible fiberoptic rhinoscopy in the diagnosis of sinusitis. J Allergy Clin Immunol 1989;83:91–4.
31. Wood RA, Phipatanakul W, Hamilton RG, et al. A comparison of skin prick tests, intradermal skin tests, and RASTs in the diagnosis of cat allergy. J Allergy Clin Immunol 1999;103:773.
32. Rondon C, Romero JJ, Lopez S, et al. Local IgE production and positive nasal provocation test in patients with persistent non-allergic rhinitis. J Allergy Clin Immunol 2007;119:899–905.
33. Demirjian M, Rumbyrt JS, Gowda VC, et al. Serum IgE and eosinophil count in allergic rhinitis – analysis using a modified Bayes' theorem. Allergol Immunopathol (Madr) 2012;40:281–7.
34. McAfee MF. Imaging of paranasal sinuses and rhinosinusitis. Clin Allergy Immunol 2007;20:185–226.
35. Bonifazi F, Bilò MB, Antonicelli L, et al. Rhinopharyngoscopy, computed tomography, and magnetic resonance imaging. Allergy 1997;52(33 Suppl.):28–31.
36. Varonen H, Mäkelä M, Savolainen S, et al. Comparison of ultrasound, radiography, and clinical examination in the diagnosis of acute maxillary sinusitis: a systematic review. J Clin Epidemiol 2000;53(9):940–8.
37. Meltzer EO, Hamilos DL, Hadley JA, et al.; American Academy of Allergy, Asthma and Immunology (AAAAI), American Academy of Otolaryngic Allergy (AAOA), American Academy of Otolaryngology – Head and Neck Surgery (AAO-HNS), American College of Allergy, Asthma and Immunology (ACAAI), American Rhinologic Society (ARS). Rhinosinusitis: establishing definitions for clinical research and patient care. J Allergy Clin Immunol 2004;114(6 Suppl.):155.
38. Hamilos DL. Chronic rhinosinusitis patterns of illness. Clin Allergy Immunol 2007;20:1.
39. Lindberg S, Malm L. Comparison of allergic rhinitis and vasomotor rhinitis patients on the basis of a computer questionnaire. Allergy 1993;48:602–7.
40. Ellis AK, Keith PK. Non-allergic rhinitis with eosinophilia syndrome. Curr Allergy Asthma Rep 2006;6:215–20.
41. Sublett JW, Bernstein DI. Occupational rhinitis. Immunol Allergy Clin North Am 2011;31:787–96.
42. Chhabra N, Houser SM. The diagnosis and management of empty nose syndrome. Otolaryngol Clin North Am 2009;42:311–30.
43. Graf PM. Rhinitis medicamentosa. Clin Allergy Immunol 2007;19:295–304.
44. *Varghese M, Glaum MC, Lockey RF. Drug-induced rhinitis. Clin Exp Allergy 2010;40:381–4.

45. Ellegård E, Hellgren M, Torén K, et al. The incidence of pregnancy rhinitis. Gynecol Obstet Invest 2000;49:98.
46. Franklin KA, Holmgren PA, Jönsson F, et al. Snoring, pregnancy-induced hypertension, and growth retardation of the fetus. Chest 2000;117:137.
47. Smith K, Edwards PC, Saini TS, et al. The prevalence of concha bullosa and nasal septal deviation and their relationship to maxillary sinusitis by volumetric tomography. Int J Dent 2010;ii:404982.
48. Santos RS, Cipolotti R, D'Avila FS, et al. Schoolchildren submitted to fiberoptic examination at school: findings and tolerance. J Pediatr (Rio J) 2005;81:443–6.
49. Persky MS, Tabaee A. Cancer of the nasal vestibule and paranasal sinus: surgical management. In: Harrison LB, Sessions RB, Hong WK, editors. Head and neck cancer. 3rd ed. Philadelphia: Lippincott Williams & Wilkins; 2009. p. 454.
50. *Kumar S. Vernal keratoconjunctivitis: a major review. Acta Ophthalmol 2009;87:133.
51. Elhers WH, Donshik PC. Giant papillary conjunctivitis. Curr Opin Allergy Clin Immunol 2008;8:445.
52. Tuft SJ, Kemeny DM, Dart JK, et al. Clinical features of atopic keratoconjunctivitis. Ophthalmology 1991;98:150.
53. Weiss A, Brinser JH, Nazar-Stewart V. Acute conjunctivitis in childhood. J Pediatr 1993;122:10.
54. Latkany R. Dry eyes: etiology and management. Curr Opin Ophthalmol 2008;19:287.
55. Nichols KK, Foulks GN, Bron AJ, et al. The international workshop on meibomian gland dysfunction: executive summary. Invest Ophthalmol Vis Sci 2011;52:1922.
56. Noecker R. Effects of common ophthalmic preservatives on ocular health. Adv Ther 2001;18:205.
57. Oltz M, Check J. Rosacea and its ocular manifestations. Optometry 2011;82:92.
58. Leibowitz HM. The red eye. N Engl J Med 2000;343:345.
59. Congdon NG, Friedman DS. Angle-closure glaucoma: impact, etiology, diagnosis, and treatment. Curr Opin Ophthalmol 2003;14:70.
60. Sheikh A, Hurwitz B, Shehata Y. House dust mite avoidance measures for perennial allergic rhinitis. Cochrane Database Syst Rev 2007;(1):CD001563.
61. *Sheikh A, Hurwitz B, Nurmatov U, et al. House dust mite avoidance measures for perennial allergic rhinitis. Cochrane Database Syst Rev 2010;(7):CD001563.
62. Bjornsdottir US, Jakobinudottir S, Runarsdottir V, et al. The effect of reducing levels of cat allergen (Fel d 1) on clinical symptoms in patients with cat allergy. Ann Allergy Asthma Immunol 2003;91:189–94.
63. Wood RA, Johnson EF, Van-Natta ML, et al. A placebo-controlled trial of a HEPA air cleaner in the treatment of cat allergy. Am J Respir Crit Care Med 1998;158:115–20.
64. *Simons FE. Advances in H_1-antihistamines. N Engl J Med 2004;351:2203–17.
65. de Blic J, Wahn U, Billard E, et al. Levocetirizine in children: evidenced efficacy and safety in a 6-week randomized seasonal allergic rhinitis trial. Pediatr Allergy Immunol 2005;16:267–75.
66. LaForce C, Dockhorn RJ, Prenner BM, et al. Safety and efficacy of azelastine nasal spray (Astelin NS) for seasonal allergic rhinitis: a 4-week comparative multicenter trial. Ann Allergy Asthma Immunol 1996;76:181.
67. Fairchild CJ, Meltzer EO, Roland PS, et al. Comprehensive report of the efficacy, safety, quality of life, and work impact of Olopatadine 0.6% and Olopatadine 0.4% treatment in patients with seasonal allergic rhinitis. Allergy Asthma Proc 2007;28:716–23.
68. *Weiner JM, Abramson MJ, Puy RM. Intranasal corticosteroids versus oral H1 receptor antagonists in allergic rhinitis: systematic review of randomized controlled trials. BMJ 1998;317:1624–9.
69. *Wilson AM, O'Byrne PM, Parameswaran K. Leukotriene receptor antagonists for allergic rhinitis: a systematic review and meta-analysis. Am J Med 2004;116:338–44.
70. Bernstein DI, Levy AL, Hampel FC, et al. Treatment with intranasal fluticasone propionate significantly improves ocular symptoms in patients with seasonal allergic rhinitis. Clin Exp Allergy 2004;34:952–7.
71. Selner JC, Weber RW, Richmond GW, et al. Onset of action of aqueous beclomethasone dipropionate nasal spray in seasonal allergic rhinitis. Clin Ther 1995;17:1099–109.
72. Jen A, Baroody F, de Tineo M, et al. As-needed use of fluticasone propionate nasal spray reduces symptoms of seasonal allergic rhinitis. J Allergy Clin Immunol 2000;105:732–8.
73. Holm AF, Fokkens WJ, Godthelp T, et al. A 1-year placebo-controlled study of intranasal fluticasone propionate aqueous nasal spray in patients with perennial allergic rhinitis: a safety and biopsy study. Clin Otolaryngol 1998;23:69–73.
74. Schenkel EJ, Skoner DP, Bronsky EA, et al. Absence of growth retardation in children with perennial allergic rhinitis after one year of treatment with mometasone furoate aqueous nasal spray. Pediatrics 2000;105:E22.
75. Philip G, Malmstrom K, Hampel FC, et al. Montelukast for treating seasonal allergic rhinitis: a randomized, double-blind, placebo-controlled trial performed in the spring. Clin Exp Allergy 2002;32:1020–8.
76. Borum P, Mygind N, Schultz LF. Intranasal ipratropium, a new treatment for perennial rhinitis. Clin Otolaryngol 1979;4:407.
77. Bronsky EA, Druce H, Findlay SR, et al. A clinical trial of ipratropium bromide nasal spray in patients with perennial non-allergic rhinitis. J Allergy Clin Immunol 1995;95:1117–22.
78. Silvers WS. The skier's nose: a model of cold-induced rhinorrhea. Ann Allergy Asthma Immunol 1991;67:32–6.
79. Katelaris CH, Ciprandi G, Missotten L, et al. A comparison of the efficacy and tolerability of olopatadine hydrochloride 0.1% ophthalmic solution and cromolyn sodium 2% ophthalmic solution in seasonal allergic conjunctivitis. Clin Ther 2002;24:1561–75.
80. Weiner JM, Abramson MJ, Puy RM. Intranasal corticosteroids versus oral H1 receptor antagonists in allergic rhinitis: systematic review of randomized controlled trials. BMJ 1998;317:1624–9.
81. Hampel FC, Ratner PH, van Bavel J, et al. Double-blind, placebo-controlled study of azelastine and fluticasone in a single nasal spray delivery device. Ann Allergy Asthma Immunol 2010;105:168–73.

82. Ratner PH, van Bavel JH, Martin BG, et al. A comparison of the efficacy of fluticasone propionate aqueous nasal spray and loratadine, alone and in combination, for the treatment of seasonal allergic rhinitis. J Fam Pract 1998;47:118–25.
83. Lanier BQ, Abelson MB, Berger WE, et al. Comparison of the efficacy of combined fluticasone propionate and olopatadine versus combined fluticasone propionate and fexofenadine for the treatment of allergic rhinoconjunctivitis induced by conjunctival allergen challenge. Clin Ther 2002;24:1161–74.
84. Wallace DV, Dykewicz MS, Bernstein DI, et al.; Joint Task Force on Practice; American Academy of Allergy; Asthma & Immunology; American College of Allergy; Asthma and Immunology; Joint Council of Allergy, Asthma and Immunology. The diagnosis and management of rhinitis: an updated practice parameter. J Allergy Clin Immunol 2008;122(2 Suppl.):S1–84.
85. James LK, Shamji MH, Walker SM, et al. Long-term tolerance after allergen immunotherapy is accompanied by selective persistence of blocking antibodies. J Allergy Clin Immunol 2011;127:509–16.
86. *Brüggenjürgen B, Reinhold T, Brehler R, et al. Cost-effectiveness of specific subcutaneous immunotherapy in patients with allergic rhinitis and allergic asthma. Ann Allergy Asthma Immunol 2008;101:316–24.
87. Turnbull GL, Rundell OH, Rayburn WF, et al. Managing pregnancy-related nocturnal nasal congestion. The external nasal dilator. J Reprod Med 1996;41:897.
88. Wilson J. Use of sodium cromoglycate during pregnancy. J Pharm Med 1982;8:45.
89. Gluck PA, Gluck JC. A review of pregnancy outcomes after exposure to orally inhaled or intranasal budesonide. Curr Med Res Opin 2005;21:1075–84.
90. Seto A, Einarson T, Koren G. Pregnancy outcome following first trimester exposure to antihistamines: meta-analysis. Am J Perinatol 1997;14:119–24.
91. Tan R, Corren J. Optimum treatment of rhinitis in the elderly. Drugs Aging 1995;7:168–75.

Key references are preceded by an asterisk.

CHAPTER 9

Drug Allergy

Oliver Hausmann

CHAPTER OUTLINE

INTRODUCTION

HISTORICAL PERSPECTIVE

EPIDEMIOLOGY

PATHOGENESIS AND ETIOLOGY

CLINICAL FEATURES (PHENOTYPES)

Urticaria and Angioedema (Immediate Type)

Maculopapular Exanthem (MPE) (Delayed Type)

Fixed Drug Eruptions (Delayed Type)

Exfoliative Dermatitis (Stevens–Johnson Syndrome and Toxic Epidermal Necrolysis) (Delayed Type)

Systemic Drug Reactions: Severe Drug Hypersensitivity Syndromes (Delayed Type)

Isolated Drug-induced Organ Damage (Delayed Type)

Pediatric Aspects in Drug Allergy

PATIENT EVALUATION, DIAGNOSIS, AND DIFFERENTIAL DIAGNOSIS

DRUG CLASSES OF SPECIAL INTEREST

Non-steroidal Anti-inflammatory Drugs (NSAIDs)

Angiotensin Converting Enzyme Inhibitor (ACE-I)

Beta-lactams

Radio Contrast Media

Biologicals

TREATMENT

Referral

CONCLUSIONS

SUMMARY OF IMPORTANT CONCEPTS

- The history and clinical presentation can aid the distinction between immediate and delayed-type reactions, which have a different diagnostic and therapeutic approach.
- During the acute reaction phase, laboratory tests are advisable in immediate-type reactions (serum tryptase) to prove mast cell involvement and in delayed-type reactions (eosinophil count, C-reactive protein (CRP), and liver enzymes) to define organ involvement and severity.
- The most common drug classes involved in hypersensitivity (immediate and delayed) reactions are antibiotics, non-steroidal anti-inflammatory drugs (NSAIDs), and anticonvulsants.
- Some drugs induce severe systemic forms of delayed-type drug hypersensitivities in patients with a certain human leukocyte antigen (HLA) class I allele (e.g., abacavir associated with HLA B*57:01). Here, HLA testing is recommended before use.
- Risk for drug hypersensitivity is increased in patients with viral infections (e.g., EBV, HIV), during or shortly after a severe drug hypersensitivity reaction ('flare up') or if high doses, prolonged or repetitive treatment courses are needed (e.g., in cystic fibrosis).
- Supporting national pharmacovigilance programs is an important contribution for general drug safety.

INTRODUCTION

Adverse drug reactions (ADR) are common and inherent to all pharmacologic therapy. Sooner or later, every practicing physician will be confronted with this phenomenon. ADRs in general have been reported to affect 10–20% of hospitalized patients and up to 25% of outpatients.[1] Drug allergy is one important subgroup of ADR. Typically,

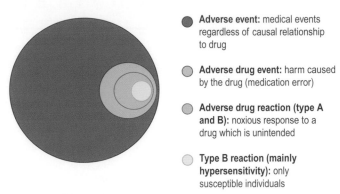

Adverse event: medical events regardless of causal relationship to drug

Adverse drug event: harm caused by the drug (medication error)

Adverse drug reaction (type A and B): noxious response to a drug which is unintended

Type B reaction (mainly hypersensitivity): only susceptible individuals

Figure 9-1 Nomenclature for drug reaction.

allergic reactions affect the skin, but organ involvement (hepatitis) and blood eosinophilia are also common in systemic forms of drug hypersensitivity and may serve as 'red flags' for a more severe course. Fortunately, the majority of drug allergic patients have only mild symptoms limited to the skin and do not progress to life-threatening organ involvement and/or anaphylaxis.

Although different classifications have been proposed, ADRs are usually classified into two subtypes (Fig. 9-1):

Type A reactions, which are predictable from known pharmacologic properties, e.g. sleepiness caused by first generation antihistamines or gastrointestinal toxicity of non-steroidal anti-inflammatory drugs (NSAIDs), and *type B reactions*, which are unpredictable or unexpected and restricted to a vulnerable subpopulation. The majority of these unexpected type B reactions are *hypersensitivity reactions*. They are responsible for about one in six of all ADRs and comprise:

1. *Allergic* (immune-mediated) reactions
2. *Pharmacological* (direct interaction with specific immune receptors [HLA, TCR], briefly termed p-i concept) reactions
3. *Non-allergic intolerance* (also called '*pseudo-allergic*') reactions without a defined genetic defect.

The term *idiosyncrasy* was previously used synonymously for all type B reactions, but is nowadays limited to non-allergic hypersensitivity reactions with a genetic background, for example, an enzyme defect such as glucose-6-phosphate dehydrogenase (G6PD) deficiency, also known as favism. This deficiency leads to hemolytic anemia upon intake of metamizol or one of the other G6PD-dependent drugs.

Use of the terms *immediate* or *delayed-type* reaction to qualify the onset of symptoms has been recommended because they indicate the probable underlying immune mechanism. They refer to the onset of symptoms within or later than 1 hour after dosing, even if this time point is set rather arbitrarily and solid data supporting it are still lacking. During the initial evaluation and together with other clinical features, the timing of the reaction might help in distinguishing whether the probable immunologic mechanism is an antibody-mediated (mostly immunoglobulin E, IgE), immediate-type or a T cell–mediated, delayed-type reaction. However, some IgE-mediated immediate reactions may start later than 1 hour after exposure, and very strong T cell–mediated delayed-type reactions, especially on repetitive exposure, may start rapidly, within hours; such examples defy the original definition of these terms. In general, delayed-type reactions are much more frequent than immediate-type reactions in drug allergy.

The risk of sensitization or immune stimulation and sometimes also the consecutive clinical severity depend on different factors, which may be drug- and/or patient-specific (Table 9-1). Of note, an atopic genetic background with an IgE-mediated response to ingested or inhaled proteins (e.g., hay fever) is not associated with an increased risk for drug hypersensitivity.

TABLE 9-1 Factors Conveying a Risk of Sensitization or Immune Stimulation by a Certain Drug and a Risk for Severe Clinical Symptoms

Patient	Drug
Immunogenetic predisposition (particularly the human leukocyte antigen, HLA alleles)	Protein binding Structure (LMW vs HMW)
Preactivated immune system (particularly chronic viral infection, e.g., EBV, HIV, ongoing drug allergy)	Cross-reactivity Dosage Route of administration
Underlying disease (particularly active systemic autoimmune diseases)	Duration of treatment

The aim of this chapter is to stress the significance and importance of drug hypersensitivity in the context of general medicine and ambulatory care. It therefore only provides a very concise review of the basic pathogenetic concepts of drug hypersensitivity. The focus is on a detailed clinical description, including the warning signs ('red flags') for a potentially severe course on initial evaluation of a patient, considering common diagnostic errors and specific pediatric aspects. The management of the acute phase of drug allergy and the necessity and optimal timing for referral to a specialist is discussed. The specialist's task is then to define the elicitor(s), the underlying mechanism, and the safety of re-administration of the same drug, as well as to provide information on safe alternative(s) for further treatment of the patient.

For general safety, most countries run their own pharmacovigilance program for the monitoring of ADRs. Electronic reporting systems such as MedWatch (www.fda.gov/Safety/MedWatch) are available and easily accessible. It is the responsibility and an important contribution of the treating physician to inform the regulatory agencies about any relevant ADR which might have been missed during the licensing process. This postmarketing surveillance has led to drug withdrawal in several cases (Table 9-2).

HISTORICAL PERSPECTIVE

Drug allergy, as is the case with modern pharmacotherapy itself, is a fairly young field of medicine. The German dermatologist Heinrich Koebner (1838–1904) was the first to coin the term 'drug exanthema' in 1877, describing a quinine-specific skin reaction in two patients, which he clearly separated from the known toxic side effects. In the following years, researchers and clinicians from different countries contributed their observations, highlighting the fact that different drugs may cause the same clinical presentation, as well as the fact that the same drug may elicit different forms of drug hypersensitivity. They could already define several distinct syndromes, which still apply today.[2] Only with the advent of modern immunology have the underlying mechanisms become apparent, sometimes more than 50 years after their first clinical description. Many aspects of drug hypersensitivity are still unclear and this therefore remains a very active field of applied immunology.

Today, regulatory agencies and a strict jurisdiction control the development and licensing process of new drugs. Protein binding properties and immunogenicity play an important role here. Most of the drugs in use are still low-molecular-weight (LMW) compounds and should actually not be recognized by our immune system. Only after binding to an endogenous carrier protein (haptenization), immunogenic complexes arise and can elicit a complex immune response with B and T cell reactions. Therefore, strong protein binding properties (leading to hapten formation) of a drug usually leads to termination in the early stages of drug development due to the risk of immune reactions in later clinical use. The highly effective beta-lactam class of antibiotics (penicillins, cephalosporins), with their strong binding to albumin, would most probably not have reached the market if invented today, or would at least struggle with the restrictive licensing requirements. In spite of these restrictions and avoidance of drugs with the potential to bind via covalent bonds to proteins, hypersensitivity reactions still persist.

TABLE 9-2   List of Drugs Withdrawn for Safety Reasons in all EU Member States between 2002 and 2011 Grouped by Adverse Drug Reaction or Safety Concern

Drug name	Drug class or use	Year first marketed	Year of withdrawal	Length of time on market (years)	Adverse reaction or safety concern
Rofecoxib	NSAID (COX-2 inhibitor)	1999	2004	5	Thrombotic events
Thioridazine	Neuroleptic (α-adrenergic and dopaminergic receptor antagonist)	1958	2005	47	Cardiac disorders
Valdecoxib	NSAID (COX-2 inhibitor)	2003	2005	2	Cardiovascular and cutaneous disorders
Rosiglitazone	Antidiabetic treatment (PPAR agonist)	2000	2010	10	Cardiovascular disorders
Sibutramine	Treatment of obesity (serotonin-noradrenaline reuptake inhibitor)	1999	2010	11	Cardiovascular disorders
Orciprenaline	Sympathomimetic (non-specific β-agonist)	1961	2010	49	Cardiac disorders
Benfluorex	Anorectic and hypolipidemic	1974	2009	35	Heart valve disease Pulmonary hypertension
Clobutinol	Cough suppressant (centrally acting)	1961	2007	46	QT prolongation
Buflomedil	Vasodilator (α1 and α2 receptor antagonist)	1974	2011	37	Neurologic and cardiac disorders (sometimes fatal)
Veralipride	Neuroleptic (and dopaminergic receptor antagonist)	1979	2007	28	Neurologic and psychiatric disorders
Rimonabant	Treatment of obesity (cannabinoid receptor antagonist)	2006	2008	2	Psychiatric disorders
Carisoprodol	Muscle relaxant	1959	2007	48	Intoxication: psychomotor impairment Addiction: misuse
Aceprometazine + Acepromazine + Clorazepate	Hypnotic	1988	2011	23	Cumulative adverse effects Misuse: fatal side effect
Dextropropoxyphene	Opioid painkiller	~1960	2009	49	Fatal overdose
Nefazodone	Antidepressant	1994	2003	9	Hepatotoxicity
Ximelagatran/ melagatran	Anticoagulant (thrombin inhibitor)	2003	2006	3	Hepatotoxicity
Lumiracoxib	NSAID (COX-2 inhibitor)	2003	2007	4	Hepatotoxicity
Sitaxentan	Antihypertensive (endothelin receptor antagonist)	2006	2010	4	Hepatotoxicity
Bufexamac	NSAID	~1970	2010	40	Contact allergic reactions

EU, European Union; NSAID, non-steroidal anti-inflammatory drug.
(McNaughton R, Huet G, Shakir S. An investigation into drug products withdrawn from the EU market between 2002 and 2011 for safety reasons and the evidence used to support the decision-making. BMJ Open 2014; 4(1):e004221.)

Most of these reactions are due to T cell stimulations and are caused by direct binding of the drug to a human leukocyte antigen (HLA) or a T cell receptor (TCR) molecule. This process of direct drug binding is summarized under the term *p-i concept* (pharmacological interaction with *i*mmune receptors).

Therapeutically applied high-molecular-weight (HMW) proteins, the so-called 'biologicals' or 'biopharmaceuticals' (e.g., antibodies or receptors), are still small in number compared with LMW classical drugs, but they represent the future of drug therapy. Most of the drugs in development or in the licensing process belong to this new drug class. They are immunogenic *per se* and immediate-type reactions dominate the clinical picture.

EPIDEMIOLOGY

Sound epidemiologic data on drug hypersensitivity reactions are still lacking. The most common drug classes causing hypersensitivity reactions are beta-lactam antibiotics and non-steroidal anti-inflammatory drugs (NSAIDs). Epidemiologic studies indicate that cutaneous reactions, such as maculopapular eruptions and urticaria, are the most common clinical manifestations of drug allergy. Rarely, drugs induce more severe and potentially life-threatening reactions such as toxic epidermal necrolysis (TEN), Stevens–Johnson syndrome (SJS), immune hepatitis or drug rash with eosinophilia and systemic symptoms (DRESS), for delayed-type reactions or anaphylaxis for immediate-type reactions. In the US, about 1 in 300 hospitalized patients dies from an ADR, and 6–10% of these reactions are most probably allergic in origin.

In the age of personalized medicine based on 'next generation' deoxyribonucleic acid (DNA) sequencing technologies, new aspects in epidemiology of drug allergy have arisen: immunogenetic studies have shown a strong genetic association between certain (HLA) alleles and severe forms of drug hypersensitivity (Table 9-3) and, in this respect, the previously postulated unpredictability of type B reactions no longer holds true. HLA screening before prescribing the drug to avoid these serious conditions is currently only recommended for *abacavir with HLA B*57:01* being the risk transferring allele, which is common in White European origin populations and for *carbamazepine with HLA B*15:02*, the risk allele for Southeast Asians. This form of primary prevention of drug hypersensitivity is one of the first great successes of personalized medicine.[3]

Limited data are available on the cost of drug allergy. A study in a hospital setting showed that penicillin-allergic patients had higher medical costs related to the use of alternative antibiotics. Alternative treatments for drug-allergic patients are commonly more expensive and often more toxic than first-line drugs.

TABLE 9-3 Associations of Different Forms of Delayed-type Drug Hypersensitivity and HLA Class I Alleles in Association with a Certain Ethnic Background (modified according to [3])

Causative drug	HLA allele	Hypersensitivity reactions	Ethnicity	Odds ratio (95% CI)
Abacavir	B*57:01	Abacavir hypersensitivity	Caucasians	117 (29–481)
Allopurinol	B*58:01	SJS/TEN/DRESS	Asians	74.18 (26.95–204.14)
			Non-Asians	101.45 (44.98–228.82)
Carbamazepine	B*15:02	SJS/TEN	Han Chinese	115.32 (18.17–732.13)
			Thai	54.43 (16.28–181.96)
			Malaysians	221.00 (3.85–12694.65)
			Indians	54.60 (2.25–1326.20)
	B*15:11		Japanese	16.3 (4.76–55.61)
			Koreans	18.0 (2.3–141.2)
			Han Chinese	31.00 (2.74–350.50)
	B*15:18		Japanese	13.58 (nd)
	A*31:01	DRESS	Han Chinese	23.0 (4.2–125)
			Europeans	57.6 (11.0–340)
		SJS/TEN	Europeans	4.4 (1.1–17.3)
			All populations	3.94 (1.4–11.5)
		SJS/TEN	Europeans	25.93 (4.93–116.18)
		DRESS	Europeans	12.41 (1.27–121.03)
		MPE	Europeans	8.33 (3.59–19.36)
		SJS/TEN/DRESS	Japanese	10.8 (5.9–19.6)
Oxcarbazepine	B*15:02	SJS/TEN	Taiwan/Han Chinese	80.7 (3.8–1714.4)
Phenytoin	B*15:02	SJS/TEN	Han Chinese	4.26 (1.93–9.39)
Dapsone	B*13:01	DRESS	Mainland China/Han Chinese	20.53 (11.55–36.48)
Lamotrigine	B*15:02	SJS/TEN	Han Chinese	3.59 (1.15–11.22)
Nevirapine	B*35:05	DRESS/MPE	Thai	18.96 (4.87–73.44)
Flucloxacillin	B*57:01	Hepatitis	Europeans/Caucasians	80,6 (22.8–284.9)

TABLE 9-4   Immunopathologic Penicillin Reactions

Gell and Coombs classification	Mechanism	Examples of adverse penicillin reactions
I	Anaphylactic (IgE-mediated)	Acute anaphylaxis Urticaria
II	Complement-dependent cytolysis (IgG/IgM)	Hemolytic anemias Thrombocytopenia
III	Immune complex damage	Serum sickness Drug fever Some cutaneous eruptions and vasculitis
IV	Delayed or cellular hypersensitivity	Contact dermatitis Morbilliform eruptions SJS/TEN Hepatitis

The Gell and Coombs classification: IgE-mediated type I drug reactions may involve acute anaphylaxis or urticaria. Cytolytic type II reactions usually are confined to drugs which bind to cell surface structures. Drug-specific immune complexes result from high-dose, prolonged therapy, and may produce drug fever, a classic type III serum sickness syndrome, as well as various forms of vasculitis. Contact dermatitis from topically applied drugs as well as maculopapular rashes involve T cell–mediated type IV reactions. Severe blistering skin reactions, such as SJS and TEN, belong to the same reaction type with involvement of drug specific cytotoxic CD8$^+$ T cells and possibly natural killer (NK) leading to keratinocyte death and the resulting widespread skin damage.

Ig, Immunoglobulin; SJS, Stevens–Johnson syndrome; TEN, toxic epidermal necrolysis.

PATHOGENESIS AND ETIOLOGY

Drug allergy syndromes (*type B reactions*) are recognized by the constellation of signs and symptoms linked to a particular mechanism. The Gell and Coombs classification is conceptually useful, even if it is unable to cover all mechanisms involved in drug allergy (Table 9-4).

The time of appearance of the first allergic symptoms is helpful to distinguish different forms of drug hypersensitivity. In an already sensitized individual and not on first contact, *IgE-mediated* reactions tend to appear rapidly, normally within minutes (with IV doses) to 1 hour (after oral intake). However, the sensitization and production of IgE antibodies to the drug or drug metabolite must have occurred earlier and clinically 'silent.' For sensitization LMW compounds need to bind to a carrier protein (haptenization) in order to be recognized by the immune system. Thus, a symptomless sensitization phase during the initial treatment is succeeded by a sudden allergic to anaphylactic reaction upon re-exposure.

On the other hand, delayed-type hypersensitivity, which is mostly *T cell–mediated*, appears later in the treatment course but may already manifest during the first treatment cycle, if it lasts long enough. In the beginning, only a few T cells seem to react with the drug and no symptoms appear. An exanthema may only arise after expansion and the migration of the drug specific effector T cells into the tissue. This explains the typical time interval between the start of treatment and the appearance of clinical symptoms, for example, in amoxicillin-induced exanthema at day 7 to 10 of treatment (Fig. 9-2). One should be aware that upon re-exposure, symptoms of these T cell reactions may appear much faster (within 2–48 hours), dependent on the amount of drug-reactive (primed) T cells and drug dosage.

T cell recognition, a cornerstone for both IgE and T cell–mediated reactions, depends upon drug presentation by antigen presenting cells (APC) on their HLA molecule and engagement of the corresponding T cell receptor (TCR) on CD4$^+$ or CD8$^+$ T lymphocytes. Again, haptenization of the presented peptide may be involved but it is no prerequisite here. The drug may also directly bind the immune receptors, namely the HLA molecule or to the TCR and stimulate T cells directly without haptenization and processing of a hapten-modified protein. This direct binding capacity is an inherent pharmacologic feature of most of the LMW drugs designed to fit into pockets of enzymes

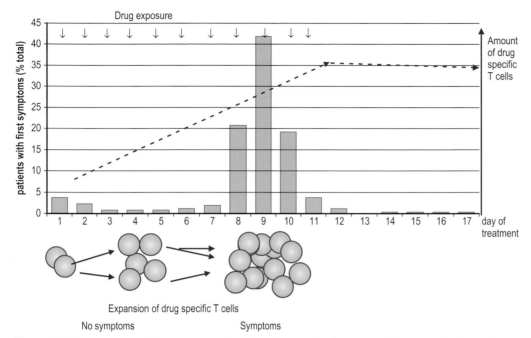

Figure 9-2 Appearance of first symptoms in delayed type drug hypersensitivity to quinolones (gemifloxacin-treated women, mainly skin rashes, n=270; Schmid DA, Campi P, Pichler WJ. Hypersensitivity reactions to quinolones. Curr Pharm Des. 2006;12(26):3313–26.)

(e.g. ACE inhibitors) and block their function. This kind of immune stimulation via *p*harmacological interaction with *i*mmune receptors (*p-i concept*) bypasses the classical control mechanisms of our immune system and can result in severe forms of hypersensitivity. This mechanism may also explain the sometimes puzzling clinical similarities to graft versus host disease (GvHD) where the same immunologic principles of direct activation of the grafted T cells by the patient (host) HLA molecules apply.[4]

In addition, a 'pre-activated' immune system is prone for mounting a drug hypersensitivity reaction, for example, a generalized viral infection (EBV or HIV), with its associated strong T-cell response, predisposes to delayed type drug hypersensitivity as well as multiple drug hypersensitivity (MDH). During or shortly after a severe drug hypersensitivity reaction, especially in DHS/DRESS (see below), T cells are highly susceptible to otherwise subthreshold stimuli, and a so-called 'flare up' reaction may arise. Under all of these highly stimulatory circumstances, even structurally unrelated drugs taken regularly may elicit allergic reactions.

On the other hand, a state of 'organ predisposition' (e.g., chronic urticaria, asthma, rhinosinusitis) with a lower local reaction threshold may also lead to clinical symptoms even without a compound-specific sensitization. A typical example is the non-allergic NSAID intolerance with either skin reactions (exacerbation of chronic urticaria) or reactions in the airways (acute rhinitis or asthma exacerbation) related to the intensity of eosinophilic inflammation in the upper and lower respiratory tract. They occur rapidly, namely as early as 15 min after oral intake, are highly dose-dependent and do not require a sensitization phase. They are based on the mode of action of all NSAIDs interfering with the arachidonic acid metabolism and ultimately leading to a prostaglandin-leukotriene imbalance. Non-allergic intolerance to radio contrast media rely on their capacity of direct mast cell activation, most probably due to their high (salt) concentration and rapid infusion rate that is needed for their optimal radiographic characteristics. Again, no sensitization phase is needed here.

The decade-long search for a specific mechanism in non-allergic drug intolerance reactions lately revealed a single receptor, known as MRGPRX2 (Mas-Related G-Protein Coupled Receptor Member X2) in humans and Mrgprb2 (Mas-related g-protein coupled receptor member b2) in mice, to be crucial for an IgE-independent, direct mast cells stimulation by certain drugs associated with systemic non-allergic ('pseudo-allergic,' 'anaphylactoid') reactions such as quinolone antibiotics and neuromuscular blocking agents (NMBA). These drugs share a common chemical motif, which might help to predict side effects of future compounds.[5] The fact that the different drugs all trigger a single receptor makes it an attractive drug target to prevent non-allergic drug intolerance reactions. True IgE-mediated allergic reactions are independent of this mechanism and remain unaffected.

CLINICAL FEATURES (PHENOTYPES)

Skin rashes are a frequent phenomenon in daily clinical practice. They may be reactive, for example, due to an underlying infection, drug-induced, or disease-specific. History and presentation alone probably overestimates the role of drug allergies in cutaneous reactions and a thorough allergological work-up to prove an allergic mechanism is advisable. Most of the drug allergic patients (>80%) suffer from skin symptoms, mostly maculopapular rashes. Acute urticaria is also common. The latter may quickly progress to anaphylaxis and needs special attention. An intense palmar and plantar itch, anxiety, and a rapid progression of symptoms from skin involvement to circulatory symptoms are warning signs for a severe, potentially lethal course. Immediate treatment with intramuscular epinephrine (0.3–0.5 mg, IM, lateral thigh) with the patient in supine position is the therapeutic cornerstone (see Ch. 13 on Anaphylaxis).

One major concern of general internists is the distinction of immediate and delayed-type drug hypersensitivity on initial clinical investigation. Besides the above-mentioned timing of the first symptoms, the morphology of the skin changes is very helpful in this respect: erythema, urticaria, and angioedema as typical signs of an immediate-type reaction, are non-fixed and without involvement of the epidermal structures (no scaling, no blistering). They may quickly change their appearance (confluence, borders) due to the underlying pathomechanism of vasodilation with or without tissue edema. In contrast, the T cell–mediated inflammation of delayed-type reactions, for example, in maculo-papular exanthema, leads to less transient skin rashes involving the epidermis, with either scaling or blister formation as well as to additional sensations such as warmth or pain besides itch, depending on the extent of tissue infiltration.

In delayed-type reaction involving effector T cells, the skin rash may only be the tip of the iceberg, and the involvement of internal organs (liver, lungs, kidney) and the extent of blood eosinophilia (>1.0 Giga/L is a good indicator of tissue infiltration) should be checked for at least once. In rare cases, drug allergic reactions are limited to the internal organs, for example, drug induced liver injury (DILI). Because recruitment and expansion of the drug reactive T cells take several days, symptoms may start as late as 7 to 10 days into therapy or even after cessation of the causative drug(s). In severe forms of drug allergy, for example, DRESS or SJS, it may even take more than 2 weeks for the first symptoms to appear. The warning signs ('red flags') on initial evaluation of a putative delayed-type hypersensitivity reaction are summarized in Table 9-5.

TABLE 9-5   Warning Signs (Red Flags) for Progression to a Severe Form of Delayed-type Drug Hypersensitivity (e.g., DRESS, SJS/TEN)

Signs and symptoms	Laboratory tests
Confluent infiltrative exanthema with progression to erythroderma	Blood eosinophilia (>10% and/or >1 Giga/L)
Bullous or pustulous lesions	Presence of lymphoblasts in the peripheral blood
Painful skin lesions	Hepatitis (elevated liver enzymes)
Mucosal involvement	Nephritis (creatinine, urine sediment)
Positive Nikolsky sign (epidermal detachment upon lateral traction of the skin)	Acute phase protein (elevated CRP, but usually <100 mg/L)
'B symptoms' (lymphadenopathy, fever, malaise)	

TABLE 9-6   Common Elicitors of Drug Hypersensitivity Reactions Corresponding to their Clinical Presentation

Immediate type (IgE, non-allergic intolerance)	Delayed type (T cell involvement)
<1 h, mostly <15 min	>6 h, mostly 7–14 days
Beta-lactam antibiotics (penicillins, cephalosporins) Vancomycin Quinolones NSAIDs (aspirin, diclofenac, ibuprofen) Neuromuscular blocking agents (NMBA) Radiocontrast media Therapeutic proteins/peptides (monoclonal antibodies)	Antibiotics (penicillins, cephalosporin, sulfonamides, quinolones, minocycline) Anticonvulsants (carbamazepine, phenytoin, lamotrigine) Allopurinol Sulfasalazine HIV drugs (nevirapine, abacavir)

Every drug may potentially be involved in a hypersensitivity reaction, but there is a fairly consistent 'hit list' of common culprits with considerable differences according to the reaction type (Table 9-6). If one of these drugs is involved, it should be stopped immediately.

Urticaria and Angioedema (Immediate Type)

IgE-mediated drug reactions may involve acute anaphylaxis or urticaria with or without accompanying angioedema (Fig. 9-3), the latter being a deeper-seated variant of urticaria mostly affecting soft tissues such as the eyelids, lips, tongue, pharyngeal, or genital tissue. Urticaria and angioedema are mostly histamine-dependent and usually accompanied by an intense itch, but are transient in nature and typically quickly change their location, as well as the extent of their skin involvement. It can occur early or late in a course of drug therapy and readily responds to antihistamines.

Maculopapular Exanthem (MPE) (Delayed Type)

MPE is the most frequent manifestation of drug hypersensitivity and is usually based on a T cell–mediated delayed-type hypersensitivity. A considerable proportion of MPE cases will be reactive due to an underlying infection and are not or not only drug-induced. Especially in children, the interaction between virus-induced and drug-induced immune stimulation seem to play an important role, illustrated by the pathognomonic maculopapular skin rash after intake of aminopenicillins in an EBV infection (Fig. 9-4).

Of interest for daily clinical practice, there are indications that cutaneous eruptions due to a drug hypersensitivity differ from reactive forms in their distribution pattern. In drug allergic skin rashes, the flexural aspects of the proximal extremities are affected first and most, whereas they are typically spared in reactive rashes. This might be consistent with an immunologic interaction of drugs or drug metabolites as well as T cell skin homing mechanisms and local factors such as friction, local skin temperature and possibly eccrine gland distribution. This would explain the typical distribution of drug allergic eruptions in the axillae, genital area, and buttocks; a phenomenon that is still poorly understood and detailed investigations are ongoing. Nevertheless, this typical distribution pattern might be helpful in daily clinical practice, especially for urgent bedside or office decisions (Fig. 9-5).

Extreme forms of this typical flexural distribution of drug allergic skin rashes are the symmetrical drug-related intertriginous and flexural exanthema (SDRIFE, formerly known as 'baboon syndrome') and acute generalized exanthematous pustulosis (AGEP). SDRIFE is quite strictly limited to the flexural surfaces and buttocks. AGEP shows the same distribution pattern in its early stages but later typically spreads over the body. They are usually diagnosed on the spot due to their typical and distinctive appearance. In SDRIFE, the flexural skin lesions are of typical maculopapular appearance, whereas in AGEP disseminated sterile pustules are seen and patients may have fever as well as an impressive blood leukocytosis (sometimes with eosinophilia). Mucous membranes are not involved. Epicutaneous patch test reactions may cause a similar pustular reaction locally (Fig. 9-6).

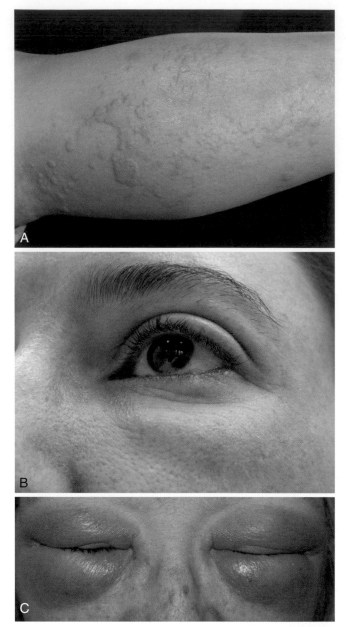

Figure 9-3 A. Urticaria. B, C. Mild and severe angioedema.

Fixed Drug Eruptions (Delayed Type)

This benign, rather unusual form of drug hypersensitivity, is characterized by immune-mediated cutaneous lesions that appear as annular, sometimes blistering, and reddish-brown to dark-red macules or plaques. Their diagnostic hallmarks include residual hyperpigmentation after healing and rapid recurrence at the previously affected site on re-exposure. Topical glucocorticoids are advisable, even prophylactically, if repetitive treatment with the same drug is necessary.

Exfoliative Dermatitis (Stevens–Johnson Syndrome and Toxic Epidermal Necrolysis) (Delayed Type)

The most severe forms of delayed-type drug hypersensitivity reactions involve wide-spread keratinocyte death and consecutive skin blistering (Fig. 9-7) and are either called Stevens–Johnson syndrome (SJS) or toxic epidermal necrolysis (TEN), depending on the

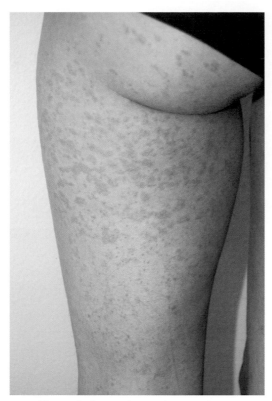

Figure 9-4 Maculopapular exanthema.

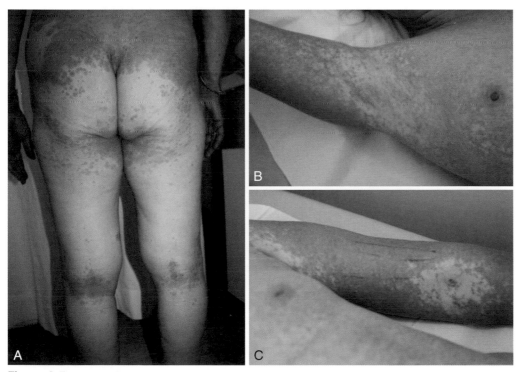

Figure 9-5 Typical flexural distribution in drug allergic exanthema (**A**) as opposed to infection-associated reactive exanthema (**B, C**).

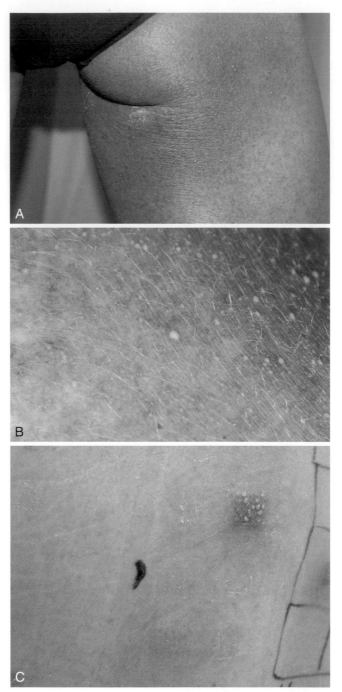

Figure 9-6 **A**. Acute generalized exanthematous pustulosis (AGEP) with typical sterile pustules (**B**) that can be reproduced in skin testing (**C**).

extent of skin involvement: SJS <10% skin detachment; TEN >30% skin detachment. The intermediate form with 10–30% skin detachment is called SJS/TEN overlap syndrome. They are rare (1 : 100 000 for SJS; 1 : 1 000 000 for TEN) and, according to the European Registry of Severe Cutaneous Adverse Reactions (RegiSCAR), are associated with a high mortality rate (SJS 13%; TEN 39%; SJS/TEN overlap 21%).

SJS/TEN has to be differentiated from erythema exsudativum multiforme (EEM), which may also have a central blister but is mainly caused by viral infection, is often recurrent, and affects younger patients (mean age 24 years). The main causes for SJS/TEN are drugs (Table 9-7), which on a global scale appear to differ in frequency due to the different genetic background. Most reactions start within the first 5 weeks of

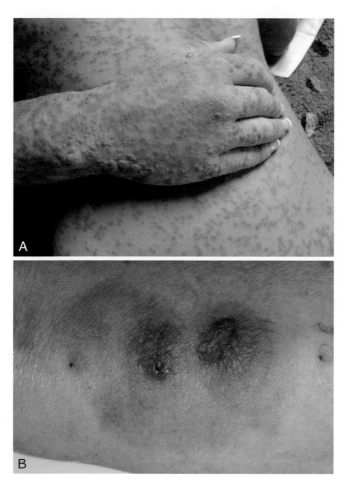

Figure 9-7 **A.** Blistering in the exanthematous skin area as an early sign of Stevens–Johnson syndrome (SJS), which may progress to toxic epidermal necrolysis (TEN), which may again be reproduced in skin testing (**B**).

TABLE 9-7   Drugs Eliciting Severe Cutaneous or Systemic Delayed-type Reactions

Acute generalized exanthematous pustulosis (AGEP)	Stevens–Johnson syndrome (SJS) and toxic epidermal necrolysis (TEN)	Drug rash with eosinophilia and systemic symptoms (DRESS)[†]
Aminopenicillins	Allopurinol*	Carbamazepine*
Cephalosporins	Phenytoin	Phenytoin
Pristinamycin	Carbamazepine*	Lamotrigine
Celecoxib	Lamotrigine	Minocycline
Quinolone	Cotrimoxazole (SMX)	Allopurinol*
Diltiazem	Nevirapine	Dapsone*
Terbinafine	Barbiturate	Sulfasalazine
Macrolides	NSAID (oxicams)	Cotrimoxazole (SMX)
		Vancomycin
		Abacavir*,†

List incomplete: the most frequent elicitors are given in **bold**.
*The type of reaction might be determined by the presence of a certain HLA-allele
†Abacavir-induced systemic reactions are classified outside of DRESS; they often lack eosinophilia and preferentially affect the respiratory and gastrointestinal tract.

treatment (mean onset of symptoms is around day 17). Important risk factors are HIV infection (low CD4/high CD8 counts), renal disease, and active systemic autoimmune diseases.

SJS/TEN can develop from an initial lesion quite rapidly: the initial purple-red maculae may become painful—an ominous sign. Within 12 to 24 hours the first bullae are seen and the Nikolsky sign becomes positive (epidermal detachment upon lateral traction of the skin; see Table 9-5, Warning signs). Stopping drug treatment at this stage of SJS might prevent further progression to a more severe form of skin detachment (TEN). Mucous membranes (mouth, genitalia) are involved with blister formation, as well as a purulent keratoconjunctivitis with formation of synechiae, which require intensive ocular care to avoid permanent eye damage.

As a rule of thumb, any drug rash involving mucosal surfaces or blistering warrants immediate drug withdrawal and often requires hospitalization (Fig. 9-7).

If no drugs are involved or they are not known to elicit SJS/TEN, paraneoplastic pemphigus (not pemphigus vulgaris) must also be considered. These forms of cancer-associated skin and mucosal detachment cannot be distinguished from drug-induced SJS/TEN clinically or by standard histology. Thus, whenever doubt prevails, a skin biopsy of the affected area should be examined by direct immunofluorescence (IF) to demonstrate or exclude intercellular immunoglobulin deposition (autoantibodies against desmosomal proteins). If positive, confirmative assays and an extended search for an underlying malignancy must follow and the involvement of an experienced dermatologist is advisable.

Systemic Drug Reactions: Severe Drug Hypersensitivity Syndromes (Delayed Type)

Some drugs are known to cause severe systemic disease, with fever, lymphadenopathy, potentially severe hepatitis, and various forms of exanthema associated with the typical facial swelling (Table 9-7). A few patients also develop colitis, pancreatitis or interstitial lung disease. More than 70% of patients have a marked blood eosinophilia (>1.5 Giga/L) and lymphoblasts (>2%) are found in differential blood count. During the last decades, this syndrome has had many names, the most frequently used ones being drug (induced) hypersensitivity syndrome (DHS or DiHS) and drug rash with eosinophilia and systemic symptoms (DRESS).

Of note, DHS/DRESS may begin up to 10 weeks after initiation of the treatment, frequently following an updosing step, and may then persist and recur for many weeks to months, even after cessation of the culprit drug. The clinical picture resembles a generalized viral infection (e.g., acute EBV infection), from which it can usually be distinguished by its prominent blood eosinophilia. Many patients have facial swelling, and some have signs of a capillary leak syndrome. As the clinical picture is quite dramatic and the disease tends to persist, in spite of stopping all drugs, many patients are not diagnosed correctly or in a timely manner. There may also be persistent intolerance to other, chemically distinct drugs, leading to flare-up reactions (e.g., acetaminophen) weeks to months after stopping the initial drug therapy, further adding to the confusion. Treatment often requires high doses of corticosteroids, particularly if the hepatitis is severe. Stopping of ALL drugs is the most important therapeutic step and requires some courage in critically ill patients, who are frequently treated in an intensive care unit. The mortality is around 10%, and some patients may even require life-saving emergency liver transplantation.

It has been shown that in many patients with this syndrome, circulating human herpes virus type 6 can be found during the third or fourth week of the disease, followed by a rising IgM antibody titer to HHV 6. Other reports document reactivation of cytomegalovirus (CMV) infection. Thus, similar to HIV, where T cell activation can also enhance virus production, a massive drug-induced immune stimulation, as in DHS/DRESS, may somehow reactivate these latent lymphotropic herpes viruses, which subsequently replicate and possibly contribute to the chronic course and persistent drug intolerance of the affected patients. Physicians using anticonvulsants should be familiar with this syndrome, as it occurs in about $1:3000$ patients treated with this drug class.

Isolated Drug-induced Organ Damage (Delayed Type)

Drugs may induce isolated hepatitis (drug-induced liver injury, DILI), or an isolated interstitial nephritis, for example, penicillins, proton pump inhibitors, and quinolones. In drug-induced interstitial nephritis, eosinophils can sometimes be detected in the urine, even in the absence of blood eosinophilia. More rarely, interstitial lung diseases (furadantin), pancreatitis, isolated fever, or blood eosinophilia are encountered as the only symptom of a drug allergy.

Pediatric Aspects in Drug Allergy

Children may also develop drug hypersensitivity. If the symptoms are acute (urticaria, angioedema, anaphylaxis), a careful diagnosis and strict avoidance is recommended as IgE-mediated reactions are potentially life-threatening. Drug sensitization may persist until adulthood.

Far more frequent are delayed-onset urticaria or maculopapular rashes. In this situation, in spite of its typical clinical presentation, provocation studies with for example, beta-lactam antibiotics could only show a low rate of reproducibility (<10%). Viral infections may be the important (co-)factor in many of these skin rashes. Intradermal skin testing and subsequent provocation testing are in most instances negative, most probably because co-factors are missing. Allergological work-up should be considered in those children who develop more severe symptoms. In milder forms, a re-exposure may be directly attempted, and if tolerated, it may help to reduce the overdiagnosis of 'penicillin allergy,' which is frequent, and leads to unnecessary use of alternative second-line antibiotics. Furthermore, during the acute phase, a high success rate with spontaneous resolution of ampicillin rashes, despite continuation of therapy, has been reported in children.[6]

PATIENT EVALUATION, DIAGNOSIS, AND DIFFERENTIAL DIAGNOSIS

Appropriate diagnosis of drug hypersensitivity reactions depends largely on careful history-taking, with special attention to prior drug exposure, route of administration, current treatment duration, and dose (Table 9-8), as well as the chronology and type of reaction that is supplemented by compatible physical and laboratory findings. Especially in anaphylaxis, differential diagnoses such as vasovagal reactions, vocal cord dysfunction, or panic reactions, need to be considered. Co-factors such as heat, alcohol, or exercise, may also play a relevant role in these acute reactions.

During the acute phase of a drug hypersensitivity reaction, it is recommended to:

1. Measure *serum tryptase* within 15 min up to 3 hours after the reaction start of a suspected IgE-mediated *immediate-type reaction* to prove mast cell involvement. Tryptase is a stable mast cell specific enzyme and samples may be kept at room temperature for at least 2 days and at 2–8°C for at least 5 days before analysis (long-term storage at −20°C is possible).

TABLE 9-8   Suggestion for a Chronologic Documentation of Drug Intake

Substance	Daily dose/route	Start	End
Amoxicillin/clavulanic acid	4×2.2 g IV	2014/11/10	2014/11/17
Amoxicillin/clavulanic acid	3×2.2 g IV	2014/11/18	2014/12/04
Levofloxacin	2×500 mg oral	2014/12/05	2014/12/16
Rifampicin	1×600 mg oral	2014/12/05	Ongoing
Piperacillin/Tazobactam	3×4.5 g IV	2014/12/16	Ongoing

2. Measure *liver enzymes*, CRP, and the *differential blood count* (eosinophilia, lymphoblasts) to define the severity of a suspected T cell–mediated *delayed-type reaction*.

In most cases, history and physical examination alone is not sufficient for establishing the diagnosis. Provocation tests from a large series of patients with a history of mostly mild drug allergy have shown that <20% are currently allergic to the previously offending drugs. Possible explanations include the presence of co-factors at the time of reaction, such as infections or other comorbid situations, and waning sensitivity to the offending drug over time. For a more accurate assessment of current allergy, subjects with a compatible history of drug allergy should be evaluated by further diagnostic tests for definite diagnosis.

In *immediate-type* reactions, patients with repetitive anaphylaxis or multiple exposures (surgery with general anesthesia, hospitalized patients), a thorough allergological work-up might reveal a common culprit such as latex, disinfectants (chlorhexidine), dyes, or excipients of soluble drugs.

Skin tests (e.g., skin-prick, intradermal, and epicutaneous/patch test) with the offending drug, and if positive, with potentially cross-reacting as well as alternative drugs are the mainstay of the allergological work-up (Fig. 9-8). Intradermal skin tests should be read at 20 min (immediate type) and after 24 hours (delayed type). All skin tests should be postponed for at least 4 weeks (immediate type) or 6 to 12 weeks (delayed type), to avoid testing during a refractory period where the involved immune cells have not regained their full reactivity. Unfortunately, sensitivity of the tests begins to fade 6 months after the acute phase of the reaction. However, T cell–mediated delayed-type reaction might still be detectable more than 20 years after the reaction. Additionally, even under optimal conditions, skin test sensitivity remains low, but is counterbalanced by a good specificity, i.e. positive skin tests are virtually always relevant, whereas negative tests do not exclude an allergic mechanism and need to be interpreted with caution. Guidelines for standardization of the skin test procedures and the optimal, non-irritative skin test concentration were recently published by the drug allergy interest group of the

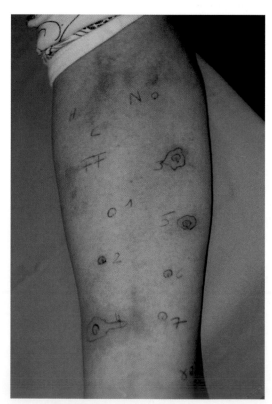

Figure 9-8 Intradermal skin test.

European Academy of Allergy and Clinical Immunology (EAACI), with the intention to harmonize the test procedure.[7]

Besides skin testing, serology (drug-specific IgE) and cellular tests such as the basophil activation test (BAT) for immediate-type hypersensitivity, and the lymphocyte transformation test (LTT) mostly for delayed-type hypersensitivity, are complementing the diagnostic allergological armamentarium. Again, these tests should not be performed within the first weeks of the reaction due to the possible anergy of the involved cell types. The combination of all test methods available (skin tests, serology, LTT, BAT) allows for an identification of the culprit drug in a majority of patients (around 70%).

Definite diagnosis of drug allergy sometimes involves provocation testing, during which gradually increasing doses of the offending drug are given. It is standardized only for immediate-type reactions and should only be performed by experienced personnel in an appropriate setting. Informed consent must be obtained from the patient before the procedure. The starting dose should be between 1:10000 and 1:100 of the therapeutic dose with sequential up-dosing every 30 min (IV) to 60 min (PO/SC). The provocation test can usually be completed within 1 day, with a maximum of 3 to 5 incremental doses and a 2-hour observation period after the provocation for a patient with history of an immediate-type reaction. Provocation tests should not be performed if an acute reaction occurred within the last 4 to 8 weeks, antihistamines or oral corticosteroids are being used, or there are active signs of underlying disease such as urticaria, uncontrolled asthma (i.e. forced expiratory volume in 1 second (FEV_1) of <70% of predicted), or uncontrolled cardiac, renal, hepatic, or infectious disease. Inclusion of a placebo is recommended to eliminate false-positive results for patients with largely subjective reactions, but is rarely performed in clinical practice.

For delayed-type reactions, provocation tests are not standardized and differ significantly between the various centers. Some centers continue treatment after reaching the full dose until the period needed for the initial reaction in delayed-type reactions is covered. They may last days to weeks, namely for a full treatment period. Re-challenge, even with incremental dosing, is contraindicated in patients with histories of SJS/TEN, DHS/DRESS, AGEP, or severe organ-specific involvement.

DRUG CLASSES OF SPECIAL INTEREST

Non-steroidal Anti-inflammatory Drugs (NSAIDs)

NSAIDs are typical elicitors of acute urticaria and angioedema, as well as exacerbations of rhinitis and asthma.[8] Two distinct clinical patterns can be identified: up to 30% of the patients with chronic urticaria (as an underlying disease) experience a *flare-up* reaction after intake of different NSAIDs as a classical dose-dependent, non-allergic intolerance reaction. As soon as the urticaria remits, this intolerance subsides. This also holds true for patients with chronic rhinitis and/or asthma, in the sense that by taking NSAIDs, an underlying prostaglandin-leukotriene imbalance is unmasked (see also 'Pathogenesis and Etiology, above). The possibility of a *truly IgE-mediated drug reaction* needs to be considered if there is no cross-sensitivity, i.e. only one specific NSAID leads to symptoms and others are well-tolerated. A typical example of a drug causing non-allergic intolerance *and* true allergic reactions is metamizol. The classical intolerance reaction is strictly dose-dependent and the eliciting NSAID doses should be documented.

Angiotensin Converting Enzyme Inhibitor (ACE-I)

A special form of angioedema (AE) without itch and accompanying urticarial lesions is angiotensin converting enzyme inhibitor (ACE-I) induced. It affects 0.1–0.7% of all ACE-I treated patients and is often seen first in the primary care setting. It is a histamine-independent form of AE, attributable to the interference of ACE-I with the metabolism of the vasoactive substance bradykinin. As with NSAID intolerance, ACE-I intolerance is based on the mode of action and not the chemical structure of the ACE-I molecule. Therefore, once established, it applies for all available ACE-I. Of note, antidiabetics of the gliptine class (inhibitors of dipeptidylpeptidase IV) not only block the metabolism

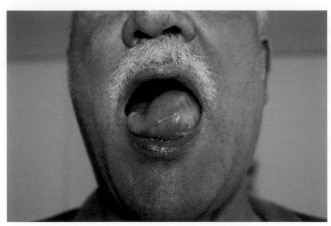

Figure 9-9 Angioedema of the tongue in ACE-I induced angioedema (AAE).

of incretins but also 'cross-inhibit' the metabolism of the vasoactive substance P. In combination with ACE-I (and only in combination), gliptines increase the risk and extent of angioedema.

ACE-I induced angioedema (AAE) may first manifest after several years of well-tolerated treatment without an obvious cause such as updosing or change in medication. AAE has no correlation to the more frequent ACE-I associated cough. Unfortunately, AAE has few prodromal symptoms compared with the tingling sensations of hereditary angioedema, or the itch of allergic angioedema. It usually progresses very quickly, which is its most critical and dangerous feature. It mainly affects the tongue, facial, and laryngeal structures, and dysarthria is an early sign indicating laryngeal involvement (Fig. 9-9). During the first hours, all patients should be referred to a hospital equipped for emergency intubation and/or tracheotomy, until remission is achieved.

Acute treatment relies on immediate withdrawal of all ACE-I and securing patency of the airways. The only causal treatment is the bradykinin receptor antagonist *icatibant*, which is currently only licensed for hereditary angioedema but has shown optimal efficacy and safety in one multicenter, double blind, randomized trial[9] and several case series of AAE. Infusions of C1-inhibitor and corticosteroids during the acute stage of AAE have also been used in this indication, with less impressive results. Emergency treatment with epinephrine (inhalations 1 mg epinephrine in 1 mL NaCl 0.9% using a nebulizer and/or 0.3–0.5 mg-wise IM, lateral thigh, supine position) has been applied as well.

If antihypertensive therapy interfering with the renin-angiotensin system is necessary, for example, for nephroprotection in diabetics, a switch-over to an angiotensin II or renin antagonist is usually possible. Neither interferes with the metabolism of bradykinin and/or substance P.

Beta-lactams

The beta-lactam antibiotic drug class consists of four major subclasses, as listed in Figure 9-10.

In the penicillin allergic patient, the matter of cross-reactivity is a frequent concern of the treating physicians. As a rule of thumb, cross-reactivities are quite frequent within the subclasses mentioned in Figure 9-10, and are usually based on side-chain similarity rather than the beta-lactam ring itself. Again, it is very important to distinguish the different reaction types, even if this clear-cut distinction is still inconsequently applied in the literature. In delayed-type reactions, cross-reactivities are less frequent because T cells recognize larger, more complex structures than IgE molecules. Common clinical examples are the tolerance of cephalosporins in penicillin-allergic subjects. IgE binds to smaller parts of the allergen, for example, a methylated side-chain, so the risk of cross-reactivity with cephalosporins is about 1–2% in amoxicillin-induced immediate-type reactions with urticaria and/or anaphylaxis. The early reports on cross-reactivity rates between penicillins and cephalosporins of up to 10% were most probably due to the

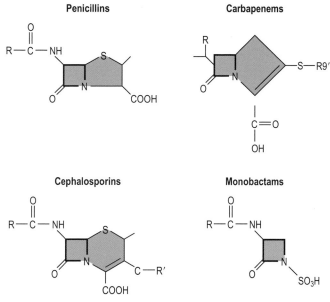

Figure 9-10 Classes of beta-lactam antibiotics.

contamination of cephalosporin antibiotics with trace amounts of penicillin. Therefore, in immediate-type reactions to a penicillin, the use of cephalosporins needs some caution and second-line, structurally non-related alternative antibiotics have to be considered. Carbapenems and monobactams (with the exception of aztreonam in ceftazidime allergic patients) are generally safe in penicillin-allergic patients.

In immediate-type reactions, the negative predictive value of intradermal skin testing with a selected set of beta-lactams using non-irritative concentrations (penicillin G, penicilloyl polylysine, minor determinant mixture (MDM), amoxicillin, cefazolin, cefuroxime and ceftriaxone) is high, and a confirmative provocation test with the beta-lactam in question is safe and recommended.[10]

Radio Contrast Media

Reactions to intravascular radio contrast media (RCM) are divided into *acute*, usually during or immediately after the examination, and *delayed* forms. The latter are typically based on a T cell–mediated sensitization and intradermal skin testing is helpful for diagnosis and definition of safe alternatives. Prophylaxis with corticosteroids is recommended for patients at risk, especially if they already experienced an episode of eczema after RCM. The acute reactions are also termed 'anaphylactoid' because they may have some or all the features of anaphylaxis from upper and lower airway obstruction to hypotensive shock. Concomitant asthma increases the risk for acute reactions to RCM. Since the introduction of non-ionic agents, which are almost exclusively used today, reactions have become less common. A direct stimulation of histamine-rich effector cells (mast cells, basophils) by the high salt content and its rapid application (in bolus form) is thought to be the underlying pathomechanism. Therefore, non-ionic agents are considered safer than ionic agents, which break down into charged and therefore more stimulatory particles when entering the bloodstream. Whether such reactions can be prevented by premedication is a subject of much debate among radiologists as well as the treating physicians.[11] Little evidence has been found to support the use of drugs to prevent serious reactions to contrast media and current guidelines emphasize the lack of evidence to support prophylaxis, as well as the safety of non-ionic agents.

Biologicals

Therapeutically applied peptides and proteins, the so-called 'biologicals' or 'biopharmaceuticals,' are today mainly used in anti-inflammatory and cancer treatment. They represent the future of pharmaceutical medicine as the majority of drugs in development or in the licensing process belong to this new drug class. Biologicals usually directly interfere with the immune system and its signaling process (cytokines, chemokines, receptors). As a result, their side effects differ significantly from synthetic drugs such as penicillin, and cannot only be explained by a substance-specific IgE- or T cell–mediated immune response. A new classification of ADR to biologicals was proposed, related but clearly distinct from the classification of side effects observed with synthetic drugs. This classification differentiates five distinct types, namely clinical reactions because of high cytokine levels (type alpha); hypersensitivity because of an immune reaction against the biological agent (type beta), including the classical IgE and T cell–mediated reactions; immune or cytokine imbalance syndromes (type gamma); symptoms because of cross-reactivity of the target structures (type delta); and symptoms that are either not immune-mediated or unclear (type epsilon), for example, the retinopathy under interferon treatment. This classification could help to better deal with the diverse clinical features of these ADR to biologicals.[12]

Acute infusion-related reactions (IRR) are the most frequently observed ADR to biologicals with an incidence of 0.1–3%. There is no clear definition of IRR (timing, symptoms), and re-exposure under slightly modified conditions (infusion rate, premedication) is possible in most of the cases. This does not fit into the picture of IgE-mediated anaphylaxis. On the other hand, sporadic anaphylactic fatalities are reported. While regulatory agencies and the pharmaceutical industry focus on immunogenicity (anti-drug antibodies, ADA), other possibly involved mechanisms should also be considered (aggregate formation, complement system, coagulation cascade, cytokine release). These additional pathophysiologic mechanisms are inadequately reflected in the Gell and Coombs classification.

TREATMENT

Management of acute allergic drug reactions involves: (1) identification by history and presentation and withdrawal of the most probable culprit drugs; (2) introduction of required supportive, suppressive, or remittive therapy; and (3) consideration of whether and how the incriminating drug should be substituted. Severe anaphylactic reactions must be treated with parenteral epinephrine (0.3–0.5 mg IM, repetitive, lateral thigh, supine position) as the therapeutic cornerstone (see Ch. 13). Exfoliative syndromes, including SJS and toxic epidermal necrolysis (TEN), and any drug rash involving mucosal surfaces, often require hospitalization.

There are a few exceptions to the rule of immediate drug withdrawal. In patients with life-threatening diseases, for example, enterococcal endocarditis, who require long-term treatment with high-dose treatment to effect a cure, 'treating through' isolated episodes of urticarial, generalized pruritus or late occurring maculopapular exanthema may be attempted. Experience suggests that most mild episodes (no blistering, no mucosal or organ involvement, no systemic symptoms) are self-limited and will remit with continuous therapy, provided there is a compelling clinical need to do so. H1-antihistamines and systemic/topical corticosteroids can be used to suppress symptoms, while careful monitoring for fever, blood eosinophilia, proteinuria, arthralgia, lymphadenopathy, and hepatitis is warranted. Prompt cessation of therapy is mandatory if new signs or symptoms appear. One should be very careful when continuing treating with drugs known to elicit DRESS (Table 9-7). When continuing treating those with mild type I reactions, it is obligatory to avoid lapses in treatment because restarting treatment after a lapse may invoke anaphylaxis.

There are three approaches to providing acceptable pharmacotherapy for the underlying condition in confirmed drug allergy: administration of (1) an unrelated alternative drug; (2) a potentially cross-reactive drug; or (3) re-administration of the offending drug.

The most common approach is administration of an unrelated alternative drug that is safe and effective for the disease requiring treatment. For the most common outpatient infections, alternative antibiotics provide a reasonable choice for the penicillin-allergic patient. Careful attention should be given to the risks of second-line therapy, especially treatment failure with antibiotics, and to the toxicity and cost of alternative regimens.

The second alternative for drug-sensitive patients is to receive a medication not identical to, but potentially cross-reactive with, the offending drug. As a rule of thumb, cross-reactivities are quite frequent within the drug class, for example, quinolones and penicillins, but the absolute risk of cross-reactions is small. If beta-lactam reactions involve an immediate-type mechanism, preliminary skin testing with the chosen alternative and slow dose escalation as standard intravenous dose at incremental rates over 4 to 6 hours under observation can minimize the potential for life-threatening anaphylaxis. Whether gradual dose escalation is advantageous for delayed-type reactions is unknown, as it has not been properly studied and should definitely be avoided in SJS/TEN or DHS/DRESS patients.

The third alternative for drug-allergic subjects is re-administration of the offending drug by desensitization. If an offending drug is irreplaceable or significantly more effective than the alternatives, the drug may need to be re-administered. Desensitization should only be performed under close supervision of a specialist experienced with this multi-step procedure, ideally in a hospital setting. Progressive doses of the offending drug are administered every 15 to 30 min for IgE-mediated reactions until a full therapeutic dose is clinically tolerated. The procedure entails the risk of acute allergic reactions, which occur in mild form in 30–80% of penicillin-allergic patients. Using recommended procedures, the success rate is high. Nevertheless, the risk:benefit ratio needs to be evaluated thoroughly, as in rare cases, death has occurred during desensitization attempts.

The mechanism by which clinical tolerance is induced during drug desensitization is complex and may involve low-level, subthreshold allergen stimulation, rendering the involved cells 'areactive' to the offending drug. Desensitization is an active process depending on the continuous presence of the drug. After the full therapeutic dose has been achieved without incident, continuous therapy should start immediately with appropriate monitoring. After drug discontinuation, the desensitized state typically gets lost after 2 to 3 days, and repetitive desensitization is usually required for subsequent treatment courses. Again, it is best studied in IgE-mediated immediate-type reactions, as well as in NSAID intolerance, whereas desensitization for delayed-type hypersensitivity reactions is still experimental.[13]

Premedication with antihistamines and corticosteroids have not been systematically studied for the prevention of IgE-mediated anaphylaxis. Numerous anecdotal reports attest their failure to prevent serious anaphylactic episodes. Premedication may mask early cutaneous symptoms and allow for a quicker updosing than advisable. Drugs reinstituted under the cover of corticosteroids may still be problematic when steroids are withdrawn. For these reasons, the regular use of premedication when undertaking drug desensitization is not recommended.

Some individuals are more vulnerable to mainly delayed-type hypersensitivity reactions as a result of genetic or metabolic abnormalities, frequent and recurrent drug exposure (e.g., antibiotics in cystic fibrosis), or certain disease states related to immune dysfunction (e.g., HIV infection). Such patients are prone to develop a drug allergy and are likely to benefit from a thorough and proactive evaluation that documents sensitizations. Ongoing re-evaluation helps to keep the list of usable drugs from becoming unacceptably limited. Prevention of recurrent infections including vaccination is a primary objective in patients with multiple antibiotic sensitivities.

Referral

When ambiguity surrounds which drug induced a severe immunologic reaction, plans should be made to pursue a definitive diagnosis after the patient's convalescence. Involving an allergologist minimizes the risk for another drug reaction without unnecessary limitations for further treatment and is especially important in certain instances:

1. In severe forms of drug hypersensitivity, e.g., anaphylaxis, DRESS, SJS/TEN, etc.
2. If multiple and/or irreplaceable drugs were involved

3. To clarify cross-reactivity patterns and define safe alternatives if re-exposure is expected (radio contrast media, neuromuscular blocking agents, antibiotics)
4. In repetitive reactions (e.g., mastocytosis)
5. If the patient needs reassuring.

Experience with the drugs in question, national and international databases, as well as specialized internet resources (an excellent example for drug induced pulmonary AE is: www.pneumotox.com) may be helpful in identifying the correct culprit. The allergologist must also consider the significance of the substance for the treatment of the patient, as well as the availability of safe alternatives in the individual setting of patient and underlying disease. This needs allergological, a broader medical and pharmacologic knowledge and an understanding of the individual situation of the patient. This ambitious task can only be addressed by a therapeutic partnership of primary care physician, specialist, and patient.

If the drug culprit is identified, the use of wallet cards, identification jewelry, and registry services (e.g., MedicAlert) should be recommended for patients with documented severe reactions. The following information should be included and clearly documented:
- Culprit drug (non-proprietary name and product name)
- Type of reaction (immediate/delayed, organ involvement, severity)
- Proof of sensitization (history only, or by skin testing, serology, LTT, BAT)
- Cross-reactive substance(s) and safe alternative(s).

Finally, again highlighting the role of the national pharmacovigilance programs, every physician is encouraged to document all relevant ADR encountered. National electronic reporting systems such as MedWatch (www.fda.gov/Safety/MedWatch) are usually easily accessible.

CONCLUSIONS

Drug hypersensitivity is a frequent phenomenon, but often presents a frustrating challenge for most practicing physicians. Because immunodiagnostic tests for drug allergy are limited in number and require some sophistication to interpret, many practitioners have concluded that the only reasonable option for drug-reactive patients is permanent and total avoidance of putative offenders. In the extreme, patients with multiple drug hypersensitivity syndromes are sometimes abandoned by their primary care physicians, or they are told to do without all drug therapy.

Armed with an understanding of the distinction between regular side effects, drug allergy and idiosyncrasy, the risk factors for drug allergy, and the pharmacoepidemiology of sensitizing drugs, physicians can safely provide useful drug therapy for a surprisingly large number of drug-allergic patients. For allergy and immunology specialists, the willingness to undertake this task is usually appreciatively obliged by other professionals, who readily refer drug-sensitive patients and are grateful for the assistance received.

Medical progress in understanding and managing drug hypersensitivity states often requires the collaborative efforts of multiple disciplines, including basic immunology, pharmacology, toxicology, genetics, biochemistry, pathology, and epidemiology. The high morbidity rates and costs associated with drug hypersensitivity make this set of disorders a high priority for future research investment.

REFERENCES

1. Suh DC, Woodall BS, Shin SK, et al. Incidence of adverse drug reactions in hospitalized patients: a meta-analysis of prospective studies. JAMA 1998;279:1200–5.
2. *Bircher AJ. Drug hypersensitivity. Chem Immunol Allergy 2014;100:120–31.
3. *Cheng CY, Su SC, Chen CH, et al. HLA associations and clinical implications in T-cell mediated drug hypersensitivity reactions: an updated review. J Immunol Res 2014;2014:565320.
4. *Hausmann O, Schnyder B, Pichler WJ. Drug hypersensitivity reactions involving skin. Handb Exp Pharmacol 2010;196:29–55.
5. *McNeil BD, Pundir P, Meeker S, et al. Identification of a mast-cell-specific receptor crucial for pseudoallergic drug reactions. Nature 2015;519(7542):237–41.

6. Caubet JC, Eigenmann PA. Diagnostic issues in pediatric drug allergy. Curr Opin Allergy Clin Immunol 2012;12(4):341–7.

7. Brockow K, Garvey LH, Aberer W, et al. Skin test concentrations for systemically administered drugs – an ENDA/EAACI Drug Allergy Interest Group position paper. Allergy 2013;68(6):702–12.

8. Kowalski ML, Asero R, Bavbek S, et al. Classification and practical approach to the diagnosis and management of hypersensitivity to non-steroidal anti-inflammatory drugs. Allergy 2013;68(10):1219–32.

9. *Baş M, Greve J, Stelter K, et al. A randomized trial of icatibant in ACE-inhibitor-induced angioedema. N Engl J Med 2015;372(5):418–25.

10. Pichichero ME, Zagursky R. Penicillin and cephalosporin allergy. Ann Allergy Asthma Immunol 2014;112(5):404–12.

11. Tramèr MR, von Elm E, Loubeyre P, et al. Pharmacological prevention of serious anaphylactic reactions due to iodinated contrast media: systematic review. BMJ 2006;333(7570):675.

12. *Pichler WJ. Adverse side-effects to biological agents. Allergy 2006;61(8):912–20.

13. Cernadas JR, Brockow K, Romano A, et al. General considerations on rapid desensitization for drug hypersensitivity – a consensus statement. Allergy 2010;65(11):1357–66.

Key references are preceded by an asterisk.

CHAPTER 10

Urticaria and Angioedema without Wheals

Clive E. H. Grattan and Sarbjit S. Saini

CHAPTER OUTLINE

INTRODUCTION AND HISTORICAL PERSPECTIVE
DEFINITIONS AND CLASSIFICATIONS
Urticaria
EPIDEMIOLOGY
NATURAL HISTORY AND PROGNOSIS
DISEASE ASSOCIATIONS
Autoimmunity
  Infections
Allergen-triggered Urticaria
Non-steroidal Anti-inflammatory Drugs (NSAIDs)
  Malignancy
PATHOGENESIS AND ETIOLOGY
Skin Histopathologic Features
Pathogenesis
  Autoimmune Hypothesis
  Skin Mast Cells
  Blood Basophils
DIAGNOSTIC APPROACH
History
Physical Examination

Laboratory Assessments
  Inducible Urticarias
Diseases Resembling Urticaria
  Differential Diagnosis
Systemic Diseases
TREATMENT OF URTICARIA
General Principles
First-line Treatments
Second-line (Targeted) Treatments
  Leukotriene Pathway Inhibitors
  Oral Corticosteroids
  Other Second-line Therapies
Third-line (Immunomodulatory) Drugs
Special Considerations
  Urticaria and Angioedema in Children
  Urticaria in Pregnancy

SUMMARY OF IMPORTANT CONCEPTS

- Urticaria is an illness characterized by itchy wheals (hives), angioedema, or both. It may be acute or chronic, depending on the duration of the whole episode.
- Acute urticaria occurs in up to 20% of the population and may be associated with a drug or food allergy, or with infection. It is, by definition, self-limiting and usually resolves over 2 to 3 weeks.
- Chronic urticaria occurs in up to 1% of the population. It is defined by continuous disease for ≥6 weeks. All cases go through an acute phase. Most have chronic spontaneous urticaria. The cause of this is often difficult to identify in the clinic but research studies indicate that up to one third of patients have functional autoantibodies that release histamine from basophils and mast cells in the laboratory (autoimmune urticaria), and a small number appear to be due to underlying infection.
- Approximately 25% of patients with chronic urticaria have a reproducible external trigger for their skin lesions, although the cause of their illness remains unknown. These patients are said to have an inducible urticaria.
- Urticaria should be managed by treatment of the cause (if one can be found), minimizing of aggravating factors that worsen spontaneous disease, avoidance of

inducing triggers, and control of symptoms with non-sedating H_1-antihistamines, until natural disease remission occurs.

- In patients in whom antihistamines are ineffective, or in those who have been dependent on oral corticosteroids for relief, several anti-inflammatory or immunomodulatory approaches can be tried, with careful monitoring for toxicity. Recent studies show that the monoclonal antibody omalizumab (anti-IgE) can be highly effective for chronic spontaneous urticaria and other treatment-refractory inducible urticarias.

INTRODUCTION AND HISTORICAL PERSPECTIVE

Urticaria affects people of all ages and is common. For the purposes of this chapter, the terms *chronic idiopathic urticaria (CIU)* and *chronic spontaneous urticaria (CSU)* are used as being directly equivalent and the term 'CSU' has been used throughout in line with recent international guidelines.[1] Nearly one in five persons will experience an episode of urticaria in their lifetime; the chronic spontaneous form of disease affects up to 1% of the general population at any one time[2] but the prevalence of all types of chronic urticaria will be higher. Because of the similarity of chronic urticaria symptoms to those seen in patients suffering allergic reactions to drugs or foods, the condition often leads to a search for an environmental (and avoidable) cause. In most cases, no identifiable cause can be identified, and the disease is managed by controlling symptoms and avoidance of triggers.

DEFINITIONS AND CLASSIFICATIONS

Urticaria

The condition is characterized by the appearance of short-lived, pruritic, pink wheals (hives) that fade rapidly without a mark. Wheals are superficial swellings of the dermis. Angioedema is a deeper swelling of the dermis or subcutaneous tissue that may occur on its own or with wheals. Angioedema swellings are pale, poorly defined, painful rather than itchy, and usually take more than a day to fade. They affect skin and submucosal tissues. *Acute* urticaria (AU) is defined by a disease duration of <6 weeks, whereas *chronic* urticaria (CU) is generally defined by the presence of urticaria on most days of the week, for a period of ≥6 weeks. Approximately 40% of patients with CU have accompanying episodes of angioedema, whereas 10% have angioedema as their main manifestation.

CU can be further classified using various criteria. Approximately 25% of patients with CU have a reproducible external trigger for their skin lesions, rather than sponta-neous swellings; this form of the disorder used to be termed 'physical urticaria,' but the term *inducible urticaria* is now preferred.[1] Inducible urticarias include physical, cholin-ergic, and contact urticaria subtypes. These cases are labeled according to the nature of the inciting stimulus (Table 10-1). In the remaining 75% of cases, no external cause or physical trigger can be identified; accordingly, the condition has historically been called 'chronic idiopathic urticaria (CIU),' implying that an etiology cannot be found. However, the clinical term *chronic spontaneous urticaria* (CSU) is now preferred because it carries no inference about etiology but serves to separate those patients with the ordinary pre-sentation of chronic urticaria from those with inducible urticarias. Some guidelines and experts identify a subset of CSU patients with an autoimmune etiology on the basis of serological evidence of functional autoantibodies targeting IgE or the high affinity IgE receptor (observed in 30–40% of these patients) and strong circumstantial evidence for having an autoimmune illness *chronic autoimmune urticaria* (CAU). Those CSU patients without evidence of an autoimmune or infectious etiology remain idiopathic. Thus, patients can have chronic spontaneous idiopathic or spontaneous autoimmune urticaria but not both.

TABLE 10-1 Physical Urticaria: Subtypes, Triggers, and Testing Procedures

Disorder	Triggering factor	Test description
Symptomatic dermographism (urticaria factitia)	Stroking, scratching, pressure	Mild stroking of skin with tip of pen or tongue blade or dermographometer at ≤ 36 g/mm^2
Delayed pressure urticaria	Application of pressure 30 min to 12 h before onset	Shoulder sling with weight of 7 kg placed for 15 min; patient records symptoms over 24 h or a dermographometer held at 100 g/mm^2 on the shoulder for 70 s
Cholinergic urticaria	Elevation of body temperature with exercise, hot water, strong emotion, or spicy food	Exercise with a stationary bike for 15 min beyond onset of sweating; or passive heating of one arm to 42°C with water bath or whole body immersion Evidence of reaction to sweat antigen
Cold contact urticaria	Exposure of skin to cold air, cold objects, or cold liquids	Ice cube test for 5 min on arm Temperature 'threshold' test if available (TempTest™)
Heat contact urticaria	Warm object in direct contact with skin	Application of test-tube containing warm water at 44°C or use of (TempTest™)
Exercise-induced urticaria	Exercise activity	Treadmill testing or exercise bicycle
Aquagenic urticaria	Skin contact with water at any temperature	Application of water compress at 35°C to the trunk or water immersion for 10 min
Solar urticaria	Exposure of skin to sunlight of specific wavelength	Exposure of skin to UVA, UVB, or visible light
Vibratory urticaria	Lawn mowing, riding a bike, exposure to vibrating machinery	Vortex platform held to forearm skin for 10 min

UVA, ultraviolet A; UVB, ultraviolet B.

EPIDEMIOLOGY

Both children and adults can acquire CU, although it appears to be more common in adults, with women with CSU being affected twice as often as men. The average age of patients suggests that the condition typically begins in the third to fifth decades of life. The coexpression of atopic disease diagnosis in patients with CU appears to be only slightly higher than in the general population.

NATURAL HISTORY AND PROGNOSIS

CU is a self-limited disorder in nearly all patients, although it not infrequently persists for years. Estimates of disease duration vary, but one study indicated that 50% of patients are better in 6 months, another 20% by 3 years, and a further 20% by 5 years, with just 8% persisting for more than 10 years.[3]

Angioedema, thyroid autoimmunity, hypertension, and increased disease severity have been identified as factors associated with longer disease duration.

DISEASE ASSOCIATIONS

Autoimmunity

An association of CSU with autoimmune thyroid disease has been confirmed in multiple publications, since it was first reported in 1983. The association is particularly strong (30%) in patients with histamine-releasing autoantibodies in their blood. Other autoimmune disorders are also more prevalent in chronic spontaneous urticaria than the general population. Furthermore, increased human leukocyte antigen (HLA) class II DR antigen expression is noted in subjects with CSU and, in particular, those with evidence of functional autoantibodies in their serum.

Infections

The topic of infections and CU has been reviewed.[4] A link between infections and CU onset has often been proposed but is difficult to prove. *Helicobacter pylori* infection of the stomach has been widely studied, but the data are conflicting. Upper respiratory viral and pyogenic bacterial infections are associated with acute urticaria, especially in children. Some pediatric series suggest that an infection is associated with disease or possibly is related to the antibiotic used to treat the illness, although it is usually the former. Acute urticaria can be observed in the early stages of hepatitis A, B, and C infection, but little evidence exists for a causative association with CU.

In the past, exhaustive stool studies to exclude parasites as a cause of urticaria have been recommended. Pathogens such as *Ancylostoma*, *Strongyloides*, *Filaria*, *Echinococcus*, *Trichinella*, *Fasciola*, *Schistosoma mansoni*, and *Blastocystis hominis* have all been associated with CSU. Stool studies for parasites probably are relevant only in persons with a history of recent travel to endemic areas and often with peripheral eosinophilia. Ingestion of fish contaminated with *Anisakis simplex* also can lead to urticaria in pre-sensitized patients.

Allergen-triggered Urticaria

Patients experiencing anaphylaxis triggered by foods, drugs, and other agents or conditions, frequently demonstrate skin symptoms within 30 min, and such allergens may be viewed as a direct cause of urticaria (see Chs. 9 and 12). Certain foods such as strawberries and tomatoes may cause skin eruptions without a clear allergic basis. Skin contact with raw fruits, certain foods, and aeroallergens in an allergic host can elicit an acute urticarial eruption.

Non-steroidal Anti-inflammatory Drugs (NSAIDs)

NSAIDs that include aspirin, ibuprofen, and naproxen, are in common use and can trigger urticaria acutely or aggravate pre-existing CSU. This reaction is related to inhibition of cyclooxygenase by these agents. The reported frequency of NSAID-induced exacerbations of skin disease ranges from 25% to 50%. In some affected patients, the period of aspirin sensitivity ends after the urticaria resolves. Genetic variability of prostaglandin E_2 receptor subtype EP4 gene in aspirin-intolerant CSU has also been described.

Malignancy

Older studies raised concern that CU may be due to an underlying malignancy. The question of whether patients with CU are at higher risk for malignancies has not been conclusively answered. Two large studies have addressed this question and reached opposite conclusions. In the first study, 1155 Swedish patients with CU were followed in an academic dermatology department for an average of 8.2 years. The incidence of malignant cancer during the observation period was compared with the expected number of cancers from the Swedish Cancer Registry, yielding a relative risk of 0.88 (95% confidence interval, 0.61–1.12).[5] In the second study, a cohort of 12 720 Taiwanese patients were identified as having CU from a national cancer registry. The rate of malignancies diagnosed in this cohort over an average follow-up period of 5 years was compared with expected rates. The standardized incidence ratio for patients with CU was 2.2 (95% CI, 2.0–2.4).[6] Younger patients appeared to be at higher risk for hematologic malignancies, including lymphoma.

PATHOGENESIS AND ETIOLOGY

Skin Histopathologic Features

Histopathologic examination of an urticarial lesion will show skin mast cells that have degranulated in the dermis, as well as a perivascular leukocyte infiltrate composed of lymphocytes, eosinophils, neutrophils, and also basophils that have migrated to the skin lesion. Both mast cells and basophils release histamine and other inflammatory mediators (e.g., prostaglandins, leukotrienes, cytokines, and kinins) on activation, which are capable of causing local vasodilation, itch, and swelling in the skin. Histamine appears to be a central mediator, as suggested by the prominent clinical symptom of pruritus and the beneficial response to H_1-antihistamines.

Current understanding of the roles for eosinophils, lymphocytes, and neutrophils in disease pathology is limited. A predominance of neutrophils in the skin lesion biopsy, the definitive feature of *neutrophilic urticaria*, should lead to a search for associated systemic diseases such as Schnitzler syndrome, adult-onset Still disease, systemic lupus erythematosus (SLE), and the hereditary autoinflammatory fever syndromes. Studies of other immune pathways involved in CSU have focused mainly on T lymphocytes and circulating serum cytokines. Increased IL-6 and C-reactive protein (CRP) levels are noted in the serum of subjects with CU plus NSAIDs sensitivity demonstrated on aspirin challenge, lending support to the concept that increased inflammatory markers reflect the urticarial disease. Immune features in patients with CSU resistant to high-dose antihistamine therapy relative to antihistamine responders include greater basopenia, higher mean platelet volume, higher levels of CRP, and higher levels of serum complement component, C3, which are features of low-grade inflammation and platelet activation. A series of studies suggest that the extrinsic coagulation pathway is activated in CU associated with increased levels of the fibrin degradation product, D-dimer, and prothrombin fragments.

Pathogenesis

Of the several theories regarding the pathogenesis of CSU, none has been conclusively established. Most studies have examined the autoimmune theory of disease and the serologic tests to establish autoimmunity. Other theories involve abnormalities in skin mast cells and basophils. Limited data on other causes such as chronic infections, provide some support for additional pathogenesis mechanisms.

Autoimmune Hypothesis

It is thought that 30–40% of patients with CSU have an autoimmune disease driven by pathogenic immunoglobulin G (IgG) autoantibodies to either IgE or the α-subunit of the high-affinity IgE receptor that activates mast cells and basophils immunologically (Fig. 10-1). The evolution of the autoimmune theory (Fig. 10-2) dates back to the 1980s when a serum factor that could elicit an immediate red wheal response on intradermal re-injection was described in over 50% of patients with CSU. This became known as the autologous serum skin test (ASST). However, a positive ASST reaction has also been described in persons with allergic airway disease and in healthy control subjects, raising issues about its specificity in CSU disease.

In parallel with early studies of ASST, non-functional IgG antibodies targeting the Fc region of IgE were found by an immunoassay, followed by a study that demonstrated IgG antibodies with properties of anti-IgE in CSU sera could release histamine from basophils of healthy donors. Subsequently, IgG autoantibodies with specificity against the alpha-chain of the high affinity IgE receptor (anti-Fc$_\varepsilon$RI$_\alpha$) were identified as the main serum factor responsible for histamine releasing activity (HRA) on basophils.[7] Early reports suggested that basophil histamine releasing activity and ASST reactions decreased in disease remission. Subsequent studies showed that IgG from CSU sera could also release histamine from neonatal foreskin slices containing mast cells, that are thought to be the primary effector cell of CU. Immunoassays that detect functional and non-functional autoantibodies have demonstrated anti-Fc$_\varepsilon$RI$_\alpha$ in other diseases and healthy controls. As yet, no simple and reproducible assay for functional autoantibodies in CSU has been developed for use in routine clinical practice. This has hampered studies on epidemiology, disease associations and establishing therapeutic relevance of histamine release autoantibodies in CSU. The concept of autoimmune urticaria is still debated.

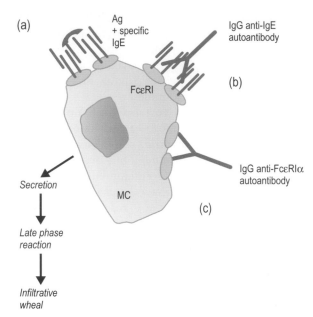

Figure 10-1 Diagrammatic representation of different modes of mast cell (MC) activation in the pathogenesis of urticaria. (a) An antigen cross-linking IgE; (b) IgG anti-IgE antibody, as seen in 5–10% of patients with CSU. (c) IgG anti-IgE receptor antibody directed to the α-subunit (FcεRIα), as seen in 40% of patients with CSU. IgE, IgG, immunoglobulins E and G. *(Modified from Kaplan AP, Greaves M. Pathogenesis of chronic urticaria. Clin Exp Allergy 2009; 39:777–787.)*

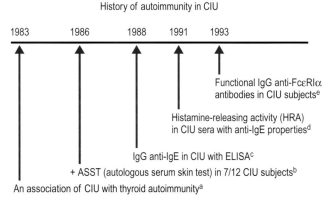

Figure 10-2 Timeline of recognition of autoimmune theory in chronic spontaneous urticaria (CSU). ELISA, Enzyme-linked immunosorbent assay; IgE, IgG, immunoglobulins E and G. *(Modified from (a) Leznoff A, Josse RG, Denburg J, et al. Association of chronic urticaria and angioedema with thyroid autoimmunity. Arch Dermatol 1983; 119:636–640. (b) Grattan CEH, Wallington TB, Warin RP, Kennedy CTC, Bradfield JW. A serological mediator in chronic idiopathic urticaria – a clinical, immunologic and histological evaluation. Br J Dermatol 1986; 114:583–90. (c) Gruber BL, Baeza ML, Marchese MJ, et al. Prevalence and functional role of anti-IgE autoantibodies in urticarial syndromes. J Invest Dermatol 1988; 90:213–217. (d) Grattan CE, Francis DM, Hide M, et al. Detection of circulating histamine releasing autoantibodies with functional properties of anti-IgE in chronic urticaria. Clin Exp Allergy 1991; 21:695–704. (e) Hide M, Francis DM, Grattan CE, et al. Autoantibodies against the high-affinity IgE receptor as a cause of histamine release in chronic urticaria. N Engl J Med 1993; 328:1599–604.)*

Skin Mast Cells

Mast cell degranulation is a central event in the development of the lesions in urticaria, and histamine levels are elevated in biopsied skin. Of note, however, the connective tissue mast cell number in patients with CU (chymase- and tryptase-positive mast cells) is not increased in either lesional or non-lesional skin in comparison with the skin of healthy control subjects. Similarly, total serum tryptase level, an indirect measure of total body mast cell numbers, is only slightly elevated in subjects with CU in comparison with healthy and atopic subjects but is still within the normal range.

Blood Basophils

A role for blood basophils in the pathogenesis of CU has emerged. Since the 1960s, it has been known that the number of circulating basophils in CSU is reduced. This basopenia is linked to the presence of serum HRA. In the 1970s, two groups of investigators demonstrated that blood basophils of patients with CU were reduced in their ability to release histamine after IgE receptor activation. Blood basophil IgE receptor responses of patients with CIU have been segregated into two basophil phenotypes: CSU responders and CSU non-responders. These two functional phenotypes are stable in active disease, are independent of the presence of autoimmune serum factors, and also reflect differences in some clinical features. Furthermore, hyporeleasability of basophil response becomes less so in disease remission. Skin biopsy studies using basophil-specific stains have provided evidence for basophil presence in both lesional sites and non-lesional skin tissues; a finding not seen in healthy skin. The degree of basopenia is correlated with disease severity and may reflect blood basophil recruitment to the skin lesions, whereas with CIU remission, basopenia remits. Collectively, this evidence suggests that altered basophil IgE receptor function and trafficking is present in CU.

DIAGNOSTIC APPROACH

Evidence-based guidelines have been published on the approach to diagnosis and the treatment of CU.[1]

History

The duration of the skin symptoms should be sought for classification of the urticaria as either acute or chronic, as well as the details of the characteristic and other lesions. Wheals are typically pruritic, and the discomfort can be severe enough to disrupt work, school, or sleep, with significant impairment of quality of life. Any area of the body may be affected, and areas in which clothing compresses the skin (e.g., waistbands) or areas of skin friction are more often affected. Patients whose symptoms have resolved can have difficulty describing urticarial lesions in a detailed manner, and in such cases, reviewing any photographs of the urticarial lesions can be helpful. The duration of an individual lesion can be useful to distinguish CU from urticarial vasculitis. In CSU, wheals typically last less than 24 hours without residual change to the skin area, whereas lesions in urticarial vasculitis generally last for days and may bruise. By contrast, the wheals of inducible urticaria (with the exception of delayed pressure urticaria that lasts up to a day) fade within an hour, and this can be a very helpful part of the history (Fig. 10-3).

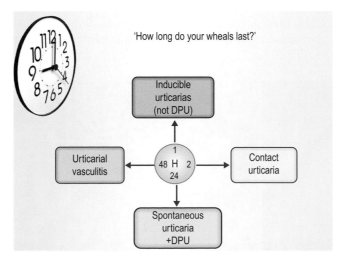

Figure 10-3 Timing of wheals is helpful in the diagnosis of the different patterns of chronic urticaria ('the urticaria clock'). DPU, delayed pressure urticaria.

The pruritus of CU is often most noticeable at night. Patients also may report more severe symptoms during periods of stress and may suffer from other emotional issues. Food allergies often are suspected by patients but are rarely substantiated. Pseudo-allergens, or chemicals in foods (histamine, natural salicylates, additives, spices, and alcohol), have been linked to CSU but appear to aggravate established disease rather than cause it. Restricted diets over a 3-week trial initially followed by stepwise re-introduction may assist patients so affected. Aspirin or other NSAIDs may exacerbate CSU in up to 30% of patients and should generally be avoided unless there is a specific indication, such as low-dose aspirin for cardiovascular prophylaxis, or severe pain. Patterns of skin symptoms such as an association with menstrual cycles should be ascertained and may suggest other diseases such as progesterone dermatitis. Physical factors such as pressure, friction, and heat can exacerbate skin manifestations. The presence (both recent and remote) of systemic signs and symptoms such as fever, weight loss, and arthralgias should lead to further investigation for an underlying disorder, such as systemic lupus or other autoinflammatory disease.

Physical Examination

The typical hive is pruritic, raised, and erythematous and may exhibit central pallor as it first comes up. The lesion can take several forms in CSU and may appear round, oval, or serpiginous, and multiple lesions may become confluent (Fig. 10-4). Wheals of symptomatic dermographism and cholinergic urticaria have a distinctive morphology: dermographic wheals are typically linear but may form large plaques where the skin has been scratched (Fig. 10-5), whereas wheals of cholinergic urticaria are small, with a pale center initially surrounded by a red flare, and often become confluent (Fig. 10-6). Coexistence of different patterns of chronic urticaria is relatively common, such as delayed pressure urticaria or dermographism with CSU or cholinergic and cold urticaria. If the patient is currently taking H_1-antihistamines, the lesions may not be itchy or raised. Wheals can range in diameter from a few millimeters to several centimeters across.

Angioedema involving the face, lips, tongue, extremities, or genitalia may occur with or without wheals at different times in the same patient (Fig. 10-7). Angioedema without wheals should prompt an investigation for underlying hereditary angioedema or acquired C1 esterase inhibitor deficiency with appropriate laboratory testing, or for drug-induced angioedema (such as that related to angiotensin-converting enzyme, ACE, inhibitors). However, recurrent angioedema presenting without wheals most commonly represents a type of idiopathic angioedema due to mast cell mediator release, rather than due to bradykinin-induced angioedema.

Laboratory Assessments

The diagnosis of CU is made clinically, on the basis of findings on the history and physical examination. No cause can be identified by routine laboratory tests in most adults

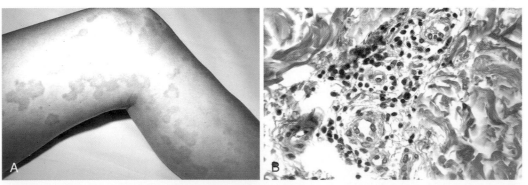

Figure 10-4 A. Typical skin lesions in a patient with chronic spontaneous urticaria. B. Skin biopsy findings from a patient with chronic spontaneous urticaria (hematoxylin eosin stain).

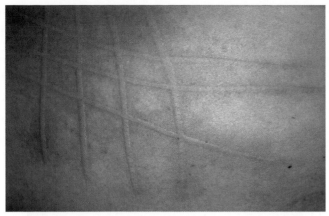

Figure 10-5 Symptomatic dermographism. Onset was within minutes of scratching. *(From Bolognia JL, Jorizzo JL, Schaffeer JV, eds. Dermatology. 3rd edn. London: Saunders; 2012. Courtesy Jean L. Bolognia, MD.)*

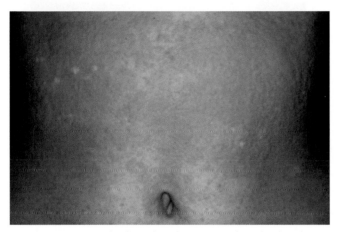

Figure 10-6 Cholinergic urticaria. Multiple and coalescing papular wheals in a patient after prolonged immersion in a hot bath to raise the body core temperature. *(From Bolognia JL, Jorizzo JL, Schaffeer JV, eds. Dermatology. 3rd edn. London: Saunders; 2012. Courtesy Clive E. Grattan.)*

and children with CU although up to one third of patients with CSU will be found to have a positive serum basophil histamine release assay, where this assay is available, and around 50% of children and adults will have a positive autologous serum skin test (ASST). Current guidelines do not recommend the ASST as a routine investigation because its significance is uncertain.[1,8] Although results on laboratory testing are rarely abnormal, consensus statements recommend limited testing; a complete blood count with differential to assess for eosinophilia associated with parasitic infection, CRP or erythrocyte sedimentation rate (ESR) determination to screen for an underlying rheumatic disease or an autoinflammatory syndrome, and measurement of thyroid autoantibodies with thyroid-stimulating hormone (TSH) level in view of the known association between CSU and autoimmune thyroiditis are suggested. Results of these laboratory studies are normal in most patients who lack signs and symptoms of systemic disease. A meta-analysis of the work-up findings in patients with CU involving 29 clinical studies and more than 6000 cases, found no association between the number of tests ordered and the diagnosis reached. An underlying disease was found in 1.6% of cases tested (105 of 6462) and included, in rank order: cutaneous vasculitis (60 cases); thyroid disease (17 cases); SLE (7 cases); connective tissue disease (16 cases); and paraproteinemia (3 cases).[9] Rarely of any value, is testing for chronic infections such as those caused by viral hepatitis or *H. pylori*, although this may be more relevant in parts of the world where these diseases are prevalent. Removal of suspected offending drugs can be

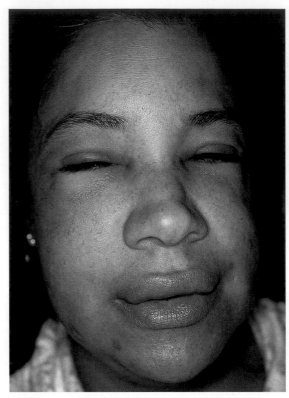

Figure 10-7 The swelling is deeper than that with typical wheals and may affect mucosal surfaces. Note the swelling of the lips and periorbital region and the lack of erythema. *(From Bolognia JL, Jorizzo JL, Schaffeer JV, eds. Dermatology. 3rd edn. London: Saunders; 2012.)*

attempted (such as non-steroidal anti-inflammatories, NSAIDs), or replacement with another class of compound can be tried.

The value of testing for thyroid autoantibodies is linked to the idea of identifying an underlying association with an autoimmune etiology for CSU, although evidence that thyroid autoimmunity can be regarded as a surrogate for functional autoantibodies is currently lacking. Patients with a positive result, however, can be given forewarning that they may be at risk of hypo- or hyperthyroidism developing over their lives. In the case of specific physical urticarias, provocation testing such as with a melting ice cube in thin polythene applied to the forearm for 5 min or TempTest™ (Moxie, GmbH) for cold contact urticaria, or exercise testing for cholinergic urticaria, may be helpful to confirm diagnostic suspicions (Table 10-1). Provocation tests for inducible urticarias are relatively simple to perform in the outpatient setting but some experience and skill are required to interpret the outcomes and there is a small, but important, risk of inducing anaphylaxis with exercise testing for cholinergic urticaria or exercise-induced anaphylaxis. Allergen skin-prick testing is of little value in CSU except in rare cases where there is a strongly suggestive history of allergic triggers, or in very young children suspected of having food allergies, and it is of no value for inducible urticarias elicited by physical triggers. A high rate of false-positive results may be expected, when dermographism is also present. Allergen testing for specific IgE may be important in acute urticaria suspected of being caused by a food allergen, immunologic contact urticaria (e.g., due to animal or vegetable protein contact) and food and exercise-induced anaphylaxis where pre-exercise ingestion of a food to which the individual is pre-sensitized; for instance, omega-5 gliadin (a gluten in wheat, barley, oats, and rye) or shrimp may act as a co-factor with exercise to precipitate anaphylaxis.

A *skin biopsy* should be performed if urticarial vasculitis is suspected or the patient fails to respond to usual treatments. Systemic lupus erythematosus (SLE) is an important differential diagnosis because urticaria and urticarial vasculitis are among the reported

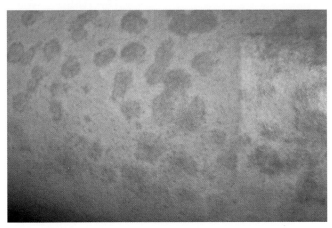

Figure 10-8 Urticarial vasculitis. Lesions look like those of spontaneous urticaria but last longer and may bruise. An incidental finding in a skin graft donor site. *(From Bolognia JL, Jorizzo JL, Schaffeer JV, eds. Dermatology. 3rd edn. London: Saunders; 2012. Courtesy Jean L. Bolognia, MD.)*

cutaneous manifestations of SLE. Urticarial vasculitis should be considered when the hives are painful rather than pruritic, last longer than 48 hours or leave residual pigmentation changes (Fig. 10-8). Neutrophil-rich biopsies involving skin appendages without vasculitis point to a possible autoinflammatory disease, such as Schnitzler syndrome, a rare disease characterized by chronic urticarial rash and periodic fever, high ESR, IgM gammopathy, leukocytosis, bone pain and joint pain (sometimes with joint inflammation). It may also be associated less commonly with weight loss, malaise, fatigue, pruritus, swollen lymph glands and enlarged spleen and liver.

Inducible Urticarias

The inducible urticarias merit classification as a separate group on the basis of their unique eliciting trigger and short attack duration, which is usually less than an hour, except in delayed pressure urticaria, where swellings can last a day or more (Table 10-1). Available evidence regarding underlying mechanisms suggests that certain physical urticarias have a basis in IgE and can be passively transferred to a non-affected individual, such as in cold contact urticaria, solar urticaria, and symptomatic dermographism.

Cold Induced Urticarias. In *cold contact urticaria*, exposure to cold will rapidly generate symptoms of pruritus, erythema, and swelling at the site of exposure. Symptoms may only appear after re-warming. Cold drinks may trigger pharyngeal symptoms. Hypotension and fatalities have been reported after whole body cold water immersion, although this is fortunately a very rare event. Alternative diagnoses, such as secondary cold contact urticaria presenting with cryoglobulinemia, must be considered, as well as familial cold inherited syndromes, which typically also manifest with systemic signs along with non-itchy wheals. Hepatitis B and C infections should be excluded in patients with cryoglobulinemia.

Cholinergic urticaria typically is related to elevation of core body temperature after active or passive overheating and is associated with the appearance of numerous intensely pruritic papular wheals that may coalesce, with or without angioedema, after hot bath challenge testing (Fig. 10-6). Recent data suggest that some cases may result from an autoantibody to a sweat antigen that consists of a protein that induces degranulation of basophils and mast cells via antigen-specific IgE.

Mechanically Induced Urticaria. Very itchy linear wheals that come up rapidly after gentle skin stroking or light scratching are known as 'symptomatic dermographism'; a non-itchy variant occurs in around 5% of the general population after skin scratching, known as simple dermographism. Delayed pressure urticaria, by contrast, appears several hours after a sustained pressure stimulus, with deep urticarial lesions that may resemble angioedema (e.g., under a shoulder strap or tight boots). In biopsied skin samples from patients with delayed pressure urticaria, evidence of neutrophils and eosinophils can be seen.

Other Inducible Urticarias. *Solar urticaria* is defined by mast cell activation by certain wavelengths of solar radiation. Classification of this form of urticaria into six different forms is based on the wavelengths of solar radiation that are implicated, or on identification of an underlying metabolic disease such as protoporphyria. Repeated exposure to the eliciting wavelength has been attempted to desensitize patients with solar urticaria.

Aquagenic urticaria is a rare form of disease that results in lesions when contact is made with any water, regardless of temperature.

Diseases Resembling Urticaria

Differential Diagnosis

A number of conditions can manifest with urticarial rash that are clinically and pathogenetically different to urticaria. Among the possibilities are a drug- or food-based reaction; unrecognized infections such as hepatitis or mononucleosis; insect bites leading to papular urticaria; the whealing response seen after rubbing urticaria pigmentosa (Darier's sign); urticarial vasculitis; familial cold autoinflammatory syndrome; hereditary and acquired angioedemas (non-histaminergic); and rare syndromes such as Muckle–Wells syndrome (MWS; periodic fever, chills, and painful joints caused by a defect in the NLRP3 (CIAS1) gene, which creates the protein cryopyrin). MWS is closely related to two other syndromes, familial cold urticaria and neonatal-onset multisystem inflammatory disease, which are related to mutations in the same gene and designated as cryopyrin-associated periodic syndromes (CAPS), Schnitzler syndrome, Gleich syndrome (episodic angioedema with eosinophilia), and Wells syndrome (eosinophilic dermatitis). Some of the more commonly encountered entities are discussed next, by etiologic category.

Systemic Diseases

Systemic diseases also may be associated with urticarial eruptions. Accompanying signs and symptoms may include fever, arthralgias, arthritis, weight change, bone pain, and lymphadenopathy. Urticarial vasculitis is usually normocomplementemic, in which case it is usually skin-limited, or hypocomplementemic, in which case it is a multisystem disorder. Urticarial vasculitis may occur in patients with other systemic inflammatory diseases, such as Sjögren syndrome, in addition to SLE and warrants testing for other autoimmune conditions. Antinuclear antibody testing and rheumatoid factor assay should be considered in this setting.

Schnitzler syndrome is a rare condition characterized by periodic fever, urticaria, and IgM monoclonal gammopathy. This syndrome has been described in patients with a monoclonal IgM or, very rarely, an IgG component (monoclonal gammopathy), who have associated fever, leukocytosis, weight loss, bone pain, adenopathy, and urticarial rash. The striking and consistent response to an interleukin 1 receptor antagonist, anakinra, implicates the inflammasome (a multiprotein complex expressed in myeloid cells and a component of the innate immune system) in its etiology.

Hypereosinophilic syndrome refers to a group of disorders characterized by persistent overproduction of eosinophils that infiltrate and damage tissues. Cutaneous symptoms include recurrent urticarial rash and angioedema.

The *cryopyrin-associated periodic syndrome* (CAPS) embraces familial cold autoinflammatory syndrome (FCAS), Muckle–Wells syndrome (MWS), and neonatal-onset multisystem inflammatory disease (NOMID). These are rare genetic disorders characterized by mutations in the NLRP3 (CIAS1) gene. *Familial cold autoinflammatory syndrome* manifests with periodic fever, urticaria, leukocytosis, conjunctivitis, and muscle and skin tenderness after exposure to cold. The onset of symptoms occurs during infancy in most cases and varies in severity between individuals and at different times of the disease. *Muckle–Wells syndrome* involves periodic urticarial eruptions without obvious cold exacerbations, sensorineural deafness, and amyloidosis that may lead to renal failure if the disease is not recognized and treated. NOMID represents the most severe form of the CAPS spectrum and often presents early in life with neurological impairment, in addition to the other features.

TREATMENT OF URTICARIA

General Principles

Recent evidence-based guidelines support that the most effective, first-line therapy for CU is the use of non-sedating, newer-generation H_1-antihistamines such as fexofenadine, loratadine, desloratadine, cetirizine, and levocetirizine. These agents alleviate the main symptom of pruritus and reduce the occurrence of wheals. Another important measure is reduction of aggravating factors (e.g., overheating, clothing pressure and, possibly, stress). In addition, avoidance of aspirin and other NSAIDs is advisable, in view of the fact that up to one third of patients will suffer skin exacerbations with use of this class of compounds.

First-line Treatments

Non-sedating H_1-antihistamines are effective at controlling the symptoms of urticaria in up to 50% of CU patients. They should be taken prophylactically while symptoms are active, rather than after an eruption of wheals, since peak absorption after a single dose in healthy volunteers ranges from 45 min to 3 hours (fastest is rupatadine; longest is desloratadine). It has been common practice to offer 'classical' sedating antihistamines (e.g., chlorpheniramine, diphenhydramine, hydroxyzine) at night to aid sleep because they often cause sedation but there is no pharmacologic advantage in updosing second-generation non-sedating H_1-antihistamines. Rapid eye movement (REM) sleep is suppressed leading to poor quality sleep and 'hangover' following day effects. Avoiding sedating antihistamines for CU is now a strong recommendation of recent international guidelines.[1] A possible link between using classical antihistamines with additional anticholinergic properties and increased incidence of dementia has also been highlighted recently.

If non-sedating antihistamines are only partially effective at their licensed doses, as may be the case in up to 50% of these patients, the dose of the non-sedating H_1-antihistamines can be increased up to four-fold, in line with current guidelines, followed by the addition of an H_2-antihistamine. Although the evidence for doing so is very limited due to lack of well-controlled published studies, clinical experience with this combination indicates that it can improve disease control in some patients and be effective for the hyperacidity that may occur in severe CSU.

Evidence of the benefits of escalating doses of selective, non-sedating antihistamines has been recently demonstrated in CSU and cold urticaria. Combination therapy approaches of various classes have limited evidence in the literature. The possibility of sedation after updosing minimally sedating H_1-antihistamines (cetirizine and levocetirizine) should be explained to patients and caution should be exercised when updosing H_1-antihistamines with potential to prolong the ECG QTc interval, including mizolastine.

Second-line (Targeted) Treatments

Leukotriene Pathway Inhibitors

Controlled studies have shown mixed results with the use of leukotriene pathway inhibitors in CU but these agents are often tried because of their favorable safety profile. In patients with CSU in association with aspirin sensitivity, montelukast was found to be superior to placebo and to cetirizine and also offered protection in aspirin challenges. In a second study in patients with CSU, no benefit was identified for montelukast as an add-on to desloratadine. In a third trial, only subjects with ASST positivity were found to benefit from the addition of zafirlukast to cetirizine, whereas monotherapy with zafirlukast offered no benefit over placebo. Studies of montelukast in combination with loratadine or desloratadine showed benefit over antihistamine therapy alone for delayed pressure urticaria.

Oral Corticosteroids

Short courses of oral corticosteroids are widely used and nearly always effective in terms of rescue therapy if the aforementioned second-line agents fail to provide relief. However, the optimal dose and duration of such rescue corticosteroid therapy are not well studied. The adverse effects of repeated courses of oral steroids should prompt consideration of an alternative treatment agent such as an immunomodulator and possibly a skin biopsy to confirm the diagnosis of CU if there is clinical uncertainty.

Other Second-line Therapies

Several agents have been demonstrated to offer benefit as alternatives to corticosteroids in antihistamine-refractory cases of CU and include sulfasalazine, dapsone, and *hydroxychloroquine*. The mechanism of action of these alternative agents in CU is unknown but may be anti-inflammatory in part. Patients should be screened for glucose-6-phosphatase deficiency before starting any of the three drugs. *Sulphasalazine* can be especially valuable for delayed pressure urticaria but should be avoided in NSAID-sensitive patients because its aminosalicylate component may aggravate associated CSU. The most frequent side effects are gastrointestinal intolerance and headache, but Stevens–Johnson syndrome (with or without toxic epidermal necrolysis) has been reported.

Although evidence on the use of *dapsone* in CU, especially in neutrophilic urticaria, is limited, it is preferred in urticarial vasculitis and in delayed pressure urticaria and angioedema. Monitoring for dapsone toxicity including anemia, neuropathy, and methemoglobinemia is required. Dapsone hypersensitivity syndrome may start within a month of drug initiation and patients should be warned of the presenting symptoms.

Doxepin has a long history of use in antihistamine-refractory CU and is positioned as a fourth-line therapy in the latest US Practice Parameter.[8] It is a tricyclic antidepressant with potent properties of an H_1- and H_2-antihistamine. It is generally given at doses considerably lower than used for its licensed indication of depression (i.e. 25–75 mg at night rather than up to 300 mg daily) but nevertheless, may not be tolerated due to sedation and its anticholinergic properties (blurred vision and dry mouth).

Other targeted drugs used for H_1-antihistamine-unresponsive CU include danazol (a derivative of the synthetic steroid ethisterone that suppresses the production of gonadotrophins and has some weak androgenic effects) for cholinergic urticaria, anticoagulants and calcium channel blockers for CSU, cyclophosphamide for severe steroid-dependent CSU and thyroxine in euthyroid CSU patients with positive thyroid autoantibodies.

Third-line (Immunomodulatory) Drugs

Immunosuppressive drugs have been used effectively for over 25 years to treat H_1-antihistamine-unresponsive CSU on the basis that severely affected patients may have an autoimmune etiology with relatively little evidence from clinical trials to support the practice. A small but controlled study supported an effect of *ciclosporin* in patients with ASST-positive CSU at 4 mg/kg per day for 1 to 2 months, with reduction of serological histamine releasing activity on basophils; reduction in size of the ASST; and control of symptoms for up to 6 months after stopping an H_1-antihistamine in 25% of patients, suggesting a possible disease-modifying effect in these patients.[10] Other studies have shown a sustained benefit from cyclosporine at much lower doses. Patients with a positive basophil histamine release assay generally respond quicker and more completely than those with a negative assay. The latter often need long-term treatment with attendant risks of adverse effects, including hypertension and renal impairment. Evidence from small open series has shown benefits from a range of immunomodulatory approaches, including intravenous immunoglobulins, plasmapheresis, tacrolimus, methotrexate, and mycophenolate mofetil but properly powered randomized controlled studies need to be done with adequate follow-up information, to determine whether these interventions have a disease modifying effect on CU or not.

The most recently licensed treatment for antihistamine-unresponsive CSU is the anti-IgE monoclonal antibody, *omalizumab*. Following a single-dose study demonstrating dose-related control of CSU symptoms,[11] further double-blind, placebo-controlled phase III licensing studies were conducted that demonstrated efficacy[12] and safety.[13] What has emerged from these studies is a novel treatment with rapid onset (often within 1 week) and a slower relapse (usually 6–8 weeks after the last dose) that controls symptoms effectively but does not appear to modify the course of the illness. Small series and anecdotal reports indicate that omalizumab can also be effective for inducible urticarias, including delayed pressure urticaria. It is likely that the landscape for treating CU patients in the near future will be based on stronger evidence with more effective therapies than in the past but, to date, no cure has emerged.

Special Considerations

Urticaria and Angioedema in Children

Most clinicians prefer to manage CU in children with non-sedating H_1-antihistamines at approved doses over older-generation compounds, out of concerns of sedation. No clear difference in total IgE levels or in specific IgE levels between children with acute and those with the chronic form of urticaria has been noted.

Urticaria in Pregnancy

Treatment of urticarial disease in pregnancy raises concerns regarding drug safety. Safety data are limited, and only loratadine and cetirizine (both FDA category B) are currently recommended for use in pregnancy.

Urticaria is a multifaceted illness with different clinical presentations and etiologies. Management strategies include removing the cause, where one can be identified, minimizing aggravating factors, and alleviating symptoms pending spontaneous remission.

REFERENCES

1. *Zuberbier T, Aberer W, Asero R, et al. European Academy of Allergy and Clinical Immunology; Global Allergy and Asthma European Network; European Dermatology Forum; World Allergy Organization. The EAASI/GA2LEN/EDF/WAO Guideline for the definition, classification, diagnosis, and management of urticaria; the 2013 revision and update. Allergy 2014;69:868–87.
2. *Maurer M, Weller K, Bindslev-Jensen C, et al. Unmet clinical needs in chronic spontaneous urticaria. A GA²LEN task force report. Allergy 2011;66:317–30.
3. Beltrani VS. An overview of chronic urticaria. Clin Rev Allergy Immunol 2002;23:147–69.
4. Wedi B, Raap U, Kapp A. Chronic urticaria and infections. Curr Opin Allergy Clin Immunol 2004;4:387–9.
5. Lindelöf B, Sigurgeirsson B, Wahlgren CF, et al. Chronic urticaria and cancer: an epidemiological study of 1155 patients. Br J Dermatol 1990;123:453–6.
6. Chen YJ, Wu CY, Shen JL, et al. Cancer risk in patients with chronic urticaria: a population-based cohort study. Arch Dermatol 2012;148:103–8.
7. *Hide M, Francis DM, Grattan CE, et al. Autoantibodies against the high-affinity IgE receptor as a cause of histamine release in chronic urticaria. N Engl J Med 1993;328:1599–604.
8. Bernstein JA, Lang DM, Khan DA, et al. The diagnosis and management of acute and chronic urticaria: 2014 update. J Allergy Clin Immunol 2014;133:1270–7.
9. *Kozel MM, Bossuyt PM, Mekkes JR, et al. Laboratory tests and identified diagnoses in patients with physical and chronic urticaria and angioedema: a systematic review. J Am Acad Dermatol 2003;48:409–16.
10. Grattan CE, O'Donnell BF, Francis DM, et al. Randomized double-blind study of cyclosporin in chronic 'idiopathic' urticaria. Br J Dermatol 2000;143:365–72.
11. Saini S, Rosen KE, Hseih H-J, et al. A randomized, placebo-controlled, dose-ranging study of single-dose omalizumab in patients with H_1-antihistamine-refratory chronic idiopathic urticaria. J Allergy Clin Immunol 2011;128:567–73.
12. *Maurer M, Rosén K, Hsieh HJ, et al. Omalizumab for the treatment of chronic idiopathic or spontaneous urticaria. N Engl J Med 2013;368:924–35.
13. Kaplan A, Ledford D, Ashby M, et al. Omalizumab in patients with symptomatic chronic idiopathic/spontaneous urticaria despite standard combination therapy. J Allergy Clin Immunol 2013;132:101–9.

Key references are preceded by an asterisk.

CHAPTER 11

Atopic Dermatitis and Allergic Contact Dermatitis

Donald Y. M. Leung and **Mark Boguniewicz**

CHAPTER OUTLINE

INTRODUCTION
HISTORICAL PERSPECTIVE
EPIDEMIOLOGY
PATHOGENESIS AND ETIOLOGY
Genetics
Atopic Diathesis
Natural History
Role of the Abnormal Epidermal Barrier
CLINICAL FEATURES (PHENOTYPE)
Complicating Features
  Ocular Problems
  Hand Dermatitis
  Infections
PATIENT EVALUATION, DIAGNOSIS, AND DIFFERENTIAL DIAGNOSIS
Psychosocial Implications
Role of Allergens
Foods
Aeroallergens
Microbial Agents
Autoantigens
Immunology
Immunopathologic Features
Cytokine Expression
Role of IgE in Cutaneous Inflammation
Skin-directed Th2-like Cell Response
TREATMENT
Conventional Therapy
  Irritants
  Allergens

Psychosocial Factors
Patient Education
Hydration
Moisturizers and Occlusives
Corticosteroids
Topical Calcineurin Inhibitors
Tar Preparations
Wet Dressings
Anti-infective Therapy
  Anti-pruritic Agents
  Recalcitrant Disease Hospitalization
  Cyclosporin A
  Mycophenolate Mofetil
  Azathioprine
  Methotrexate
Phototherapy and Photochemotherapy
  Allergen Immunotherapy
Experimental and Unproven Therapies
  Intravenous Immune Globulin
  Omalizumab
  Recombinant Human Interferon-γ
  Probiotics
  Rituximab
  Dupilumab
Other Investigational Agents
CONCLUSIONS

SUMMARY OF IMPORTANT CONCEPTS

- Atopic dermatitis is the most common chronic skin disease of young children, with lifetime prevalence in US schoolchildren of up to 17%.
- Abnormal skin barrier differentiation and immune response genes play key roles in atopic dermatitis.
- Colonization and infection by microbial organisms (e.g., *Staphylococcus aureus*, herpes simplex virus) in atopic dermatitis patients reflect its complex skin pathophysiology.
- Treatment for most patients with chronic atopic dermatitis includes avoidance of irritants and allergens, hydration and moisturizers to maintain a healthy epidermis, antimicrobial therapy for acute infections, and topical anti-inflammatory agents

(e.g., corticosteroids, calcineurin inhibitors). Systemic immunomodulatory agents should be reserved for patients with recalcitrant disease.

- Because non-lesional skin in atopic dermatitis patients is not normal with respect to skin barrier and immune abnormalities, proactive (maintenance) therapy may be appropriate for a subgroup of patients with relapsing disease.

INTRODUCTION

Atopic dermatitis (AD) is a chronically relapsing inflammatory skin disease usually associated with respiratory allergy.[1] In the 1930s, Hill and Sulzberger[2] suggested the name 'atopic dermatitis' to describe both the weeping eczema of early childhood and the chronic xerosis and lichenified lesions more typical of older patients. Before that time, however, a number of other terms were used to describe this disease, with the earliest illustrations consistent with AD dating back to the late 1700s and early 1800s (Fig. 11-1).[3] Of note, the term *atopic dermatitis* recognized the close relationship among AD, asthma, and allergic rhinitis. In support of this observation, in the largest cross-sectional study of a cohort of 2270 children with physician-confirmed AD, Kapoor and colleagues[4] showed that almost 66% had symptoms of at least one additional form of atopy (particularly asthma or allergic rhinitis) by the third year of life. Although significant progress has been made in the understanding of AD, its cause is still unknown, and much remains to be learned about the complex interrelationship of genetic, environmental, immunologic, and epidermal factors in this disease.[1,5]

HISTORICAL PERSPECTIVE

Descriptions of illness consistent with AD can be found dating back to the ancient Roman Empire. In the 1800s, clinical descriptions of skin disorders by Willan and others included terms such as *strophulus confertus*, *lichen agrius*, *porrigo larvalis*, and *eczema rubrum*, whose images are consistent with the diagnosis of AD on retrospective review. Besnier's *diathetic prurigo* established an association between pruritic skin disease and respiratory as well as gastrointestinal symptoms. The discovery of the concept of allergy in the early 1900s was followed by descriptions of 'atopy' in the 1920s, which in turn eventually led to introduction of the term 'atopic dermatitis' in the 1930s.[2] The role of allergens in AD was demonstrated by Tuft in the 1940s, whilst the role of *Staphylococcus aureus* was shown in the 1970s. The 1980s saw important insights into immune abnormalities associated with the disease, including recognition of the role of IgE

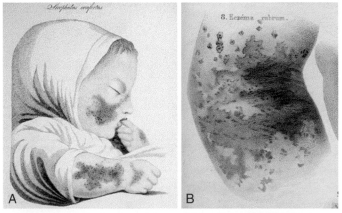

Figure 11-1 Early historical drawings of atopic dermatitis. **A.** Strophulus confertus, 1796; **B.** Eczema rubrum, 1835. *(From Wallach D, Coste J, Tilles G, Taïeb A. The first images of atopic dermatitis: an attempt at retrospective diagnosis in dermatology. J Am Acad Dermatol 2005;53:684–689.)*

molecules on epidermal Langerhans cells. In the 1990s, Leung and colleagues demonstrated a role for Th2 cytokines and staphylococcal toxins as novel allergens in AD as well as important immunologic distinctions between uninvolved, acutely involved, and chronically involved skin at the lesional level. In addition, the concept of T cell homing to the skin via a unique skin-selective receptor, cutaneous lymphocyte-associated antigen, was described in AD. The following decade started with the FDA's approval in 2000 of tacrolimus ointment, the first topical calcineurin inhibitor indicated for AD, described as *"a new milestone in the management of AD."* The publication of a landmark study in 2006 established a strong association between loss-of-function mutations in the gene encoding filaggrin, a skin barrier protein and risk for AD. Of note, the authors also found that mutations in the filaggrin gene were associated with increased risk for asthma in patients with AD, suggesting a mechanism for the atopic march. Further investigation into uninvolved skin in AD pointed to broad terminal differentiation abnormalities along with previously described immune abnormalities. These studies provided a rationale for a paradigm shift in treating AD patients with a relapsing course by changing from reactive to proactive management. Studies addressing both skin barrier and immune abnormalities, utilizing a molecular signature for AD provide a rationale for the next generation of biologic therapies in this disease.

EPIDEMIOLOGY

A number of studies suggest an increasing prevalence of AD. In Denmark, Schultz Larsen[6] demonstrated a cumulative incidence rate (up to 7 years) of 12% for twins born between 1975 and 1979 versus 3% for twins born from 1960 to 1964. A 1992 cross-sectional questionnaire confirmed this increased prevalence with a frequency of AD of 15.6% in 3000 children age 7 years from Denmark, Germany, and Sweden.[7] Questionnaire data from US schoolchildren age 5 to 9 years found a lifetime prevalence of AD up to 17%.[8] More recent data derived from the 2003 National Survey of Children's Health found prevalence ranging by state from 8.7% to 18.1% in a sample of 102 353 children age 17 years and younger.[9] A Japanese study used skin examinations rather than questionnaires to ascertain the prevalence of childhood and adolescent AD.[10] More than 7000 patients were examined, and AD was documented in 24% of those age 5 to 6 years; 19% of those 7 to 9 years; 15% of those 10 to 12 years; 14% of those 13 to 15; and 11% of those age 16 to 18 years. Importantly, the prevalence of AD in 9- to 12-year-old children was twice that in children of similar ages examined 20 years earlier, and for 18-year-old adolescents it was five times higher. A subsequent study in 23 719 children aged 6 to 7 and 11 to 12 years, examined by dermatologists in eight prefectures of Japan randomly selected from urban and rural districts, found a point prevalence of AD of 11.2% (7.4–15.0%).[11] Of the patients, 74% were classified with mild; 24% with moderate; 1.6% with severe; and 0.3% with more severe AD. Prevalence in the younger cohort was slightly higher than in the older patients (11.8% vs 10.5%; $p < 0.01$). No apparent difference was seen in prevalence between urban and rural districts or between boys and girls.

Increased exposure to pollutants and indoor allergens (especially house-dust mites) and a decline in breastfeeding, along with a greater awareness of AD, have been suggested as reasons for the increased frequency of AD.[12] In a prospective study, Zeiger and associates[13,14] found that restricting the pregnant mother's diet during the third trimester and lactation, and the child's diet during the first 2 years of life, resulted in decreased prevalence of AD in the prophylaxis group compared with a control group at age 12 months but not at 24 months. Follow-up through 7 years of age showed no difference between the prophylaxis and control groups for AD or respiratory allergy.[14] In a large study of an ethnically and socially diverse group of children in suburban Birmingham, England, Kay and coworkers[15] found that breastfeeding did not affect the lifetime AD prevalence rate of 20%. A study of prevalence of childhood eczema found a correlation with increased socioeconomic class that did not result from heightened parental awareness.[16] The National Survey of Children's Health analysis by Shaw and associates[9] also found increased prevalence of eczema to be related to metropolitan living, along with black race and higher education level.

The effects of genetic and environmental factors on allergic diseases were studied in two Japanese cities with differing climates.[17] The prevalence of allergic diseases and AD in the city with a temperate climate was significantly higher than in the one with a subtropical climate, even after controlling for genetic and environmental factors. In both cities, children from atopic families had a significantly higher risk of contracting respiratory allergies and AD. In a global survey of the prevalence of asthma, allergic rhinoconjunctivitis, and AD, 463 801 children age 13 to 14 years from 155 centers in 56 countries participated.[18] The highest prevalence of AD was reported from scattered centers, including sites in Scandinavia and Africa, that were not among centers with the highest prevalence of asthma. On the other hand, the lowest prevalence rates for AD occurred in centers with the lowest prevalence of asthma and allergic rhinoconjunctivitis. Thus, the ultimate presentation of an atopic disease may depend on a complex interaction of environmental exposures with end-organ response in a genetically predisposed individual.

Updated data from the International Study of Asthma and Allergies in Childhood (ISAAC phase III) on 385 853 participants age 6 to 7 years from 143 centers in 60 countries showed that the prevalence of current AD ranged from 0.9% in India to 22.5% in Ecuador, with new data showing high values in Asia and Latin America.[19] Prevalence in 663 256 participants age 13 to 14 years from 230 centers in 96 countries ranged from 0.2% in China to 24.6% in Columbia, with the highest occurrence in Africa and Latin America. These data emphasize the importance of AD as a global health problem in both developed and developing countries.

PATHOGENESIS AND ETIOLOGY

Genetics

The genetics of atopic disease is complex and an area of active research.[20] A number of genes are likely involved in the development of AD, but skin barrier/epidermal differentiation genes[21] and immune response/host defense genes have been proposed as playing a key role. An important advance in understanding the contribution of skin barrier abnormalities was recognizing loss-of-function mutations of the gene encoding the epidermal barrier protein filaggrin as a major predisposing factor for AD.[22] Patients with *FLG* gene mutations have early-onset, severe, and persistent AD,[23] although most appear to outgrow their disease, just more slowly than those without *FLG* mutations.[24] Importantly, AD patients with *FLG* mutations are at increased risk for development of asthma, as well as food and inhalant allergies[22] (see 'Role of the Abnormal Epidermal Barrier,' below).

Studies of gene and protein expression of the skin barrier proteins loricrin and involucrin showed that both were significantly decreased in involved and uninvolved skin of AD patients.[25] Candidate-gene approaches have implicated variants in the *SPINK5* gene, which is expressed in the uppermost epidermis, where its product, LEKTI-1, inhibits two serine proteases (stratum corneum tryptic and chymotryptic enzymes) involved in desquamation and inflammation.[5] Thus, an imbalance of protease versus protease inhibitor activity may contribute to skin barrier breakdown and staphylococcal colonization in AD. These observations establish a key role for impaired skin barrier function in AD pathogenesis, allowing increased transepidermal water loss and, importantly, increased entry of allergens, antigens, and chemicals from the environment, resulting in skin inflammatory responses (Fig. 11-2).

Atopic Diathesis

Most patients with AD have a genetic predisposition to develop an IgE response to common environmental allergens. Abnormal IgE responses are associated with cellular abnormalities resulting in overproduction of helper T type 2 (Th2)-type cytokines, which also contribute to the eosinophilia seen in these diseases. Early onset of AD is associated

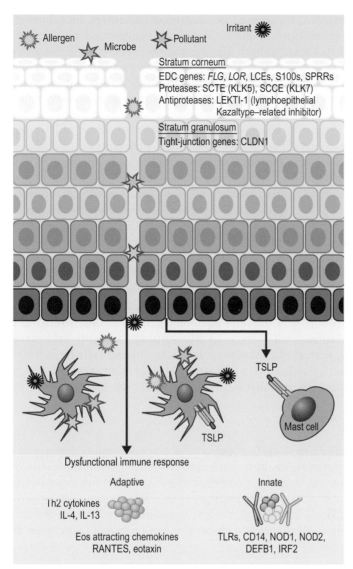

Figure 11-2 Epidermal barrier abnormalities and immune dysregulation. SCCE, stratum corneum chymotryptic enzyme; SCTE, stratum corneum tryptic enzyme; TLRs, Toll-like receptors; TSLP, thymic stromal lymphopoietin. *(From Barnes KC. An update on the genetics of atopic dermatitis: scratching the surface in 2009. J Allergy Clin Immunol 2010;125:16–29.)*

with an increased risk for respiratory allergy. The highest incidence of asthma at a given age has been observed in children with onset of AD before 3 months, in those with severe AD and a family history of asthma. An association of increased risk for asthma and/or rhinoconjunctivitis with early onset of AD has been confirmed.[26] Respiratory allergy occurred in 50% of children who had onset of AD during the first 3 months of life and two or more atopic family members, compared with 12% of children who had onset of AD after 3 months of age and no atopic family members.

In a prospective study of 94 children with AD observed through 7 years of age, only 14 had experienced no signs or symptoms of asthma or allergic rhinoconjunctivitis.[27] In addition, children with AD have more severe asthma than asthmatic children without AD, suggesting that epidermal allergen sensitization may predispose to more severe and persistent respiratory disease through effects on the systemic allergic response. In support of this hypothesis, mouse studies have shown that epicutaneous sensitization with protein antigen can elicit a localized dermatitis, along with elevated serum IgE, airway eosinophilia, and hyperresponsiveness to methacholine.[28] Importantly, epidemiologic studies in AD patients with *FLG* mutations have also shown a strong association with asthma and allergies (as discussed previously). In addition, in a murine model of filaggrin deficiency, cutaneous sensitization leads to systemic allergic responses.[29]

Patients with AD react to both allergic and non-specific triggers, similarly to patients with asthma and allergic rhinitis. Skin hyperreactivity to irritants such as sodium lauryl sulfate (SLS) has been shown in patients with both active and inactive AD, as well as patients with allergic respiratory disease even with no skin involvement, compared with non-atopic subjects.[30] An abnormal intrinsic hyperreactivity of inflammatory cells in atopic individuals may predispose them to a lower threshold of irritant responsiveness. Confirming and extending these (individuals) observations, Tabata and associates[31] showed that the stratum corneum abnormalities in non-involved AD skin were associated with increased transepidermal water loss, even 7 days after application of SLS.[31] Of note, atopy can be transferred through bone marrow transplantation.[32] These observations suggest that the cutaneous abnormality in AD results from a complex interaction of resident and infiltrating cells.

Furthermore, a study of bronchial and cutaneous reactivity in asthmatic patients with and without AD found a latent predisposition for bronchial asthma and implicated circulating activated eosinophils as the common effector cells.[33] Because the ability of eosinophils to reach their target organ depends partly on eosinophil-specific chemotactic factors, increased expression of eotaxin and monocyte chemotactic protein-4 (MCP-4), structurally homologous eosinophil chemoattractants acting through a common CCR3 receptor, has been reported in the respiratory mucosa of both asthma patients[34] and AD patients.[35] Also, increased numbers of IgE+ Langerhans cells have been shown in both active AD and active asthma versus inactive AD and inactive asthma, suggesting systemic regulation of active allergic disease, further aggravated by local inflammation in atopic skin lesions.[36]

Natural History

AD typically manifests in early childhood, with onset before 5 years of age in approximately 90% of patients. In adults with new-onset dermatitis, especially without a history of childhood eczema, asthma, or allergic rhinitis, other diseases need to be considered (Table 11-1).

Although Vickers's 20-year follow-up[37] suggested that 84% of children outgrow their AD by adolescence, more recent data present less optimistic outcomes. In one study, AD

TABLE 11-1   Differential Diagnosis in Patients with Atopic Dermatitis

Differential category	Diagnostic examples
Congenital disorders	Netherton syndrome
Chronic dermatoses	Seborrheic dermatitis Contact dermatitis (allergic or irritant) Nummular eczema Lichen simplex chronicus
Infections and infestations	Scabies Human immunodeficiency virus–associated dermatitis
Malignancy	Cutaneous T cell lymphoma (mycosis fungoides/Sézary syndrome)
Immunodeficiencies	Wiskott–Aldrich syndrome Severe combined immunodeficiency Immune dysregulation, polyendocrinopathy, enteropathy, X-linked (IPEX) syndrome Hyper-IgE syndrome DOCK8 mutation associated immunodeficiency
Metabolic disorders	Zinc deficiency Pyridoxine (vitamin B_6) and niacin deficiency Multiple carboxylase deficiency Phenylketonuria
Proliferative disorders	Letterer–Siwe disease

had disappeared in only 18% of children observed from infancy until age 11 to 13 years, although it had become less severe in 65%.[38] In another study, 72% of patients diagnosed during the first 2 years of life continued to have AD 20 years later.[39] In a prospective study from Finland, 77–91% of adolescent patients treated for moderate to severe AD had persistent or frequently relapsing dermatitis as adults, although only 6% had severe disease.[40] In addition, more than half the adolescents treated for mild dermatitis experienced a relapse of disease as adults. Often, adults whose childhood AD has been in remission for a number of years present with hand dermatitis, especially if daily activities require repeated hand wetting. In a prospective study of children with AD observed through age 7 years, Gustafsson and associates[27] found that, although most had milder eczema by 7 years, only approximately one third had no evidence of disease activity.

The Multicenter Allergy Study, a German birth cohort, followed 1314 children from birth to age 7 years with physical examinations and parental interviews on atopic symptoms and diagnoses, along with determination of specific IgE levels.[41] The cumulative prevalence of AD in the first 2 years of life was 21.5%. Of these children with early AD, 43.2% were in complete remission by age 3 years; 38.3% had an intermittent pattern of disease; and 18.7% had symptoms of AD every year. Severity and atopic sensitization were major determinants of prognosis. Of note, the insights into the genetics of AD previously discussed provide new information regarding risk factors for persistent AD into adulthood.[23]

Role of the Abnormal Epidermal Barrier

Atopic dermatitis is associated with abnormalities in skin barrier function that include increased transepidermal water loss, increased levels of endogenous proteolytic enzymes, and reduced ceramide levels. Use of soaps can increase skin pH, increasing activity of endogenous proteases and leading to breakdown of epidermal barrier function.[5] The epidermal barrier may be further damaged by exogenous proteases from house-dust mites and *S. aureus*. This is worsened by the lack of endogenous protease inhibitors in the skin of patients with AD. These epidermal changes likely contribute to increased allergen absorption into the skin and microbial colonization. As previously discussed, mutations in the *FLG* gene, located in the epidermal differentiation complex on chromosome 1q21, have been shown to result in complete or partial decrease of expression of a key epidermal protein, filament-aggregating protein (filaggrin), involved in formation of the epidermal barrier.[21] In addition, Th2 cytokines such as interleukins 4 and 13 (IL-4, IL-13), which are upregulated in AD, were shown to downregulate *FLG* expression.[42] More recently, a distinct subpopulation of IL-22-producing 'Th22' CD4+ and CD8+ cells has been reported in the skin of AD patients, and IL-22-regulated genes include those implicated in epidermal barrier abnormalities in AD such as *FLG*, as well as the proteins loricrin and involucrin.[43]

The growing number of mutations reported includes many unique for Caucasians of European ancestry and others for Asian populations.[22] Importantly, *FLG* mutations were a major risk factor for eczema-associated asthma. Importantly, because epicutaneous sensitization to allergens results in a greater immune response than sensitization via the airway,[28] decreased epidermal barrier function could act as a site for allergen sensitization and predispose such children to the development of respiratory allergy later in life.[44] Meta-analyses support the association of *FLG* mutations with increased risk for both asthma[45] and allergies.[46]

De Benedetto and colleagues[47] pointed to a role of a second barrier defect in AD. Tight junctions (TJs) located directly below the stratum corneum regulate the selective permeability of the paracellular pathway. Reduced expression of the tight-junction proteins claudin-1 and claudin-23 were observed only in patients with AD, validated at the messenger RNA (mRNA) and protein levels. Claudin-1 expression inversely correlated with Th2 biomarkers. CLDN1 haplotype-tagging SNPs were associated with AD. These data suggest that an impairment in TJs contributes to the barrier dysfunction and immune dysregulation observed in AD patients, which may be mediated in part by reduction in claudin-1 (Fig. 11-2).

In a novel approach, Broccardo and associates[48] used a non-invasive, semiquantitative profiling method to identify proteins involved in the pathogenesis of AD. Proteins related to the skin barrier (filaggrin-2, corneodesmosin, desmoglein-1, desmocollin-1, transglutaminase-3) and generation of natural moisturizing factor (arginase-1, caspase-14, γ-glutamylcyclotransferase) were expressed at significantly lower levels in lesional versus non-lesional sites of AD patients. Epidermal fatty acid-binding protein was expressed at significantly higher levels in patients with MRSA. The lower expression of skin barrier proteins and enzymes involved in the generation of natural moisturizing factor could further exacerbate barrier defects and perpetuate water loss from the skin. The greater expression of epidermal fatty acid-binding protein, especially in patients colonized with MRSA, might perpetuate the inflammatory response through eicosanoid signaling.

CLINICAL FEATURES (PHENOTYPE)

Atopic dermatitis has no pathognomonic skin lesions or unique laboratory parameters. Therefore, the diagnosis is based on the presence of major and associated clinical features (Box 11-1).[49] Attempts to standardize signs and symptoms of AD include severity scoring of atopic dermatitis (SCORAD) and the eczema area and severity index (EASI).[50,51] The principal features include severe pruritus, a chronically relapsing course, typical morphology and distribution of the skin lesions, and a history of atopic disease. The presence of pruritus is critical to the diagnosis of AD, and patients with AD have a reduced threshold for pruritus.

Acute AD is characterized by intensely pruritic, erythematous papules associated with excoriations, vesiculations, and serous exudate. Subacute AD is characterized by erythematous, excoriated, scaling papules, whereas chronic AD is characterized by thickened skin with accentuated markings (lichenification) and fibrotic papules. Patients with chronic AD may have all three types of lesions. In addition, patients usually have dry skin. Significant differences can be observed in pH, capacitance, and transepidermal water loss between AD lesions and uninvolved skin in the same patient and on skin of normal controls.

During infancy, AD involves primarily the face, scalp, and extensor surfaces of the extremities. The diaper area is usually spared; if involved, it may be secondarily infected with *Candida* species, in which case the dermatitis does not spare the inguinal folds. In contrast, infragluteal involvement is a common distribution in children. In older patients with longstanding disease, the flexural folds of the extremities are the predominant location of lesions. In the Copenhagen Prospective Study on Asthma in Childhood, arm

---

Box 11-1   Clinical Features of Atopic Dermatitis

MAJOR FEATURES

- Pruritus
- Facial and extensor involvement in infants and children
- Flexural lichenification in adults
- Chronic or relapsing dermatitis
- Personal or family history of atopic disease

MINOR FEATURES

- Xerosis
- Cutaneous infections
- Non-specific dermatitis of hands or feet
- Ichthyosis, palmar hyperlinearity, keratosis pilaris
- Pityriasis alba
- Nipple eczema
- White dermatographism and delayed blanch response
- Anterior subcapsular cataracts
- Elevated serum IgE levels
- Positive immediate-type allergy skin tests

(Modified from Hanifin JM, Rajka G. Diagnostic features of atopic dermatitis. Acta Derm Venereol (Stockh) 1980;92:44–47.)

and joint involvement carried the highest predictive value for the development of AD at age 3 years.[52] Localization of AD to the eyelids may be an isolated manifestation but should be differentiated from allergic contact dermatitis.

Complicating Features

Ocular Problems

Increased numbers of IgE-bearing Langerhans cells are found in the conjunctival epithelium of patients with AD. These cells can capture aeroallergens and present them to infiltrating T cells, thus contributing to ocular inflammation. Ocular complications associated with AD can result in significant morbidity.

Atopic keratoconjunctivitis is always bilateral, and symptoms include itching, burning, tearing, and copious mucoid discharge.[53] It is frequently associated with eyelid dermatitis and chronic blepharitis and may result in visual impairment from corneal scarring. Keratoconus is a conical deformity of the cornea that is thought to result from persistent rubbing of the eyes in patients with AD and allergic rhinitis. Anterior subcapsular cataracts may develop during adolescence or early adult life.

Hand Dermatitis

Patients with AD often have non-specific hand dermatitis that is frequently irritating and aggravated by repeated wetting, especially in the occupational setting. A history of past or present AD at least doubles the effects of irritant exposure and doubles the risk in occupations where hand eczema is a common problem.

Infections

Patients with AD have an increased susceptibility to infection or colonization with a variety of organisms.[54] These include viral infections with herpes simplex virus (HSV), molluscum contagiosum, and human papillomavirus (HPV). Important insights into our understanding of the unique susceptibility that AD patients have to eczema herpeticum (EH) and eczema vaccinatum (a potentially lethal complication of smallpox vaccine) include the demonstration of an acquired defect in the cutaneous antimicrobial peptide response.[55] Beck and colleagues[56] showed that AD patients with EH had more severe disease based on scoring systems, body surface area affected, and biomarkers (e.g., circulating eosinophil counts, serum IgE, TARC, CTACK), than AD patients without a history of EH. AD patients with EH also had more cutaneous infections with *Staphylococcus aureus* or molluscum contagiosum virus and were also more likely to have a history of asthma and food and inhalant allergies. Leung and associates[57] showed that AD patients with eczema herpeticum have reduced interferon-γ (IFN-γ) production, and that IFN-γ and receptor (IFN-γR1) single-nucleotide polymorphisms (SNPs) are significantly associated with AD and EH and may contribute to an impaired immune response to HSV. In addition, genetic variants in interferon regulatory factor 2 were also shown to be associated with AD and EH and may contribute to abnormal immune responses to HSV.[58]

Superimposed dermatophytosis may cause AD to flare. The opportunistic yeast *Malassezia sympodialis* (formerly *Pityrosporum ovale*) has also been associated with a predominantly head and neck distribution of AD and reported to occur in both extrinsic and intrinsic subtypes of AD.[59]

A number of studies have elucidated the importance of *S. aureus* in AD.[54] Preferential adherence of *S. aureus* may be related to expression of adhesins such as fibronectin and fibrinogen in inflamed skin.[60] *S. aureus* can be cultured from the skin of more than 90% of patients with AD, compared with only 5% of normal subjects.[61] The higher rate of *S. aureus* colonization in AD lesions compared with lesions from other skin disorders may also be associated with colonization of the nares, with the hands serving as the vector of transmission.[62] Patients without obvious superinfection may have a better response to combined anti-staphylococcal and topical corticosteroid therapy than to corticosteroids alone.[63] Recurrent pustulosis has become a significant problem for a number of patients, especially with the emergence of methicillin-resistant *S. aureus* (MRSA) as an important pathogen in AD.[64]

PATIENT EVALUATION, DIAGNOSIS, AND DIFFERENTIAL DIAGNOSIS

A number of diseases may be confused with AD (Table 11-1). In infants, immunodeficiency, including immune dysregulation, polyendocrinopathy, enteropathy, and X-linked (IPEX) syndrome, need to be considered. IPEX is a rare disorder associated with dermatitis, enteropathy, type 1 diabetes, thyroiditis, hemolytic anemia, and thrombocytopenia.[65] IPEX results from mutations of *FOXP3*, a gene located on the X chromosome that encodes the DNA-binding forkhead box P3 protein required for development of regulatory T cells.

Wiskott–Aldrich syndrome is an X-linked recessive disorder characterized by an eczematous rash, associated with thrombocytopenia, along with variable abnormalities in humoral and cellular immunity and severe bacterial infections. Hyper-IgE syndrome (HIE) with mutations in the gene encoding signal transducer and activator of transcription 3 (*STAT3*) is a multisystem autosomal dominant disorder characterized by recurrent deep-seated bacterial infections, including cutaneous cold abscesses and pneumonias caused by *S. aureus*.[66] Patients with mutations in the gene encoding dedicator of cytokinesis 8 protein (*DOCK8*) have a unique combined primary immunodeficiency that accounts for most cases of autosomal recessive HIE.[67] These patients have an eczematous dermatitis with recurrent viral skin infections but lack the coarse facies of autosomal dominant HIE.

Scabies can present as a pruritic skin disease. However, distribution in the genital and axillary areas, the presence of linear lesions, and the finding of mites, ova, and scybala in epithelial debris from skin scrapings help distinguish scabies from AD. An adult who has eczematous dermatitis with no history of childhood eczema and without other atopic features may have contact dermatitis, but more importantly, cutaneous T cell lymphoma needs to be ruled out. Ideally, biopsies should be obtained from three separate sites to increase the yield in identifying abnormal Sézary cells. In addition, eczematous rash suggestive of AD can be seen in patients with human immunodeficiency virus (HIV) infection.

Contact dermatitis should be considered in patients whose AD does not respond to appropriate therapy.[68] It is caused by the interaction of substances with the skin and includes allergic and irritant contact dermatitis, photoallergic contact dermatitis, phototoxic dermatitis, contact urticaria, and protein contact dermatitis. Allergic contact dermatitis, however, complicating AD may appear as an acute flare of the underlying disease rather than the more typical vesiculobullous eruption following direct contact with the injurious substance. People with an atopic diathesis are more likely to experience irritant contact dermatitis, especially in the workplace. Proper diagnosis depends on confirmation of a suspected allergen with patch testing.

Psychosocial Implications

Patients with AD may have high levels of anxiety and problems dealing with anger and hostility.[69] Although not a cause, these emotions can exacerbate AD. Patients often respond to stress or frustration with itching and scratching.[70] Stimulation of the central nervous system may intensify cutaneous vasomotor and sweat responses and contribute to the itch–scratch cycle. In some patients, scratching is associated with significant secondary gain or with a strong component of habit. Severe disease can have a significant impact on patients, leading to problems with social interactions and self-esteem. Importantly, sleep disturbance is common in this chronic disease and significantly impacts the quality of life of patients and family members.[71]

Role of Allergens

Although elevated serum IgE levels can be demonstrated in 80–85% of patients with AD, particularly those seen in tertiary care/specialist centers, and a similar number have immediate skin test response or positive in-vitro tests to food and inhalant allergens, the relationship between the course of AD and implicated allergens has been difficult to establish. Nevertheless, well-controlled studies suggest that allergens can impact the course of this disease.[72]

Foods

May[73] first recognized that patients with AD and positive food allergen skin tests could have negative food challenges to the implicated allergen, distinguishing between symptomatic and asymptomatic hypersensitivity. Thus, triggers for clinical disease cannot be predicted simply by performing allergy testing. However, double-blind, placebo-controlled food challenges have demonstrated that food allergens can cause exacerbations in a subset of patients with AD.[74] Approximately 33% of infants and young children with AD will show clinically relevant reactivity to a food allergen.[75]

Although lesions induced by single positive challenges are usually transient, repeated challenges, more typical of real-life exposure, can result in eczematous lesions. Food-specific T cells have been cloned from lesional skin and peripheral blood of patients with AD.[76,77] Furthermore, elimination of food allergens results in amelioration of skin disease and a decrease in spontaneous basophil histamine release.[78]

Aeroallergens

The evidence supporting a role for aeroallergens in AD includes the finding of both allergen-specific IgE antibodies and allergen-specific T cells.[79] Exacerbation of AD can occur with exposure to allergens such as house-dust mites, animal danders, and pollens. In the 1940s, Tuft[80] demonstrated that introduction of aeroallergens intranasally could exacerbate AD. Subsequently, in a double-blind, randomized, placebo-controlled trial (RCT), a subgroup of patients with AD who underwent bronchoprovocation with a standardized house-dust mite extract developed unequivocal cutaneous lesions after inhalation of dust mite.[81] All the patients with dust mite–induced dermatitis had a history of asthma, and in eight of these nine patients, the skin reaction was preceded by an early bronchial reaction. Therefore, the respiratory route may be important in the induction and exacerbation of AD. Direct contact with inhalant allergens can also result in eczematous skin eruptions.[82] Using the atopy patch test, Langeveld–Wildschut and coworkers[83] showed that positive reactions to house-dust mites were associated with IgE+ Langerhans cells in the epidermis of AD patients.

In addition, the severity of AD has been correlated with the degree of sensitization to aeroallergens.[84] Most importantly, environmental control measures aimed at reducing dust mite allergen have been shown to result in clinical improvement in AD patients.[85,86] These studies suggest that inhalation or contact with aeroallergens may be involved in the pathogenesis of AD.

Microbial Agents

In addition to their role as infectious agents, both the lipophilic yeast *Malassezia sympodialis*[59] and the superficial dermatophyte *Trichophyton rubrum* have been associated with elevated specific-IgE levels. Patients with AD predominantly of the head and neck, compared with a group without this distribution and with a group of normal controls, more often demonstrated IgE testing, and specific histamine release to *M. sympodialis*. These findings are of clinical significance because patients improve after antifungal therapy.

Leung and colleagues[87] showed that exotoxins secreted by *S. aureus* are superantigens that can result in persistent inflammation or exacerbations of AD. More than half of the AD patients studied had *S. aureus* cultured from their skin; the organisms secreted primarily enterotoxins A and B and toxic shock syndrome toxin-1. In addition, almost half of the patients had specific IgE antibodies directed against the staphylococcal toxins found on their skin. AD patients are unique in that they can be colonized by *S. aureus* bacteria that secrete more than one superantigen compared with patients with other superantigen-mediated disease such as toxic shock syndrome.[64] Basophils from patients with antitoxin IgE released histamine on exposure to the relevant toxin but not in response to toxins to which they had no specific IgE. Other investigators have confirmed these observations.[88,89] In addition, analysis of the peripheral blood skin-homing (CLA[+]) T cells of superantigen-positive patients, as well as their skin lesions, revealed that they had undergone expansion of the T cell receptor (TCR) variable-domain β-chain (Vβ), consistent with superantigenic stimulation.[90,91] A correlation also has been found between the presence of IgE against superantigens and severity of AD.[88] Furthermore, superantigens have an additive effect with conventional allergens in inducing cutaneous inflammation.[92] Superantigens can also augment allergen-specific IgE synthesis,[93] subvert T regulatory (Treg) cell function,[94] and induce corticosteroid resistance,[95] suggesting several mechanisms by which superantigens could aggravate the severity of AD. In addition, staphylococcal enterotoxin B (SEB) applied to the skin induced erythema and induration, with the infiltrating T cells selectively expanded in response to the specific superantigen.[96,97]

Autoantigens

Several groups have suggested a role for autoantigens in chronic AD. Valenta and associates[98] reported that the majority of sera from patients with severe AD contain IgE antibodies directed against human proteins. One of these IgE-reactive autoantigens, a 55-kD cytoplasmic protein in skin keratinocytes, has been cloned from a human epithelial complementary DNA (cDNA) expression library and designated Hom s 1.[99] Although the autoallergens characterized to date have mainly been intracellular proteins, they have been detected in IgE immune complexes of AD sera, suggesting that release of these autoallergens from damaged tissues could trigger IgE or T cell-mediated responses. In another study, 30% of sera from patients with AD had both IgG and IgE autoantibodies that reacted with an autoantigen called dense fine speckled 70 (DFS70).[100]

These data suggest that skin inflammation in AD, especially in severe cases, could be maintained by endogenous human antigens. Because these autoantigens are primarily nuclear or microsomal in origin, damage to the skin by infectious organisms or scratching could release intracellular antigens that in turn could elicit and perpetuate IgE and T cell responses in AD. Of interest, human manganese superoxide dismutase (MnSOD) may play a role as an autoallergen in a subset of patients with AD.[101] By molecular mimicry leading to cross-reactivity, such sensitization might be induced primarily by exposure to MnSOD of the skin-colonizing yeast *M. sympodialis*.

Immunology

A number of immunoregulatory abnormalities have been described in AD (Box 11-2).[102] B cells from patients with AD synthesize high levels of IgE. T cells from these patients produce increased amounts of IL-4 and express abnormally high levels of IL-4 receptor. Peripheral blood mononuclear cells (PBMCs) isolated from patients with AD have a decreased capacity to make IFN-γ, which is inversely correlated with serum IgE levels.

Box 11-2   Immunoregulatory Abnormalities in Atopic Dermatitis

- Increased synthesis of IgE
- Increased levels of specific IgE to multiple allergens, including foods, aeroallergens, microorganisms, and enterotoxins
- Increased expression of CD23 on B cells and monocytes
- Increased surface expression of FcεRI on antigen-presenting cells in the skin
- Increased levels of cutaneous T cell-attracting chemokine (CTACK) and thymus- and activation-regulated chemokine (TARC)
- Increased secretion of interleukin-4 (IL-4), IL-5, and IL-13 by T helper type 2 (Th2) cells
- Decreased secretion of interferon-γ by Th1 cells
- Decreased CD4[+]/CD25[+] regulatory T (Treg) cell immunosuppressive activity after superantigen stimulation
- Decreased secretion of antimicrobial peptides by keratinocytes
- Increased levels of monocyte cyclic adenosine monophosphate phosphodiesterase, with increased IL-10 and prostaglandin E_2.

Among differences noted between the intrinsic and extrinsic forms of AD, skin-derived T cells from extrinsic AD interacted with B cells to support IgE synthesis, whereas T cells from the intrinsic form of AD did not.[103]

Studies have shown an increased frequency of both circulating[104,105] and lesional allergen-specific Th2 cells secreting IL-4, IL-5, and IL-13 in patients with AD.[103,106] Furthermore, an increased frequency of circulating skin-homing (CLA+) type 2 cytokine-producing cells and decreased frequency of CLA+ type 1 cytokine-producing cells have been reported in the peripheral blood of AD patients.[107] In addition to acting as an IgE isotype-specific switch, IL-4 also inhibits the production of IFN-γ and downregulates the differentiation of Th1 cells.[108] The importance of Th2 cytokines in driving AD skin inflammation is strongly supported by the observation that a humanized monoclonal antibody that blocks the action of IL-4 and IL-13 was found to reduce the skin severity of AD.[109]

Immunopathologic Features

Routine histologic examination of clinically normal-appearing skin in AD reveals mild epidermal hyperplasia and a sparse, predominantly lymphocytic infiltrate in the dermis.[102] Acute eczematous lesions are characterized by both intercellular edema of the epidermis (spongiosis) and intracellular edema. A sparse lymphocytic infiltrate may be observed in the epidermis, whereas a marked perivenular infiltrate consisting of lymphocytes and some monocytes with rare eosinophils, basophils, and neutrophils is seen in the dermis. In chronic lichenified lesions, the epidermis has prominent hyperkeratosis with increased numbers of epidermal Langerhans cells and predominantly monocytes/macrophages in the dermal infiltrate.

Immunohistochemical staining of acute and chronic skin lesions in AD shows that the lymphocytes are predominantly CD3, CD4, and CD45RO memory T cells; that is, the lymphocytes previously encountered antigen (Fig. 11-3).[1] These cells also express CD25 and human leukocyte antigen (HLA)-DR on their surface, indicative of intralesional activation. In addition, almost all the T cells infiltrating into atopic skin lesions express high levels of the skin lymphocyte-homing receptor cutaneous lymphocyte antigen (CLA).

The role of keratinocytes in skin inflammation in AD has been increasingly recognized.[1] Keratinocytes are an important source of thymic stromal lymphopoietin (TSLP), which activates dendritic cells to prime naive T cells to produce IL-4 and IL-13 (Th2 cell differentiation). Mice genetically engineered to overexpress TSLP in the skin develop AD-like skin inflammation.[110] Recently, S. aureus membrane-derived lipopeptides were shown to induce TSLP in keratinocytes through the Toll-like receptor 2 (TLR2)-TLR6 pathway.[111]

Besides producing proinflammatory cytokines, keratinocytes also play a vital role in the cutaneous innate immune responses by secreting antimicrobial peptides, including human β-defensins and β-cathelicidins, in response to microbial insult or tissue injury. Their keratinocytes produce reduced amounts of antimicrobial peptides, which may predispose AD patients to their frequent colonization and infection by S. aureus, viruses, and fungi.[112] Vitamin D has been found to be involved in the regulation of antimicrobial peptides in keratinocytes,[113] and the treatment with oral vitamin D in AD patients supports this hypothesis.[114] Patients with AD receiving oral vitamin D supplementation showed prevention of winter time exacerbation of eczema.[115]

Cytokine Expression

Cytokine expression in AD lesions reflects the nature of the underlying inflammation (Fig 11-4). Hamid and associates[116] used in situ hybridization to study IL-4, IL-5, and IFN-γ mRNA expression in acute and chronic skin lesions as well as uninvolved skin of patients with AD. Biopsies from uninvolved atopic skin showed a significant increase in the number of cells expressing IL-4 mRNA, but not IL-5 or IFN-γ mRNA. Both acute and chronic lesions had significantly greater numbers of cells positive for IL-4 and IL-5 than did uninvolved or normal skin. Neither acutely involved nor uninvolved atopic

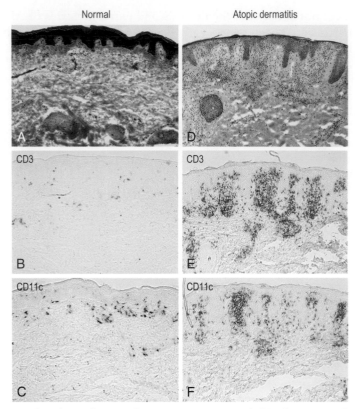

Normal   Atopic dermatitis

Figure 11-3 Immunohistology of atopic dermatitis versus normal skin showing epidermal hyperplasia with T cells (CD3) and dendritic cells (CD11c) in the superficial dermis. *(From Guttman-Yassky E, Nograles KE, Krueger JG. Contrasting pathogenesis of atopic dermatitis and psoriasis. Part I. Clinical and pathologic concepts. J Allergy Clin Immunol 2011;127:1110–1118.)*

skin showed significant numbers of IFN-γ mRNA-expressing cells. In contrast, chronic AD skin lesions had significantly fewer IL-4 mRNA-expressing cells and significantly more IL-5 mRNA-expressing cells than acute lesions. T cells made up the majority of IL-5-expressing cells in both acute and chronic lesions. Activated eosinophils were found in significantly greater numbers in chronic than in acute lesions. These data suggest that although both acute and chronic lesions in AD are associated with increased IL-4 and IL-5 gene activation, acute skin inflammation is associated with predominantly IL-4 expression, whereas chronic inflammation is associated with IL-5 expression and eosinophil infiltration.

Interleukin-13 expression was also found to be higher in acute AD lesions than in chronic AD or psoriatic lesions.[117] These data suggest that IL-13 may be involved in the pathogenesis of AD and further support the hypothesis that acute inflammation in AD is mediated by Th2-type cytokines. Chronic lesions had increased numbers of IL-12 mRNA-positive cells compared with acute or uninvolved skin. IL-12 is a potent inducer of IFN-γ synthesis, and consistent with this observation, increased IFN-γ expression has been reported in chronic AD lesions.[118] At a clonal level, T cells from AD patients with cow's milk allergy showed significantly greater production of IL-4, whereas IFN-γ production was greater in the milk-tolerant patients.[119] IL-5 and IL-13 cytokine production strongly correlated with IL-4 production.

Pruritus is a hallmark of AD, and the underlying processes involved are complex.[120] Mice that overexpress the T cell–derived cytokine IL-31 develop intense pruritus and dermatitis, and patients with AD have CLA⁺ T cells that produce higher levels of IL-31.[121] In patients with AD as well as allergic contact dermatitis (ACD, another pruritic dermatosis), expression of IL-31 is associated with expression of IL-4 and IL-13, which are Th2 cytokines that characterize the atopic phenotype.[122] In addition, *S. aureus* superantigen rapidly induces IL-31 expression in atopic individuals, and because patients

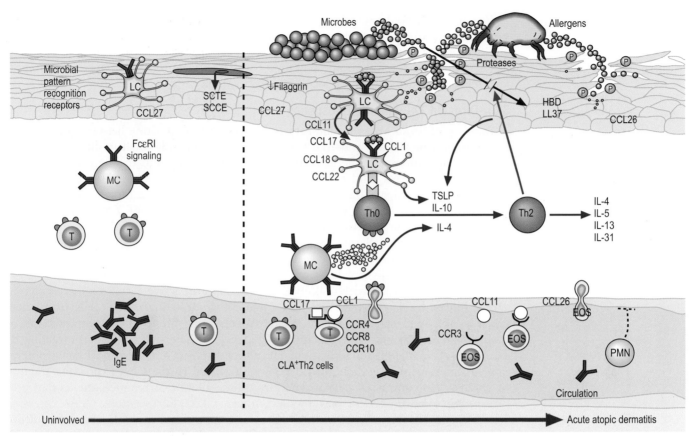

Figure 11-4 Immunologic abnormalities in the progression of atopic dermatitis. MC, mast cell; PMN, polymorphonuclear neutrophil; T, T lymphocyte, Th, helper T cell. *(Reproduced from J Allergy Clin Immunol 2006;118:cover.)*

with AD are heavily colonized with toxin-producing *S. aureus*, this can further contribute to their pruritus.[123] Calcineurin inhibitors and other agents that target T cells are effective at reducing pruritus in AD patients, and new insights into the role of IL-31 in AD may reveal new targets for anti-pruritic therapy.

Increasingly, as previously discussed, the keratinocyte-derived cytokine TSLP has been recognized as the 'master switch' for allergic inflammation.[124] In AD the TSLP-induced Th2 cytokine milieu can participate in a vicious cycle impacting the skin barrier and microbial colonization.[111] Genetic variants in TSLP have been shown to be associated with AD and eczema herpeticum.[125,126]

Role of IgE in Cutaneous Inflammation

In AD patients, IgE may play an important role in allergen-induced, cell-mediated reactions involving Th2-type cells that are distinct from conventional delayed-type hypersensitivity reactions mediated by Th1-type cells.[127] IgE-dependent biphasic reactions are frequently associated with clinically significant allergic reactions and may contribute to the inflammatory process of AD. Immediate-type reactions related to mediator release by mast cells bearing allergen-specific IgE may result in the pruritus and erythema that occur after exposure to relevant allergens. IgE-dependent late-phase reactions can then lead to more persistent symptoms. The T cell infiltrate in cutaneous allergen-induced late-phase reactions has increased mRNA for IL-3, IL-4, IL-5, and GM-CSF, but not for IFN-γ. These cells are therefore similar to the Th2-type cells found in AD lesions. In addition, the cutaneous late-phase reaction is associated with a pattern of cell adhesion molecule (CAM) expression similar to that in AD. Therefore, a sustained IgE-dependent late-phase reaction may be part of the chronic inflammatory process in AD patients.

Furthermore, epidermal LCs in AD skin express IgE on their cell surface and are significantly more efficient than IgE-negative LCs at presenting allergen to T cells.[128] In addition, LCs from atopic individuals have a much higher level of FcεRI expression.[129] Efficient allergen capture and presentation to Th2 cells in atopic skin may be an important mechanism for sustaining local T cell activation.

Skin-Directed Th2-Like Cell Response

A number of studies have demonstrated important similarities between the allergic inflammation of asthma and AD. Common features include local infiltration of Th2-type cells in response to allergens, development of specific IgE to allergens, a chronic inflammatory process, and organ-specific hyperreactivity. In both diseases, IL-4- and IL-5-secreting memory Th2-type cells have a central role in the induction of local IgE responses and recruitment of eosinophils.[116] The recognition of T cell heterogeneity based on expression of tissue-selective homing receptors suggests that an individual's propensity for specific allergic disease may be a function of end-organ targeting by effector T cells. In this respect, T cells migrating to the skin express CLA, whereas most memory/effector T cells isolated from asthmatic airways do not.

In a study of patients with milk-induced AD, casein-reactive T cells expressed significantly higher levels of CLA than did *Candida albicans*–reactive T cells from these patients or casein-reactive T cells from patients with milk-induced enterocolitis or eosinophilic gastroenteritis.[130] As further evidence for selective end-organ targeting by T cell subsets in allergic inflammation, data show that dust mite–specific T cell proliferation in mite-sensitized patients with AD was localized to the CLA-expressing fraction of T cells.[131] In contrast, T cells isolated from mite-allergic asthmatic patients that proliferated on exposure to the relevant allergen were CLA⁻. Furthermore, CLA-expressing T cells isolated from patients with AD, but not from normal controls, showed evidence of activation (HLA-DR expression) and also spontaneously produced IL-4 but not IFN-γ. This suggests that T cell effector function in AD is closely linked to CLA expression.

TREATMENT

Conventional Therapy

Current understanding of the pathophysiology of AD supports the concept that assessing the role of allergens, infectious agents, irritants, physical environment, and emotional stressors is as important as initiating therapy with first-line agents. The acute and chronic aspects of AD need to be considered when designing an individualized treatment plan. Patients should understand that therapy is not curative, but that avoidance of exacerbating factors together with proper daily skin care can control symptoms and improve the long-term outcome. Management of patients with AD has been comprehensively reviewed (Fig. 11-5).[132-134]

Irritants

Patients with AD have a lowered threshold of irritant responsiveness. Therefore, recognition and avoidance of irritants are integral to successful management of this disease. Irritants include detergents, soaps, chemicals, pollutants, and abrasive materials, as well as extremes of temperature and humidity. Cleansers with minimal defatting activity and a neutral pH should be used rather than soaps. A number of mild cleansers are available in sensitive skin formulations. New clothing should be laundered before it is worn, to reduce the content of formaldehyde and other chemicals. Residual laundry detergent in clothing may be irritating, and although changing to a milder detergent can be helpful, using liquid rather than powder detergent and adding an extra rinse cycle are more beneficial. Occlusive clothing should be avoided, and cotton or cotton blends should be used.

Ideally, the temperature in the home and work environments should be temperate to minimize sweating. Swimming is usually well tolerated; however, because swimming

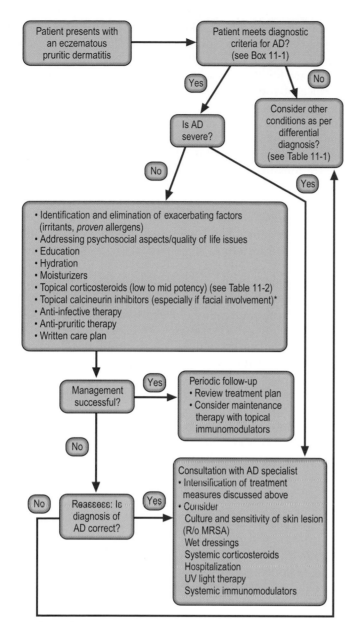

Figure 11-5 Approach to the patient with atopic dermatitis (AD). R/o MRSA, rule out methicillin-resistant *Staphylococcus aureus*; UV, ultraviolet. *Per boxed warning*: second-line, intermittent therapy for patients ≥2 years of age.

pools are treated with chlorine or bromine, it is important for patients to shower and use a mild soap immediately afterward, to remove these potentially irritating chemicals, and then to apply moisturizers or occlusives. Although sunlight may be beneficial to some patients with AD, non-sensitizing sunscreens should be used to avoid sunburn. Products developed for use on the face are often best tolerated by patients with AD. Prolonged sun exposure can cause evaporative losses, overheating, and sweating, which can be irritating.

Allergens

Identification of allergens involves taking a careful history and doing selective immediate-hypersensitivity skin tests or in-vitro tests when appropriate. Negative skin tests with proper controls have a high predictive value for ruling out a suspected allergen. Positive skin tests have a lower correlation with clinical symptoms in suspected food allergen-induced AD and should be confirmed with double-blind, placebo-controlled food challenge, unless the patient has a history of anaphylaxis to the suspected food. In children who have undergone such a challenge, milk, egg, peanut, soy, wheat, and fish account for approximately 90% of the food allergens found to exacerbate AD. More importantly, avoidance of foods implicated in controlled challenges results in clinical improvement.[74,78]

Extensive elimination diets, which may be both extremely burdensome and at times nutritionally unsound, are almost never warranted, because even patients with multiple positive allergy tests are rarely clinically sensitive to more than three foods on challenge. Specific IgE concentrations in response to four food allergens measured by the Phadia ImmunoCAP assay—*egg*, 7 kU$_A$/L (2 kU$_A$/L age ≤2 years); *milk*, 15 kU$_A$/L (5 kU$_A$/L age ≤2 years); *peanut*, 14 kU$_A$/L; and *fish*, 20 kU$_A$/L—have been shown to be associated with a >95% probability of clinical reaction.

However, these levels do not identify the type or severity of reaction.[135] The atopy patch test has revealed sensitization in some patients with AD but remains an investigational tool.[136]

Environmental control measures aimed at reducing dust mite load may improve AD in patients who demonstrate specific IgE to dust mite allergen.[85] These measures include using dust mite–proof encasings on pillows, mattresses, and box springs; washing linens in hot water weekly; removing bedroom carpeting; and decreasing indoor humidity levels. Adult AD patients not sensitized to house-dust mite benefited from allergy-proof covers as much as sensitized patients, suggesting that impermeable covers may reduce exposure to other allergens, irritants, or infectious organisms.[137]

Psychosocial Factors

Recognizing and addressing sleep disturbance problems in both patients and caregivers are critical in a chronic, relapsing disease such as AD.[71] Counseling is often helpful in dealing with the frustrations associated with AD. Relaxation, behavioral modification, and biofeedback may all be of benefit, especially for patients with habitual scratching.[69]

Patient Education

Learning about the chronic nature of AD, exacerbating factors, and appropriate treatment options is important for both patients and caregivers.[138] In addition, patients and their families should be counseled about the natural history and prognosis and receive appropriate vocational counseling. The International Study of Life with Atopic Eczema (ISOLATE) found that patients and caregivers often delay initiation of treatment for AD flares and have concerns about their prescribed medications.[139] Clinicians should provide patients and their families with detailed written skin care recommendations and should review this information on follow-up. Educational materials may be obtained from the National Eczema Association (www.nationaleczema.org), a not-for-profit, patient-oriented organization. In addition, written information and a DVD on skin care are available from the Office of Professional Education, National Jewish Health (http://www.nationaljewish.org/professionals/education/pro-ed/overview).

Hydration

Atopic dry skin shows enhanced transepidermal water loss and reduced water-binding capacity. Patients may also have decreased ceramide levels in their skin, resulting in reduced water-binding capacity, higher transepidermal water loss, and decreased water content.[35,140] Therefore, skin hydration is an essential component of therapy. The best way to re-establish the skin's barrier function is to soak the affected area or bathe for approximately 10 min in warm (not lukewarm) water and then apply an occlusive agent to retain the absorbed water. Substances such as oatmeal or baking soda added to the bathwater may feel soothing to certain patients but do not affect water absorption. Hydration of the face or neck can be achieved by applying a wet facecloth or towel to the involved area. A wet washcloth may be more readily accepted if holes are cut out for the eyes and mouth, allowing the patient to remain functional. Hand or foot dermatitis can be treated by soaking the limb in a basin. Baths may need to be taken several times a day during flares of AD, whereas showers may be adequate for patients with mild disease. It is essential to use an occlusive preparation within a few minutes after hydrating the skin to prevent evaporation, which is damaging to the epidermis. Patients and their families need to understand proper hydration techniques.

Bathing may also remove allergens from the skin surface and reduce colonization by *S. aureus*. Bleach baths with dilute sodium hypochlorite have been recommended to reduce skin infections (¼ to ½ cup of household bleach per full tub of water), but this approach may lead to skin irritation and should be used with caution. In a small, controlled study of diluted bleach baths, Huang and associates[141] showed that patients who received both dilute bleach baths and intranasal mupirocin treatment had significantly greater mean reductions from baseline in EASI scores than the placebo group at 1- and 3-month visits. However, patients remained colonized by *S. aureus*.

Moisturizers and Occlusives

The use of an effective emollient, especially when combined with hydration therapy, helps to restore and preserve the stratum corneum barrier and can decrease the need for topical corticosteroids.[142] Moisturizers are available as lotions, creams, and ointments. Lotions contain more water than creams and may be more drying because of an evaporative effect. Both lotions and creams can cause skin irritation secondary to added preservatives and fragrances. Because moisturizers usually need to be applied several times daily on a long-term basis, they should be obtained in 1-pound (0.45 kg) jars if available. Vegetable-oil shortening (e.g., Crisco) can be used if an inexpensive moisturizer is needed. Petroleum jelly (e.g., Vaseline) is an effective occlusive when used to seal in water after bathing.

Alpha-hydroxy acids affect keratinization through corneocyte cohesion and stratum corneum formation and increase dermal mucopolysaccharides and collagen formation. Assessment of 12% ammonium lactate emulsion by clinical criteria and by non-invasive methods showed a significant increase in electrical capacitance, skin surface lipids, dermal extensibility and firmness, and improvement in the skin barrier function and skin surface topography in all patients.[143] Ammonium lactate mitigated the epidermal and dermal atrophy associated with topical corticosteroid use.[144]

In contrast to changes in sphingolipid metabolism caused by aging, the enzyme SM deacylase is highly expressed in the epidermis of AD patients and competes with sphingomyelinase or β-glucocerebrosidase for the common substrate SM or glucosylceramide.[145] This in turn leads to ceramide deficiency of the stratum corneum in AD. Whereas an equimolar ratio of ceramides, cholesterol, and either the essential fatty acid linoleic acid or the non-essential palmitic or stearic fatty acids allows normal repair of damaged human skin, further acceleration of barrier repair occurs as the ratio of any of these ingredients is increased up to three-fold.[146] Non-steroidal creams (e.g., Atopiclair, EpiCeram, MimyX) marketed as 'medical devices' have unique formulations and have not been compared; although not regulated by the US Food and Drug Administration (FDA), these creams do require a prescription.[147]

Corticosteroids

Corticosteroids reduce inflammation and pruritus and are effective for both the acute and chronic components of AD. They affect multiple resident and infiltrating cells primarily through suppression of inflammatory genes, reducing inflammation and pruritus. Topical corticosteroids are available in a wide variety of formulations, ranging from extremely high-potency (group 1) to low-potency (group 7) preparations (Table 11-2). The vehicle in which the product is formulated can alter the potency of the corticosteroid and move it up or down in this classification. Generic formulations of topical corticosteroids are required to have the same active ingredient and the same concentration as the original product. However, many generics do not have the same vehicle formulation, and the bioequivalence of the product can vary significantly.

TABLE 11-2   Select Topical Corticosteroid Preparations*

Group	Preparations
1	Clobetasol propionate (Temovate) 0.05% ointment/cream Betamethasone dipropionate (Diprolene) 0.05% ointment/cream
2	Mometasone furoate (Elocon) 0.1% ointment Halcinonide (Halog) 0.1% cream Fluocinonide (Lidex) 0.05% ointment/cream Desoximetasone (Topicort) 0.25% ointment/cream
3	Fluticasone propionate (Cutivate) 0.005% ointment Halcinonide (Halog) 0.1% ointment Betamethasone valerate (Valisone) 0.1% ointment
4	Mometasone furoate (Elocon) 0.1% cream Triamcinolone acetonide (Kenalog) 0.1% ointment/cream Fluocinolone acetonide (Synalar) 0.025% ointment
5	Fluocinolone acetonide (Synalar) 0.025% cream Hydrocortisone valerate (Westcort) 0.2% ointment
6	Desonide (DesOwen) 0.05% ointment/cream/lotion/gel Alclometasone dipropionate (Aclovate) 0.05% ointment/cream
7	Hydrocortisone (Hytone) 2.5% and 1% ointment/cream

*Representative corticosteroids are listed by group from 1 (superpotent) through 7 (least potent).
(Modified from Stoughton RB. Vasoconstrictor assay-specific applications. In: Maibach HI, Surber C, eds. Topical corticosteroids. Basel, Switzerland: Karger; 1992:42–53.)

Choice of a particular product depends on the severity and distribution of skin lesions. In general, an effective topical corticosteroid of the lowest potency should be used. However, choosing a preparation that is too weak may result in persistent or worsening AD. Resistant lesions may respond to a potent topical corticosteroid under occlusion, although this needs to be used cautiously to prevent irreversible atrophic changes. When treating pediatric patients, clinicians should be aware of age-appropriate indications (e.g., fluticasone 0.05% cream, up to 28 days in children age ≥3 months; fluticasone lotion, ≥12 months of age; mometasone cream/ointment, ≥2 years of age).

With appropriately used low- to medium-potency topical corticosteroids, side effects are infrequent. Thinning of the skin with telangiectasias, bruising, hypopigmentation, acne, striae, and secondary infections may occur. The face, particularly the eyelids, and the intertriginous areas are especially sensitive to these adverse effects, and only low-potency preparations should be used routinely on these areas. Perioral dermatitis, characterized by erythema, scaling, and follicular papules and pustules that occur around the mouth, in the alar creases, and sometimes on the upper lateral eyelids, can occur with the use of topical corticosteroids on the face. 'Steroid addiction' describes an adverse effect primarily of the face of adult women treated with topical corticosteroids, who complain of a burning sensation. Patients improve with total discontinuation of the corticosteroid therapy.[148] High-potency topical corticosteroids must be used cautiously, especially under occlusion, because they may lead to significant atrophic changes and systemic side effects.

Topical corticosteroids are available in a variety of bases, including ointments, creams, lotions, solutions, gels, sprays, oil, and even tape (Table 11-2). Therefore, no need exists to compound these medications. Ointments are most occlusive and as a rule provide better delivery of the medication while preventing evaporative losses. In addition, ointments spread more evenly than other creams or solutions. In a humid environment, creams may be better tolerated than ointments because the increased occlusion can cause itching or even folliculitis. In general, however, creams and lotions, although easier to spread, are less effective and can contribute to skin dryness and irritation. Solutions can be used on the scalp and hirsute areas, although the alcohol content can be irritating, especially if used on inflamed or open lesions, and additives used to formulate the different bases can cause sensitization. Furthermore, allergic contact dermatitis to the corticosteroid molecule is being recognized with increasing frequency.[149] This diagnosis is often difficult to establish clinically because it can present as acute or chronic eczema. Patch testing has been done primarily with tixocortol pivalate and budesonide. Expanded testing has been associated with both false-positive and false-negative reactions.

An inadequate prescription size often contributes to suboptimally controlled AD, especially when patients have widespread, chronic disease. Approximately 30 g of medication is needed to cover the entire body of an average adult. The *fingertip unit* (FTU) has been proposed as a measure for applying topical corticosteroids and has been studied in children with AD.[150] This is the amount of topical medication that extends from the tip to the first joint on the palmar aspect of the index finger. It takes approximately 1 FTU to cover the hand or groin; 2 FTUs for the face or foot; 3 FTUs for an arm; 6 FTUs for the leg; and 14 FTUs for the trunk. Patients need to be instructed in the proper use of topical corticosteroids.

Application of an emollient immediately before or over a topical corticosteroid preparation may decrease the effectiveness of the corticosteroid. Patients often assume that the potency of their prescribed corticosteroid is based solely on the percentage noted after the compound name (e.g., they believe that hydrocortisone 2.5% is more potent than clobetasol 0.05%) and therefore may apply the preparations incorrectly. In addition, patients are often given a high-potency corticosteroid and told to discontinue it after a time without being given a lower-potency corticosteroid; this can result in rebound flaring of the AD, similar to that often seen with oral corticosteroid therapy for AD. A stepwise care approach with a midrange or high-potency preparation (although usually not to face, axillae, or groin) followed by low-potency preparations may be more successful.

Once-daily treatment may help with patient adherence to the regimen and has been effective for fluticasone propionate, a molecule with an increased binding affinity for the corticosteroid receptor.[151] Topical mometasone has been studied in children with AD and is also approved for once-daily use.[152] Topical corticosteroids usually have been discontinued after the inflammation resolves, while hydration and moisturizers are continued. An important concept to recognize is that normal-appearing skin in AD shows evidence of immunologic dysregulation,[116] and more recently, skin barrier abnormalities have been demonstrated in non-lesional skin.[153] These data provide a rationale for the use of topical corticosteroids as 'proactive' or maintenance therapy.[154]

In several studies with fluticasone, after control of AD with a once-daily regimen was achieved, long-term control could be maintained with twice-weekly applications of the topical corticosteroid to areas that had previously been involved but now appeared normal. This approach has resulted in fewer relapses and less need for topical corticosteroids than has 'reactive' eczema therapy.

In addition to their anti-inflammatory properties, topical corticosteroids can decrease *S. aureus* colonization in patients with AD. In a double-blind, randomized, 1-week trial of desonide compared with a vehicle in children with AD, clinical scores improved and *S. aureus* density significantly decreased within the desonide group but not in the vehicle group.[155]

A number of AD patients may not show clinical improvement with topical corticosteroids, perhaps the result of superinfection complication or inadequate drug potency. In addition, allergen-induced immune activation can alter the T cell response to glucocorticoids by inducing cytokine-dependent abnormalities in glucocorticoid receptor-binding affinity.[156] PBMCs from patients with chronic AD have reduced glucocorticoid receptor-binding affinity, which can be sustained with the combination of IL-2 and IL-4 in-vitro. In addition, corticosteroid unresponsiveness may contribute to treatment failure in some patients.[131] Endogenous cortisol levels have been found to control the magnitude of cutaneous allergic inflammatory responses, suggesting that an impaired response to corticosteroids could contribute to chronic AD.[157] Alternatively, Blotta and associates[158] suggested that chronic corticosteroid therapy can have deleterious but insidious immunologic effects in allergic patients. These results are based on in-vitro data that may not recreate the complex milieu in allergic inflammation. A much more common reason for failure of corticosteroid therapy is non-adherence to the treatment regimen. Patients or parents often expect a quick and permanent resolution of the AD and become disillusioned by the lack of cure with current therapy. A significant number of patients and caregivers also admit to non-adherence to prescribed topical corticosteroid therapy because of fear of using this class of medications.[139,159] These findings emphasize the need for both education and alternative therapies.

Systemic corticosteroids, including oral prednisone, should be avoided in the management of a chronic, relapsing disorder such as AD.[133] Often, patients or parents demand immediate improvement of the disease and find systemic corticosteroids more convenient to use than topical therapy. However, the dramatic improvement observed with systemic corticosteroids may be associated with an equally dramatic flaring of AD after discontinuation. If a short course of *oral* corticosteroids is given, topical skin care should be intensified during the taper to suppress rebound flaring of AD.

Topical Calcineurin Inhibitors

The approval of the topical calcineurin inhibitors (TCIs) tacrolimus ointment 0.03% and 0.1% and pimecrolimus cream 1% represented a milestone in AD management.[160] Both non-steroidal drugs have proved effective, with a good safety profile for treatment up to 4 years with tacrolimus ointment[161] and up to 2 years with pimecrolimus cream.[162] A fairly common side effect with TCIs is a transient burning sensation of the skin, although a few patients may complain of more prolonged burning or stinging. TCIs are not associated with skin atrophy and thus are particularly useful on the face and intertriginous regions. TCIs may be particularly useful in the treatment of steroid-insensitive patients.[163] Ongoing surveillance and recent reports have shown no trend for increased frequency of viral superinfections, especially eczema herpeticum, and no problems with response to childhood vaccinations.[164]

Currently, tacrolimus ointment 0.03% is approved for intermittent treatment of moderate to severe AD in children 2 years and older; tacrolimus ointment 0.1% for intermittent treatment of moderate to severe AD in adults; and pimecrolimus cream 1% for intermittent therapy of patients 2 years and older with mild to moderate AD.

Although there is no evidence of a causal link between cancer and TCIs, the FDA has issued a boxed warning for tacrolimus ointment 0.03% and 0.1% (Protopic, Astellas) and pimecrolimus cream 1% (Elidel, Novartis) because of a lack of long-term safety data (see US package inserts for Protopic, Astellas; and Elidel, Novartis). Further, the new labeling states that these drugs are recommended as second-line treatments and that their use in children under the age of 2 years is currently not recommended. Long-term safety studies with TCIs in patients with AD, including infants and children, are ongoing. A joint task force of the American College of Allergy, Asthma and Immunology and the American Academy of Allergy, Asthma and Immunology reviewed the available data and concluded that the risk : benefit ratios of tacrolimus ointment 0.03% and 0.1% and pimecrolimus cream 1% are similar to those of most conventional therapies for the treatment of chronic relapsing eczema.[165] In addition, a nested case–control study of a large database ($n = 293\,253$) did not find an increased risk of lymphoma in AD patients treated with TCIs.[166]

Ongoing studies with TCIs have shown that pimecrolimus cream 1% is well tolerated and effective in infants 3 to 23 months of age with AD.[167,168] Given the chronic and relapsing nature of AD, the question of whether TCI therapy for early signs or symptoms of disease could influence long-term outcomes was addressed in clinical trials up to 1 year in duration with pimecrolimus cream 1%.[169] The primary efficacy parameter was the incidence of flares and need for topical corticosteroid rescue. In the infant study, 64% of the pimecrolimus group versus 35% of the vehicle group did not require topical corticosteroids during the study.[168] Subgroup analysis showed significantly fewer flares in the pimecrolimus-treated children of all degrees of clinical severity, including severe AD. These studies suggest that earlier use of a TCI can lead to better long-term disease control with fewer flares and significantly less need for topical corticosteroid rescue therapy. Similar to the proactive use of topical corticosteroids, several studies of tacrolimus ointment in both adults and children have shown efficacy with this approach.[154] Proactive therapy with tacrolimus ointment has been approved for use in Europe for up to 12 months in patients 2 years or older.

Tar Preparations

Crude coal tar extracts have anti-inflammatory properties that are not as pronounced as those of topical corticosteroids. Nevertheless, in a study using the atopy patch test, tar performed similar to a topical corticosteroid in its ability to inhibit the influx of proinflammatory cells and in the expression of cell adhesion molecules (CAMs) in response to epicutaneous allergen challenge.[170] Tar preparations used with topical corticosteroids in chronic AD may reduce the need for more potent corticosteroid preparations. Tar shampoos are often beneficial for scalp involvement. The use of tar preparations on acutely inflamed skin should be avoided because it may result in skin irritation. Other than dryness or irritation, side effects associated with tar products are rare but include photosensitivity reactions and a pustular folliculitis.

Wet Dressings

Wet-wrap dressings reduce pruritus and inflammation, act as a barrier to trauma associated with scratching, and improve penetration of topical corticosteroids.[133] In addition, wet-wrap therapy can aid with epidermal barrier recovery that persists even after wrap therapy is discontinued.[171] In one study, children with severe AD showed significant clinical improvement after 1 week of treatment using tubular bandages applied over diluted topical corticosteroids.[172] No significant differences were demonstrated among several dilutions of a midpotency corticosteroid, suggesting that clinical benefit can be achieved with this approach in more severely affected patients even with the use of lower-potency corticosteroids. Although long-term studies with wet-wrap therapy are lacking, most of the improvement in the latter study occurred during the first week. An alternative approach employs clothing, using wet pajamas or long underwear, with dry pajamas or a sweatsuit on top.[133] Hands and feet can be covered by wet tube socks under dry tube socks. Alternatively, the face, trunk, or extremities can be covered by wet gauze then dry gauze and secured in place with an elastic bandage or pieces of tube socks. Dressings may be removed when dry or may be rewetted. Dressings are often best tolerated at bedtime.

Overuse of wet-wrap dressings can result in chilling, maceration of the skin, or, infrequently, secondary infection. Because this approach can be labor intensive, it is best reserved for acute exacerbations of AD, along with selective use in areas of resistant dermatitis. The package inserts recommend that TCIs not be used under any occlusive dressing.

Anti-Infective Therapy

Systemic antibiotics may be necessary to treat AD when a secondary infection with *S. aureus* is present.[133] Therapy with semisynthetic penicillins or first- or second- generation cephalosporins for 7 to 10 days is usually effective. Erythromycin-resistant organisms are fairly common, making macrolides less useful alternatives. Unfortunately, recolonization after a course of antistaphylococcal therapy occurs rapidly.[173] Maintenance antibiotic therapy should be avoided, however, because it may result in colonization by methicillin-resistant organisms. The topical antistaphylococcal antibiotic mupirocin (Bactroban), applied three times daily to affected areas for 7 to 10 days, may be effective for treating localized areas of involvement. Twice-daily treatment for 5 days with a nasal preparation of mupirocin may reduce nasal carriage of *S. aureus*, which may result in clinical benefit in AD patients. Although effective in reducing bacterial skin flora, antibacterial cleansers can cause significant skin irritation. However, a double-blind, placebo-controlled study found that daily bathing with an antimicrobial soap containing 1.5% triclocarban resulted in reductions in *S. aureus* colonization and significantly greater clinical improvement than with the placebo soap[174] (see earlier discussion of bleach baths).

Patients with disseminated eczema herpeticum, also called Kaposi varicelliform eruption, usually require treatment with systemic acyclovir.[54] Recurrent cutaneous herpetic infections can be controlled with daily prophylactic oral acyclovir. Superficial dermatophytosis and *M. sympodialis* infections can be treated with topical (or rarely with systemic) antifungal drugs.[54]

Anti-pruritic Agents

Pruritus is the most common and usually the worst-tolerated symptom of AD. Even partial reduction of pruritus can significantly improve quality of life for patients with severe AD. The participation of histamine in the pruritus of AD has been questioned, and a dermal microdialysis study of mast cell degranulation concluded that mediators other than histamine cause pruritus.[175] Neuropeptides or cytokines may be important mediators because centrally acting agents such as opioid receptor antagonists have been effective against the itch of AD.[176] Use of cyclosporin A, which results in decreased transcription of several proinflammatory cytokines, leads to rapid improvement in pruritus for many AD patients.[177]

Systemic antihistamines and anxiolytics may be most useful through their tranquilizing and sedative effects and can be used primarily in the evening to avoid daytime drowsiness. The tricyclic antidepressant doxepin, which has both histamine H_1 and H_2 receptor-binding affinity as well as a long half-life, may be given as a single 10- to 50-mg dose in the evening in adults. If nocturnal pruritus remains severe, short-term use of a sedative to allow adequate rest may be appropriate. Although reportedly ineffective in treating the pruritus associated with AD, second-generation antihistamines have shown modest clinical benefit in at least some AD patients.[178]

Treatment of AD with topical antihistamines and topical anesthetics should be avoided because of potential sensitization. Although in a 1-week study, topical 5% doxepin cream resulted in significant reduction of pruritus and no sensitization,[179] re-challenge with the drug after the 7-day course of therapy was not evaluated. Later case reports have documented reactions to topical doxepin.[180]

Recalcitrant Disease Hospitalization

Patients with AD who are erythrodermic or who appear toxic may need to be hospitalized. Hospitalization may also be appropriate for patients with severe disseminated AD resistant to first-line therapy. Often, removing the patient from environmental allergens or stressors, together with intense education and assurance of compliance with therapy, results in marked clinical improvement. In this setting, the patient can also undergo appropriately controlled provocative challenges to help identify potential triggering factors. This can be done in a day hospital model.[133]

Cyclosporin A

The benefit of oral cyclosporin A in severe AD in adults has been demonstrated in placebo-controlled studies.[181,182] A 1-year study of cyclosporin A (5 mg/kg per day) in a pediatric population using either intermittent or continuous treatment showed no significant differences between these two approaches with respect to efficacy or safety parameters, and a subset of patients remained in remission after treatment was stopped.[183] In addition, children as young as 22 months responded to low-dose (2.5 mg/kg per day) cyclosporin A.[184] A meta-analysis of 15 studies that included 602 patients with AD found that cyclosporin A consistently decreased disease severity in all studies.[185]

Short-term oral cyclosporin A therapy can result in increased serum urea, creatinine, and bilirubin concentrations, but these values normalize after treatment is discontinued. Because of the concern for progressive or irreversible nephrotoxicity with extended treatment, few patients receiving maintenance therapy have been evaluated. In one study, patients with severe AD treated with oral cyclosporin A, 5 mg/kg per day for 6 weeks, were monitored until relapse, then treated with a second 6-week course.[186]

Although this regimen did not result in lasting remission for most patients, a subset appeared to receive extended clinical benefit. In another prospective, open multicenter study, 100 adults with severe AD were treated for up to 48 weeks.[187] For the first 8 weeks, cyclosporin A was administered at 2.5 mg/kg per day, then adjusted according to clinical response. Cyclosporin A produced rapid and highly significant improvements in all indices of disease activity, including signs and symptoms, body surface area, pruritus, and sleep disturbance.

Mycophenolate Mofetil

Mycophenolate mofetil (MMF), a purine biosynthesis inhibitor, has been used for inflammatory skin disorders. The drug has been well tolerated, although herpes retinitis has been reported. An observer-blinded RCT compared enteric-coated MMF (1440 mg) with cyclosporin A (5 mg/kg) as long-term treatment in 55 adult patients with severe AD.[188] During maintenance phase, disease activity was comparable in both study arms. Side effects in both groups were mild and transient. After study medication withdrawal, disease activity of the cyclosporin A patients significantly increased compared with MMF patients. In a retrospective analysis of 14 AD children treated with MMF as systemic monotherapy, four achieved complete clearance, four had >90% improvement, five had 60–90% improvement, and one failed to respond.[189] Initial responses occurred within 8 weeks (mean 4 weeks) with maximal effects attained after 8 to 12 weeks (mean 9 weeks) at MMF doses of 40 to 50 mg/kg per day in younger children and 30 to 40 mg/kg per day in adolescents. MMF was well-tolerated in all patients, with no infectious complications or laboratory abnormalities.

Azathioprine

Azathioprine is a systemic immunosuppressive agent affecting purine nucleotide synthesis and metabolism shown to be effective for dermatologic diseases such as severe recalcitrant AD.[134] A systematic review of patients with refractory AD showed an overall decrease in disease severity after active treatment with azathioprine.[190]

Azathioprine has a number of side effects, including myelosuppression, hepatotoxicity, gastrointestinal disturbances, increased susceptibility to infections, and risk of skin cancer. The drug is metabolized by the enzyme thiopurine methyltransferase; TPMT deficiency should be excluded before starting oral immunosuppressive therapy with azathioprine. The recommended dosage of azathioprine for dermatologic indications is 1 to 3 mg/kg daily but should be adjusted based on TPMT levels, and routine screening blood tests should be performed. The onset of action is usually slow, and benefit may not be apparent for several months after starting treatment.

Methotrexate

Methotrexate, a folic acid antagonist that interferes with purine and pyrimidine synthesis, has been effective in moderate to severe AD. In an open-label dose-ranging study (median dose 15 mg/week), disease activity decreased by 52% from baseline after 24 weeks.[191] A group of patients had continued improvement more than 12 weeks after discontinuing therapy. In a retrospective study, 75% of patients treated with weekly doses of 7.5 to 25 mg of methotrexate intramuscularly had clinical improvement of >70% after 3 months of therapy.[192] In another retrospective study of methotrexate (10–25 mg) given weekly (8–12 weeks), 80% of patients with moderate to severe AD had a mean decrease in AD severity score (SCORAD) of 44%.[193] A randomized assessor-blinded trial in patients with severe AD found methotrexate (10–22.5 mg/week) to be comparable in clinical efficacy to azathioprine (1.5–2.5 mg/kg per day) after 12 weeks of treatment.[190]

Symptom improvement in responders can be seen as early as 2 weeks and up to 3 months after initiating therapy, and patients not responding to 15 mg of methotrexate weekly after 3 months are unlikely to improve with further dose escalation.[191] Nausea and liver enzyme elevation are the most common adverse events, resulting in transient or complete discontinuation of methotrexate therapy.

Phototherapy and Photochemotherapy

Ultraviolet (UV) light therapy can be a useful treatment for chronic recalcitrant AD, but should be done under the supervision of an experienced dermatologist. The most common phototherapy modalities are narrowband UVB, broadband UVB, and UVA1.[194–196] Short-term adverse effects from phototherapy may include erythema, skin pain, pruritus, and pigmentation. Potential long-term adverse effects include premature skin aging and cutaneous malignancies.

In an open trial in patients with moderate to severe chronic AD, all patients had a ≥50% reduction in SCORAD with narrowband UVB phototherapy three times weekly for up to 12 weeks.[197] Gene expression and immunohistochemistry studies of both lesional and non-lesional skin showed that Th2, Th22, and Th1 immune pathways were suppressed and measures of epidermal hyperplasia and differentiation normalized. Clinical improvement was associated with decrease in Th2/Th22 associated cytokines and chemokines and importantly, normalized expression of epidermal barrier proteins. A retrospective review of children with severe eczema who had undergone narrowband UVB found that of those who completed more than 10 exposures, complete clearance, or minimal residual activity was achieved in 40%; good improvement in 23%; and moderate improvement in 26%.[198] Overall, the treatment was well tolerated, and the median length of remission was 3 months. A prospective analysis of narrowband UVB phototherapy found that it was an effective and well-tolerated treatment modality in children.[199] A systematic review of phototherapy in AD found that UVA1 should be used to control acute flares of AD, whereas UVB modalities, especially narrowband, should be used for management of chronic AD.[200] However, a 6-week course of medium-dose UVA1 and narrowband UVB in a double-blind crossover RCT showed no significant difference between treatments with respect to clinical scores, pruritus score, or health-related quality of life.[201] In a randomized, investigator-blinded, half-sided comparison study between narrowband UVB and medium-dose UVA1 in adults with AD, both modalities significantly decreased clinical severity and dermal cellular infiltrate.[202] Importantly, UVB phototherapy has been shown to significantly decrease levels of toxin producing *S. aureus* on the skin of pediatric AD patients.[203]

Photochemotherapy with oral methoxypsoralen therapy followed by UVA (PUVA) may be indicated in patients with severe AD, although studies comparing it with other modes of phototherapy are limited. In one randomized observer-blinded crossover trial, PUVA was shown to provide better short-term and long-term response than medium-dose UVA1 in patients with severe AD.[204] Short-term adverse effects may include erythema, pruritus, and pigmentation, whereas long-term adverse effects include premature skin aging and cutaneous malignancies. Topical psoralens combined with UVA may be equally effective. PUVA therapy in children with severe AD and growth suppression has resulted in accelerated growth.[205] However, the long-term risk of cutaneous malignancies has usually precluded treatment of children with PUVA.

Allergen Immunotherapy

Uncontrolled trials have suggested that desensitization to specific allergens may improve AD. In a double-blind controlled trial of desensitization with tyrosine-adsorbed *Dermatophagoides pteronyssinus* (house-dust mite) extract (Der p 1), children with AD and immediate hypersensitivity to *D. pteronyssinus* failed to demonstrate any clinical benefit from desensitization compared with placebo after an 8-month course of treatment.[206] In a second phase, children to whom *D. pteronyssinus* extract was initially administered were randomly assigned to continue on active treatment or placebo for an additional 6 months. The clinical scores suggested that extended desensitization was more effective than placebo, but the numbers were too small to permit confident conclusions. A high placebo effect may have concealed any additional therapeutic effect from active treatment. In a systematic review of immunotherapy for AD that included four comparable placebo-controlled studies involving a small number of patients, statistical analysis showed significant improvement in symptoms in patients with AD who received subcutaneous immunotherapy.[207]

A multicenter 1-year RCT of dust mite–pecific immunotherapy in sensitized AD patients showed a dose-dependent effect on disease symptoms.[208] An open-label study of patients with dust mite allergy and AD treated with subcutaneous dust mite allergoid demonstrated serologic and immunologic changes consistent with tolerance, in addition to significant reductions in objective and subjective SCORAD.[209] One double-blind, placebo-controlled study of children with AD treated with dust mite sublingual immunotherapy reported a significant difference from baseline values in visual analog scores, SCORAD, and medication use in the mild to moderate severity group, whereas patients with severe disease had only a marginal benefit.[210] Based on a review of available studies, the most recent practice parameter states that some data indicate immunotherapy can be effective for patients with AD when it is associated with aeroallergen sensitivity.[211]

Experimental and Unproven Therapies

Intravenous Immune Globulin

Because chronic inflammation and T cell activation appear to play a critical role in the pathogenesis of AD, high-dose intravenous immune globulin (IVIG) could have immunomodulatory effects in this disease. IVIG could also interact directly with infectious organisms or toxins involved in the pathogenesis of AD. IVIG has been shown to contain high concentrations of staphylococcal toxin-specific antibodies that inhibit the in-vitro activation of T cells by staphylococcal toxins.[212] The mechanism of inhibition by IVIG was direct blocking of toxin binding to, or presentation by, antigen-presenting cells. In addition, IVIG has been shown to reduce IL-4 protein expression in AD patients.[213]

Treatment of severe refractory AD with IVIG has yielded conflicting results. Studies have not been controlled and have involved small numbers of patients. In a study of nine patients with severe AD treated with IVIG (Venoglobulin-I, Alpha Therapeutic), 2 g/kg monthly for seven infusions, skin disease improved slightly in six patients, but their average daily prednisone dosage did not change significantly.[214] Mean serum IgE levels did not decrease significantly during IVIG therapy, and in-vitro IgE production by PBMCs after IL-4 and anti-CD40 stimulation was not significantly reduced. In contrast, a review of 32 AD patients treated with high-dose IVIG found clinical improvement in 61% of the patients.[215] Adults were less likely to respond (48%) than children (90%), and duration of response was also more prolonged in children.

Adjunctive therapy in adults was more effective than monotherapy (59% vs 0%), whereas monotherapy was effective in 90% of children. In a randomized placebo-controlled study, 48 children with moderate to severe AD were treated with three injections of 2.0 g/kg IVIG or placebo at 1-month intervals.[216] Assessments were conducted after each injection and at 3 and 6 months after completion of treatment. The disease severity index was significantly decreased at 3 months after treatment compared with baseline. However, improvement declined by 6 months after therapy.

Additional controlled studies are needed to answer the question of IVIG efficacy in a more definitive manner.

Omalizumab

Case reports and small case series in AD patients treated with omalizumab have shown both clinical benefit and lack of improvement.[217–223] Belloni and associates[222] could find no specific markers to identify responders to omalizumab. A prospective analysis assessed efficacy of omalizumab in 21 patients age 14 to 64 years with moderate to severe persistent allergic asthma and concomitant AD.[224] AD severity was assessed at 0, 1, 3, 6, and 9 months by Investigator Global Assessment; pretreatment serum IgE levels ranged from 18.2–8396 IU/mL (mean 1521 IU/mL). All 21 patients showed clinical and statistically significant improvement of their skin disease. However, a placebo-controlled trial of omalizumab given for 16 weeks to 20 patients with AD showed no significant clinical benefit.[225]

Recombinant Human Interferon-γ

Interferon-γ suppresses IgE synthesis and inhibits Th2 cell function. Treatment with subcutaneous recombinant human interferon-γ (rhIFN-γ) results in reduced clinical severity and decreased total circulating eosinophil counts in patients with AD.[226] Clinical improvement has also been shown to correlate with reduction in white blood cell, eosinophil, and lymphocyte counts and normalization of the CD4/CD8 ratio among large lymphocytes. Patients may show continued improvement several months after discontinuation of therapy. Two open, long-term studies showed clinical efficacy in AD patients receiving $50\,\mu g/m^2$ of rhIFN-γ daily or every other day for at least 22 months.[227,228] These studies demonstrated that patients with AD can be treated on a long-term basis with rhIFN-γ without deterioration of their disease or significant adverse effects. This is noteworthy because IFN-γ has proinflammatory effects in some clinical settings. Importantly, effective dosing with rhIFN-γ is associated with a decrease in eosinophil counts, suggesting that rhIFN-γ acts primarily on the allergic inflammatory response, as opposed to IgE synthesis. Therefore, a subset of patients treated with rhIFN-γ might respond to individualized titration of their treatment dose.[229]

Probiotics

Lactobacilli and *bifidobacteria* are gut microorganisms hypothesized to educate the neonatal immune system by converting the Th2-biased prenatal responses into balanced immune responses. Lactobacilli have been shown to prime monocyte-derived DCs to drive the development of T regulatory cells.[230] These Tregs produced increased levels of IL-10 and were capable of inhibiting the proliferation of bystander T cells in an IL-10-dependent manner. The mechanism was shown to be binding of the C-type lectin dendritic cell (DC)-specific intercellular adhesion molecule-3-grabbing non-integrin (DC-SIGN). Blocking antibodies to DC-SIGN inhibited the induction of the Tregs by these probiotic bacteria, stressing that ligation of DC-SIGN can actively prime DCs to induce Tregs and might explain their beneficial effect in AD.

Clinical trials in patients with AD have had varying results, and in addition, these supplements are currently not FDA regulated.[231–233] Administration of probiotics to pregnant women and subsequently to at-risk newborns to prevent AD or even to treat established AD was addressed in a review of therapeutic attempts to shift the presumed Th2 response early in life to a Th1 response.[234] Although one meta-analysis suggested a modest role for probiotics in children with moderately severe disease in reducing SCORAD,[235] another found that current evidence is more convincing for the efficacy of probiotics in the prevention rather than treatment of pediatric AD.[236] Furthermore, a study designed to reproduce earlier beneficial effects of probiotics in AD patients found that supplementation with *Lactobacillus* GG during pregnancy and early infancy neither reduced the incidence of AD nor altered the severity of AD in affected children, but was associated with an increased rate of recurrent episodes of wheezing bronchitis.[237]

A Cochrane review concluded that probiotics are not an effective treatment for AD in children, and that probiotic treatment carries a small risk of adverse events.[238] Salfeld and Kopp[239] pointed to flaws in the methodology of some analyses and the heterogeneity of treatment protocols, concluding that selection of the most beneficial probiotic strain or strains, use of probiotics with or without prebiotics, and timing of supplementation, along with optimal dose and delivery, remain to be determined. More recently, a meta-analysis of RCTs through 2011 that attempted to overcome some of the limitations of prior reviews found a reduction of approximately 20% in the incidence of AD and IgE-associated AD in infants and children with probiotic use.[240] Although these results are encouraging, probiotics for the prevention of AD remain investigational.

Rituximab

Rituximab, a chimeric anti-CD20 mAb developed for treatment of B cell malignancies was given to six patients with severe AD in an open trial.[241] Patients received two intravenous infusions of rituximab (1000 mg) 2 weeks apart, with all patients showing clinical improvement within 4 to 8 weeks. Histology of skin biopsies showed significant improvement in spongiosis and acanthosis, and dermal T cell and B cell infiltrates also decreased. Whereas circulating B cells were below detectable levels, lesional B cells were reduced by approximately 50%. Expression of IL-5 and IL-13 was also reduced after rituximab therapy. Although total serum IgE levels were reduced, allergen-specific IgE levels were not affected.

Dupilumab

Dupilumab®, a humanized anti-IL-4 receptor alpha mAb that blocks the action of IL-4 and IL-13, was recently reported to cause rapid reduction in clinical severity of AD and reduce pruritus in these patients.[109] Assessment of AD skin biopsies revealed that the abnormal molecular signatures characteristic of AD were reversed after treatment with dupilumab.[242]

Other Investigational Agents

Experimental and unproven therapies for AD include antifungals, traditional Chinese herbal therapy, essential fatty acids, and leukotriene receptor antagonists.

CONCLUSIONS

Although the diagnosis of AD continues to be based on the recognition of characteristic signs and symptoms, significant advances have been made in understanding the role of epidermal barrier defects and immune abnormalities in this increasingly prevalent disease. These studies have identified new mutations of key stratum corneum proteins and a deficiency in antimicrobial peptide synthesis by keratinocytes contributing to skin colonization and infection in AD. Other studies have revealed a multifunctional role for IgE in atopic skin inflammation. Furthermore, Th2-type cells with skin-homing capability, newly discovered Th22 cells, Langerhans cells, other dendritic cells, keratinocytes, mast cells, and eosinophils all contribute to the complex inflammatory process in AD. These observations have provided the rationale for development of immunomodulatory and anti-inflammatory agents in the treatment of chronic AD.[243] Identification of a specific biochemical or genetic marker could not only improve diagnostic capabilities but also lead to more specific strategies for studying the epidemiology and genetics of AD. Undoubtedly, the new insights into pathogenesis of AD will lead to more specific therapeutic agents and, perhaps eventually, to prevention of this disease.

REFERENCES

1. *Leung DYM, Guttman-Yassky E. Deciphering the complexities of atopic dermatitis: shifting paradigms in treatment approaches. J Allergy Clin Immunol 2014;134:769–79.
2. Hill LW, Sulzberger MB. Evolution of atopic dermatitis. Arch Dermatol Syph 1935;32:451–63.
3. Wallach D, Coste J, Tilles G, et al. The first images of atopic dermatitis: an attempt at retrospective diagnosis in dermatology. J Am Acad Dermatol 2005;53:684–9.
4. Kapoor R, Menon C, Hoffstad O, et al. The prevalence of atopic triad in children with physician-confirmed atopic dermatitis. J Am Acad Dermatol 2008;58:68–73.
5. *Elias PM, Wakefield JS. Mechanisms of abnormal lamellar body secretion and the dysfunctional skin barrier in patients with atopic dermatitis. J Allergy Clin Immunol 2014;134:781–91.
6. Schultz Larsen F. Atopic dermatitis: a genetic-epidemiologic study in a population-based twin sample. J Am Acad Dermatol 1993;28:719–23.
7. Schultz Larsen F, Diepgen T, Svensson A. The occurrence of atopic dermatitis in north Europe: an international questionnaire study. J Am Acad Dermatol 1996;34:760–4.
8. Laughter D, Istvan JA, Tofte SJ, et al. The prevalence of atopic dermatitis in Oregon schoolchildren. J Am Acad Dermatol 2000;43:649–55.
9. Shaw TE, Currie GP, Koudelka CW, et al. Eczema prevalence in the United States: data from the 2003 National Survey of Children's Health. J Invest Dermatol 2011;131:67–73.
10. Sugiura H, Umemoto N, Deguchi H, et al. Prevalence of childhood and adolescent atopic dermatitis in a Japanese population: comparison with the disease frequency examined 20 years ago. Acta Derm Venereol 1998;78:293–4.

11. Saeki H, Iizuka H, Mori Y, et al. Prevalence of atopic dermatitis in Japanese elementary schoolchildren. Br J Dermatol 2005;152:110–14.
12. Williams HC. Is the prevalence of atopic dermatitis increasing? Clin Exp Dermatol 1992;17:385–91.
13. Zeiger RS, Heller S, Mellon M, et al. Genetic and environmental factors affecting the development of atopy through age 4 in children of atopic parents: a prospective randomized study of food allergen avoidance. Pediatr Allergy Immunol 1992;3:110–27.
14. Zeiger RS, Heller S. The development and prediction of atopy in high-risk children: follow-up at age seven years in a prospective randomized study of combined maternal and infant food allergen avoidance. J Allergy Clin Immunol 1995;95:1179–90.
15. Kay J, Gawkrodger DJ, Mortimer MJ, et al. The prevalence of childhood atopic eczema in a general population. J Am Acad Dermatol 1994;30:35–9.
16. Williams HC, Strachan DP, Hay RJ. Childhood eczema: disease of the advantaged? Br Med J 1994;308:1132–5.
17. Hayashi T, Kawakami N, Kondo N, et al. Prevalence of and risk factors for allergic diseases: comparison of two cities in Japan. Ann Allergy Asthma Immunol 1995;75:525–9.
18. International Study of Asthma and Allergies in Childhood (ISAAC) Steering Committee. Worldwide variation in prevalence of symptoms of asthma, allergic rhinoconjunctivitis, and atopic eczema: ISAAC. Lancet 1998;351:1225–32.
19. Odhiambo JA, Williams HC, Clayton TO, et al. Global variations in prevalence of eczema symptoms in children from ISAAC Phase Three. J Allergy Clin Immunol 2009;124:1251–8.
20. *Barnes KC. An update on the genetics of atopic dermatitis: scratching the surface in 2009. J Allergy Clin Immunol 2010;125:16–29.
21. Palmer CN, Irvine AD, Terron-Kwiatkowski A, et al. Common loss-of-function variants of the epidermal barrier protein filaggrin are a major predisposing factor for atopic dermatitis. Nat Genet 2006;38:441–6.
22. *Irvine AD, McLean WH, Leung DY. Filaggrin mutations associated with skin and allergic diseases. N Engl J Med 2011;365:1315–27.
23. Brown SJ, Sandilands A, Zhao Y, et al. Prevalent and low-frequency null mutations in the filaggrin gene are associated with early-onset and persistent atopic eczema. J Invest Dermatol 2008; 128:1591–4.
24. Henderson J, Northstone K, Lee SP, et al. The burden of disease associated with filaggrin mutations: a population-based, longitudinal birth cohort study. J Allergy Clin Immunol 2008;121:872–7.
25. Kim BE, Leung DY, Boguniewicz M, et al. Loricrin and involucrin expression is down-regulated by Th2 cytokines through STAT-6. Clin Immunol 2008;126:332–7.
26. Bergmann RL, Edenharter G, Bergmann KE, et al. Atopic dermatitis in early infancy predicts allergic airway disease at 5 years. Clin Exp Allergy 1998;28:965–70.
27. Gustafsson D, Sjoberg O, Foucard T, et al. Development of allergies and asthma in infants and young children with atopic dermatitis: a prospective follow-up to 7 years of age. Allergy 2000;55:240–5.
28. Spergel JM, Mizoguchi E, Brewer JP, et al. Epicutaneous sensitization with protein antigen induces localized allergic dermatitis and hyperresponsiveness to methacholine after single exposure to aerosolized antigen in mice. J Clin Invest 1998;101:1614–22.
29. Fallon PG, Sasaki T, Sandilands A, et al. A homozygous frameshift mutation in the mouse *Flg* gene facilitates enhanced percutaneous allergen priming. Nat Genet 2009;41:602–8.
30. Nassif A, Chan SC, Storrs FJ, et al. Abnormal skin irritancy in atopic dermatitis and in atopy without dermatitis. Arch Dermatol 1994;130:1402–7.
31. Tabata N, Tagami H, Kligman AM. A twenty-four-hour occlusive exposure to 1% sodium lauryl sulfate induces a unique histopathologic inflammatory response in the xerotic skin of atopic dermatitis patients. Acta Derm Venereol 1998;78:244–7.
32. Bellou A, Kanny G, Fremont S, et al. Transfer of atopy following bone marrow transplantation. Ann Allergy Asthma Immunol 1997;78:513–16.
33. Brinkman L, Raajimakers JA, Bruijnzeel-Koomen C, et al. Bronchial and skin reactivity in asthmatic patients with and without atopic dermatitis. Eur Respir J 1997;10:1033–40.
34. Taha RA, Minshall EM, Miotto D, et al. Eotaxin and monocyte chemotactic protein- 4 mRNA expression in small airways of asthmatic and non-asthmatic individuals. J Allergy Clin Immunol 1999;103:476–83.
35. Taha RA, Leung DY, Minshall E, et al. Evidence for increased expression of eotaxin and monocyte chemotactic protein-4 in atopic dermatitis. J Allergy Clin Immunol 2000;105:1002–7.
36. Semper A, Heron K, Woollard A, et al. Surface expression of FεRI on Langerhans cells of clinically uninvolved skin is associated with disease activity in atopic dermatitis, allergic asthma, and rhinitis. J Allergy Clin Immunol 2003;112:411–19.
37. Vickers CF. The natural history of atopic eczema. Acta Derm Venereol 1980;92:113–15.
38. Linna O, Kokkonen J, Lahtela P, et al. Ten-year prognosis for generalized infantile eczema. Acta Paediatr 1992;81:1013–16.
39. Kissling S, Wuthrich B. Sites, types of manifestations and micromanifestations of atopic dermatitis in young adults: a personal follow-up 20 years after diagnosis in childhood. Hautarzt 1994;45:368–71.
40. Lammintausta K, Kalimo K, Raitala R, et al. Prognosis of atopic dermatitis: a prospective study in early adulthood. Int J Dermatol 1991;30:563–8.
41. Illi S, von Mutius E, Lau S, et al. The natural course of atopic dermatitis from birth to age 7 years and the association with asthma. J Allergy Clin Immunol 2004;113:925–31.
42. Howell MD, Kim BE, Gao P, et al. Cytokine modulation of atopic dermatitis filaggrin skin expression. J Allergy Clin Immunol 2007;120:150–5.
43. Nograles KE, Zaba LC, Shemer A, et al. IL-22-producing 'T22' T cells account for upregulated IL-22 in atopic dermatitis despite reduced IL-17-producing TH17 T cells. J Allergy Clin Immunol 2009;123:1244–52.

44. Bisgaard H, Simpson A, Palmer CN, et al. Gene-environment interaction in the onset of eczema in infancy: filaggrin loss-of-function mutations enhanced by neonatal cat exposure. PLoS Med 2008;5: e131.

45. Rodriguez E, Baurecht H, Herberich E, et al. Meta-analysis of filaggrin polymorphisms in eczema and asthma: robust risk factors for atopic disease. J Allergy Clin Immunol 2009;123:1361–70.

46. Van den Oord RA, Sheikh A. Filaggrin gene defects and risk of developing allergic sensitization and allergic disorders: systematic review and meta-analysis. BMJ 2009;339:b2433.

47. De Benedetto A, Rafaels NM, McGirt LY, et al. Tight junction defects in patients with atopic dermatitis. J Allergy Clin Immunol 2011;127:773–86.

48. Broccardo CJ, Mahaffey S, Schwarz J, et al. Comparative proteomic profiling of patients with atopic dermatitis based on history of eczema herpeticum infection and Staphylococcus aureus colonization. J Allergy Clin Immunol 2011;127:186–93.

49. *Hanifin JM, Rajka G. Diagnostic features of atopic dermatitis. Acta Derm Venereol (Stockh) 1980;92:44–7.

50. European Task Force on Atopic Dermatitis. Severity scoring of atopic dermatitis: the SCORAD index. Dermatology 1993;186:23–31.

51. Hanifin JM, Thurston M, Omoto M, et al. The eczema area and severity index (EASI): assessment of reliability in atopic dermatitis. EASI Evaluator Group. Exp Dermatol 2001;10:11–18.

52. Brydensholt HL, Loland L, Buchvald FF, et al. Development of atopic dermatitis during the first 3 years of life. Arch Dermatol 2006;142:561–6.

53. Bielory B, Bielory L. Atopic dermatitis and keratoconjunctivitis. Immunol Allergy Clin North Am 2010;30:323–36.

54. *Boguniewicz M, Leung DY. Recent insights into atopic dermatitis and implications for management of infectious complications. J Allergy Clin Immunol 2010;125:4–13.

55. Howell MD, Wollenberg A, Gallo RL, et al. Cathelicidin deficiency predisposes to eczema herpeticum. J Allergy Clin Immunol 2006;117:836–41.

56. Beck LA, Boguniewicz M, Hata T, et al. Phenotype of atopic dermatitis subjects with a history of eczema herpeticum. J Allergy Clin Immunol 2009;124:260–9.

57. Leung DY, Gao PS, Grigoryev DN, et al. Human atopic dermatitis complicated by eczema herpeticum is associated with abnormalities in gamma interferon response. J Allergy Clin Immunol 2011;127:965–73.

58. Gao PS, Leung DY, Rafaels NM, et al. Genetic variants in interferon regulatory factor 2 (IRF2) are associated with atopic dermatitis and eczema herpeticum. J Invest Dermatol 2012;132:650–7.

59. Casagrande BF, Fluckiger S, Linder MT, et al. Sensitization to the yeast Malassezia sympodialis is specific for extrinsic and intrinsic atopic eczema. J Invest Dermatol 2006;126:2414–21.

60. Cho SH, Strickland I, Boguniewicz M, et al. Fibronectin and fibrinogen contributes to the enhanced binding of S. aureus to atopic skin. J Allergy Clin Immunol 2001;108:269–74.

61. Leyden JE, Marples RR, Kligman AM. Staphylococcus aureus in the lesions of atopic dermatitis. Br J Dermatol 1974;90:525–30.

62. Williams J, Vowels B, Honig P, et al. S. aureus isolation from the lesions, the hands, and the anterior nares of patients with atopic dermatitis. Pediatr Dermatol 1998;15:194–8.

63. Leyden J, Kligman A. The case for steroid-antibiotic combinations. Br J Dermatol 1977;96:179–87.

64. Schlievert PM, Strandberg KL, Lin YC, et al. Secreted virulence factor comparison between methicillin-resistant and methicillin-sensitive Staphylococcus aureus, and its relevance to atopic dermatitis. J Allergy Clin Immunol 2010;125:39–49.

65. Torgerson TR, Ochs HD. Immune dysregulation, polyendocrinopathy, enteropathy, X-linked: Forkhead box protein 3 mutations and lack of regulatory T cells. J Allergy Clin Immunol 2007;120:744–50.

66. Holland SM, DeLeo FR, Elloumi HZ, et al. STAT3 mutations in the hyper-IgE syndrome. N Engl J Med 2007;357:1608–19.

67. Zhang Q, Davis JC, Lamborn IT, et al. Combined immunodeficiency associated with DOCK8 mutations. N Engl J Med 2009;361:2046–55.

68. *Nixon RL, Diepgen T. Contact dermatitis. In: Adkinson NF, Bochner BS, Burks AW, et al., editors. Middleton's allergy, principles and practice. 8th ed. Philadelphia: Elsevier; 2014. p. 565–74.

69. Kelsay K, Klinnert M, Bender B. Addressing psychosocial aspects of atopic dermatitis. Immunol Allergy Clin North Am 2010;30:385–96.

70. Koblenzer CS. Itching and the atopic skin. J Allergy Clin Immunol 1999;104:S109–13.

71. Kelsay K. Management of sleep disturbance associated with atopic dermatitis. J Allergy Clin Immunol 2006;118:198–201.

72. Caubet JC, Eigenmann PA. Allergic triggers in atopic dermatitis. Immunol Allergy Clin North Am 2010;30:289–307.

73. May CE. Objective clinical laboratory studies of immediate hypersensitivity reactions to foods in asthmatic children. J Allergy Clin Immunol 1976;58:500–15.

74. Sampson HA, McCaskill CC. Food hypersensitivity and atopic dermatitis: evaluation of 113 patients. J Pediatr 1985;107:669–75.

75. Sicherer SH, Sampson HA. Food hypersensitivity and atopic dermatitis: pathophysiology, epidemiology, diagnosis, and management. J Allergy Clin Immunol 1999;104:S114–22.

76. Van Reijsen FC, Felius A, Wauters EA, et al. T-cell reactivity for a peanut-derived epitope in the skin of a young infant with atopic dermatitis. J Allergy Clin Immunol 1998;101:207–9.

77. Schade RP, van Ieperen-van Dijk AG, Van Reijsen FC, et al. Differences in antigen-specific T-cell responses between infants with atopic dermatitis with and without cow's milk allergy: relevance of TH2 cytokines. J Allergy Clin Immunol 2000;106:1155–62.

78. Sampson HA, Broadbent K, Bernhisel-Broadbent J. Spontaneous basophil histamine release and histamine-releasing factor in patients with atopic dermatitis and food hypersensitivity. N Engl J Med 1989;321:228–32.

79. Van der Heijden F, Wierenga EA, Bos JD, et al. High frequency of IL-4 producing CD4[+] allergen-specific T lymphocytes in atopic dermatitis lesional skin. J Invest Dermatol 1991;97:389–94.
80. Tuft L. Importance of inhalant allergens in atopic dermatitis. J Invest Dermatol 1949;12:211–19.
81. Tupker RA, De Monchy JG, Coenraade PJ, et al. Induction of atopic dermatitis by inhalation of house dust mite. J Allergy Clin Immunol 1996;97:1064–70.
82. Clark RA, Adinoff AD. The relationship between positive aeroallergen patch test reactions and aeroallergen exacerbations of atopic dermatitis. Clin Immunol Immunopathol 1989;53:S132–40.
83. Langeveld-Wildschut EG, Bruijnzeel PL, Mudde GC, et al. Clinical and immunologic variables in skin of patients with atopic eczema and either positive or negative atopy patch test reactions. J Allergy Clin Immunol 2000;105:1008–16.
84. Schafer T, Heinrich J, Wjst M, et al. Association between severity of atopic eczema and degree of sensitization to aeroallergens in schoolchildren. J Allergy Clin Immunol 1999;104:1280–4.
85. Tan BB, Weald D, Strickland I, et al. Double-blind controlled trial of effect of housedust-mite allergen avoidance on atopic dermatitis. Lancet 1996;347:15–18.
86. Holm L, Ohman S, Bengtsson A, et al. Effectiveness of occlusive bedding in the treatment of atopic dermatitis: a placebo-controlled trial of 12 months' duration. Allergy 2001;56:152–8.
87. *Leung DY, Harbeck R, Bina P, et al. Presence of IgE antibodies to staphylococcal exotoxins on the skin of patients with atopic dermatitis: evidence for a new group of allergens. J Clin Invest 1993;92:1374–80.
88. Bunikowski R, Mielke M, Skarabis H, et al. Prevalence and role of serum IgE antibodies to the *Staphylococcus aureus*-derived superantigens SEA and SEB in children with atopic dermatitis. J Allergy Clin Immunol 1999;103:119–24.
89. Nomura I, Tanaka K, Tomita H, et al. Evaluation of the staphylococcal exotoxins and their specific IgE in childhood atopic dermatitis. J Allergy Clin Immunol 1999;104:441–6.
90. Strickland I, Hauk PJ, Trumble AE, et al. Evidence for superantigen involvement in skin homing of T cells in atopic dermatitis. J Invest Dermatol 1999;112:249–53.
91. Bunikowski R, Mielke ME, Skarabis H, et al. Evidence for a disease-promoting effect of *Staphylococcus aureus*-derived exotoxins in atopic dermatitis. J Allergy Clin Immunol 2000;105:814–19.
92. Herz U, Schnoy N, Borelli S, et al. A human-SCID mouse model for allergic immune response bacterial superantigen enhances skin inflammation and suppresses IgE production. J Invest Dermatol 1998;110:224–31.
93. Hofer MF, Harbeck RJ, Schlievert PM, et al. Staphylococcal toxins augment specific IgE responses by atopic patients exposed to allergen. J Invest Dermatol 1999;112:171–6.
94. Cardona ID, Goleva E, Ou L-S, et al. Staphylococcal enterotoxin B inhibits regulatory T cells by inducing glucocorticoid induced TNF receptor-related protein ligand on monocytes. J Allergy Clin Immunol 2006;117:688–95.
95. Hauk PJ, Hamid QA, Chrousos GP, et al. Induction of corticosteroid insensitivity in human PBMCs by microbial superantigens. J Allergy Clin Immunol 2000;105:782–7.
96. Strange P, Skov L, Lisby S, et al. Staphylococcal enterotoxin B applied on intact normal and intact atopic skin induces dermatitis. Arch Dermatol 1996;132:27–33.
97. Skov L, Olsen JV, Giorno R, et al. Application of staphylococcal enterotoxin B on normal and atopic skin induces upregulation of T cells via a superantigen- mediated mechanism. J Allergy Clin Immunol 2000;105:820–6.
98. Valenta R, Seiberler S, Natter S, et al. Autoallergy: a pathogenetic factor in atopic dermatitis? J Allergy Clin Immunol 2000;105:432–7.
99. Valenta R, Natter S, Seiberler S, et al. Molecular characterization of an autoallergen, Hom s 1, identified by serum IgE from atopic dermatitis patients. J Invest Dermatol 1998;111:1178–83.
100. Ochs RL, Muro Y, Si Y, et al. Autoantibodies to DFS 70 kd/transcription coactivator p75 in atopic dermatitis and other conditions. J Allergy Clin Immunol 2000;105(1211–1220).
101. Schmid-Grendelmeier P, Fluckiger S, Disch R, et al. IgE-mediated and T cell-mediated autoimmunity against manganese superoxide dismutase in atopic dermatitis. J Allergy Clin Immunol 2005;115:1068–75.
102. Leung DYM, Boguniewicz M, Howell M, et al. New insights into atopic dermatitis. J Clin Invest 2004;113:651–7.
103. Akdis CA, Akdis M, Simon D, et al. T cells and T cell-derived cytokines as pathogenic factors in the non-allergic form of atopic dermatitis. J Invest Dermatol 1999;113:628–34.
104. Kimura M, Tsuruta S, Yoshida T. Unique profile of IL-4 and IFN-γ production by peripheral blood mononuclear cells in infants with atopic dermatitis. J Allergy Clin Immunol 1998;102:238–44.
105. Kimura M, Tsuruta S, Yoshida T. Correlation of house dust mite-specific lymphocyte proliferation with IL-5 production, eosinophilia, and the severity of symptoms in infants with atopic dermatitis. J Allergy Clin Immunol 1998;101:84–9.
106. Van Reijsen FC, Bruijnzeel-Koomen CA, Kalthoff FS, et al. Skin-derived aeroallergen-specific T-cell clones of Th2 phenotype in patients with atopic dermatitis. J Allergy Clin Immunol 1992;90:184–93.
107. Teraki Y, Hotta T, Shiohara T. Increased circulating skin-homing cutaneous lymphocyte-associated antigen (CLA)[+] type 2 cytokine-producing cells, and decreased CLA[+] type 1 cytokine-producing cells in atopic dermatitis. Br J Dermatol 2000;143:373–8.
108. Vercelli J, Jabara HH, Lauener RP, et al. IL-4 inhibits the synthesis of IFN-γ and induces the synthesis of IgE in human mixed lymphocyte cultures. J Immunol 1990;144:570–3.
109. *Beck LA, Thaci D, Hamilton JD, et al. Dupilumab treatment in adults with moderate-to-severe atopic dermatitis. N Engl J Med 2014;371:130–9.
110. Yoo J, Omori M, Gyarmati D, et al. Spontaneous atopic dermatitis in mice expressing an inducible thymic stromal lymphopoietin transgene specifically in the skin. J Exp Med 2005;202:541–9.
111. Vu AT, Baba T, Chen X, et al. *Staphylococcus aureus* membrane and diacylated lipopeptide induce thymic stromal lymphopoietin in keratinocytes through the Toll- like receptor 2-Toll-like receptor 6 pathway. J Allergy Clin Immunol 2010;126:985–93.

112. Ong PY, Ohtake T, Brandt C, et al. Endogenous antimicrobial peptides and skin infections in atopic dermatitis. N Engl J Med 2002;347:1151–60.

113. Schauber J, Gallo RL. Antimicrobial peptides and the skin immune defense system. J Allergy Clin Immunol 2008;122:261–6.

114. Hata TR, Kotol P, Jackson M, et al. Administration of oral vitamin D induces cathelicidin production in atopic individuals. J Allergy Clin Immunol 2008;122:829–31.

115. Camargo CA Jr, Ganmaa D, Sidbury R, et al. Randomized trial of vitamin D supplementation for winter-related atopic dermatitis in children. J Allergy Clin Immunol 2014;134:831–5.

116. Hamid Q, Boguniewicz M, Leung DY. Differential in situ cytokine gene expression in acute versus chronic atopic dermatitis. J Clin Invest 1994;94:870–6.

117. Hamid Q, Naseer T, Minshall EM, et al. In vivo expression of IL-12 and IL-13 in atopic dermatitis. J Allergy Clin Immunol 1996;98:225–31.

118. Thepen T, Langeveld-Wildschut EG, Bihari IC, et al. Biphasic response against aeroallergen in atopic dermatitis showing a switch from an initial TH2 response to a TH1 response in situ: an immunocyto-chemical study. J Allergy Clin Immunol 1996;97:828–37.

119. Schade RP, van Ieperen-van Dijk AG, van Reijsen FC, et al. Differences in antigen-specific T-cell responses between infants with atopic dermatitis with and without cow's milk allergy: relevance of TH2 cytokines. J Allergy Clin Immunol 2000;106:1155–62.

120. Steinhoff M, Bienenstock J, Schmelz M, et al. Neurophysiological, neuroimmunological, and neuroen-docrine basis of pruritus. J Invest Dermatol 2006;126:1705–18.

121. Bilsborough J, Leung DY, Maurer M, et al. IL-31 is associated with cutaneous lymphocyte antigen-positive skin homing T cells in patients with atopic dermatitis. J Allergy Clin Immunol 2006;117:418–25.

122. Neis MM, Peters B, Dreuw A, et al. Enhanced expression levels of IL-31 correlate with IL-4 and IL-13 in atopic and allergic contact dermatitis. J Allergy Clin Immunol 2006;118:930–7.

123. Sonkoly E, Muller A, Lauerma AI, et al. IL-31: a new link between T cells and pruritus in atopic skin inflammation. J Allergy Clin Immunol 2006;117:411–17.

124. Ziegler SF, Artis D. Sensing the outside world: TSLP regulates barrier immunity. Nat Immunol 2010;11:289–93.

125. Gao PS, Rafaels NM, Mu D, et al. Genetic variants in thymic stromal lymphopoietin are associated with atopic dermatitis and eczema herpeticum. J Allergy Clin Immunol 2010;125:1403–7.

126. Laberge S, Ghaffar O, Boguniewicz M, et al. Association of increased CD4$^+$ T-cell infiltration with increased IL-16 gene expression in atopic dermatitis. J Allergy Clin Immunol 1998;102:645–50.

127. Muller KM, Jaunin F, Masouye I, et al. Th2 cells mediate IL-4-dependent local tissue inflammation. J Immunol 1993;150:5576–84.

128. Mudde GC, van Reijsen FC, Boland GJ, et al. Allergen presentation by epidermal Langerhans cells from patients with atopic dermatitis is mediated by IgE. Immunology 1990;69:335–41.

129. Jürgens M, Wollenberg A, Hanau D, et al. Activation of human epidermal Langerhans cells by engage-ment of the high affinity receptor for IgE, FcεRI. J Immunol 1995;155:5184–9.

130. Abernathy-Carver KJ, Sampson HA, Picker LJ, et al. Milk-induced eczema is associated with the expan-sion of T cells expressing cutaneous lymphocyte antigen. J Clin Invest 1995;95:913–18.

131. Santamaria Babi LF, Picker LJ, Soler MT, et al. Circulating allergen-reactive T cells from patients with atopic dermatitis and allergic contact dermatitis express the skin-selective receptor, the cutaneous lymphocyte-associated antigen. J Exp Med 1995;181:1935–40.

132. *Schneider L, Lio P, Boguniewicz M, et al. Atopic dermatitis: a practice parameter update 2012. J Allergy Clin Immunol 2013;131:295–9.

133. Boguniewicz M, Nicol N, Kelsay K, et al. A multidisciplinary approach to evaluation and treatment of atopic dermatitis. Semin Cutan Med Surg 2008;27:115–27.

134. Akdis CA, Akdis M, Bieber T, et al. Diagnosis and treatment of atopic dermatitis in children and adults. European Academy of Allergology and Clinical Immunology/American Academy of Allergy, Asthma and Immunology/PRACTALL Consensus Report. J Allergy Clin Immunol 2006;118:152–69.

135. Sicherer SH, Sampson HA. Food allergy. J Allergy Clin Immunol 2006;117:S470–5.

136. Mehl A, Rolinck-Werninghaus C, Staden U, et al. The atopy patch test in the diagnostic workup of suspected food-related symptoms in children. J Allergy Clin Immunol 2006;118:923–9.

137. Holm L, Ohman S, Bengtsson A, et al. Effectiveness of occlusive bedding in the treatment of atopic dermatitis: a placebo-controlled trial of 12 months' duration. Allergy 2001;56:152–8.

138. Nicol NH, Ersser SJ. The role of the nurse educator in managing atopic dermatitis. Immunol Allergy Clin North Am 2010;30:369–83.

139. Zuberbier T, Orlow SJ, Paller AS, et al. Patient perspectives on the management of atopic dermatitis. J Allergy Clin Immunol 2006;118:226–32.

140. Imokawa G, Abe A, Jin K, et al. Decreased level of ceramides in stratum corneum of atopic dermatitis: an etiologic factor in atopic dry skin? J Invest Dermatol 1991;96:523–6.

141. Huang JT, Abrams M, Tlougan B, et al. Treatment of *Staphylococcus aureus* colonization in atopic dermatitis decreases disease severity. Pediatrics 2009;123:e808–14.

142. Lucky AW, Leach AD, Laskarzewski P, et al. Use of an emollient as a steroid- sparing agent in the treat-ment of mild to moderate atopic dermatitis in children. Pediatr Dermatol 1997;14:321–4.

143. Vilaplana J, Coll J, Trullas C, et al. Clinical and non-invasive evaluation of 12% ammonium lactate emulsion for the treatment of dry skin in atopic and non-atopic subjects. Acta Derm Venereol 1992;72:28–33.

144. Lavker RM, Kaidbey K, Leyden J. Effects of topical ammonium lactate on cutaneous atrophy from a potent topical corticosteroid. J Am Acad Dermatol 1992;26:535–44.

145. Hara J, Higuchi K, Okamoto R, et al. High expression of sphingomyelin deacylase is an important determinant of ceramide deficiency leading to barrier disruption in atopic dermatitis. J Invest Dermatol 2000;115:406–13.

146. Chamlin SL, Kao J, Frieden IJ, et al. Ceramide-dominant barrier repair lipids alleviate childhood atopic dermatitis: changes in barrier function provide a sensitive indicator of disease activity. J Am Acad Dermatol 2002;47:198–208.

147. Boguniewicz M, Zeichner JA, Eichenfield LF, et al. MAS063DP is effective monotherapy for mild to moderate atopic dermatitis in infants and children: a multicenter, randomized, vehicle-controlled study. J Pediatr 2008;152:854–9.

148. Rapaport MJ, Rapaport V. Eyelid dermatitis to red face syndrome to cure: clinical experience in 100 cases. J Am Acad Dermatol 1999;41:435–42.

149. Matura M, Goossens A. Contact allergy to corticosteroids. Allergy 2000;55:698–704.

150. Long CC, Mills CM, Finlay AY. A practical guide to topical therapy in children. Br J Dermatol 1998;138:293–6.

151. Wolkerstorfer A, Strobos MA, Glazenburg EJ, et al. Fluticasone propionate 0.05% cream once daily versus clobetasone butyrate 0.05% cream twice daily in children with atopic dermatitis. J Am Acad Dermatol 1998;39:226–31.

152. Lebwohl M. A comparison of once-daily application of mometasone furoate 0.1% cream compared with twice-daily hydrocortisone valerate 0.2% cream in pediatric atopic dermatitis patients who failed to respond to hydrocortisone. Mometasone Furoate Study Group. Int J Dermatol 1999;38:604–6.

153. Suarez-Farinas M, Tintle SJ, Shemer A, et al. Non-lesional atopic dermatitis skin is characterized by broad terminal differentiation defects and variable immune abnormalities. J Allergy Clin Immunol 2011;127:954–64.

154. Schmitt J, von Kobyletzki L, Svensson A, et al. Efficacy and tolerability of proactive treatment with topical corticosteroids and calcineurin inhibitors for atopic eczema: systematic review and meta-analysis of randomized controlled trials. Br J Dermatol 2011;164:415–28.

155. Stalder JF, Fleury M, Sourisse M. Local steroid therapy and bacterial skin flora in atopic dermatitis. Br J Dermatol 1994;131:536–40.

156. Nimmagadda SR, Szefler SJ, Spahn JD, et al. Allergen exposure decreases glucocorticoid receptor binding affinity and steroid responsiveness in atopic asthmatics. Am J Respir Crit Care Med 1997;155:87–93.

157. Herrscher RF, Kasper C, Sullivan TJ. Endogenous cortisol regulates immunoglobulin E-dependent late phase reaction. J Clin Invest 1992;90:596–603.

158. Blotta MH, DeKruyff RH, Umetsu DT. Corticosteroids inhibit IL-12 production in human monocytes and enhance their capacity to induce IL-4 synthesis in CD4+ lymphocytes. J Immunol 1997;158:5589–95.

159. Charman CR, Morris AD, Williams HC. Topical corticosteroid phobia in patients with atopic eczema. Br J Dermatol 2000;142:931–6.

160. Boguniewicz M, Eichenfield LF, Hultsch T. Current management of atopic dermatitis and interruption of the atopic march. J Allergy Clin Immunol 2003;112:S140–50.

161. Hanifin JM, Paller AS, Eichenfield L, et al. Efficacy and safety of tacrolimus ointment treatment for up to 4 years in patients with atopic dermatitis. J Am Acad Dermatol 2005;53:S186–94.

162. Papp KA, Werfel T, Folster-Holst R, et al. Long-term control of atopic dermatitis with pimecrolimus cream 1% in infants and young children: a two-year study. J Am Acad Dermatol 2005;52:240–6.

163. Leung DY, Hanifin JM, Pariser DM, et al. Effects of pimecrolimus cream 1% in the treatment of patients with atopic dermatitis who demonstrate a clinical insensitivity to topical corticosteroids: a randomized, multicentre vehicle-controlled trial. Br J Dermatol 2009;161:435–43.

164. Paul C, Cork M, Rossi AB, et al. Safety and tolerability of 1% pimecrolimus cream among infants: experience with 1133 patients treated for up to 2 years. Pediatrics 2006;117:e118.

165. Fonacier L, Spergel J, Charlesworth EN, et al. Report of the Topical Calcineurin Task Force of the American College of Allergy, Asthma and Immunology and the American Academy of Allergy, Asthma and Immunology. J Allergy Clin Immunol 2005;115:1249–53.

166. Arellano FM, Wentworth CE, Arana A, et al. Risk of lymphoma following exposure to calcineurin inhibitors and topical steroids in patients with atopic dermatitis. J Invest Dermatol 2007;127:808–16.

167. Ho VC, Gupta A, Kaufmann R, et al. Safety and efficacy of non-steroid pimecrolimus cream 1% in the treatment of atopic dermatitis in infants. J Pediatr 2003;142:155–62.

168. Kapp A, Papp K, Bingham A, et al. Long-term management of atopic dermatitis in infants with topical pimecrolimus, a non-steroid anti-inflammatory drug. J Allergy Clin Immunol 2002;110:277–84.

169. Wahn U, Bos JD, Goodfield M, et al. Efficacy and safety of pimecrolimus cream in the long-term management of atopic dermatitis in children. Pediatrics 2002;110:e2.

170. Langeveld-Wildschut EG, Riedl H, Thepen T, et al. Modulation of the atopy patch test reaction by topical corticosteroids and tar. J Allergy Clin Immunol 2000;106:737–43.

171. Lee JH, Lee SJ, Kim D, et al. The effect of wet dressing on epidermal barrier in patients with atopic dermatitis. J Eur Acad Dermatol Venereol 2007;21:1360–8.

172. Wolkerstorfer A, Visser RL, de Waard-van der Spek FB, et al. Efficacy and safety of wet-wrap dressings in children with severe atopic dermatitis: influence of corticosteroid dilution. Br J Dermatol 2000;143:999–1004.

173. Boguniewicz M, Sampson H, Harbeck R, et al. Effects of cefuroxime axetil on S. aureus colonization and superantigen production in atopic dermatitis. J Allergy Clin Immunol 2001;108:651–2.

174. Breneman DL, Hanifin JM, Berge CA, et al. The effect of antibacterial soap with 1.5% triclocarban on Staphylococcus aureus in patients with atopic dermatitis. Cutis 2000;66:296–300.

175. Rukwied R, Lischetzki G, McGlone F, et al. Mast cell mediators other than histamine induce pruritus in atopic dermatitis patients: a dermal microdialysis study. Br J Dermatol 2000;142:1114–20.

176. Metze D, Reimann S, Beissert S, et al. Efficacy and safety of naltrexone, an oral opiate receptor antagonist, in the treatment of pruritus in internal and dermatological diseases. J Am Acad Dermatol 1999;41:533–9.

177. Berth-Jones J, Graham-Brown RA, Marks R, et al. Long-term efficacy and safety of cyclosporin in severe adult atopic dermatitis. Br J Dermatol 1997;136:76–81.

178. Diepgen TL. Long-term treatment with cetirizine of infants with atopic dermatitis: a multi-country, double-blind, randomized, placebo-controlled trial (the ETAC trial) over 18 months. Early Treatment of the Atopic Child Study Group. Pediatr Allergy Immunol 2002;13:278–86.

179. Drake LA, Fallon JD, Sober A, et al. Relief of pruritus in patients with atopic dermatitis after treatment with topical doxepin cream. J Am Acad Dermatol 1994;31:613–16.

180. Shelley WB, Shelley ED, Talanin NY. Self-potentiating allergic contact dermatitis caused by doxepin hydrochloride cream. J Am Acad Dermatol 1996;34:143–4.

181. Sowden JM, Berth-Jones J, Ross JS, et al. Double-blind, controlled, crossover study of cyclosporin in adults with severe refractory atopic dermatitis. Lancet 1991;338:137–40.

182. Van Joost T, Heule F, Korstanje M, et al. Cyclosporin in atopic dermatitis: a multicentre placebo-controlled study. Br J Dermatol 1994;130:634–40.

183. Harper JI, Ahmed I, Barclay G, et al. Cyclosporin for severe childhood atopic dermatitis: short course versus continuous therapy. Br J Dermatol 2000;142:52–8.

184. Bunikowski R, Staab D, Kussebi F, et al. Low-dose cyclosporin A microemulsion in children with severe atopic dermatitis: clinical and immunologic effects. Pediatr Allergy Immunol 2001;12:216–23.

185. Schmitt J, von Kobyletzki L, Svensson A, et al. Efficacy and tolerability of proactive treatment with topical corticosteroids and calcineurin inhibitors for atopic eczema: systematic review and meta-analysis of randomized controlled trials. Br J Dermatol 2011;164:415–28.

186. Granlund H, Erkko P, Sinisalo M, et al. Cyclosporin in atopic dermatitis: time to relapse and effect of intermittent therapy. Br J Dermatol 1995;132:106–12.

187. Berth-Jones J, Graham-Brown RA, Marks R, et al. Long-term efficacy and safety of cyclosporin in severe adult atopic dermatitis. Br J Dermatol 1997;136:76–81.

188. Haeck IM, Knol MJ, Ten Berge O, et al. Enteric-coated mycophenolate sodium versus cyclosporin A as long-term treatment in adult patients with severe atopic dermatitis: a randomized controlled trial. J Am Acad Dermatol 2011;64:1074–84.

189. Heller M, Shin HT, Orlow SJ, et al. Mycophenolate mofetil for severe childhood atopic dermatitis: experience in 14 patients. Br J Dermatol 2007;157:127–32.

190. Schram ME, Borgonjen RJ, Bik CM, et al. Off-label use of azathioprine in dermatology: a systematic review. Arch Dermatol 2011;147:474–88.

191. Weatherhead SC, Wahie S, Reynolds NJ, et al. An open-label, dose-ranging study of methotrexate for moderate-to-severe adult atopic eczema. Br J Dermatol 2007;156:346–51.

192. Goujon C, Berard F, Dahel K, et al. Methotrexate for the treatment of adult atopic dermatitis. Eur J Dermatol 2006;16:155–8.

193. Lyakhovitsky A, Barzilai A, Heyman R, et al. Low-dose methotrexate treatment for moderate-to-severe atopic dermatitis in adults. J Eur Acad Dermatol Venereol 2010;24:43–9.

194. Krutmann J, Diepgen TL, Luger TA, et al. High-dose UVA1 therapy for atopic dermatitis: results of a multicenter trial. J Am Acad Dermatol 1998;38:589–93.

195. Krutmann J, Czech W, Diepgen T, et al. High-dose UVA1 therapy in the treatment of patients with atopic dermatitis. J Am Acad Dermatol 1992;26:225–30.

196. Abeck D, Schmidt T, Fesq H, et al. Long-term efficacy of medium-dose UVA1 phototherapy in atopic dermatitis. J Am Acad Dermatol 2000;42:254–7.

197. Tintle S, Shemer A, Suarez-Farinas M, et al. Reversal of atopic dermatitis with narrowband UVB phototherapy and biomarkers for therapeutic response. J Allergy Clin Immunol 2011;128:583–93.

198. Clayton TH, Clark SM, Turner D, et al. The treatment of severe atopic dermatitis in childhood with narrowband ultraviolet B phototherapy. Clin Exp Dermatol 2007;32:28–33.

199. Tan E, Lim D, Rademaker M. Narrowband UVB phototherapy in children: a New Zealand experience. Australasian J Dermatol 2010;51:268–73.

200. Meduri NB, Vandergriff T, Rasmussen H, et al. Phototherapy in the management of atopic dermatitis: a systematic review. Photodermatol Photoimmunol Photomed 2007;23:106–12.

201. Gambichler T, Othlinghaus N, Tomi NS, et al. Medium-dose ultraviolet (UV) A1 vs. narrowband UVB phototherapy in atopic eczema: a randomized crossover study. Br J Dermatol 2009;160:652–8.

202. Majoie IM, Oldhoff JM, van Weelden H, et al. Narrowband ultraviolet B and medium-dose ultraviolet A1 are equally effective in the treatment of moderate to severe atopic dermatitis. J Am Acad Dermatol 2009;60:77–84.

203. Silva SH, Guedes AC, Gontijo B, et al. Influence of narrow-band UVB phototherapy on cutaneous microbiota of children with atopic dermatitis. J Eur Acad Dermatol Venereol 2006;20:1114–20.

204. Tzaneva S, Kittler H, Holzer G, et al. 5-Methoxypsoralen plus ultraviolet (UV) A is superior to medium-dose UVA1 in the treatment of severe atopic dermatitis: a randomized crossover trial. Br J Dermatol 2010;162:655–60.

205. Sheehan MP, Atherton DJ, Norris P, et al. Oral psoralen photochemotherapy in severe childhood atopic eczema: an update. Br J Dermatol 1993;129:431–6.

206. Glover MT, Atherton DJ. A double-blind controlled trial of hyposensitization to Dermatophagoides pteronyssinus in children with atopic eczema. Clin Exp Allergy 1992;22:440–6.

207. Bussmann C, Bockenhoff A, Henke H, et al. Does allergen-specific immunotherapy represent a therapeutic option for patients with atopic dermatitis? J Allergy Clin Immunol 2006;118:1292–8.

208. Werfel T, Breuer K, Rueff F, et al. Usefulness of specific immunotherapy in patients with atopic dermatitis and allergic sensitization to house dust mites: a multi-centre, randomized, dose-response study. Allergy 2006;61:202–5.

209. Bussmann C, Maintz L, Hart J, et al. Clinical improvement and immunologic changes in atopic dermatitis patients undergoing subcutaneous immunotherapy with a house dust mite allergoid: a pilot study. Clin Exp Allergy 2007;37:1277–85.

210. Pajno GB, Caminiti L, Vita D, et al. Sublingual immunotherapy in mite-sensitized children with atopic dermatitis: a randomized, double-blind, placebo-controlled study. J Allergy Clin Immunol 2007;120:164–70.

211. Cox L, Nelson H, Lockey R, et al. Allergen immunotherapy: a practice parameter, third update. J Allergy Clin Immunol 2011;127:S1–55.
212. Takei S, Arora YK, Walker SM. Intravenous immunoglobulin contains specific antibodies inhibitory to activation of T cells by staphylococcal toxin superantigens. J Clin Invest 1993;91:602–7.
213. Jolles S, Hughes J, Rustin M. Intracellular interleukin-4 profiles during high-dose intravenous immunoglobulin treatment of therapy-resistant atopic dermatitis. J Am Acad Dermatol 1999;40:121–3.
214. Wakim M, Alazard M, Yajima A, et al. High dose intravenous immunoglobulin in atopic dermatitis and hyper-IgE syndrome. Ann Allergy Asthma Immunol 1998;81:153–8.
215. Jolles S. A review of high-dose intravenous immunoglobulin treatment for atopic dermatitis. Clin Exp Dermatol 2002;27:3–7.
216. Jee SJ, Kim JH, Baek HS, et al. Long-term efficacy of intravenous immunoglobulin therapy for moderate to severe childhood atopic dermatitis. Allergy Asthma Immunol Res 2011;3:89–95.
217. Krathen RA, Hsu S. Failure of omalizumab for treatment of severe adult atopic dermatitis. J Am Acad Dermatol 2005;53:338.
218. Lane JE, Cheyney JM, Lane TN, et al. Treatment of recalcitrant atopic dermatitis with omalizumab. J Am Acad Dermatol 2006;54:68–72.
219. Park SY, Choi MR, Na JI, et al. Recalcitrant atopic dermatitis treated with omalizumab. Ann Dermatol 2010;22:349–52.
220. Amrol D. Anti-immunoglobulin E in the treatment of refractory atopic dermatitis. South Med J 2010;103:554–8.
221. Caruso C, Gaeta F, Valluzzi RL, et al. Omalizumab efficacy in a girl with atopic eczema. Allergy 2010;65:278–9.
222. Belloni B, Ziai M, Lim A, et al. Low-dose anti-IgE therapy in patients with atopic eczema with high serum IgE levels. J Allergy Clin Immunol 2007;120:1223–5.
223. Vigo PG, Girgis KR, Pfuetze BL, et al. Efficacy of anti-IgE therapy in patients with atopic dermatitis. J Am Acad Dermatol 2006;55:168–70.
224. Sheinkopf LE, Rafi AW, Do LT, et al. Efficacy of omalizumab in the treatment of atopic dermatitis: a pilot study. Allergy Asthma Proc 2008;29:530–7.
225. Heil PM, Maurer D, Klein B, et al. Omalizumab therapy in atopic dermatitis: depletion of IgE does not improve the clinical course – a randomized, placebo- controlled and double-blind pilot study. J Dtsch Dermatol Ges 2010;8:990–8.
226. Boguniewicz M, Jaffe HS, Izu A, et al. Recombinant γ interferon in treatment of patients with atopic dermatitis and elevated IgE levels. Am J Med 1990;88:365–70.
227. Schneider LC, Baz Z, Zarcone C, et al. Long-term therapy with recombinant interferon-γ (rIFN-γ) for atopic dermatitis. Ann Allergy Asthma Immunol 1998;80:263–8.
228. Stevens SR, Hanifin JM, Hamilton T, et al. Long-term effectiveness and safety of recombinant human interferon-γ therapy for atopic dermatitis despite unchanged serum IgE levels. Arch Dermatol 1998;134:799–804.
229. Boguniewicz M, Leung DY. Atopic dermatitis: a question of balance. Arch Dermatol 1998;134:870–1.
230. Smits HH, Engering A, van der Kleij D, et al. Selective probiotic bacteria induce IL- 10-producing regulatory T cells in-vitro by modulating dendritic cell function through dendritic cell-specific intercellular adhesion molecule 3-grabbing non-integrin. J Allergy Clin Immunol 2005;115:1260–7.
231. Kalliomaki M, Salminen S, Poussa T, et al. Probiotics and prevention of atopic disease: 4-year follow-up of a randomised placebo-controlled trial. Lancet 2003;361:1869–71.
232. Rosenfeldt V, Benfeldt E, Nielsen SD, et al. Effect of probiotic Lactobacillus strains in children with atopic dermatitis. J Allergy Clin Immunol 2003;111:389–95.
233. Weston S, Halbert A, Richmond P, et al. Effects of probiotics on atopic dermatitis: a randomised controlled trial. Arch Dis Child 2005;90:892–7.
234. Jung T, Stingl G. Atopic dermatitis: therapeutic concepts evolving from new pathophysiologic insights. J Allergy Clin Immunol 2008;122:1074–81.
235. Michail SK, Stolfi A, Johnson T, et al. Efficacy of probiotics in the treatment of pediatric atopic dermatitis: a meta-analysis of randomized controlled trials. Ann Allergy Asthma Immunol 2008;101:508–16.
236. Lee J, Seto D, Bielory L. Meta-analysis of clinical trials of probiotics for prevention and treatment of pediatric atopic dermatitis. J Allergy Clin Immunol 2008;121:116–21.
237. Kopp MV, Hennemuth I, Heinzmann A, et al. Randomized, double-blind, placebo-controlled trial of probiotics for primary prevention: no clinical effects of Lactobacillus GG supplementation. Pediatrics 2008;121:e850–6.
238. Boyle RJ, Bath-Hextall FJ, Leonardi-Bee J, et al. Probiotics for treating eczema. Cochrane Database Syst Rev 2008;(4):CD006135.
239. Salfeld P, Kopp MV. Probiotics cannot be generally recommended for primary prevention of atopic dermatitis. J Allergy Clin Immunol 2009;124:170.
240. Pelucchi C, Chatenoud L, Turati F, et al. Probiotics supplementation during pregnancy or infancy for the prevention of atopic dermatitis: a meta-analysis. Epidemiology 2012;23:402–14.
241. Simon D, Hosli S, Kostylina G, et al. Anti-CD20 (rituximab) treatment improves atopic eczema. J Allergy Clin Immunol 2008;121:122–8.
242. Hamilton JD, et al. Dupilumab improves the molecular signature in skin of patients with moderate-to-severe atopic dermatitis. J Allergy Clin Immunol 2014;134:1293–300.
243. *Noda S, Krueger JG1, Guttman-Yassky E. The translational revolution and use of biologics in patients with inflammatory skin diseases. J Allergy Clin Immunol 2015;135(2):324–36.

Key references are preceded by an asterisk.

CHAPTER 12

Food Allergy and Gastrointestinal Syndromes

Anna Nowak-Węgrzyn, A. Wesley Burks, and Hugh A. Sampson

CHAPTER OUTLINE

INTRODUCTION

HISTORICAL PERSPECTIVE

EPIDEMIOLOGY

Children

Adults

Prevalence of Food Allergy

Natural History of Food Allergy

Food Allergy in Adults

Food Allergy as a Marker of Atopic Predisposition

Pathogenesis and Etiology

Normal Immune Response to the Ingested Food Antigens

Food Allergens

Cross-reactivity

Pathophysiologic Mechanisms of Food Allergy

IgE-mediated Food Allergy

Augmentation Factors

CLINICAL FEATURES

Gastrointestinal Food Allergy

   Gastrointestinal IgE-mediated Food Allergy

   Mixed IgE- and Non-IgE-mediated Gastrointestinal Food Allergy

   Non-IgE-mediated Gastrointestinal Food Allergy

Cutaneous Food Allergy

   Cutaneous IgE-mediated Food Allergy

   Mixed IgE- and Non-IgE-mediated Cutaneous Food Allergy

   Non-IgE-mediated Cutaneous Food Allergy

Respiratory Food Allergy

   Non-IgE-mediated Respiratory Food Allergy

Food-induced Generalized Anaphylaxis

Food-dependent, Exercise-induced Anaphylaxis

Delayed Anaphylaxis Caused by Mammalian Meat

Other Food-induced Hypersensitivity Reactions

PATIENT EVALUATION, DIAGNOSIS, AND DIFFERENTIAL DIAGNOSIS

Unproven Tests for Food Allergy

FOOD ALLERGY TREATMENT

Practical Management

Food Allergen Avoidance Strategies

   General Approach to Avoidance

   Labeling of Manufactured Products

   Cross-contact

Manner of Exposure

   Restaurants, Food Establishments, Travel

   Avoidance for Schools and Camp

   Nutritional Issues

EMERGENCY MANAGEMENT

Recognition of Reactions

Treatment with Epinephrine and Antihistamines

Emergency Plans and Special Considerations for School

Prevention of Food Allergy

Trials Using Oral Tolerance Induction to Prevent Food Allergies

FUTURE THERAPEUTIC STRATEGIES

Oral Immunotherapy

Extensively Heated Milk and Egg Protein

Sublingual Immunotherapy

Epicutaneous Immunotherapy

CONCLUSIONS

SUMMARY OF IMPORTANT CONCEPTS

- Food allergy affects 6% of US children younger than 5 years of age and 3.5–4% of the general population, and the incidence of peanut allergy has quadrupled over the past decade in the US.
- Sensitization to food allergens may occur in the gastrointestinal tract (traditional or class 1 food allergy), through the inflamed skin in atopic dermatitis, or it may result from sensitization to cross-reacting inhalant allergens (secondary or class 2 food allergy).

- Food reactions may have immunoglobulin E (IgE)-mediated, non-IgE-mediated, or a combination of IgE- and non-IgE-mediated pathophysiologic mechanisms involving the skin, gastrointestinal tract, respiratory tract, and/or cardiovascular system.
- Foods are the most common triggers of anaphylaxis in children and major triggers in adults.
- Increasing levels of food-specific serum IgE antibodies or skin-prick test wheal diameters correlate with increasing probabilities of clinical reactivity, although the double-blind, placebo-controlled food challenge remains the gold standard for diagnosing food allergy.
- Avoidance of food allergens requires educating patients and caregivers about reading ingredient labels, avoiding cross-contact with allergen, and obtaining safe meals in various circumstances.
- Appropriate management of food-induced anaphylaxis requires education about recognizing symptoms and treating promptly with epinephrine.
- Strategies to prevent food allergy such as delayed weaning and delayed exposure to food allergens have recently been called into question.
- Evidence suggests early cutaneous exposure to food protein through a disrupted skin barrier leads to allergic sensitization, and early oral exposure to food allergen may induce tolerance.
- New therapies for food allergy employ both allergen-specific and allergen-non-specific approaches, with great promise for effective desensitization associated with successful immunomodulation.
- Because of safety concerns and long-term efficacy parameters that are still being evaluated, therapies for food allergy are considered investigational.

INTRODUCTION

Box 12-1 gives brief definitions of food allergies, food intolerances, and food aversions.

HISTORICAL PERSPECTIVE

In the past two decades, food allergy has emerged as an important public health problem affecting people of all ages in societies with a Western lifestyle, such as the United States, Canada, UK, Australia, and Western Europe.[1-3] The overall prevalence of food allergy in American children increased by 18% from 1997 to 2007.[4] Peanut allergy quadrupled during a similar period in the US, Canada, UK, and Australia.[5,6] Food allergy is the most common cause of anaphylaxis in the outpatient setting for all ages, and it can lead to fatalities. The diagnosis of food allergy requires labor-intensive, medically supervised oral food challenges (OFCs) that carry a risk for anaphylaxis and are not readily available to all patients. There is no cure for food allergy. Current management relies on

---

Box 12-1   Definitions

- *Food allergy* is defined as an adverse health effect arising from a specific immune response that occurs reproducibly following exposure to a given food.[1] Non-allergic adverse reactions to foods may be the result of food intolerances or adverse physiologic reactions.
- *Food intolerances* are thought to comprise most adverse reactions to foods. They can be caused by factors inherent in the food ingested, such as toxic contaminants, toxins, pharmacologic properties of the food (e.g., caffeine in coffee), and host characteristics such as metabolic disorders (e.g., lactase deficiency) and idiosyncratic responses.
- *Food aversions* may mimic adverse food reactions, but they typically cannot be reproduced when the patient ingests the food in a blinded fashion. Food allergy must be distinguished from a variety of adverse reactions to foods that do not have an immune basis, but whose clinical manifestations may resemble food allergy. Examples of adverse food reactions are presented in Table 12-1.

TABLE 12-1   Non-allergic Adverse Reactions to Consider in the Differential Diagnosis of Food Allergy

Condition	Symptoms	Mechanism and comments
Enzyme deficiencies		
Lactose intolerance	Bloating, abdominal pain, diarrhea (dose dependent)	Lactase deficiency
Fructose intolerance	Emesis, poor feeding, jaundice, hypoglycemia, seizures	Hereditary fructose aldolase B deficiency; rare
Fructose malabsorption	Bloating, abdominal pain, diarrhea (dose dependent)	Deficiency of fructose carrier GLUT5 in the enterocytes in small intestines; 10% prevalence in Asia, up to 30% in Western Europe and Africa
Pancreatic insufficiency	Malabsorption	Deficiency of pancreatic enzymes, acquired or congenital (e.g., cystic fibrosis, Schwachman–Diamond syndrome)
Alcohol	Nasal congestion, flushing, vomiting	Polymorphism of the aldehyde dehydrogenase gene (*ALDH*), resulting in deficiency of ALDH, which metabolizes alcohol in the liver; common in Asians
Gallbladder or liver disease	Malabsorption	Deficiency of liver enzymes
Gastrointestinal disorders		
Gastroesophageal reflux disease	Nausea, emesis, abdominal pain, heartburn, dysphagia	Chronic symptom of mucosal damage caused by stomach acid refluxing into the esophagus
Peptic ulcer disease	Abdominal pain, bloating, loss of appetite, weight loss, melena	Ulcer of the gastrointestinal tract (commonly duodenum); 70–90% are associated with *Helicobacter pylori* infection
Anatomic defects		
Hiatal hernia	Abdominal pain, shortness of breath, nausea, emesis	Protrusion (or herniation) of the upper part of the stomach into the thorax through a tear or weakness in the diaphragm
Pyloric stenosis	Severe, non-bilious, projectile vomiting in the first few months of life	Stenosis due to hypertrophy of muscle around pylorus, which spasms when stomach empties; rare case reports of eosinophilic infiltrates in pylorus and reported resolution of muscle hypertrophy with hypoallergenic formula or steroids
Hirschsprung disease	Delayed passage of meconium, constipation, ileus, emesis	Failure of neural crest cells to migrate completely during fetal development of the intestine, causing aganglosis; usually affects short segment of the distal colon
Tracheoesophageal fistula	Copious salivation associated with choking, coughing, vomiting, and cyanosis coincident with the onset of feeding in newborns and young infants	*Congenital*: failed fusion of tracheoesophageal ridges during third week of embryologic development *Acquired*: usually sequela of surgical procedures (e.g., laryngectomy)
Physiologic effects of active substances		
Caffeine	Tremors, cramps, diarrhea	Xanthine alkaloid acts as stimulant drug; found in seeds, leaves, and fruit of some plants, where it acts as a natural pesticide; consumed in coffee, tea, and drinks containing kola nut, yerba mate, guarana berry, or guayusa derivatives
Theobromine	Sleeplessness, tremors, restlessness, anxiety, increased urination, loss of appetite, nausea, vomiting	Bitter alkaloid in cocoa bean and tea leaves; elderly more susceptible
Tyramine	Migraine	Naturally occurring monoamine compound derived from tyrosine; acts as a catecholamine-releasing agent; pharmacologic effects in susceptible individuals; found in pickled, aged, smoked, fermented, or marinated foods (e.g., hard cheeses, tofu, sauerkraut, fava beans)
Histamine	Flushing, headache, nausea	Naturally occurring in fermented foods and beverages (e.g., fish, sauerkraut) due to a conversion from histidine to histamine performed by fermenting bacteria or yeasts; sake contains histamine in the 20–40 mg/L range and wines in the 2–10 mg/L range
Serotonin	Flushing, diarrhea, palpitations	Monoamine neurotransmitter derived from tryptophan; found in nuts, mushrooms, fruits, and vegetables; highest values (25–400 mg/kg) in nuts of walnut and hickory genera; concentrations of 3–30 mg/kg found in plantain, pineapple, banana, kiwi, plums, and tomatoes

Continued on following page

TABLE 12-1   Non-allergic Adverse Reactions to Consider in the Differential Diagnosis of Food Allergy (Continued)

Condition	Symptoms	Mechanism and comments
Food additives and contaminants		
Sodium metabisulfite	Rare reports of bronchospasm in sensitive individuals	Antioxidant and preservative in food, also known as E223
Monosodium glutamate (MSG)	Chinese restaurant syndrome begins 15–20 min after the meal and lasts for about 2 h; symptoms include numbness at the back of the neck and gradually radiating to the arms and back, general weakness, and palpitations	Naturally occurring non-essential amino acid; flavor enhancer; in a DBPCFC study, objective reactions to MSG were observed in only 2 of 130 self-selected MSG-reactive adult volunteers[2]
Accidental contaminants	Abdominal pain, diarrhea, nausea	Include heavy metals (e.g., mercury, copper), pesticides, antibiotics (e.g., penicillin), dust or storage mites
Infectious agents	Pain, fever, nausea, emesis, diarrhea	Include bacteria (e.g., *Salmonella*, *Shigella*, *Escherichia coli*, *Yersinia*, *Campylobacter*); parasites (e.g., *Giardia*, *Trichinella*); viruses (e.g., hepatitis, rotavirus, enterovirus)
Neurologic disorders		
Auriculotemporal syndrome (Frey syndrome)	Facial flush in trigeminal nerve distribution associated with spicy foods	Neurogenic reflex, frequently associated with birth trauma to trigeminal nerve (forceps delivery)
Gustatory rhinitis	Profuse watery rhinorrhea associated with spicy foods	Neurogenic reflex
Conditions confused with food reactions		
Panic disorder	Subjective reactions, fainting on smelling or seeing the food; tachycardia, perspiration, dyspnea, shivers, uncontrollable fear (fear of dying)	Psychological; anxiety disorder affects children and adults; usually leads to extensive medical testing; controlled with medications and behavioral therapy

(Modified from Nowak-Węgrzyn A, Sampson HA. Adverse reactions to foods. Med Clin North Am 2006; 90:97–127.)

food avoidance and timely treatment of acute reactions. To facilitate diagnosis and management of food allergy, the first official US guidelines for food allergy were published in 2010, and European guidelines were published in 2014.[7] The growing recognition of the burden of food allergies and the challenges in diagnosis and management are driving multifaceted research approaches with the ultimate goal of finding a cure.

EPIDEMIOLOGY

Children

Food allergies are most common in the first few years of life. Cow's milk (CM), hen's egg, soybean, wheat, peanut, tree nuts, fish, and shellfish allergies cause more than 90% of food allergy in children.[8,9] These foods have relatively high protein contents and are introduced at early stages. Local dietary habits often result in the increased presence of various food allergens in the diet. Examples include sesame in Israel, buckwheat in Japan, and mustard and lupine in France. Most allergies to CM, egg, soybean, and wheat are outgrown, whereas most allergies to peanut, nuts, seeds, and seafood persist into adulthood.[10]

Prospective studies from several countries indicate that about 2.5% of newborn infants experience hypersensitivity reactions to CM in the first year of life.[11] IgE-mediated reactions account for about 60% of these milk-allergic reactions. Hen's egg allergy is estimated to affect about 1.6% of young children in the US and UK. A rigorous, population-based study found an 8.9% prevalence of egg allergy diagnosed by oral food challenge (OFC) to raw egg in children younger than 12 months of age in Australia, suggesting that food allergies continue to increase in the youngest age groups.[5]

Most infants with non-IgE-mediated CM allergy outgrow their sensitivity by the third year of life, but about 10–25% of infants with IgE-mediated CM and egg allergies retain

TABLE 12-2   Prevalence of Allergy to Specific Foods

Food	General population	Children (<5 years)	Adults
Cow's milk	0.4–0.9%	0.5% (Israel) to 3.8% (US, UK)	
Hen's egg white	0.2%	≈2–8.9% (<12 months) (Australia)	
Soybean	0%; 0.7%	1.4%	0–0.7%
Wheat	0–1.2%	≈0.5%	0–1.2%
Peanut	0.75–1.3%	0.2% (Israel) to 1.9% (US, Canada, UK)	0.7%
Tree nuts	0.6–1.1%	1.1–1.6%	0.5–1%
Sesame oil or seeds	Overall: 0.1–<1%	0.6%	
Fish	Overall: 0.3–0.5%	0.2%; 0.5%	≈0.6%
Shellfish	0.6–2%	0.5%; 14–16 years: 5.2% (Singapore)	1.7–2.5%
Fruits	Up to 4.2% (SPT); up to 8.5% (symptoms)	0.4% (UK)	
Vegetables	0.1–0.3%, up to 2.7% (SPT); up to 13.7% (symptoms)	1.2%	
Oral allergy (raw fruits or vegetables)			22 years: 17% (Denmark)

SPT, skin-prick test.
(Modified from Sicherer SH. Epidemiology of food allergy. J Allergy Clin Immunol 2011; 127:594–602.)

their sensitivity into the second decade of life, and about 50% develop allergic reactions to other foods.[12,13]

Large, population-based studies have addressed the prevalence of peanut allergy (Table 12-2) and determined that peanut allergy affects more than 1–4% of children in Canada, the US, Australia, and the UK.[5,6] Adverse reactions to food additives affect 0.5–1% of children, especially those with atopic disorders, who have a higher prevalence of food allergy. About 35% of children with moderate to severe atopic dermatitis have IgE-mediated food allergies, many of whom exhibit skin symptoms provoked by ingestion of the food allergen.

About 6% of asthmatic children attending a general pulmonary clinic reportedly had food-induced wheezing. Among children with eosinophilic esophagitis, 50% have food-responsive disease (i.e. symptoms improve or resolve on elimination of the offending food).

Adults

Food allergy in adults is less common than in children.[1] Peanut and tree nut allergy together affect 1.2% of American adults, and seafood allergy affects about 2.3%, giving an overall estimate of 3.5–4%.[14] A survey from the UK identified 1.4–1.8% of adults reporting adverse food reactions, and a study in the Netherlands concluded that about 2% of the adult Dutch population was affected by adverse food reactions. The estimates of pollen-related food allergy are considerably higher. Among pollen-allergic individuals, 74% report symptoms (most had oral symptoms) to the pollen-associated foods (e.g., fruits, vegetables). Overall, 16.7% of young adults report pollen–food allergy symptoms.

Prevalence of Food Allergy

Studies of the prevalence of food allergy are hampered by the requirement of a physician-supervised OFC for the ultimate confirmation of food allergy. Food challenges are expensive, labor-intensive, and impractical in large-scale, population-based cohorts. For this reason, many studies use surrogate markers, such as evidence of specific IgE to food or self-reported food allergy to estimate prevalence figures. Several studies that applied similar methods over time showed a two- to three-fold increase in peanut allergy and peanut-IgE sensitization in children in the US, UK, Canada, and Australia over the past 10 to 20 years. Many studies reported rates of peanut allergy of 1–4% among young children.[1]

Food-induced anaphylaxis also appears to have increased.[15] In the US, data from one geographic region in Minnesota from 1983 to 1987, and 1993 to 1997, show a 71–100% increase.[16,17] Studies focusing on pediatric food-related ambulatory and emergency department visits or food-induced anaphylaxis also suggest increases. In the UK, there was almost a doubling of anaphylaxis, from 5.6 to 10.2 cases per 100 000 hospital discharges over the 4 years from 1991 to 1995 ($p < 0.001$).[18] The proportion of cases attributed to food-induced anaphylaxis also increased over the same period.[19]

The reasons for increased cases of food allergy are unknown. There appears to be a strong genetic contribution to peanut allergy. Monozygotic twins have 64% concordance for peanut allergy; dizygotic twins have 7% concordance. However, the rapid rate of increase suggests that environmental factors play a more important role, likely by affecting the expression of genetic susceptibility. Potential genetic and environmental risk factors contributing to the increase in prevalence of food allergy are discussed in Table 12-3.

Natural History of Food Allergy

The prevalence of food hypersensitivity is greatest in the first few years of life. Most young children outgrow their food hypersensitivity (i.e. become tolerant) within a few years, except in most cases of peanut, tree nut, and seafood allergy.

Most children outgrow CM allergy, and those with a milder phenotype of CM allergy become tolerant by school age. In a prospective, population-based study, most CM-allergic children lost their CM allergy by 3 years of age: 50% by 1 year, 70% by 2 years, and 85% by 3 years.[20] All children with negative skin-prick test results to CM at 1 year of age lost their sensitivity by their third birthday, whereas 25% of those with positive skin test results remained CM-allergic at 3 years of age. In contrast, among children with a more severe phenotype (i.e. multiple food allergies, asthma, and allergic rhinitis), 21% remained allergic to CM by 16 years of age.[13] The highest serum concentration of CM-specific IgE for each patient (defined as the peak CM-IgE level), was highly predictive of outcome ($p < 0.001$), with few children whose peak CM-specific IgE concentration exceeded $50\,kU_A/L$ outgrowing milk allergy by their teenage years. Clinically, reactivity to baked milk appears to be a useful marker of a more severe CM allergy. Children who were initially reactive to baked milk were 28 times less likely to become tolerant to unheated milk compared with children tolerant to baked milk over a median of 37 months (range, 8–75 months; $p < 0.001$).[21,22]

Similar to milk allergy, 66% of egg-allergic children become egg tolerant by 5 years of age.[12] However, among those with a more severe phenotype, 32% continued to avoid egg at the age of 16 years. A patient's highest recorded egg IgE level, presence of other atopic disease, and presence of other food allergy were significantly related to the persistence of egg allergy. In contrast to milk allergy, children reactive to baked egg have excellent chances of outgrowing their egg allergy.[23,24]

Approximately 20% of children with peanut allergy and 9% of children with tree nut allergy become tolerant to these foods with age.[25,26] Unlike milk and egg allergy, peanut allergy occasionally recurs in children who appear to have outgrown their reactivity.[27] Risk of recurrence appears to be approximately 10% among children who refuse to eat peanuts on a regular basis, compared with rare recurrences in children eating peanuts regularly. The possibility of peanut allergy recurrence should be discussed before undertaking the OFC to peanut and before indicating that patients should ingest peanut frequently after a negative OFC result. Epinephrine should be carried for several months after a negative result until the patient has proven tolerance to multiple ingestions of regular servings of peanuts and peanut-containing foods. It appears that the natural

TABLE 12-3 Potential Genetic and Risk Factors for Food Allergy Development

Potential risk factor for food allergy	Mechanism/comments
Genetic	
Gender	Several studies report that gender could be related to food allergy, particularly peanut and tree nut allergies. Peanut allergy is significantly higher in male children; this ratio reverses during and after adolescence, possibly mediated through endocrine changes.
Ethnicity	The risk of possible and likely food allergy is increased in non-Hispanic blacks compared with white individuals. Black children were more likely to be sensitized to multiple foods than white children. As assessed by genetic ancestry informative markers, African ancestry is a notable risk factor for increased risk of peanut sensitization at levels associated with clinical reactivity.
Genetic polymorphism	Gene polymorphisms in interleukin-10 (IL-10) and IL-13 have been identified in association with food allergy, but these studies will need to be replicated in different populations. Variations in the two important SNPs of CD14 (rs2569190 and rs2569193) were associated with the presence of peanut allergy. More recent studies point to important gene–environment interactions in the development of food sensitization. In a prospective birth cohort study of 970 children, children who were ever breastfed (including exclusively breastfed children) were at 1.5 times higher risk of food sensitization than never-breastfed children. However, the association was altered by rs425648 in the IL-12 receptor β_1 gene (IL-12 rβ_1). Breastfeeding increased the risk of food sensitization in children carrying the GG genotype but significantly decreased the risk of food sensitization in breastfed infants carrying the GT/TT genotype. Similar interactions were observed for SNPs in the TSLP gene and the Toll-like receptor gene (TLR9).
Atopic dermatitis and filaggrin loss-of-function mutations	There is greater frequency of sensitization and allergy to foods with increasing severity of atopic dermatitis (AD); relative risk (RR) of 5.9 for IgE-mediated food allergy in an infant with severe eczema. The loss-of-function mutations within the filaggrin (*FLG*) gene are associated with development of AD. *FLG* was also studied as a candidate gene in the etiology of peanut allergy. The association of *FLG* mutation with peanut allergy is highly significant ($p = 0.0008$) even after controlling for coexistent AD. This indicates a role for epithelial barrier dysfunction in the pathogenesis of peanut allergy.
Environmental	
Lack of microbial exposure	The *hygiene hypothesis* suggests that the lack of early life exposures to infectious agents (e.g., bacteria, parasites) may lead to a faulty programming of tolerogenic mechanisms, increasing the host's susceptibility to allergic diseases. Limited data for the hygiene hypothesis exist with respect to food allergy.
C-section	A meta-analysis of six studies showed a mild effect of cesarean delivery increasing the risk of food allergy (odds ratio [OR] = 1.32; 95% confidence interval [CI], 1.12–0.55). The pro-allergy skewing effect of cesarean section may be explained by the abnormal bacterial colonization of a newborn's gut in the absence of exposure to the protective bacterial flora in the birth canal. Alternatively, cesarean section is associated with higher maternal age, a higher number of first-born infants, and a higher number of male births, which all have been identified as independent risk factors for atopy.
Season of birth/vitamin D	Epidemiologic findings, such as the observations that season of birth is a risk factor, that food-induced pediatric anaphylaxis is more common in northern areas of the US (i.e. less sunlight exposure than in the southern states), and that maternal intake of vitamin D during pregnancy was associated with a decreased risk of food sensitization, support the hypothesis that relative deficiency of vitamin D may predispose offspring to development of atopy and food allergy. However, two independent studies showed that infants who received vitamin D supplementation were at increased risk of food allergy.
Obesity	The coinciding trend in increasing atopy with increasing childhood obesity has been well studied, especially in the context of asthma. Obesity induces an inflammatory state associated with an increased risk of atopy and could theoretically lead to an increased risk for food allergy. Atopy (defined by any positive specific IgE measurement) is increased in obese compared with normal-weight children. This association is driven primarily by allergic sensitization to foods (OR for food sensitization = 1.59; 95% CI, 1.28–1.98). Elevated C-reactive protein levels as a measure of inflammation were associated with total IgE levels, atopy, and food sensitization.
n-3-polyunsuturated fatty acids (n-3- PUFA)	The typical Western diet is characterized by the reduced consumption of n-3 PUFAs (found in oily fish) and increased consumption of pro-inflammatory omega-6 polyunsaturated fatty acids (found in margarine and vegetable oils) led to the increased production of prostaglandin E_2 (PGE_2). This presumably results in reduced production of interferon-γ (IFN-γ) by T cells and increased production of IgE by B cells, amplifying the risk of atopy and asthma.
Timing of food allergen introduction into the diet	Timing of exposure to food allergens may be critical for the development of oral tolerance. A review of 13 studies (only one was controlled) found a consistent association between the persistence of eczema and the introduction of solid foods before 4 months of age but not with an increased risk of asthma, food allergy, allergic rhinitis, or animal allergies. Several reports suggested that early introduction of peanut, cow's milk, egg, and wheat into the infant diet was associated with decreased risk of allergy to these foods. Countries in Asia, Africa, and the Middle East have low rates of peanut allergy, and peanut consumption is unrestricted during pregnancy and early childhood. A questionnaire-based study found that the prevalence of peanut allergy in the UK was 1.85% and the prevalence in Israel was 0.17% ($p < 0.001$). The adjusted risk ratio for peanut allergy between countries was 9.8 (95% CI, 3.1–30.5) in primary English school children. The only difference identified between the two populations was the timing of introduction of peanuts, which in Israel occurs during early weaning. Randomized clinical trials are underway to determine whether early introduction of peanuts and other solid foods protects against food allergy.

history of allergy to seeds, fish, and shellfish is similar to nuts. Among 133 children with soy allergy evaluated in a food allergy referral center and followed for a median time of 5 years (range, 1–19 years), rates of resolution were 25% by 4 years, 45% by 6 years, and 69% by 10 years of age.[28]

In a population of 103 children with IgE-mediated wheat allergy in a food allergy referral center, rates of resolution were 29% by 4 years, 56% by 8 years, and 65% by 12 years of age. Higher wheat IgE levels were associated with poorer outcomes. The peak wheat IgE level recorded was a useful predictor of persistent allergy ($p < 0.001$), although many children, even those with the highest levels of wheat IgE, outgrew wheat allergy.[29]

Food Allergy in Adults

Although younger children are more likely to outgrow their food allergies, older children and adults also may lose their reactivity if the responsible food allergen is identified and eliminated from the diet. Approximately one third of children and adults lose their clinical reactivity after 1 to 2 years of allergen avoidance. Skin-puncture test results typically remain positive and do not predict which patients will lose their clinical reactivity. Monitoring food allergen-specific IgE levels may be useful in predicting when patients outgrow their allergy. A significant drop in the specific IgE level to CM and egg by 50% over 1 to 2 years has been identified as a favorable prognostic factor in children.[30] The severity of the initial reaction does not appear to correlate with the ultimate likelihood of losing clinical reactivity, but the degree of compliance with the allergen avoidance diet and the food responsible for the reaction do affect the outcome.

Most non-IgE-mediated gastrointestinal food allergies occur in infants and are outgrown in the first 2 to 3 years of life. However, allergic eosinophilic esophagitis is frequently seen in adults, and the number of young children and adolescents affected appears to be increasing. Long-term studies have not been completed, and the prognosis of this disorder is unknown. Although most cases of dietary protein-induced enteropathy are outgrown, celiac disease is a lifelong sensitivity, and gluten-containing grains must be avoided for life. No formal studies on the natural history of non-IgE-mediated cutaneous or respiratory disorders have been undertaken, but these sensitivities are thought to be long-lasting.

Food Allergy as a Marker of Atopic Predisposition

In many children, food allergy coexists with other atopic conditions, such as atopic dermatitis, asthma, and allergic rhinitis. Sensitization to egg white in children with atopic dermatitis and a family history of atopy is associated with a 70% risk for respiratory allergic disease (i.e. asthma or allergic rhinitis) at 5 years of age. Individuals with past and current food allergy should be considered at high risk for asthma and environmental allergy.

Pathogenesis and Etiology

The gastrointestinal tract processes ingested food into a form that can be absorbed and used for energy and cell growth. This requires the intestinal immune system to discriminate between harmful and harmless foreign proteins.[31] As shown in Table 12-4, a variety of immunologic and non-immunologic factors may destroy or block antigens from entering the body. However, developmental immaturity of these mechanisms in infants reduces the efficiency of their mucosal barriers and likely plays a major role in the increased prevalence of gastrointestinal infections and food allergy seen in the first few years of life.

Normal Immune Response to the Ingested Food Antigens

Low concentrations of serum IgG, IgM, and IgA food-specific antibodies are commonly found in normal individuals. The younger an infant when a food antigen is introduced into the diet, the more pronounced the antibody response is likely to be. After introduction of CM, serum levels of CM protein-specific IgG antibodies rise over the first month,

TABLE 12-4   Gastrointestinal Barriers to Ingested Food Antigens

Barriers	Food allergy predisposition in newborns and infants
Immunologic Barriers	
Block penetration of ingested antigens Antigen-specific sIgA in gut lumen	Newborn lacks IgA and IgM in exocrine secretions. Salivary sIgA is absent at birth, and levels remain low during early months of life

Clear antigens penetrating GI barrier
  Serum antigen-specific IgA and IgG
  Reticuloendothelial system
	Immaturity of the humoral immune system, low
	 levels of circulating antibodies

Physiologic Barriers	

Breakdown of ingested antigens
  Gastric acid and pepsins
  Pancreatic enzymes
  Intestinal enzymes
  Intestinal epithelial cell lysozyme activity
	Low basal acid output during first month of life
	 Immaturity of the intestinal proteolytic activity
	 until about 2 years of age

Block penetration of ingested antigens
  Intestinal mucous coat (i.e. glycocalyx)
  Intestinal microvillus membrane composition
  Intestinal peristalsis
	Intestinal microvillus membranes are immature in
	 infants, resulting in altered antigen binding and
	 transport through mucosal epithelial cells.

GI, gastrointestinal; IgM, immunoglobulin M; sIGA, secretory immunoglobulin A.

achieving peak antibody levels after several months, and they then decline, even though CM proteins continue to be ingested.

Individuals with various inflammatory gastrointestinal disorders (e.g., celiac disease, food allergy, inflammatory bowel disease) frequently have high levels of food-specific IgG and IgM antibodies. However, these antibodies do not indicate that the patient is allergic to these foods. The increased levels of food-specific antibodies (not IgE) appear to result from increased gastrointestinal permeability to food antigens and reflect dietary intake.

Food Allergens

Among 399 described food allergens, only 71 of 14 831 (0.5%) protein families are represented, and the top 20 (0.13%) protein families account for 80% of all described food allergens, suggesting that food allergens share common characteristics that render them allergenic.[32] Functionally, based on the ability to induce allergic sensitization in the gastrointestinal tract, food proteins can be classified as class I (traditional) food allergens or as class II food allergens that do not have the capacity to sensitize in the gastrointestinal tract but become allergenic as a consequence of sensitization to inhalant allergens.[33] The major food allergens that have been identified in class I allergy are water-soluble glycoproteins, which have molecular masses ranging from 10 to 70 kD and are more stable to treatment with heat, acid, and proteases. However, there are no obvious physicochemical properties common to the class II food allergens. The mostly plant-derived proteins are highly heat labile and difficult to extract intact, often making standardized extracts for diagnostic purposes unsatisfactory. Several class I and II food allergens have been identified, cloned, sequenced, and expressed as recombinant proteins. Many of the plant-related allergens are homologous to pathogenesis-related (PR) proteins, which are expressed by the plant in response to infections or other stress factors, or comprise seed-storage proteins, profilins, peroxidases, or protease inhibitors common to many plants (Table 12-4).

Food additives and colorings derived from natural sources that contain proteins may induce allergic reactions. They include colors derived from turmeric, paprika, seeds (e.g., annatto), and insects (e.g., carmine, cochineal).[34] Chemical additives are not likely to cause IgE-mediated food allergy, but some may have drug effects that cause adverse reactions, including allergy-like symptoms, or they may invoke immune responses.[35] Tartrazine (yellow #5) is a synthetic color that has been extensively investigated because

Box 12-2 **Categories of Food Additives with Examples**

Starches/Complex Carbohydrates	*Cornstarch, Modified Starch*
Preservatives (antimicrobials)	Potassium sorbate, sodium benzoate
Preservatives (antioxidants)	Butylated hydroxyanisole/hydroxytoluene (BHA/BHT)
Preservatives (antibrowning)	Potassium metabisulfite, sulfur dioxide
Nutrients	Vitamin A, ferrous sulfate
Flavors	Ethyl vanillin, cinnamic aldehyde
Anticaking agents	Sodium aluminosilicate
Emulsifying agents	Lecithin
Sequestrants	Citric acid
Stabilizers and gums	Tragacanth gum, xanthan gum
Acidulents	Phosphoric acid, hydrochloric acid
Flavor enhancers	Monosodium glutamate
Colors	Tartrazine, annatto
Enzymes	Papain
Leavening agents	Sodium bicarbonate

of concerns that it may trigger urticaria, allergic reactions, and asthma. However, well-conducted studies have not validated these concerns. Sulfites are added to foods as a preservative, an anti-browning agent, or for its bleaching effect. In sensitive persons, sulfites may induce asthma (Box 12-2).

Cross-Reactivity

Structural homology among allergens underlies immunologic and clinical cross-reactivity. More than 70% identity in the primary sequence is considered necessary for clinical cross-reactivity. However, the expression of clinical cross-reactivity is modulated by additional factors, including protein solubility and digestibility, concentration and affinity of the specific IgE antibodies, and the dose and route of allergen exposure. High rates of clinical cross-reactivity are observed among milks from cows, goats, and sheep (>90%); melons (90%); crustacean shellfish (75%); fruits from the Rosaceae family, such as apple, pear, peach (55%); and bony fish (50%). Lower rates are observed among tree nuts (37%), grains (20%), CM and beef (10%), and peanuts and other legumes (5%). The rates of pollen-fruit cross-reactivity are about 50% for birch pollen and Rosaceae (e.g., apple, peach, pear, cherry) fruits. The rate of reactions to kiwi, banana, or avocado among latex-allergic individuals is about 11%. The risk of latex allergy among kiwi-, banana-, or avocado-allergic individuals is about 35%.[36]

Pathophysiologic Mechanisms of Food Allergy

In the susceptible host, a failure to develop or a breakdown in oral tolerance, commonly as a result of heavy occupational exposure or sensitization to cross-reactive allergens, may result in allergic responses to ingested food antigens.[1] The extended Gell and Coombs classification provides a framework for discussing hypersensitivity reactions, but food-allergic disorders usually involve more than one of the classic mechanisms described in Table 12-5.

IgE-Mediated Food Allergy

The best characterized food allergic reactions involve IgE antibodies that bind to high-affinity receptors on mast cells and basophils as well as low-affinity receptors on macrophages, monocytes, lymphocytes, and platelets. When food allergens penetrate mucosal barriers and reach IgE, antibodies bind to mast cells or basophils, mediators are released that induce vasodilatation, smooth muscle contraction, and mucus secretion, producing the symptoms of immediate hypersensitivity. IgE-mediated allergic reactions are associated with a variety of symptoms: generalized (e.g., hypotension, shock); cutaneous (e.g., urticaria, angioedema, pruritic morbilliform rash); oral and gastrointestinal (e.g., lip, tongue, and palatal pruritus and swelling, laryngeal edema, vomiting, diarrhea); and upper and lower respiratory systems (e.g., ocular pruritus and tearing, nasal congestion, pharyngeal edema, wheezing). A rise in plasma histamine has been associated with the

TABLE 12-5 Classification of Food-Allergic Disorders Based on Pathophysiology

Disorder	IgE-mediated response	IgE- and cell-mediated response	Non-IgE-mediated response
Generalized	Food-dependent, exercise-induced anaphylaxis		
Cutaneous	Urticaria, angioedema, flushing, acute morbilliform rash, acute contact urticaria	Atopic dermatitis, contact dermatitis	Contact dermatitis, dermatitis herpetiformis
Gastrointestinal	Oral allergy syndrome, gastrointestinal anaphylaxis	Allergic eosinophilic esophagitis, allergic eosinophilic gastroenteritis	Allergic proctocolitis, food protein-induced enterocolitis syndrome, celiac disease, infantile colic
Respiratory	Acute rhinoconjunctivitis, acute bronchospasm	Asthma	Pulmonary hemosiderosis (Heiner syndrome)

(Modified from Nowak-Węgrzyn A, Sampson HA. Adverse reactions to foods. Med Clin North Am 2006; 90:97–127.)

development of these symptoms after blinded food challenges. In contrast, serum β-tryptase levels are usually not elevated.

In one study, increased levels of serum platelet-activating factor (PAF) were reported for subjects with peanut-induced anaphylaxis who presented to the emergency department.[37] Serum PAF acetylhydrolase activity was significantly lower in patients with fatal peanut anaphylaxis than in control patients, which suggested that impaired ability to break down PAF might contribute to severe anaphylaxis. However, these findings require replication.

Augmentation Factors

Several factors have been associated with increased risk of developing food allergy and with increased severity of food-allergic reactions. Drugs lowering the gastric acidity predisposed to de novo sensitization to food allergen (i.e. hazelnut and codfish) in a mouse model and in treated humans.[38–40] In allergic individuals, antacids increased the severity of codfish-induced anaphylaxis.[41] Exercise, ingestion of alcohol and nonsteroidal anti-inflammatory drugs are associated with increased severity of food-induced anaphylaxis.

CLINICAL FEATURES

Classification of food hypersensitivity disorders into those primarily involving IgE-mediated reactions, those not involving IgE-mediated mechanisms, and those that may involve IgE- and non-IgE-mediated mechanisms is most useful for clinical and diagnostic purposes, as depicted in Table 12-6.[1]

Gastrointestinal Food Allergy

Gastrointestinal IgE-Mediated Food Allergy

Pollen-food allergy syndrome (*oral allergy syndrome*) is elicited by a variety of plant proteins, especially PR proteins cross-reacting with airborne allergens. Sensitization to inhaled pollen is the primary event, with secondary reactions occurring following ingestion of the cross-reactive plant foods. It is estimated that pollen-food allergy syndrome affects 50–70% of adults suffering from pollen allergy, especially to birch, ragweed, and mugwort pollens. Symptoms are provoked almost exclusively in the oropharynx and rarely involve other target organs. Little is known regarding its prevalence among children. Local contact induces IgE-mediated mast cell activation and provokes the rapid onset of pruritus, tingling, and angioedema of the lips, tongue, palate, and throat, and it occasionally elicits a sensation of pruritus in the ears or tightness in the throat. Symptoms are usually induced by raw fruits and vegetables and are short-lived due to exquisite susceptibility of the allergens to digestion. The cooked forms of these foods typically are not capable of inducing symptoms.

TABLE 12-6   Gastrointestinal Food-Allergic Disorders

Disorder	Age group	Characteristics	Diagnosis	Prognosis and course
IgE-mediated disorders				
Acute gastrointestinal hypersensitivity	Any	Onset: minutes to 2 h; nausea, abdominal pain, emesis, diarrhea; typically in conjunction with cutaneous and/or respiratory symptoms	History, positive SPT, and/or serum food-IgE level; confirmatory OFC	Varies, food-dependent; milk, soy, egg, and wheat typically outgrown; peanut, tree nuts, seeds, and shellfish typically persistent
Pollen-food allergy syndrome (oral allergy syndrome)	Any; most common in young adults (50% of birch pollen-allergic adults)	Immediate symptoms on contact of raw fruit with oral mucosa: pruritus, tingling, erythema, or angioedema of the lips, tongue, oropharynx; throat pruritus/tightness	History, positive SPT with raw fruits or vegetables; OFC positive with raw fruit, negative with cooked	Severity of symptoms varies with pollen season; may improve in a subset of patients with pollen immunotherapy
IgE- and Non-IgE-mediated disorders				
Eosinophilic esophagitis	Any, but especially infants, children, and adolescents	*Children*: chronic or intermittent symptoms of gastroesophageal reflux, emesis, dysphagia, abdominal pain, and irritability *Adults*: abdominal pain, dysphagia, and food impaction	History, positive SPT, and/or food-IgE level in 50% but poor correlation with clinical symptoms; patch testing may be of value; elimination diet and OFC; endoscopy or biopsy provides conclusive diagnosis and information about treatment response	Varies, not well established; improvement with elimination diet within 6–8 weeks; elemental diet may be required; often responds to swallowed topical steroids
Allergic eosinophilic gastroenteritis	Any	Chronic or intermittent abdominal pain, emesis, irritability, poor appetite, failure to thrive, weight loss, anemia, protein-losing gastroenteropathy	History, positive SPT, and/or food-IgE level in 50% but poor correlation with clinical symptoms, elimination diet, and OFC; endoscopy or biopsy provides conclusive diagnosis and information about treatment response	Varies, not well established; improvement with elimination diet within 6–8 weeks; elemental diet may be required
Non-IgE-mediated disorders				
Food protein-induced allergic proctocolitis	Young infants (<6 months), frequently breastfed	Blood-streaked or heme-positive stools; otherwise healthy appearing	History, prompt response (resolution of gross blood in 48 h) to allergen elimination; biopsy conclusive but not necessary for most	Most able to tolerate milk or soy by 1–2 years
Food protein-induced enterocolitis syndrome	Young infants	*Chronic*: emesis, diarrhea, failure to thrive on chronic exposure *Subacute*: repetitive emesis, dehydration (15% shock), diarrhea on repeat exposure after elimination period; breastfeeding protective	History, response to dietary restriction; OFC	Most have resolution in 1–3 years; rarely persists into late teenage years
Food protein-induced enteropathy	Young infants; incidence has decreased	Protracted diarrhea, (steatorrhea), emesis, failure to thrive, anemia in 40%	History, endoscopy and biopsy; response to dietary restriction	Most have resolution in 1–2 years
Celiac disease (gluten-sensitive enteropathy)	Any	Chronic diarrhea, malabsorption, abdominal distention, flatulence, failure-to-thrive or weight loss; may be associated with oral ulcers and/or dermatitis herpetiformis	Biopsy diagnostic, shows villous atrophy; screening with serum IgA anti-tissue transglutaminase and antigliadin; resolution of symptoms with gluten elimination and relapse on oral challenge	Lifelong

IgE, immunoglobulin E; OFC, oral food challenge; SPT, skin-prick test.
(Modified from Nowak-Węgrzyn A, Sampson HA. Adverse reactions to foods. Med Clin North Am 2006; 90:97–127.)

Ragweed-allergic patients may experience pollen-food allergy syndrome after contact with raw melons (e.g., watermelon, cantaloupe, honeydew) and bananas. Symptoms may vary throughout the year, as shown for birch pollen-related food allergies. Symptoms are more prominent during the birch pollen season, corresponding to the seasonal rise in birch-specific IgE levels. Birch pollen–allergic patients may develop symptoms after the ingestion of raw carrots, celery, apples, pears, hazelnuts, and kiwi. Cross-reactivity between birch pollen and various fruits and vegetables is due to homology among various PR proteins. For example, Mal d 1, the major apple allergen, is 63% homologous with the major birch pollen allergen, Bet v 1 (Table 12-6).

Immediate gastrointestinal food allergy (i.e. *gastrointestinal anaphylaxis*) is a form of IgE-mediated gastrointestinal hypersensitivity that often accompanies allergic manifestations in other target organs and results in a variety of symptoms. Symptoms usually develop within minutes to 2 hours of consuming the responsible food and consist of nausea, abdominal pain, cramps, vomiting, and diarrhea. In food-allergic children with atopic dermatitis, frequent ingestion of a food allergen appears to induce partial desensitization of gastrointestinal mast cells, resulting in less pronounced symptoms, such as occasional minor complaints of poor appetite and periodic abdominal pain. A similar diminution of symptoms is seen in young infants with frequent vomiting, leading to a loss of consistent vomiting immediately after feeding.

Diagnosis is established by clinical history, determination of food-specific IgE antibodies (i.e. skin-prick tests or in-vitro IgE measurement), complete elimination of the suspected food allergen for up to 2 weeks with resolution of symptoms, and OFC. OFCs usually provoke typical symptoms if the allergen has been strictly eliminated from the patient's diet for 10 to 14 days.

Mixed IgE- and Non-IgE-Mediated Gastrointestinal Food Allergy

Mixed IgE- and non-IgE-mediated disorders may involve both IgE- and cell-mediated mechanisms. Allergic eosinophilic esophagitis, gastritis, and gastroenteritis are characterized by infiltration of the esophagus, stomach, and intestinal walls with eosinophils, basal zone hyperplasia, papillary elongation, absence of vasculitis, and peripheral eosinophilia in about 50% of patients. Eosinophilic esophagitis (EoE) is increasingly seen during infancy through adolescence, although the diagnosis appears to be occurring more frequently in adults. EoE typically manifests with symptoms of chronic gastroesophageal reflux disease, intermittent emesis, food refusal, abdominal pain, dysphagia, irritability, sleep disturbance, and failure to respond to conventional reflux medications. In adults, abdominal discomfort, dysphagia, and food impaction are more common. Diagnosis depends on the gastrointestinal biopsy demonstrating a characteristic eosinophilic infiltration, typically more than 15 eosinophils per high-power field (×40).[42]

Elimination of the responsible food allergens from the diet for up to 8 weeks may be necessary to bring about resolution of symptoms and for up to 12 weeks to bring about normalization of intestinal histology. This diet often requires the use of an amino acid–derived formula or an oligoantigenic diet. To identify the responsible foods, challenges are required that consist of reintroducing the suspect food allergen and demonstrating recurrence of symptoms and a significant eosinophilic infiltrate on biopsy.

Dietary intervention is effective, and about 50% of children respond favorably to dietary modifications. However, an elemental diet (e.g., amino acid–based formulas) may be necessary to identify the food allergens that provoke symptoms. A six-food elimination diet was effective in eliminating symptoms and esophageal pathology in more than 70% of patients treated.[43] An alternative approach is to use inhaled or oral corticosteroids, which usually bring about rapid symptomatic relief.

Infantile colic is an ill-defined syndrome of paroxysmal fussiness characterized by inconsolable agonized crying, drawing up of the legs, abdominal distention, and excessive gas. It usually develops in the first 2 to 4 weeks of life and persists through the third or fourth month. Although a variety of psychosocial and dietary factors have been implicated, it is difficult to establish the cause of infantile colic. Double-blind, crossover trials of bottle-fed and breast-fed infants suggest that IgE-mediated hypersensitivity may be a pathogenic factor in some infants. Allergic mechanisms probably account for only 10–15% of colicky infants. Diagnosis of food-induced colic can be established by implementation of several brief trials of hypoallergenic formula. Symptoms should resolve when the child is placed on the hypoallergenic formula and recur when the regular formula or breastfeeding resumes.

Non-IgE-Mediated Gastrointestinal Food Allergy

Several gastrointestinal disorders are thought to result from cell-mediated hypersensitivities (Table 12-6). *Food protein–induced enterocolitis syndrome (FPIES)* is a disorder most commonly seen in infants between 1 week and 3 months of age who present with protracted vomiting and diarrhea, which may result in dehydration.[44] A study from Israel reported a prevalence for milk-induced FPIES of 0.34% in a large (>14 000 infants), population-based birth cohort.[45] Vomiting usually occurs 1 to 4 hours after feeding, and continued exposure may result in watery or bloody diarrhea, anemia, abdominal distention, and failure to thrive. Symptoms are most commonly provoked by CM or soy protein-based formulas.

FPIES has been reported in older infants and children due to rice, oatmeal, egg, wheat, oat, peanut, nuts, chicken, turkey, and fish. Hypotension occurs in about 15% of cases after allergen ingestion, and 10–15% of patients present with methemoglobinemia. In adults, shellfish sensitivity may provoke a similar syndrome, with symptoms of severe nausea, abdominal cramps, and protracted vomiting. After an acute reaction, there is a prominent increase in the number of peripheral blood neutrophils, peaking at 4 to 6 hours from the onset of symptoms. Stools often contain occult blood, neutrophils, eosinophils, and Charcot–Leyden crystals. Skin-prick test results for the suspected foods are negative. Jejunal biopsies reveal flattened villi, edema, and increased numbers of lymphocytes, eosinophils, and mast cells.

Diagnosis can be established when elimination of the responsible allergen leads to resolution of symptoms within 72 hours and oral challenge provokes symptoms. However, secondary disaccharidase deficiency may uncommonly persist longer and may result in ongoing diarrhea for up to 2 weeks. OFCs consist of administering 0.3 to 0.6 g/kg of body weight of the suspected food protein.[46] Vomiting usually develops within 1 to 4 hours of administering the challenge food, often accompanied by pallor and lethargy. Diarrhea or loose stools may develop after 4 to 8 hours. In conjunction with a positive food challenge result, the peripheral blood absolute neutrophil count increases to at least 3500 cells/mm^5 within 4 to 6 hours of developing symptoms, and neutrophils and eosinophils may be found in the stools. Because about 15% of OFC lead to profuse vomiting, dehydration and hypotension, they must be performed under medical supervision.[47]

Food protein–induced allergic proctocolitis usually manifests in the first few months of life. Although such reactions are often caused by CM or soy protein hypersensitivity, most occur in breastfeeding infants.[48] They typically appear well, often have normally formed stools, and usually are discovered because of the presence of blood (gross or occult) in their stools. Blood loss is usually minor but occasionally can produce anemia. The diagnosis can be established when elimination of the responsible allergen leads to resolution of gross blood passage (hematochezia), usually with dramatic improvement within 72 hours of appropriate food allergen elimination, but complete clearance and resolution of mucosal lesions may take up to 1 month. Reintroduction of the allergen leads to recurrence of symptoms within several hours to days. Lesions are confined to the distal large bowel. Sigmoidoscopy findings vary, ranging from areas of patchy mucosal injection to severe friability with small, aphthoid ulcerations and bleeding.[49] Colonic biopsy reveals a prominent eosinophilic infiltrate in the surface and crypt epithelia and the lamina propria. In severe lesions with crypt destruction, neutrophils are prominent.

CM and soy protein–induced proctocolitis usually resolve within 6 months to 2 years of allergen avoidance, but occasional refractory cases are seen.

Food protein–induced enteropathy (excluding celiac disease) usually manifests in the first several months of life with diarrhea (mild to moderate steatorrhea in about 80%)

and poor weight gain. Symptoms include protracted diarrhea, vomiting in up to two thirds of patients, failure to thrive, and malabsorption, which is demonstrated by the presence of reducing substances in the stools, increased fecal fat, and abnormal D-xylose absorption. CM hypersensitivity is the most frequent cause of this syndrome, but it also has been associated with sensitivity to soy, egg, wheat, rice, chicken, and fish.[50]

Diagnosis requires the identification and exclusion of the responsible allergen from the diet, which brings about a resolution of symptoms within several days to weeks. On endoscopy, a patchy villous atrophy is evident, and biopsy reveals a prominent mononuclear round cell infiltrate and a small number of eosinophils, which is not unlike celiac disease but usually is much less extensive. Colitis-like features are usually absent, but anemia occurs in about 40% of affected infants, and protein loss occurs in most. Complete resolution of the intestinal lesions may require 6 to 18 months of allergen avoidance. Unlike celiac disease, loss of clinical reactivity frequently occurs, but the natural history of this disorder has not been well studied.

Celiac disease is an extensive enteropathy that leads to malabsorption.[51] The disease occurs in adults and children at rates approaching 1% of the population. Total villous atrophy and extensive cellular infiltrates are associated with sensitivity to gliadin, the alcohol-soluble portion of gluten found in wheat, rye, and barley. Celiac disease represents an interplay between the environment and genetics, with a strong association with human leukocyte antigen (HLA)-DQ2 ($\alpha 1^*0501$, $\beta 1^*0201$), which is present in more than 90% of patients. The incidence of celiac disease is 1 case per 250 people in the US, according to the Celiac Disease Foundation. Introduction of gluten into infant diets before 4 months of age has been identified as a risk factor for celiac disease by some studies, whereas introduction after 6 months has been identified as a risk factor for wheat allergy. The intestinal inflammation in celiac disease is precipitated by exposure to gliadin. Gluten-specific T cells are found in the biopsies of these patients, and without exception, they respond to gluten-derived peptides bound to the disease-associated HLA-DQ2 or HLA-DQ8 molecules. Most patients develop IgA antibodies against gliadin and tissue transglutaminase (tTGase). Virtually all celiac disease patients possess autoantibodies to distinct epitopes on the tTGase molecule, but the antibodies do not appear to be responsible for the pathology.[52]

Initial symptoms often include diarrhea or frank steatorrhea, abdominal distention and flatulence, weight loss, and occasionally nausea and vomiting. Oral ulcers and other extra-intestinal symptoms caused by malabsorption are not uncommon. Villous atrophy of the small bowel is a characteristic feature of celiac patients who ingest gluten. IgA antibodies to gluten are present in more than 80% of adults and children with untreated celiac disease. Patients usually have increased levels of IgG antibodies to a variety of foods, which is presumably the result of increased food antigen absorption. Diagnosis depends on demonstrating biopsy evidence of villous atrophy and inflammatory infiltrate, resolution of biopsy findings after 6 to 12 weeks of gluten elimination, and recurrence of biopsy changes after a gluten challenge. Revised diagnostic criteria have eliminated the requirement for a gluten challenge and instead place a greater focus on serologic studies.

Quantification of IgA anti-gliadin and IgA anti-endomysial antibodies may be used for screening with IgA anti-tTGase antibodies in patients older than 2 years of age. After the diagnosis of celiac disease is established, lifelong elimination of gluten-containing foods is necessary to control symptoms and to avoid the increased risk of malignancy.

Cutaneous Food Allergy

The skin is a frequent target organ in IgE- and non-IgE-mediated food hypersensitivity reactions (Table 12-7). Ingestion of food allergens may lead to the rapid onset of cutaneous symptoms or aggravate chronic conditions.[1]

Cutaneous IgE-Mediated Food Allergy

Urticaria and angioedema are the most common acute symptoms of food-allergic reactions, although the prevalence of these reactions is unknown. Because the onset of

TABLE 12-7   Cutaneous Food-Allergic Disorders

Disorder	Age group	Characteristics	Diagnosis	Prognosis and course
IgE-mediated disorders				
Acute urticaria and angioedema	Any	Pruritic, evanescent skin rash (hives) and swelling within minutes to 2 h after food ingestion; food identified as a culprit in 20%	History, positive SPT, and/ or serum food-IgE level; confirmed by OFC if necessary	Varies, food-dependent; milk, soy, egg, and wheat typically outgrown; peanut, tree nuts, seeds, and shellfish typically persistent
Chronic urticaria and angioedema (rare)	Any	Hives and swelling for >6 weeks; approximately 2% caused by food	History, positive SPT, and/ or serum food-IgE level; confirmed by OFC if necessary	Varies
IgE- and Non-IgE-mediated disorders				
Atopic dermatitis	Infant and child; 90% start <5 years	Relapsing pruritic vesiculopapular rash; generalized in infants, localized to flexor areas in older children; food allergy in about 35% of children with moderate to severe atopic dermatitis	History, SPT, and/or serum food-IgE level; elimination diet and OFC	60–80% improve significantly or allergy resolves by adolescence
Non-IgE-mediated disorders				
Contact dermatitis	Any; more common in adults	Relapsing pruritic eczematous rash, often on hands or face; often occurs in occupational contact with food stuff	History, patch testing	Varies
Dermatitis herpetiformis	Any	Intensely pruritic vesicular rash on extensor surfaces and buttocks	Biopsy diagnostic, shows IgA granule deposits at the dermal-epidermal junction; resolves with dietary gluten avoidance	Lifelong

Ig, Immunoglobulin; OFC, oral food challenge; SPT, skin-prick test.
(Modified from Nowak-Węgrzyn A, Sampson HA. Adverse reactions to foods. Med Clin North Am 2006; 90:97–127.)

symptoms follows within minutes of ingesting the responsible allergen, the cause-and-effect nature of the reaction is often obvious. Most individuals with these reactions do not seek medical assistance or necessarily report these to their physicians. The foods most commonly incriminated in adults are fish, shellfish, tree nuts, and peanut, and in children, they include egg, milk, peanut, and nuts.

Acute contact urticaria has been reported with raw meats, fish, shellfish, milk, raw egg, vegetables, and fruits. Most studies of patients with chronic urticaria and angioedema (i.e. symptoms lasting >6 weeks) indicate that allergy to foods or food additives are rarely (2–4%) implicated. Diagnosis is based on the demonstration of food-specific IgE antibodies (i.e. skin test or in-vitro IgE), resolution of skin symptoms with complete elimination of the putative food from the diet, and development of symptoms after challenge.

Mixed IgE- and Non-IgE-Mediated Cutaneous Food Allergy

Atopic dermatitis usually begins in early infancy (90% younger than 1 year of age). It is characterized by a typical distribution, extreme pruritus, chronically relapsing course, and association with asthma and allergic rhinitis.[53]

In one study, 35–40% of children with moderate to severe atopic dermatitis presenting to a university-based dermatologist were found to be food allergic after allergy evaluations and DBPCFCs.[54] An earlier study demonstrated a direct correlation between disease severity and the likelihood of food allergy. In a follow-up study of 34 children with atopic dermatitis, 17 children with food allergy placed on an appropriate allergen elimination diet experienced marked, significant improvement in their eczematous rash over the 4-year follow-up period compared with non-food-allergic children and food-allergic children not adhering to an allergen-elimination diet. In a series of almost 500 children with atopic dermatitis and food allergy, approximately one third of symptomatic food hypersensitivities were outgrown in 2 to 3 years. The probability of developing tolerance appeared to depend on the food antigen responsible; development of tolerance to soy was common, whereas development of tolerance to peanut was rare. Results of skin-prick tests often became negative or remained unchanged, but concentrations of allergen-specific IgE dropped significantly. The pathogenic role of food allergy in adults with atopic dermatitis requires further investigation.

Diagnosis is based on demonstration of food-specific IgE antibodies or occasionally on food-specific patch tests, elimination diets, and OFCs. At the time of first evaluation, skin symptoms provoked by a DBPCFC usually consist of a markedly pruritic, erythematous, morbilliform rash that develops in sites for which atopic dermatitis has a predilection. Urticarial lesions are rarely seen. However, urticaria is frequently seen in follow-up challenges conducted 1 to 2 years later in patients who had adhered to an appropriate allergen elimination diet and had experienced clearing of their eczema but who remained food sensitive. Attempts at reintroducing food should be under a physician's supervision.[55] Although the history may not suggest other food-induced complaints, food challenges can provoke intestinal symptoms (e.g., nausea, abdominal cramping, vomiting, diarrhea) in almost half of patients; upper respiratory symptoms (e.g., laryngeal edema, sensation of itching and tightness in the throat; persistent throat clearing with a dry, hacking cough; hoarseness) in about one third; and wheezing in about 10% of positive challenges. When absorption studies are performed (e.g., lactulose-rhamnose, lactulose-mannitol), most patients are found to have malabsorption, even though gastrointestinal complaints are minimal.

Non-IgE-Mediated Cutaneous Food Allergy

Food-induced contact dermatitis is seen frequently among food handlers, especially among those who handle raw fish, shellfish (e.g., snow crabs), meats, and eggs. Patch tests can be used if necessary to confirm the diagnosis.

Dermatitis herpetiformis (DH) is a chronic, blistering skin disorder associated with a gluten-sensitive enteropathy.[56,57] It is characterized by a chronic, intensely pruritic papulovesicular rash symmetrically distributed over the extensor surfaces and buttocks. The histology of the intestinal lesion is virtually identical to that seen in celiac disease, but villous atrophy and inflammatory infiltrates are usually milder. As in patients with celiac disease, virtually all DH patients have circulating IgA antibodies against tTGase, the quantity of which appears to correlate with the extent of the jejunal mucosal lesions.

Diagnosis of DH depends on the presence of the characteristic skin lesions and demonstration of IgA deposition at the dermal-epidermal junction of the skin. Although many patients have minimal or no gastrointestinal complaints, biopsy of the small bowel usually reveals intestinal involvement. Elimination of gluten from the diet usually leads to resolution of skin symptoms and normalization of intestinal findings over several months. Administration of sulfones, the mainstay of therapy, leads to rapid resolution of skin symptoms but has virtually no effect on intestinal symptoms.

Respiratory Food Allergy

Acute respiratory symptoms caused by food allergy represent pure IgE-mediated reactions, whereas chronic respiratory symptoms represent a mix of IgE-mediated and non-IgE-mediated symptoms (Table 12-8). Upper and lower respiratory reactions have been provoked in some children by double-blind, placebo-controlled food challenges (DBPCFCs), with spirometry demonstrating significant reductions in forced vital capacity (FVC), forced expiratory volume in 1 second (FEV_1), and maximum end-expiratory flow (MMEF) values during positive food challenges.[58]

Rhinoconjunctivitis alone is infrequently a manifestation of food allergy, and when present, it is typically accompanied by other allergic symptoms. Within minutes to 2 hours of ingestion, food allergens may induce typical signs and symptoms of rhinoconjunctivitis, including periocular erythema, pruritus, and tearing; nasal congestion, pruritus, and sneezing; and rhinorrhea.

TABLE 12-8   Respiratory Food-Allergic Disorders

Disorder	Age group	Characteristics	Diagnosis	Prognosis and course
IgE-mediated disorders				
Allergic rhinoconjunctivitis	Any	Ocular pruritus, conjunctival injection and watery discharge, nasal pruritus, congestion, rhinorrhea, sneezing within minutes to 2 h after food ingestion or inhalation; cutaneous and gastrointestinal manifestations typical	History, SPT, and/or serum food-IgE level; OFC	Varies
Acute bronchospasm	Any	Cough, wheezing, dyspnea on food ingestion or inhalation; possible risk factor for severe anaphylaxis; cutaneous and gastrointestinal manifestations typical	History, SPT, and/or serum food-IgE level; OFC	Varies
IgE- and Non-IgE-mediated disorders				
Asthma	Any	Chronic cough, wheezing, dyspnea; food allergy is risk factor for intubation in children who have asthma	History, SPT, and/or serum food-IgE level; OFC	Varies
Non-IgE-mediated disorders*				
Pulmonary hemosiderosis (Heiner syndrome)	Infants, children (rare)	Chronic cough, hemoptysis, lung infiltrates, wheezing, anemia; described in cow's milk– and buckwheat-allergic infants	History, SPT, and serum food-IgE negative, but milk and buckwheat IgG precipitins positive; lung biopsy with deposits of IgG and IgA	Unknown

Ig, Immunoglobulin; OFC, oral food challenge; SPT, skin-prick test.
*Presumed.
(Modified from Nowak-Węgrzyn A, Sampson HA. Adverse reactions to foods. Med Clin North Am 2006; 90:97–127.)

Approximately 25% of 112 patients with histories of adverse food reactions occurring after 10 years of age developed respiratory symptoms after an OFC, and most were nasal symptoms caused by fruit or vegetable sensitivities.[59] Despite the notion that milk ingestion frequently leads to nasal congestion in young infants, the objective evidence from oral milk challenges shows that only 0.08–0.2% of infants develop nasal symptoms after a milk challenge.

In children with atopic dermatitis, nasal symptoms typically develop within 15 to 90 min of initiating the DBPCFC and last about 0.5 to 2 hours. Nasal and periocular pruritus are commonly followed by prolonged bursts of sneezing and copious rhinorrhea.

Asthma or isolated wheezing alone is an infrequent manifestation of food allergy. Although ingestion of food allergens is rarely the main aggravating factor in chronic asthma, some evidence suggests that food antigens can provoke bronchial hyperreactivity. In surveys of children with asthma attending pulmonary clinics, food-induced respiratory reactions were demonstrated in about 6–8.5% of children.[60] About 25% of 279 children referred for evaluation with histories of food-induced wheezing or asthma experienced wheezing as one of the symptoms during a DBPCFC. Asthmatic reactions to airborne food allergens have been reported when susceptible individuals are exposed to vapors or steam emitted from cooking food (e.g., milk, fish, mollusks, crustaceans, eggs, garbanzo beans).[61] One study suggested that children with asthma who are sensitized to food allergens are at greater risk for severe asthma, as judged by hospitalizations, emergency visits, days missed from school, and rescue medication use.

Diagnosis of food-induced respiratory disease is based on a patient's history, evidence of food-specific IgE (e.g., positive skin test results, in-vitro IgE tests to food antigens), and OFCs. DBPCFCs after strict elimination of suspected food allergens are usually the only way to confirm the diagnosis of food-induced wheezing. Because many factors can exacerbate wheezing, elimination diets alone typically are not useful.

Non-IgE-Mediated Respiratory Food Allergy

Food-induced pulmonary hemosiderosis (Heiner syndrome) is a rare syndrome of recurrent episodes of pneumonia associated with pulmonary infiltrates and hemorrhage, hemosiderosis, gastrointestinal blood loss, iron-deficiency anemia, and failure to thrive. Hemosiderin-laden macrophages may be found in morning aspirates of the stomach or seen in biopsy specimens of the lung.[1] Heiner syndrome is most often associated with a non-IgE-mediated hypersensitivity to CM, but reactivity to egg, pork, and buckwheat have also been reported. Although peripheral blood eosinophilia and multiple serum precipitins to CM are a relatively constant feature, the immunologic mechanisms responsible for this disorder are unknown. Diagnosis is based on the elimination of the precipitating allergen and subsequent resolution of symptoms. Characteristic laboratory data, including precipitating IgG antibodies to CM (or the responsible antigen), are also necessary for diagnosis.

Food-Induced Generalized Anaphylaxis

Food allergies are the single leading cause of generalized anaphylaxis seen in hospital emergency departments in the US and account for at least one third of cases.[62] In addition to the cutaneous, respiratory, and gastrointestinal symptoms described earlier, patients may develop cardiovascular symptoms, including hypotension, vascular collapse, and cardiac dysrhythmias, presumably due to massive mediator release by mast cells. However, most food-induced anaphylactic reactions are not associated with major increases in serum levels of β-tryptase. In a series of 12 fatal or near-fatal food-induced anaphylactic reactions, all patients experienced severe respiratory compromise, 10 of 12 had nausea and vomiting, and only 7 of 12 patients (or 1 of 6 fatal reactions) had cutaneous symptoms.[63] About one third of patients developed a biphasic reaction and one quarter experienced prolonged symptoms, typically lasting 2 to 3 days.

Factors that appear to be associated with severe reactions include the presence of asthma; a history of severe reactions; denial of symptoms; and failure to initiate therapy expeditiously. Surveys of food-induced anaphylactic deaths found that anaphylactic reactions to foods affected both sexes equally, most victims were adolescents or young adults, and almost all individuals with a food allergy had a history of some type of reaction to the food culprit that caused the fatal reaction.[64] Among the subjects for whom data were available, virtually all were known to have asthma, very few had epinephrine available for use at the time of their reaction, and about 10% of those who received epinephrine in a timely fashion did not survive. Peanuts or tree nuts were responsible for more than 85% of the fatalities in the US.

Food-Dependent, Exercise-Induced Anaphylaxis

Food-dependent, exercise-induced anaphylaxis (FDEIA) occurs only when the patient exercises within 2 to 4 hours of ingesting a food, but in the absence of exercise, the patient can ingest the food without any apparent reaction.[1] Amongst patients with exercise-induced anaphylaxis, approximately 30–50% report associated food triggers. Patients usually have asthma and other atopic disorders, positive skin-prick test results for the food that provokes their symptoms, and occasionally a history of reacting to the food when they were younger. This disorder appears to be more common in females than males and most prevalent in the late teens to mid-30s. The exact mechanism of this disorder is unknown, but several foods have been implicated, including wheat (i.e. omega-5 gliadin portion), shellfish, fruit, milk, celery, and fish. Diagnosis is based on an unequivocal history of food ingestion followed by exercise, the rapid onset (within 1–2 h) of classic IgE-mediated symptoms, and the demonstration of food-specific IgE antibodies by skin-prick testing or in-vitro tests for IgE. Lacking this evidence, a physician-supervised food challenge is usually warranted to ensure that the suspected food is truly responsible for the anaphylactic reaction. Challenges should be done in a hospital setting by a physician experienced in the treatment of anaphylactic reactions.[65]

Delayed Anaphylaxis Caused by Mammalian Meat

Galactose-α-1,3-galactose (α-gal) has been identified as a cause of serious, even fatal, anaphylaxis.[66] In contrast to previously described cross-reactive carbohydrate determinants expressed in plants and insects, the oligosaccharide α-gal is abundantly expressed on cells and tissues of non-primate mammals. This expression pattern makes α-gal potentially clinically relevant as a food allergen (e.g., beef, pork, lamb) or as an inhaled allergen (e.g., cat, dog). IgE antibodies to α-gal are associated with an unusual form of delayed anaphylaxis, which occurs 3 to 6 hours after ingestion of mammalian meat that carries α-gal. Patients with IgE to α-gal describe generalized urticaria or frank anaphylaxis starting 3 to 6 hours after eating beef, pork, or lamb and have a consistent pattern of skin testing (likelihood of positive results is increased by testing with freshly ground meat or with intradermal testing) and serum IgE antibody results.

Most patients developed anaphylaxis to red meat in adulthood; some reported receiving multiple tick bites, suggesting that tick bites, especially the lone star tick (*Amblyomma americanum*) in the US, may predispose to sensitization to α-gal.

Other Food-Induced Hypersensitivity Reactions

Ingestion of pasteurized, whole CM by infants, especially those younger than 6 months of age, frequently leads to occult gastrointestinal blood loss and occasionally to *iron-deficiency anemia*. Substitution of infant formula (including CM-derived formulas that have been subjected to extensive heating) for whole CM usually normalizes fecal blood loss within 3 days.

PATIENT EVALUATION, DIAGNOSIS, AND DIFFERENTIAL DIAGNOSIS

Food Allergy Guidelines (Table 12-9) are available online (http://www.niaid.nih.gov/topics/foodallergy)[67] in a full format, with an executive summary, and a lay-language summary for patients, families, and caregivers. The European Academy of Allergy and Clinical Immunology (EAACI) have also published guidelines for anaphylaxis and food allergy.[65]

The diagnostic approach to food allergy begins with the medical history and physical examination.[1] These assessments guide the selection of the laboratory tests (Fig. 12-1).

The value of the medical history largely depends on the patient's recollection of symptoms and the examiner's ability to differentiate between disorders provoked by food hypersensitivity and other causes (Table 12-1). In some cases, it may be useful in diagnosing food allergy (e.g., acute events such as systemic anaphylaxis after isolated ingestion of shrimp), but history alone should never be used to make a diagnosis.

In several series, <50% of reported food-allergic reactions could be verified by DBPCFCs. Information required to establish that a food-allergic reaction occurred and to construct an appropriate blinded challenge at a later date include the following: the food presumed to have provoked the reaction; the quantity of the suspected food ingested; the length of time between ingestion and development of symptoms; whether similar symptoms developed on other occasions when the food was eaten; whether other factors (e.g., exercise, alcohol, drugs) are necessary; and how long since the last reaction to the food occurred. In chronic disorders (e.g., atopic dermatitis, asthma, chronic urticaria), the history is often an unreliable indicator of the offending allergen.

Diet diaries are frequently discussed as an adjunct to history. Patients are instructed to keep a chronologic record of all foods ingested over a specified period, including items placed in the mouth but not swallowed, such as chewing gum. Any symptoms experienced by the patient are also recorded. The diary is then reviewed to determine whether there are any relationships between foods ingested and symptoms experienced. Occasionally, this method detects an unrecognized association between a food and a patient's symptoms. Unlike the medical history, it collects information on a prospective basis and does not depend on a patient's memory. This approach should be used selectively because it often causes patients and families to focus obsessively on foods instead of other potential triggers of their reactions.

TABLE 12-9 National Institute of Allergy and Infectious Diseases: Sponsored Expert Panel Report on the Diagnosis and Management of Food Allergy in the United States

Key points	Guidelines and comments
Definitions	Food allergy is an adverse health effect arising from a specific immune response. Food allergies result in immunoglobulin E (IgE)-mediated, immediate reactions (i.e. anaphylaxis) and a variety of chronic diseases (e.g., eosinophilic esophagitis, food protein-induced enterocolitis syndrome) in which IgE may not play an important role.
Epidemiology and natural history	
Children	Food allergy is more common in children than adults. Among the most common food allergies in children, milk, egg, wheat, and soy allergies often resolve in childhood; peanut, tree nut, fish, and shellfish allergies can resolve but are more likely to persist. Peanut allergy prevalence has increased over several decades and now affects 1–2% of young children.
Adults	Adult food allergies can reflect persistence of childhood allergies or de novo sensitization to food allergens encountered after childhood. A food allergy that starts in adult life tends to persist. Among adults, shellfish (2.5%), fish (0.5%), peanut (0.6%), and tree nut (0.5%) allergies are the most common. Adults and some children experience cross-reactivity between certain aeroallergens and foods (e.g., oral allergy/pollen food allergy syndrome) detailed in the guidelines. Milk, egg, wheat, and soy allergies often resolve in childhood; peanut, tree nut, fish, and shellfish allergies can resolve but more likely persist.
Comorbidities	Food allergies may coexist with asthma, atopic dermatitis, eosinophilic esophagitis, and exercise-induced anaphylaxis. Food allergy is associated with severe asthma, increased risk of severe exacerbations, and increased hospitalization rates. Food allergies disrupt the quality of life. Food allergy is not a common trigger of eczema in adults. Eosinophilic esophagitis, which involves localized eosinophilic inflammation of the esophagus, is a chronic, remitting-relapsing condition associated with sensitization to foods. In some patients, avoidance of specific foods results in normalization of histopathology. In children, it manifests with feeding disorders, vomiting, reflux symptoms, and abdominal pain. In adolescents and adults, it most often manifests with dysphagia and esophageal food impactions. One third of patients with exercise-induced anaphylaxis report reactions triggered by foods; exercise-induced anaphylaxis has natural history marked by frequent recurrence of episodes.
Risk factors for severe anaphylaxis	Fatal food-allergic reactions are usually caused by peanut, tree nuts, and seafood but also have resulted from milk, egg, seeds, and other foods. Fatalities have been associated with age (teenagers and young adults), delayed treatment with epinephrine, and comorbid asthma. Severity of future allergic reactions is not accurately predicted by the history. There are no laboratory tests to predict severity of future reactions. Food taken on empty stomach, exercise, alcohol, non-steroidal antiinflammatory drugs, and antacid agents may increase severity of an allergic reaction. Therapy with β-blockers may decrease effectiveness of epinephrine in anaphylaxis.
Diagnosis	Food allergy is suspected when typical symptoms (e.g., urticaria, edema, wheezing, mouth itch, cough, nausea, vomiting, anaphylaxis) occur within minutes to hours of food ingestion. A detailed history of the reaction to each incriminated food is essential for proper diagnosis. Children younger than 5 years of age with moderate to severe atopic dermatitis should be considered for evaluation for milk, egg, peanut, wheat, and soy allergies if one or both of the following conditions are present: Persistent atopic dermatitis despite optimized management and topical therapy Reliable history of an immediate reaction after ingestion of a specific food A medically supervised food challenge is considered the most specific test for food allergy. Tests for food-specific IgE levels assist in the diagnosis but should not be relied as the sole means to diagnose food allergy. The medical history and examination are recommended to aid in the diagnosis. Food-specific IgE testing has limitations: Positive test results are not intrinsically diagnostic, and reactions sometimes occur despite negative test results. Testing food panels without considering the history is often misleading. Several tests are not recommended, including food-specific IgG/IgG4, total IgE, applied kinesiology, and electrodermal testing.
Prevention	The recommendations follow the 2008 American Academy of Pediatrics clinical report. Breastfeeding is encouraged for all infants, hydrolyzed infant formulas are suggested for infants at risk,* and complementary foods, including potential allergens, are not restricted after 4–6 months of age (not applicable for infants experiencing allergic reactions). Maternal diet during pregnancy should be healthy and balanced; evidence to support avoidance of potential food allergens is lacking.
Management[†]	
Avoidance	Education about food avoidance is essential to prevent reactions.
Immunizations	Patients with egg allergy can be immunized with influenza vaccines containing a low dose of egg protein. Yellow fever and rabies vaccines are contraindicated in persons with a history of urticaria, angioedema, asthma, or anaphylaxis to egg proteins. Allergy evaluation and testing can provide insight into the potential risk for an individual.

Continued on following page

TABLE 12-9   National Institute of Allergy and Infectious Diseases: Sponsored Expert Panel Report on the Diagnosis and Management of Food Allergy in the United States (Continued)

Key points	Guidelines and comments
Anaphylaxis	Management of anaphylaxis relies on prompt administration of epinephrine, observation for 4–6 h or longer after treatment, education on avoidance, early recognition and treatment, medical identification jewelry, and follow-up with a primary healthcare provider and consideration of consultation with an allergist-immunologist. Prescription for epinephrine auto-injectors and advice for patient education include having two doses available, switching from 0.15–0.3 mg fixed-dose auto-injectors at approximately 25 kg (55 lb) in the context of patient-specific circumstances, having a written emergency plan, and providing supporting educational material.

*At-risk infants are defined as having one or more immediate family members (e.g., parent, sibling) with atopic disorder.

†Several Web-based resources on food allergies are available for medical professionals and patients: National Institute of Allergy and Infectious Diseases (www.niaid.nih.gov/topics/foodAllergy); National Institute for Health and Clinical Excellence (http://guidance.nice.org.uk/CG116); World Allergy Association (WAO) Diagnosis and Rationale for Action against Cow's Milk Allergy (DRACMA) Guidelines (http://www.worldallergy .org/publications/WAO_DRACMA_guidelines.pdf); Consortium of Food Allergy Research (https://web.emmes.com/study/cofar/Education Program.htm); Food Allergy Research and Education (http://www.foodallergy.org); Kids with Food Allergies Foundation Community (www .kidswithfoodallergies.org).

(Modified from Boyce J, Assa'ad AH, Burks AW, et al. Guidelines for the diagnosis and management of food allergy in the United States: summary of the NIAID-sponsored expert panel report. J Allergy Clin Immunol 2010; 126(Suppl):S1–S58.)

Elimination diets are frequently used in the diagnosis and management of food allergy. Suspected foods are completely omitted from the diet. The success of these diets depends on the identification of the correct allergens, the ability of the patient to maintain a diet free of all forms of the offending allergens, and the assumption that other factors do not provoke similar symptoms during the period of study. Unfortunately, these conditions are rarely met. In a young infant reacting to CM-formula, resolution of symptoms after substitution with a soy formula or casein hydrolysate (e.g., Alimentum, Nutramigen) or with an elemental amino acid-based formula (e.g., Neocate, EleCare) is highly suggestive of CM or other food allergy, respectively, but it also could be caused by lactose intolerance. Although avoidance of suspected food allergens is recommended before blinded challenges, elimination diets alone are rarely diagnostic of food allergy, especially in chronic disorders such as atopic dermatitis or asthma.

Skin-prick tests are reproducible and frequently used to screen patients with suspected IgE-mediated food allergies. Glycerinated food extracts (1:10 or 1:20) and appropriate positive (e.g., histamine) and negative (e.g., saline) controls are applied by the prick or puncture technique.

Any food allergens eliciting a wheal with a diameter at least 3 mm greater than the negative control are considered to be positive; all other results are considered to be negative. A positive skin-prick test should be interpreted as indicating the *possibility* that the patient has symptomatic reactivity to the specific food, whereas negative skin test results confirm the absence of IgE-mediated reactions (negative predictive accuracy is >95%) if good-quality food extracts are used. The skin-prick test may be considered an excellent means of excluding IgE-mediated food allergies, but it can only suggest the presence of clinical food allergies. There are some exceptions to this general statement. First, IgE-mediated allergy to several fruits and vegetables (e.g., apples, oranges, bananas, pears, melons, potatoes, carrots, celery) is frequently not detected with commercially prepared reagents, presumably due to the lability of the responsible allergen. Second, commercial extracts sometimes lack the appropriate allergen to which an individual is reactive, as demonstrated by the use of fresh foods for skin test reagents. Third, children younger than 1 year of age may have IgE-mediated food allergy in the absence of positive skin test results, and infants younger than 2 years of age may have smaller wheals, presumably due to a lack of skin reactivity. Fourth, a positive skin test result for a food, that when ingested in the absence of other foods provokes a serious systemic anaphylactic reaction, may be considered diagnostic. In general, the larger the skin-prick test wheal diameter, the higher the likelihood of a reaction upon ingestion of the food. For some foods, the diagnostic decision points have been established, above which there is more than a 95% likelihood that the patient is allergic. The examples are cow milk wheal size ≥10 mm and peanut wheal size ≥8 mm in children.[68]

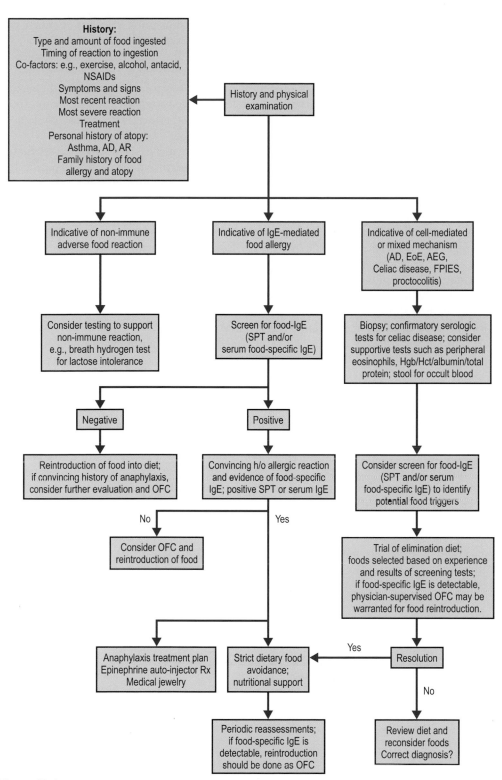

Figure 12-1 Current approach to the diagnosis and management of food allergy. AD, atopic dermatitis; AEG, allergic eosinophilic gastroenteritis; AR, allergic rhinitis; EoE, eosinophilic esophagitis; FPIES, food protein-induced enterocolitis syndrome; Hct, hematocrit; Hgb, hemoglobin; IgE, immunoglobulin E; NSAIDs, non-steroidal anti-inflammatory drugs; OFC, oral food challenge; Rx, treatment; SPT, skin-prick test. *(Modified from Nowak-Węgrzyn A, Sampson HA. Adverse reactions to foods. Med Clin North Am 2006; 90:97–127.)*

Intradermal skin testing is more sensitive than the skin-prick test but is much less specific than a DBPCFC. Intradermal skin testing increases the risk of inducing a systemic reaction compared with skin-prick testing and is therefore not recommended.

There has been increasing interest in the use of the atopy patch test for the diagnosis of non-IgE-mediated food allergy in several disorders. The lack of standardized reagents and method limits the utility of this approach. In one large study of children with atopic dermatitis, the investigators concluded that the patch test added little diagnostic benefit compared with standard diagnostic tests.[69]

In-vitro allergen-specific IgE tests are used for measuring serum for IgE-mediated food allergies. In the past 10 years, the quantitative measurement of food-specific IgE antibodies (i.e. CAP System FEIA or UniCAP) has been shown to be more predictive of symptomatic IgE-mediated food allergy than other methods. Food-specific IgE levels exceeding the diagnostic values (Table 12-10) indicate that patients are >95% likely to experience an allergic reaction if they ingest the specific food.[1,70,71] The IgE levels can be monitored, and if they fall to <2 kU_A/L for egg, milk, or peanut, the patient without recent severe reactions should be challenged again to determine whether he or she has outgrown the food allergy.

Periodic evaluations should be offered to children with peanut allergy, and an OFC for peanut should be considered in patients who have not had reactions in the past 1–2 years and who have a serum peanut-IgE level of <2.0 kU_A/L.

Component-resolved diagnosis (CRD) is based on individual natural or recombinant allergens that are purified. Using advanced microtechnology, qualified amounts of allergens can be spotted on activated biochip (e.g., ISAC microarray) surfaces, and minute quantities of serum are needed to detect IgE antibody to almost any number of specific allergens in a single-step process. CRD potentially offers superior specificity due to the purity of the components compared with wholefood extracts. OFCs were used in several studies to evaluate the clinical applications of CRD in cases of food allergy. Patients with IgE antibodies directed exclusively against birch Bet v 1 cross-reactive components in peanut Ara h 8 and hazelnut Cor a 1, are at low risk for systemic reaction to peanut and hazelnut; many may ingest these nuts without any allergic symptoms and therefore such patients are excellent candidates for supervised oral food challenges.[72] In contrast, patients with IgE directed against Ara h 2 or Cor a 9 and/or 14, are at higher risk for systemic reactions.[73,74] High levels of IgE against heat stable casein in CM and ovomucoid in egg white are associated with higher risk of reactions to baked milk and egg products.[75,76]

TABLE 12-10   Food-Specific IgE Serum Concentrations Highly Predictive of Clinical Reactivity

Allergen	Diagnostic decision level (kU_A/L)*	Sensitivity (%)	Specificity (%)	Positive predictive value (%)	Negative predictive value (%)
Egg white	7	61	95	98	38
Infants ≤2 years	0.35	91	77	95	68
Ovomucoid for baked egg	10.8	55	96	88	80
Milk	15	57	94	95	53
Infants ≤1 year	5	30	99	95	64
Peanut	14	57	99	99	36
Fish	20	25	100	99	89
Soybean	30	44	94	73	82
Wheat	26	61	92	74	87
Tree nuts	15	Other values were not calculated and are not available		95	

*kU_A/L = allergen specific kilo units per liter.

Oral food challenges are an important element in the management of food allergies in patients, and they remain the most accurate tests for the diagnosis of food allergy.[77] Food challenges may be conducted at home without medical supervision only if the physician determines that there is no risk of a severe reaction. This approach may be appropriate for patients who present with complaints that are usually not associated with food allergy and when skin or in-vitro testing results have been negative. It may also be appropriate to do a home reintroduction of a food that has been temporarily discontinued as part of an elimination diet but had been present in the diet previously. However, if there has been prolonged avoidance lasting weeks to a few months, the pattern of reactivity might have changed, and a home introduction may no longer be safe. In the majority of the cases, OFCS are performed under physician supervision.

The DBPCFC has been labeled the gold standard for the diagnosis of food allergies.[1,67,78] Many investigators have used DBPCFCs successfully in children and adults to examine a variety of food-related complaints. In clinical practice, open (unblinded) and single-blinded OFCs are frequently used. The selection of foods to be tested in an OFC is usually based on history and skin test or in-vitro IgE test results. The basic methodology underlying all oral food challenges is administration of the suspect food in gradually increasing doses under close observation in a medical setting. Challenges should be terminated and treatment administered at the first sign that a reaction is occurring. Oral food challenges carry the potential for significant risk, but these risks can be minimized by appropriate dosing and by performing challenges in a controlled setting with experienced personnel (Box 12-3). Oral challenge testing should be considered for clinical and research purposes. As shown in the algorithm in Figure 12-2, in the clinical setting, challenges are typically done for three major reasons. First, OFCs are used to establish an accurate diagnosis when the diagnosis remains unclear after other standard diagnostic methods have been tried, including obtaining the patient's history, skin testing, measurement of specific immunoglobulin E (IgE) levels, and elimination diets. Second, to determine the role food allergy plays in chronic conditions, such as atopic dermatitis or eosinophilic esophagitis. Third, OFCs are frequently used to determine whether a patient with a known food allergy has developed tolerance to that food.

Unproven Tests for Food Allergy

There are no controlled trials supporting the diagnostic value of food-specific IgG or IgG_4 antibody levels, food antigen-antibody complexes, evidence of lymphocyte activation (e.g., ^{3}H-uptake, IL-2 production, leukocyte inhibitory factor production), or sublingual or intracutaneous provocation.[1]

FOOD ALLERGY TREATMENT

Practical Management

Management of food allergies requires avoidance of the offending allergens and prompt treatment of allergic reactions.[1,65,67] Food allergen avoidance is challenging because food is necessary for sustenance and allergens are ubiquitous. Patients and caregivers must

---

| Box 12-3 | **Steps to Minimize Challenge Risks** |

- Adjust the starting dose and challenge protocol for individual patients who may be at higher risk for severe reactions.
- Use experienced observers who have been trained to do food challenges and are present throughout the challenge, continually interacting with and re-examining the patient at regular intervals.
- Stop the challenge as soon as the observer is convinced that a reaction is occurring. Prepare all medications that may be needed before the challenge so that they can be administered without delay.
- Perform challenges only in settings where all measures that might be needed to treat a severe reaction are readily available.

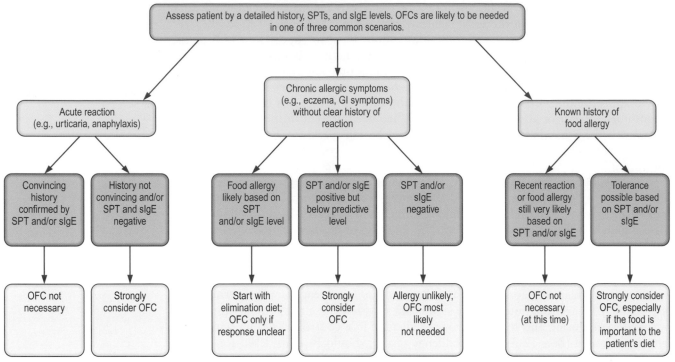

Figure 12-2 Oral food challenge decision-making algorithm. GI, gastrointestinal; OFC, oral food challenge; SPT, skin-prick test; sIgE, specific IgE.

understand food-labeling laws, prevention of cross-contact of safe foods with allergens, and means of acquiring safe meals in settings such as restaurants and schools. Adding to the complexity of avoidance is the possibility of exposure to food allergens in occupational settings, in non-food items such as cosmetics and medications, and through noningestion exposures by skin contact or inhalation. Nutritional concerns arise when multiple foods are removed from the diet. Successful emergency management requires prompt recognition and treatment of an allergic reaction or anaphylaxis.

The daily burden of managing food allergies seriously impacts quality of life.[11] Successful management requires detailed education of patients and caregivers about avoidance and treatment.

Food Allergen Avoidance Strategies

General Approach to Avoidance

Allergen avoidance should be prescribed based on a confirmed diagnosis. Avoidance education must include all persons responsible for obtaining or preparing foods. Educational materials are available through a variety of resources, including Food Allergy Research & Education (www.foodallergy.org) and the Consortium of Food Allergy Research (www.cofargroup.org); the latter organization has validated materials addressing avoidance of specific foods (e.g., CM, egg, wheat, soy) and general approaches to avoidance in different settings.

Strict avoidance is typically prescribed to avoid any risk of allergic reaction, although it may not always be necessary. Examples where ingestion of the allergenic protein may be acceptable include raw fruits and vegetables in persons with mild symptoms of pollen-food-related syndrome; extensively heated forms of milk or egg (e.g., bakery goods) in persons who tolerate them, despite reacting to whole forms; and maternal ingestion of allergens when breastfeeding allergic infants who show no evidence of reactions. Patients who tolerate these forms of exposure are identified through their medical history or by medically supervised OFC. Caution is needed because anaphylaxis can occur in some persons. The risk or benefit of allowing exposure to tolerated forms of the allergen should be individualized. There is no evidence that strict food avoidance (compared

TABLE 12-11   Options for Allergen Avoidance in Select Circumstances

Circumstance	Options	Risk or benefit*
Raw fruits and vegetables causing oral symptoms (pollen-related)	Allow ingestion on case-by-case basis based on preference and severity	Small risk of systemic reaction or anaphylaxis
Products with extensively heated (baked-in) egg or milk in persons with allergy to whole forms	Allow ingestion if tolerated by history or challenge (caution for possible anaphylaxis)	Unclear whether this approach speeds, hinders, or has no influence on recovery. Risk of reaction despite initial apparent tolerance. Possible risk of chronic inflammation from exposure
Maternal ingestion of an allergen while breastfeeding, when same allergen caused a reaction when ingested by infant	Allow mother to continue previously ingested amounts if infant showed no sign of acute or chronic reaction	May risk reaction. No data on influence on natural course. Variations in dose ingested may alter the risk
Allergy to peanut, not tree nuts	Allow ingestion of tolerated tree nuts	Cross-contact or misidentification may lead to reactions. New onset of allergy to allowed food is possible, although degree of risk uncertain
Allergy to some but not all tree nuts	Allow peanut in forms that are free from tree nuts. Allow ingestion of tolerated tree nuts	As above, with less risk for commercial peanut butter and various commercial products with isolated nut ingredients (e.g., almond in almond milk)
Allergy to some but not all fish	Allow tolerated fish. Allow canned fish that are tolerated	Risk of cross-contact, misidentification, or new onset of allergy. Less risk for processed (canned) fish
Allergy to some but not all shellfish	Allow tolerated shellfish	Risk of cross-contact, misidentification, or new onset of allergy
Allergy to some but not all botanically related foods (e.g., fruits, legumes, vegetables, grains)	Allow tolerated types	Many options to ingest 'related' foods if proved tolerated with lower risk of cross-contact, misidentification, or new onset of allergy

*Individual quality of life or nutritional benefits are assumed. Decisions are individualized based on patient preferences, physician judgment, risk assessment, and past history.

with less strict avoidance) has an effect on the rate of natural remission.[79] Avoidance of foods that are related and may have cross-reactive proteins can be individualized according to risk of clinical cross-reactivity. Table 12-11 summarizes options for the approach to avoidance of dietary allergens.

Labeling of Manufactured Products

In the US, the Food Allergen Labeling and Consumer Protection Act (FALCPA) of 2004 requires that milk, egg, peanut, tree nuts, fish, crustacean shellfish, wheat, and soy, be declared on ingredient labels using plain English words. These foods and food categories are often referred to as 'major allergens.' The law does not apply to any other foods or to non-crustacean seafood. The common names used to identify the foods may be listed within the ingredient list or in a separate statement (e.g., 'contains peanut'). Although not required, if a 'contains statement' is used, all the major allergens must be included. The law also requires that the specific type of allergen within a category be named, such as 'walnut' or 'shrimp.'

FALCPA applies to foods manufactured in or imported into the US; it does not apply to agricultural products (e.g., fresh meat, eggs, poultry, fruits, vegetables) or alcoholic beverages, which may use food proteins as ingredients or processing agents. The law is subject to revisions, as described at http://www.fda.gov/Food/FoodSafety/FoodAllergens.

Labeling laws vary among countries, and some have none. Many countries have laws that include more than just the eight food allergen groups currently covered by US laws. For example, the European Union (EU) enacted legislation in 2005 requiring that six allergens not covered in US laws be listed: rye, barley, oats, celery, mustard, and sesame seeds.

TABLE 12-12   Examples of Food Allergens in Unexpected and Non-food Items

Product type	Examples	Relevance
Cosmetics	Almond or milk in shampoos or ointments	Contact urticaria or dermatitis is possible. Some derivatives (e.g., shea nut butter) may have negligible protein
Pet food	Milk, egg, fish, soy, etc.	Animal lick may cause contact urticaria. Fish food on fingers may transfer to eyes or mouth causing symptoms
Medications	Lactose in dry powder inhaler (DPI) or tablets may have trace milk. Soy lecithin, egg lecithin	Case reports of reactions to casein identified in DPI, relevance in pills/pharmaceutical grade lactose unclear. Relevance of potential trace protein in lecithin (fatty derivative) unclear, likely low risk
Vaccines	Egg (influenza, yellow fever), possibly milk (DPT)	See Table 12-9
Nutrition supplements	glucosamine-chondroitin supplements (shark cartilage or shrimp shell), chitosan or chitin products (derived from crustacean shell)	Relevance uncertain, likely low risk
Saliva (kissing)	Residual protein from meals	Relevant for intimate contact
Transfusion	Packed red blood cells, plasma (containing allergens from donor ingestion)	Risk presumably low, theoretically higher for products that include serum proteins rather than washed blood products

The FALCPA of 2004 does not regulate the use of advisory labeling, including statements describing the potential presence of unintentional ingredients in food products; such declarations are done voluntarily in the US, and approaches are evolving internationally.[80] Although many terms are used (e.g., 'may contain,' 'manufactured on equipment with') to describe possible cross-contact, these do not convey risk. Therefore, general advice is to avoid products with these advisories. Non-etheless, there may be lower thresholds that would pose virtually no risk, and improved labeling based on studies of thresholds and adequate testing of final products may be possible. Consumers should be aware that food proteins might be a component of non-food items (Table 12-12).

Cross-Contact

Cross-contact (cross-contamination) of an otherwise safe food with an allergen is a concern for food preparation in commercial facilities, in restaurants and food establishments, and at home. Examples of cross-contact include a knife used to spread peanut butter then contaminating jelly; shared grills, pans, food processors, and other equipment used without thorough cleaning between preparation of different foods; dipping ice cream scoops from one flavor to the next; using a fryer for both shrimp and potatoes; and preparing foods in a workspace not cleaned between preparations. Patients and caregivers must be educated about these concerns and address them when obtaining or preparing meals.

Manner of Exposure

The three primary manners of exposure are skin contact, inhalation, and ingestion. The primary concern regarding avoidance of an allergen relates to *ingestion*. Although exposures through skin contact or inhalation are unlikely to cause anaphylaxis, skin rashes and respiratory symptoms may occur.[81] For young children, there is a concern that skin contact could lead to ingestion (e.g., sucking fingers). Food odors may be caused by volatile organic compounds that lack appreciable proteins and present minimal allergic risk (e.g., odor of peanut butter would not trigger anaphylaxis) or may include proteins when the food is aerosolized (e.g., during cooking, dust from powdery forms). In the latter case (e.g., in proximity to boiling milk, frying fish, or powdered milk), respiratory or skin symptoms could occur.[82] Noningestion reactions occur in occupational settings as well (e.g., food handlers, see Ch. 14). Baker's asthma describes airborne sensitivity to wheat flour. Individuals with baker's asthma can typically tolerate wheat ingestion. Persons with occupational allergy caused by foods may need to wear gloves and masks or find alternative employment. Aside from occupational exposures, individuals with food allergies may need to avoid situations where the food allergen is aerosolized nearby. Young children may need to be supervised around food allergens to avoid hand-to-mouth contact. Standard cleaning procedures (soap and water and wiping with friction) should suffice to remove allergens from surfaces. Antibacterial foams and gels do not remove allergens from hands. Minor allergic reactions from kissing are common because allergen can be transferred in saliva or residual protein on the lips. Skin contact with the saliva is unlikely to cause a severe reaction, but intimate kissing is similar in risk to ingestion, and a partner may need to avoid the allergen.[83]

Restaurants, Food Establishments, Travel

Restaurants and other food establishments, such as bakeries or ice cream stores, present challenges for food-allergic individuals.[1] Consumers should identify themselves as allergic so that instructions about avoidance are not misperceived as being taste preferences. Clear communication is crucial because those preparing the foods may have limited understanding of the needs of an allergic consumer. It may be prudent for consumers to review concerns such as cross-contact and hidden ingredients with the relevant personnel. All persons handling the food should be involved in discussions about meal preparation. This could prevent errors, such as a 'prep' worker adding butter to a food that appears dry. Consumers may present written materials that describe the allergies ('chef cards'), and food establishments may follow guidelines; both are available from several sources, including Food Allergy Research & Education (www.foodallergy.org). Buffets or specialty or ethnic restaurants (e.g., seafood, Asian) may pose high risks and should be avoided depending on the consumer's specific allergies. Traveling with food allergies requires considerations beyond obtaining meals safely in restaurants. Allergic reactions to peanut and tree nuts have been reported on commercial airliners, but the studies rely heavily on self-report.[84,85] Overall, exposure to the cabin air seems unlikely to trigger severe reactions for most persons with food allergies. Travelers with food allergies should avoid eating potentially unsafe airline foods and carry safe alternatives. Adults traveling with young children with food allergies might inspect crevices around their seats and wipe surfaces to avoid ingestion of residual allergens by toddlers. Some airlines may provide additional accommodations when requested in advance (e.g., flight with no peanuts served).[86] Vacation choices, including all-inclusive resorts, cruises, and international travel, are circumstances in which advance planning is required because meals are prepared by others.

Potentially less risky alternatives include accommodations with a kitchenette so that some meals can be self-prepared.

Avoidance for Schools and Camp

School-based strategies must be practical and must focus on policies to avoid ingestion of the allergen and promptly recognize and treat anaphylaxis.[87] Allergen avoidance may vary depending on the age of the children, with more supervision, cleaning, and containment of allergen needed for younger children. Risk-taking behaviors among adolescents with food allergy, such as eating unsafe foods and delaying treatment of a reaction, are likely contributing factors to the observation that this age-group is at increased risk for fatal allergic reactions.

Therefore, peer and patient education is suggested to improve safety for adolescents. Physicians can encourage parents to request to meet with key school staff members who have responsibility for the care of their child and to work cooperatively with schools to ensure their child's safety. Key staff members may include the school nurse, principal, and directors of transportation and food service, and classroom teachers. Avoidance strategies and emergency management must also be communicated to personnel who may not have primary responsibilities for the student, such as coaches, specialty teachers (art, music), substitute teachers, and field trip personnel. These individuals should also be familiar with emergency plans, should be trained to use epinephrine auto-injectors, and should recognize indicators for activating the emergency medical response system.

It may be helpful to counsel parents about the degree and manner of exposure that might be dangerous for a specific child, such as ingestion versus inhalation or touching food residues, so that parents are appropriately vigilant without becoming needlessly hypervigilant or anxious about avoidance strategies. Care must be taken not to ostracize or physically separate the child with food allergies. For example, an 'allergen-aware' table should include the child's friends who are eating safe meals. Experts have not espoused blanket 'bans' on foods, particularly because peanut butter, milk, egg, and other common allergens may be a protein staple of another child's diet. In specific cases, individual schools or classrooms might pursue these options. For example, removal of highly allergenic foods from the vicinity of very young children or children with significant developmental disabilities might be warranted when transfer of the allergen among the children is likely. Schools may choose to ban children from bringing food from home to share with classmates for celebratory functions and may offer acceptable alternative options. Table 12-13 provides suggestions to reduce accidental ingestion of allergens. Management of food allergy is similar for schools and camps. However, the persons providing supervision in camps may be young and inexperienced, necessitating additional safeguards, such as additional supervision at mealtimes or having more experienced supervisors available when away from first-aid and nursing services.

Nutritional Issues

Allergen avoidance diets can result in failure to thrive and deficiencies in specific macronutrients and micronutrients. These concerns, in addition to the daily lifestyle impact of following avoidance diets, underscore the importance of having an accurate diagnosis to allow the broadest diet possible.[88,89] Additionally, food aversion and anxiety may result in insufficient nutrient intake. Food allergy–related disorders such as eosinophilic esophagitis may be associated with poor appetite and early satiety, and children with untreated food allergy–related atopic dermatitis may experience malabsorption and increased energy needs from skin damage. Therefore, addressing nutritional concerns may require a multifaceted approach, including consultation with a registered dietitian. Nutritional counseling and regular growth monitoring are recommended for children with food allergies.[1]

Nutritional deficits caused by allergen-restricted diets include poor caloric intake (proteins, carbohydrates, fats) and insufficient vitamins, minerals, and trace elements. Many sources of protein, including milk, egg, soy, fish, shellfish, peanut, and tree nuts, are also common allergens. The *acceptable macronutrient distribution range* (AMDR) for protein is 5–20% for children 1 to 3 years of age, 10–30% for children 4 to 18

TABLE 12-13	Preventive Measures to Reduce Risk of Allergen Ingestion in School Settings
Setting	**Measures**
School-wide	Institute policy on no food sharing or trading. Educate teachers, including substitutes, coaches, special program teachers, and cafeteria staff. Consider allergen-safe cafeteria tables or schools, depending on student ages and needs (supervision, selective allergen exclusion). Enforce strict no-bullying policies.
Selected classroom	Allow no food in craft projects. Reduce food rewards, and provide a substitute. Maintain safe, nonperishable snacks as substitute, if needed. Consider 'bans,' depending on food (peanut) and age. Encourage handwashing.
School bus	Permit no eating or food parties. Have communication device for emergency calls. Allow younger child to sit at front.

years of age, and 10–35% for adults. Quality proteins that include essential amino acids are typically obtained from meats. Complementary foods (e.g., rice, beans) may be needed for those who are vegetarian or meat allergic. The AMDR for fat is 25–35% of total energy intake for older children and adults (30–40% for children 1 to 3 years of age). Essential fatty acids (linoleic and linolenic) are found in fish. However, essential fatty acids are also available in vegetable oils such as canola, corn, soy, and olive. The diet should consist of a blend of saturated fats, which are usually obtained from animal origin, but also monosaturated and polyunsaturated fats, which are components of vegetable oils. The AMDR for carbohydrate is 45–65% of total caloric intake. Carbohydrates, particularly grains, contribute to dietary fiber, iron, thiamine, niacin, riboflavin, and folic acid. Micronutrients include vitamins, minerals and trace elements.[88,89] The Department of Agriculture maintains documents regarding dietary recommendations via www.usda.gov or www.choosemyplate.gov. Table 12-14 describes nutritional concerns and possible solutions for diets devoid of some of the key common allergens.

EMERGENCY MANAGEMENT

The emergency management of food-induced anaphylaxis is similar to the treatment of anaphylaxis from any cause (see Ch. 13). Any food can potentially trigger anaphylaxis, but peanut, tree nuts, milk, fish, and shellfish appear to account for most of the episodes leading to fatalities.[62,64] Prompt recognition of anaphylaxis and treatment with epinephrine are crucial for a good outcome. In a study of 45 episodes of anaphylaxis in children, those who received epinephrine early were less likely to require hospital admission (14% vs 47%, respectively; $p < 0.05$).[90] Box 12-4 lists risk factors for fatal food-induced anaphylaxis and comorbid conditions that increase risk. The treatment of severe reactions caused by FPIES is different and involves intravenous hydration and corticosteroids, although proof for the efficacy of the latter is lacking.

TABLE 12-14   Nutritional Concerns and Substitutions for Diets Devoid of Select Allergens*

Allergen	Key nutrients	Substitutions
Milk	Protein, fat, calcium, vitamin A, vitamin D, vitamin B_{12}	Meats, fish, or poultry (protein, fat, vitamin B_{12}); fortified soy drinks (calcium, protein, vitamins D and B_{12}), legumes (protein), avocado (fat), enriched milks from rice, almond, oat or fortified juices (calcium; vitamins D, A, and B_{12}), dark-green leafy vegetables (vitamin A)[†]
Soy	Protein, thiamine, folate, magnesium, phosphorus, zinc, riboflavin, iron	Meat (protein, thiamine, phosphorus, iron); other legumes (protein, thiamine, folate, iron); fish (protein, phosphorus, iron); dark-green leafy vegetables (riboflavin, folate); whole grains (thiamine, riboflavin, folate, magnesium, iron); alternative fortified 'milks' (see above)
Wheat	Carbohydrates, fiber, niacin, riboflavin, iron, folate	Enriched flours, including rice, oat, corn, and potato (carbohydrates, niacin, thiamine, riboflavin, iron, folate); fruits and vegetables (fiber, carbohydrates); meat (niacin, iron, thiamine); leafy green vegetables (riboflavin, folate)
Egg	Protein, vitamin B_{12}, selenium, biotin	Meat/fish (protein, vitamin B_{12}, selenium), soy (protein, biotin)

*Table 12-14 cannot be used in isolation to construct adequate nutritional plans.
†Adults can obtain calcium and vitamin D from nondairy sources (fortified juices, alternative 'milks' and supplements). However, infants and children require a replacement source of fat and protein and fortified juices or rice milk are otherwise insufficient; complete fortified nutritional formulas (soy, casein hydrolysates, amino acid-based, etc.) may suffice, but children avoiding milk/soy may benefit from more complete dietary assessments. A diet devoid of egg, peanut, fish, or shellfish is typically easily substituted with other protein sources.

Box 12-4   Risks for Fatal Food Anaphylaxis and Comorbid Conditions

RISKS ASSOCIATED WITH FATAL FOOD ANAPHYLAXIS

- Delayed treatment with epinephrine
- Allergy to peanut, tree nuts, fish, or shellfish
- Adolescent or young adult
- Asthma
- Cardiovascular disease in middle-aged or older patient
- Lack of skin symptoms

COMORBID CONDITIONS ASSOCIATED WITH INCREASED FOOD ANAPHYLAXIS RISK OR THAT AFFECT SEVERITY OR TREATMENT

- Asthma
- Mastocytosis
- Chronic lung disease
- Medications
- β-Adrenergic antagonists
- Angiotensin-converting enzyme (ACE) inhibitors
- α-Adrenergic blockers

Recognition of Reactions

Patients diagnosed with potentially severe food allergies, and their caretakers, must be educated regarding recognition of reactions. Signs, symptoms, and time course should be reviewed, as well as when and how to inject epinephrine and alert emergency services. Anaphylaxis caused by food allergy may occur without urticaria or skin symptoms in up to 20% of patients, which may account for delays in treatment leading to poor outcomes.[63] Additionally, biphasic reactions, with recurrence of symptoms several hours after resolution of initial reactions, are described in 1–20% of patients.[1] Given the possibility of biphasic reactions, victims of food-induced anaphylaxis should remain under medical observation for 4 to 6 hours or longer after anaphylaxis to ensure that symptoms have subsided.

Treatment with Epinephrine and Antihistamines

Although antihistamines are indicated to treat symptoms such as urticaria or oral pruritus, dependence on antihistamines is a common reason for delaying anaphylaxis treatment with epinephrine, which may result in an increased risk of a progressively severe reaction. Patients and caregivers should be counseled on the appropriate use of self-injectable epinephrine and not to depend on antihistamines or bronchodilators for treatment of anaphylaxis. Repeated doses of epinephrine may be needed in 10–20% of episodes of food-induced anaphylaxis.[91] Prompt transfer to a facility capable of managing anaphylaxis should be sought. Patients and families should understand that although subsequent reactions are not necessarily more severe than initial reactions, they can be. For example, initial mild reactions to peanut may be followed by more severe reactions on subsequent exposures. Similarly, specific IgE levels do not predict the severity of a reaction. Epinephrine auto-injectors may be prescribed for anyone diagnosed with a food allergy but definitely *should* be prescribed for patients with a prior history of anaphylaxis, those with food allergy and asthma, and those with a known food allergy to potent allergens such as peanut, tree nuts, fish, and shellfish. In a survey of whether an epinephrine auto-injector is required for persons with pollen-food-related syndrome, of 122 allergists, 67% prescribed on a case-by-case basis depending on symptoms.[92]

Emergency Plans and Special Considerations for School

Patients with potentially severe food allergies should be given a written emergency plan that describes when to inject epinephrine and instructions on how to self-inject. (The prescriptions of epinephrine, plans for monitoring expiration dates of auto-injectors, avoidance measures, and follow-up instructions are detailed in Chapter 13.) Auto-injector dosing is limited because only two doses are available in the US (an 0.5 mg auto-injector is available in Europe for those weighing >45 kg), but generally, the

0.15 mg dose is recommended for children weighing 10 to 25 kg (22–55 lb) and the 0.3 mg dose for those over 25 kg.

There are special considerations for treating children in schools or camps. The family must notify the school about the child's potentially life-threatening food allergy and provide written treatment plans, including the child's name, identifying information (child's photograph, if possible), specifics about the food allergies, symptoms and treatments, instructions to activate emergency services, and medical and family contact information. In some circumstances, a child may be allowed to carry auto-injectors and to self-inject, but a supervising adult should have the primary responsibility to recognize and treat anaphylaxis. In the school setting, this is ideally a health professional, but a delegate might be needed. Epinephrine auto-injectors should be available promptly in the event of anaphylaxis. Children should be encouraged to wear medical identification jewelry. Because 25% of anaphylaxis episodes in schools occur without a previous diagnosis, a prescription for unassigned epinephrine for general use, consistent with district regulations and state laws, should be considered. When to inject epinephrine can be confusing for lay personnel. The safety of the drug should be emphasized such that injections should be given if there is suspicion of anaphylaxis. It may be advisable to inject epinephrine at the time of first symptoms if an allergen was ingested that previously caused anaphylaxis, or before symptoms if an allergen was ingested that previously caused severe anaphylaxis with cardiovascular collapse.

Prevention of Food Allergy

Given the known benefits of breastfeeding, it is globally recommended as the preferred infant nutrition in the first 4 to 6 months of life in the absence of other contraindications. In 2012, the American Academy of Pediatrics (AAP) and The European Academy of Asthma and Clinical Immunology (EAACI) recommend exclusive breastfeeding for approximately 6 months of life, followed by gradual introduction of complementary foods between 4 and 6 months of life, and continuation of breastfeeding until 1 year of age or longer as mutually desired by both mother and infant (AAP Policy Statement, at http://pediatrics.aappublications.org/content/early/2012/02/22/peds.2011-3552.full.pdf html). The current WHO guideline on breastfeeding was implemented in 2001 and confirmed last in 2010, and recommends exclusive breastfeeding until 6 months of life (WHO Assembly Resolution 2001 and 2010; accessed online January 7th 2015, at http://www.who.int/nutrition/topics/wha_nutrition_iycn/en/).

Infants at risk are defined as infants who have at least one first-degree relative (parent or sibling) with an atopic condition. In children who are at risk but cannot be exclusively breastfed during the first 4 to 6 months of life, 'hypoallergenic' formulas (e.g., partially or extensively hydrolyzed whey or casein amino acid based) were shown to be beneficial over conventional cow's milk–based formulas.

Current recommendations by both American and European expert committees are to wait to introduce solid foods into the infants' diet until 4 to 6 months of age but then allow gradual introduction of all food groups.[93,94] This reflects a change from previous guidelines recommending delaying certain allergenic foods in high-risk infants: CM until age 1 year; eggs until age 2 years; and peanut, tree nuts, fish, and shellfish until age 3 years. This change was implemented after initial reports were published suggesting a disadvantage of delayed introduction of allergens (Table 12-15).

Trials Using Oral Tolerance Induction to Prevent Food Allergies

Some theories suggest that early introduction of foods such as peanut or egg leads to tolerance and protects against developing food allergy.[95] These theories are being tested in two RCTs, summarized in Box 12-5. The LEAP study is given in further detail below.

The recent randomized trial of early introduction of dietary peanut (LEAP study; see Box 12-5) randomized 640 infants between the ages of 4 and 11 months with severe eczema, egg allergy, or both to consume or avoid peanut until 60 months of age.[96] Severe eczema and egg allergy have been previously identified as risk factors for development of peanut allergy. The primary outcome was the proportion of participants with peanut

TABLE 12-15   Changes in Notions about Allergy Prevention through Diet

Prior notion/recommendation (for those at risk for atopy)	Recent notions/recommendations
Avoid peanut during pregnancy	No proof of effectiveness
Avoid food allergens during lactation	Possible reduction in atopic dermatitis, no evidence regarding food allergy
Breastfeeding exclusively for 3–4 months	May protect for atopy, but evidence is modest; lack of evidence for food allergy prevention
Alternative hypoallergenic formulas	May protect for atopy, but evidence is modest; lack of evidence for food allergy prevention
Delay complementary foods until 4–6 months	Lack of evidence to prevent atopic disease
Avoid allergens: milk to age 1 year; egg to 2 years; and peanut, nuts, and fish to 3 years	Early introduction of allergenic foods at 4–6 months may protect against development of food allergy, but firm evidence is lacking

---

Box 12-5   Allergy Prevention Studies

LEAP STUDY (LEARNING EARLY ABOUT PEANUT ALLERGY: WWW.LEAPSTUDY.CO.UK)

- In total, 640 high-risk children were enrolled at age 4–11 months
- Each child was randomized to an avoidance group (complete avoidance of peanut-containing foods) or a consumption group (consume a peanut snack three times a week; 6 g of peanut protein/week)
- Among 530 infants in the intention-to-treat population who initially had negative results on the skin-prick test, the prevalence of peanut allergy at 60 months of age was 13.7% in the avoidance group and 1.9% in the consumption group ($p < 0.001$).
- Among 98 participants in the intention-to-treat population who initially had positive test results, the prevalence of peanut allergy was 35.3% in the avoidance group and 10.6% in the consumption group ($p = 0.004$).

EAT STUDY (ENQUIRING ABOUT TOLERANCE: WWW.EATSTUDY.CO.UK)

- Infants ($n = 1302$) were randomized to one of two groups
- In one group ($n = 651$), six allergenic foods were introduced from 3 months of age, while the infant continued to breastfeed (early introduction group)
- The other group ($n = 651$) followed current UK government weaning advice: aim for exclusive breastfeeding for 6 months (standard weaning group)
- The children will be monitored until 3 years of age to see whether early diet has an effect in reducing the prevalence of food allergy, as determined by double-blind, placebo-controlled food challenges.

---

allergy at 60 months of age. Among the 530 infants in the intention-to-treat population who initially had negative results on the skin-prick test, the prevalence of peanut allergy at 60 months of age was 13.7% in the avoidance group and 1.9% in the consumption group ($p < 0.001$). Among the 98 participants in the intention-to-treat population who initially had small positive skin test results (1- to 4-mm wheal diameter), the prevalence of peanut allergy was 35.3% in the avoidance group and 10.6% in the consumption group ($p = 0.004$). There was no significant difference in the incidence of serious adverse events in children who were ingesting peanut and those avoiding peanut. Increases in levels of peanut-specific IgG4 antibody occurred predominantly in the consumption group; a greater percentage of participants in the avoidance group had elevated titers of peanut-specific IgE antibody. A larger wheal on the skin-prick test and a lower ratio of peanut-specific IgG4:IgE were associated with peanut allergy. The early introduction of peanut significantly decreased the frequency of the development of peanut allergy among children at high risk for this allergy and modulated immune responses to peanut. The significant risk reduction observed in this study provides evidence for the benefits of early introduction of dietary peanut in infants with severe eczema and egg allergy. Early introduction of peanut takes advantage of the oral tolerance pathways activated by ingestion that precedes the potential sensitization to peanut via the disrupted skin barrier. (Figure 12-3) This exciting study opens the door to an effective early intervention for the at risk population. At this time, the optimal practical implementation of the study findings remains to be determined. It is unclear how to translate the

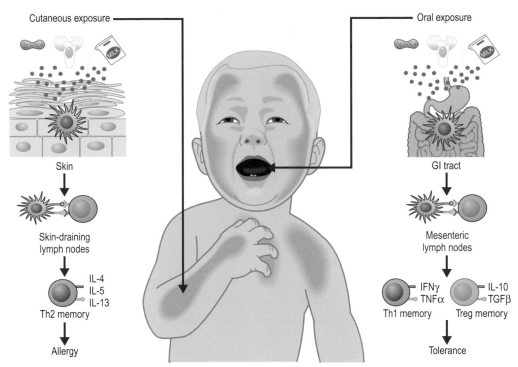

Figure 12-3 Dual-allergen-exposure hypothesis for pathogenesis of food allergy. Tolerance occurs as a result of oral exposure to food, and allergic sensitization results from cutaneous exposure. GI, gastrointestinal; IFN-γ, interferon-γ; TGF-β, transforming growth factor beta; Th2, T helper type 2 lymphocyte; TNF-α, tumor necrosis factor alpha; Treg, T regulatory lymphocyte. *(Modified from Lack G. Epidemiologic risks of food allergy. J Allergy Clin Immunol 2008; 121:1331–1336.)*

study findings to the populations of infants with milder forms of eczema or no eczema and those in the countries where peanut consumption is generally less common than in the UK, US, Canada, and Australia. The study enforced regular ingestion of peanut products, either peanut snack or peanut butter, three times per week for 5 years. This may not be practical for many families at large; the absolute minimum of peanut consumption sufficient to maintain tolerance remains to be determined.

FUTURE THERAPEUTIC STRATEGIES

The apparent rising prevalence of food allergies, lack of effective prevention strategies, and inadequate treatment that relies on allergen avoidance and injection of epinephrine for anaphylaxis have considerably increased the urgency to develop effective treatments. There are no therapies proven to accelerate the development of oral tolerance or provide effective protection from accidental exposures. However, novel allergen-specific and allergen-non-specific approaches to food allergy therapy are being developed and studied.[97] Both allergen-specific therapies and more generalized immunomodulatory approaches are under investigation in animal and human models of food allergy (Table 12-16).

Because it is important to delineate the responses to therapeutic interventions, the terms *desensitization* and *tolerance* are often used to better define the clinical and immunologic state during therapy (Box 12-6). The overall goal of effective immunotherapy is long-term tolerance induction through active immunomodulation to promote regulatory T cell development and immunologic skewing away from the classic Th2 response seen with many of the emerging therapies (Fig. 12-4).

Oral Immunotherapy

Oral immunotherapy (OIT) has been studied for several years in clinical trials and has the largest evidence base for effectiveness among emerging therapies for food allergy.[98]

TABLE 12-16   Emerging Therapies for Food Allergy*

Therapy	Use	Stage of study	Allergen studied
Allergen-non-specific therapy			
Anti-IgE therapy	Treatment	Human phase I–II	Peanut, milk
Traditional Chinese medicine	Treatment	Human phase I–II	Peanut, tree nut, fish, shellfish, sesame
Probiotics	Prevention	Longitudinal study	Non-specific
Prebiotics	Prevention	Longitudinal study	Non-specific
Trichuris suis egg therapy	Treatment	Preclinical	Peanut
Lactococcus lactis expressing IL-10 or IL-12	Treatment	Preclinical	Milk
Toll-like receptor 9	Treatment	Preclinical	Peanut
Allergen-specific therapy			
Subcutaneous IT	Treatment	Human phase I (aborted due to safety)	Peanut
Oral IT	Treatment	Human phase I–III	Peanut, milk, egg, fish, fruits
Heated antigen	Treatment	Human phase I–II	Egg, milk
Sublingual IT	Treatment	Human phase I–II	Peanut, milk, hazelnut, kiwi, peach
Epicutaneous IT	Treatment	Human phase I–II	Peanut, milk
Recombinant protein IT with adjuvants	Treatment	Human phase I	Peanut
Recombinant protein IT	Treatment	Preclinical	Peanut
Plasmid DNA IT	Treatment	Preclinical	Peanut
Peptide IT	Treatment	Preclinical	Peanut, egg
ISS-ODN IT	Treatment	Preclinical	Peanut
Human Fc-FC fusion proteins	Treatment	Preclinical	Peanut
Engineered allergen	Treatment	Preclinical	Egg, peanut, milk, fish, fruits
Mannoside-conjugated BSA	Treatment	Preclinical	BSA
Antigen-fixed leukocytes	Treatment	Preclinical	Peanut

IL, interleukin; IT, immunotherapy.
*For detailed information on clinical trials, see clinicaltrials.gov.

Box 12-6   The Clinical Outcomes of Food Immunotherapy

DESENSITIZATION
- A change in threshold dose of ingested allergen required to induce allergic symptoms after food exposure occurring while on therapy
- This is a reversible state typically induced by allergen exposure, in which effector cells are rendered less reactive or nonreactive by administration of allergen.

TOLERANCE
- The long-lasting effects of treatment, presumably due to effects on T cell responsiveness that persist after the treatment is stopped.
- The immunomodulatory effects of desensitization can be seen early in the course of immunotherapy; however, evidence suggests that the length of time to reach tolerance varies with the type and amount of specific allergen, the duration of therapy, and the individual patient.

Although still investigational, OIT is associated with a robust response to therapy, but with limitations related to its side effects profile. Early open-label trials have shown a beneficial response to OIT with a variety of allergens, including milk, egg and fish, with evidence of clinical desensitization in up to 80% of patients treated.

The concepts of clinical desensitization and tolerance have been more fully explored in recent studies. Current OIT protocols are typically conducted using an allergen flour ingested in a food vehicle and consist of the following three phases:

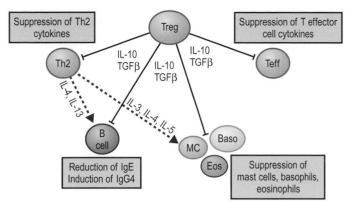

Figure 12-4 Food allergy treatments modulate the food allergic response through activation of regulatory T cells and suppression of a variety of effector cell types. Baso, basophil; Eos, eosinophil; IL, interleukin; MC, mast cell; Teff, T effector lymphocyte; TGF-β, transforming growth factor beta; Th2, T helper type 2 lymphocyte; Treg, T regulatory lymphocyte.

TABLE 12-17   Immunologic Changes in IgE-Mediated Food Allergy Compared with Effective Immunotherapy

Immune parameters	Food allergy	Effective immunotherapy
Serum IgE	↑	↓
Serum IgG4	↔	↑
Mast cell reactivity	↑	↓
Basophil activation	↑	↓
Helper T cell (Th2) cytokines	↑	↓
Regulatory T cell activation	↓	↑

1. Modified rush desensitization, with 6 to 8 doses of allergen given under observation in rapid succession during day 1 to obtain a relative 'desensitized state.'
2. Dosing buildup, with a daily dose of the food protein at home with scheduled dose escalations under observation every 1 to 2 weeks until a target dose is reached.
3. Home maintenance therapy, with daily ingestion of a target dose (typically for years).

These phases are usually followed by OFC to assess clinical desensitization (while receiving therapy) and functional tolerance (while off therapy on diet restriction). Clinical desensitization has been well documented in open-label studies for peanut, milk, and egg, with success rates ranging from 75% to 100% after 1 to 2 years of therapy. Desensitization has been associated with immunomodulation with reduced markers of mast cell (skin tests) and basophil activation, changes in IgE and IgG profiles, reduced Th2 cytokine profile, and activation of Tregs (Table 12-17).

The prevailing question is whether OIT induces *tolerance*, not just desensitization. The longest study of peanut-OIT treated 50 subjects with daily maintenance dose of 4 mg peanut protein for an average 3 years. At the end of the treatment period, 50% of the subjects were able to safely ingest a full serving of peanut (5 g of peanut protein) after 1 month of stopping the daily dosing.[99]

In combination, the results from several studies suggest sustained unresponsiveness is possible in at least a portion of participants; however, further study is needed to determine the duration of unresponsiveness and the persistence of immunomodulation.

Clinical trials using OIT have focused primarily on single-allergen delivery to impact single-food allergy. In a multi-sensitized mouse model of tree nut allergy, OIT with a single tree nut had efficacy in causing desensitization to multiple tree nuts.[100] Clinical studies are ongoing to evaluate this approach and OIT with multiple allergens.

Box 12-7   Side Effects Reported in the Trials of Food Oral Immunotherapy

- *Common*: Mild to moderate, predominantly oropharyngeal and gastrointestinal (discomfort, pain, nausea, diarrhea, vomiting) side-effects are most common, and easily treated.
- *Rare*: More severe reactions have been rarely reported, including generalized urticaria/angioedema, wheezing/respiratory distress, laryngeal edema, and repetitive emesis.
- *Discontinuation of therapy*: Of participants treated with OIT, about 20% experienced dose-limiting GI side effects, preventing continuation of therapy.
- *Augmentation factors*: Viral infections, menses, and exercise have been associated with lowering the reaction threshold for subjects receiving stable OIT dosing. These often require dose adjustments to compensate for illness.

Although OIT has demonstrated significant clinical successes, safety remains a concern for wide-scale implementation (Box 12-7).[101] Additional studies are needed to improve the safety profile before OIT can be sanctioned for widespread use.[1,102]

Extensively Heated Milk and Egg Protein

A possible alternative or treatment adjunct to OIT is the use of crude, heat-denatured allergen. Because high-temperature cooking of egg and milk proteins results in conformational changes of native protein structure and reduced IgE binding, some children with milk or egg allergy may tolerate baked products.

Two clinical trials have been conducted in milk-allergic and egg-allergic children. The results suggest that up to 80% of milk-allergic or egg-allergic children can safely ingest extensively heated milk products in a muffin or egg products in a waffle.[21,23] OFC was done to confirm the allergy and ability to tolerate the baked product. Children assigned to consume 1 to 3 servings of heated product daily were noted to experience accelerated tolerance development compared with an age-matched allergic cohort. Side effects were negligible, and no subjects who tolerated the baked product required epinephrine during OFC, although 35% of baked milk-reactive subjects and 19% of baked egg-reactive subjects did. Clinical successes were associated with reduced allergen-specific IgE and SPT, increased allergen-specific IgG4, and activated Tregs. Similar findings were noted in ovalbumin-sensitized mice treated with heated OVA or ovomucoid. Heat treatment reduced allergenicity of the egg antigens through enhanced GI digestibility and reduced absorption in a form capable of triggering basophils.

These findings suggest that ingestion of extensively heated egg or milk products may serve as a safe and efficacious treatment modality.[22,24] Questions remain about the dose required for efficacy, degree of heating needed, role of the food matrix in the observed response, ability of extensively heated proteins to induce lasting tolerance, and the role of heated allergens as treatment adjuncts to other forms of immunotherapy.

Sublingual Immunotherapy

Sublingual immunotherapy has shown efficacy for treatment of inhalant allergies and asthma. In the treatment of aeroallergens, SLIT has clinical advantages similar to SCIT but lower risks for severe, fatal reactions.[103] Minor side effects, consisting of oral pruritus and swelling, are often reported but are rarely of significance. SLIT employs a liquid concentrate administered sublingually in small, increasing doses in a controlled setting coupled with home dosing to reach a target maintenance dose. SLIT-Tablet preparations are in frequent use for inhalant allergies in Europe and Australia. Although the mechanism of action is not fully elucidated, data suggest that it is similar to that in other forms of immunotherapy.

Although both OIT and SLIT can confer benefits to patients, the therapies differ in dosing limitations, effectiveness, side effects, and immunomodulation (Table 12-18).[104] Further study is needed to improve antigen delivery using SLIT whilst maintaining its preferable safety profile, with better understanding of nuances in antigen delivery to the gut-associated lymphoid tissue (via OIT) compared with the submucosal lymphoid tissue (via SLIT). Even when effective, these forms of therapy will not likely be applicable

TABLE 12-18 Comparison of Oral Immunotherapy (OIT) and Sublingual Immunotherapy (SLIT)

	OIT	SLIT
Typical daily dose	300–4000 mg	2–7 mg
Predominant side effects	Oral, gastrointestinal (systemic increases with infection, exercise, menses)	Oropharyngeal
Desensitization	Large effect	Lesser effect
Functional tolerance	Effective in subset of patients	Unknown to date
Immunomodulation	Significant	Modest

across all ages and risk categories of food allergies, and thus specific paradigms and alternate treatments are needed.

Epicutaneous Immunotherapy

Epicutaneous immunotherapy (EPIT) has been used safely and effectively for grass pollen-induced allergic rhinitis. EPIT acts by delivering a small dose of allergenic protein directly to the epidermal layer of the skin. The current evidence base for the use of EPIT in food allergy is derived from preclinical studies using allergic mouse models and to one trial in milk-allergic infants and children and one multicenter trial in peanut allergic children. A 3-month double-blind, placebo-controlled pilot study of EPIT was conducted in milk-allergic infants and children (3 months to 15 years).[105] A total of 19 participants were randomized to milk or placebo EPIT; 16 were evaluable by a second OFC on day 90. The cumulative dose of CM consumed during OFC trended higher in the milk EPIT group (1.77 ± 2.98 mL to 23.61 ± 28.61 mL) versus the placebo group (4.36 ± 5.87 mL to 5.44 ± 5.88 mL) ($p = 0.13$). Adverse events, without anaphylaxis, were reported more often in the milk EPIT group compared with controls (24 vs 8 events, respectively) and were mostly mild skin reactions. In a multicenter double-blind, placebo-controlled phase IIb trial, 221 subjects (6–55 years) reacting at a peanut protein eliciting dose (ED) <300 mg during DBPCFC were randomized to 1 year Viaskin Peanut (VP), at different doses (50 mg, 100 mg, 250 mg p/p), or Viaskin placebo.[106] The primary efficacy endpoint at 1 year was the proportion of responders with a p/p ED 10-fold greater than the peanut protein ED at entry or achieving a post-treatment ED >1000 mg. Cumulative reacting dose of peanut protein was also measured. Immunologic studies were performed at entry, 3, 6, and 12 months. The overall primary efficacy endpoint was met, with VP250 showing best results: 50.0% responders vs 25.0% with placebo, $p = 0.0108$; children (6–11 years) exhibited 53.6% responders vs 19.4% for placebo, $p = 0.0076$. In children, the mean cumulative reacting dose showed a VP dose-dependent response: +61 mg, +471 mg, +570 mg and +1121 mg for placebo, VP50, VP100, and VP250, respectively. Children treated with VP250 – PN-IgE exhibited a median increase >50 kUA/L at 3 months and decreased back to baseline at 12 months; median PN-IgG4 at 12 months increased in a dose-dependent fashion: 5.5-, 7.2-, and 19.1-fold for VP50, VP100, and VP250, respectively. Compliance was >95%, dropout for adverse events <1%, and there were no serious adverse events related to treatment. In peanut allergy, EPIT appears safe and effective; the CRD was dose-dependent and maximum efficacy was seen with VP250.

CONCLUSIONS

Ingested foods represent the greatest foreign antigenic load confronting the human immune system. In the vast majority of individuals, tolerance develops to food antigens, which are constantly gaining access to the body proper. However, when tolerance fails to develop, the immune system responds with an allergic reaction. Allergic reactions to milk have been first described by Hippocrates more than 2000 years ago; however it is only the past two decades that food allergy has emerged as an important public health problem affecting people of all ages in societies with a western life style, such as US, Canada, UK, Australia, and Western Europe. Allergies to food affect up to 8% of children under 5 years of age and approximately 3.5% of the general population. Inadvertent ingestion of food allergens may provoke various gastrointestinal, cutaneous, respiratory symptoms, and/or systemic anaphylaxis with shock.

Food Allergy Guidelines have been established to facilitate uniform approaches to diagnosis and management. While oral food challenges remain the standard for food allergy diagnosis, skin-prick testing, and detection of specific IgE directed against complete foods and specific allergenic components are useful non-invasive tools.

Current therapy for food allergy requires education about avoidance in a variety of settings and instructions on when and how to treat inevitable allergic reactions. These approaches require constant vigilance and affect quality of life. Increasing attention has therefore focused on primary prevention and improved therapies, with a shift in our approach to the prevention of food allergy. Previous guidelines on food allergen avoidance during pregnancy, breastfeeding, and infancy have been questioned. The relationship between allergen exposure and development of food allergy is complex. Allergen exposure through a disrupted skin barrier may be involved in establishing allergy, whereas allergen exposure through the gastrointestinal mucosa may be involved in establishing tolerance. Immune responses to such allergen exposures are likely to be modulated by non-specific factors, such as GI microflora, infectious exposure, other dietary factors, and possibly sunlight exposure.

Interventional trials are in progress and in the next few years should help to determine the relative contribution of these different factors and allow us to reduce the burden caused by food allergy. Advances in our understanding of the immunologic mechanisms underlying food allergy and the complexities of the mucosal immune response have resulted in substantial progress toward definitive therapeutic options for food-allergic individuals. Current therapeutic strategies are focused on harnessing oral tolerance to modulate the allergic response using antigen-specific and antigen-non-specific approaches. Although significant gains and positive clinical and immunomodulatory insights have been appreciated, these approaches are often associated with significant risk and unanswered long-term safety and efficacy questions. Ongoing studies will fill our current therapeutic knowledge gaps and carefully move toward broader clinical application in the future.

REFERENCES

1. *Sampson HA, Aceves S, Bock SA, et al. Food allergy: a practice parameter update-2014. J Allergy Clin Immunol 2014;134:1016–25.
2. Burks AW, Tang M, Sicherer S, et al. ICON: Food allergy. J Allergy Clin Immunol 2012;129: 906–20.
3. Sicherer SH, Sampson HA. Food allergy: Epidemiology, pathogenesis, diagnosis, and treatment. J Allergy Clin Immunol 2014;133:291–307.
4. *Branum AM, Lukacs SL. Food allergy among children in the United States. Pediatrics 2009; 124:1549–55.
5. Osborne NJ, Koplin JJ, Martin PE, et al. Prevalence of challenge-proven IgE- mediated food allergy using population-based sampling and predetermined challenge criteria in infants. J Allergy Clin Immunol 2011;127:668–76.
6. Bunyavanich S, Rifas-Shiman SL, Platts-Mills TA, et al. Peanut allergy prevalence among school-age children in a US cohort not selected for any disease. J Allergy Clin Immunol 2014;134:753–5.
7. European Academy of Allergy and Clinical Immunology (EAACI). Food Allergy and Anaphylaxis Guidelines. Zurich, Switzerland: EAACI; 2014.
8. Gupta RS, Springston EE, Smith B, et al. Geographic variability of childhood food allergy in the United States. Clin Pediatr (Phila) 2012;51:856–61.
9. Gupta RS, Lau CH, Sita EE, et al. Factors associated with reported food allergy tolerance among US children. Ann Allergy Asthma Immunol 2013;111:194–8.
10. Warren CM, Jhaveri S, Warrier MR, et al. The epidemiology of milk allergy in US children. Ann Allergy Asthma Immunol 2013;110:370–4.
11. Sicherer SH. Epidemiology of food allergy. J Allergy Clin Immunol 2011;127:594–602.
12. Savage JH, Matsui EC, Skripak JM, et al. The natural history of egg allergy. J Allergy Clin Immunol 2007;120:1413–17.
13. Skripak JM, Matsui EC, Mudd K, et al. The natural history of IgE-mediated cow's milk allergy. J Allergy Clin Immunol 2007;120:1172–7.

14. *Kamdar TA, Peterson S, Lau CH, et al. Prevalence and characteristics of adult-onset food allergy. J Allergy Clin Immunol Pract 2015;3:114–15.

15. Lin RY, Anderson AS, Shah SN, et al. Increasing anaphylaxis hospitalizations in the first 2 decades of life: New York State, 1990–2006. Ann Allergy Asthma Immunol 2008;101:387–93.

16. Yocum MW, Butterfield JH, Klein JS, et al. Epidemiology of anaphylaxis in Olmsted County: A population-based study. J Allergy Clin Immunol 1999;104:452–6.

17. Decker WW, Campbell RL, Manivannan V, et al. The etiology and incidence of anaphylaxis in Rochester, Minnesota: a report from the Rochester Epidemiology Project. J Allergy Clin Immunol 2008;122: 1161–5.

18. Sheikh A, Alves B. Hospital admissions for acute anaphylaxis: time trend study. BMJ 2000;320: 1441.

19. Sheikh A, Alves B. Age, sex, geographical and socio-economic variations in admissions for anaphylaxis: analysis of four years of English hospital data. Clin Exp Allergy 2001;31:1571–6.

20. Wood RA, Sicherer SH, Vickery BP, et al. The natural history of milk allergy in an observational cohort. J Allergy Clin Immunol 2013;131:805–12.

21. Nowak-Węgrzyn A, Bloom KA, Sicherer SH, et al. Tolerance to extensively heated milk in children with cow's milk allergy. J Allergy Clin Immunol 2008;122:342–7.

22. Kim JS, Nowak-Węgrzyn A, Sicherer SH, et al. Dietary baked milk accelerates the resolution of cow's milk allergy in children. J Allergy Clin Immunol 2011;128:125–31.

23. Lemon-Mule H, Sampson HA, Sicherer SH, et al. Immunologic changes in children with egg allergy ingesting extensively heated egg. J Allergy Clin Immunol 2008;122:977–83.

24. Leonard SA, Sampson HA, Sicherer SH, et al. Dietary baked egg accelerates resolution of egg allergy in children. J Allergy Clin Immunol 2012;130:473–80.

25. Skolnick HS, Conover-Walker MK, Koerner CB, et al. The natural history of peanut allergy. J Allergy Clin Immunol 2001;107:367–74.

26. Fleischer DM, Conover-Walker MK, Matsui EC, et al. The natural history of tree nut allergy. J Allergy Clin Immunol 2005;116:1087–93.

27. Fleischer DM, Conover-Walker MK, Christie L, et al. Peanut allergy: recurrence and its management. J Allergy Clin Immunol 2004;114:1195–201.

28. Savage JH, Kaeding AJ, Matsui EC, et al. The natural history of soy allergy. J Allergy Clin Immunol 2010;125:683–6.

29. Keet CA, Matsui EC, Dhillon G, et al. The natural history of wheat allergy. Ann Allergy Asthma Immunol 2009;102:410–15.

30. Shek LP, Soderstrom L, Ahlstedt S, et al. Determination of food specific IgE levels over time can predict the development of tolerance in cow's milk and hen's egg allergy. J Allergy Clin Immunol 2004; 114:387–91.

31. Vickery BP, Scurlock AM, Jones SM, et al. Mechanisms of immune tolerance relevant to food allergy. J Allergy Clin Immunol 2011;127:576–84, quiz 85–86.

32. Radauer C, Bublin M, Wagner S, et al. Allergens are distributed into few protein families and possess a restricted number of biochemical functions. J Allergy Clin Immunol 2008;121:847–52.

33. Breiteneder H, Radauer C. A classification of plant food allergens. J Allergy Clin Immunol 2004;113:821–30, quiz 31.

34. Lucas CD, Hallagan JB, Taylor SL. The role of natural color additives in food allergy. Adv Food Nutr Res 2001;43:195–216.

35. Gultekin F, Doguc DK. Allergic and immunologic reactions to food additives. Clin Rev Allergy Immunol 2013;45:6–29.

36. Sicherer SH. Clinical implications of cross-reactive food allergens. J Allergy Clin Immunol 2001;108:881–90.

37. Vadas P, Gold M, Perelman B, et al. Platelet-activating factor, PAF acetylhydrolase, and severe anaphylaxis. N Engl J Med 2008;358:28–35.

38. Untersmayr E, Jensen-Jarolim E. The effect of gastric digestion on food allergy. Curr Opin Allergy Clin Immunol 2006;6:214–19.

39. Scholl I, Untersmayr E, Bakos N, et al. Antiulcer drugs promote oral sensitization and hypersensitivity to hazelnut allergens in BALB/c mice and humans. Am J Clin Nutr 2005;81:154–60.

40. Untersmayr E, Bakos N, Scholl I, et al. Anti-ulcer drugs promote IgE formation toward dietary antigens in adult patients. FASEB J 2005;19:656–8.

41. Untersmayr E, Poulsen LK, Platzer MH, et al. The effects of gastric digestion on codfish allergenicity. J Allergy Clin Immunol 2005;115:377–82.

42. Liacouras CA, Furuta GT, Hirano I, et al. Eosinophilic esophagitis: updated consensus recommendations for children and adults. J Allergy Clin Immunol 2011;128:3–20.

43. Kagalwalla AF, Sentongo TA, Ritz S, et al. Effect of six-food elimination diet on clinical and histologic outcomes in eosinophilic esophagitis. Clin Gastroenterol Hepatol 2006;4:1097–102.

44. Caubet JM, Ford LS, Sickles L, et al. Clinical features and resolution of food protein-induced enterocolitis syndrome: 10-year experience. J Allergy Clin Immunol 2014.

45. Katz Y, Goldberg MR, Rajuan N, et al. The prevalence and natural course of food protein-induced enterocolitis syndrome to cow's milk: a large-scale, prospective population-based study. J Allergy Clin Immunol 2011;127:647–53.

46. Sicherer SH. Food protein-induced enterocolitis syndrome: case presentations and management lessons. J Allergy Clin Immunol 2005;115:149–56.

47. Jarvinen K, Nowak-Węgrzyn A. Food protein-induced enterocolitis syndrome: Current management strategies. J Allergy Clin Immunol Pract 2013;1:317.

48. Lake AM. Food-induced eosinophilic proctocolitis. J Pediatr Gastroenterol Nutr 2000;30(Suppl.) :S58–60.

49. Odze RD, Bines J, Leichtner AM, et al. Allergic proctocolitis in infants: a prospective clinicopathologic biopsy study. Hum Pathol 1993;24:668–74.

50. Savilahti E. Food-induced malabsorption syndromes. J Pediatr Gastroenterol Nutr 2000;30(Suppl.):S61–6.
51. Green PH, Cellier C. Celiac disease. N Engl J Med 2007;357:1731–43.
52. *Ludvigsson JF, Bai JC, Biagi F, et al. Diagnosis and management of adult coeliac disease: guidelines from the British Society of Gastroenterology. Gut 2014;63:1210–28.
53. Novak N, Leung DY. Advances in atopic dermatitis. Curr Opin Immunol 2011;23:778–83.
54. Eigenmann PA, Sicherer SH, Borkowski TA, et al. Prevalence of IgE-mediated food allergy among children with atopic dermatitis. Pediatrics 1998;101:E8.
55. Flinterman AE, Knulst AC, Meijer Y, et al. Acute allergic reactions in children with AEDS after prolonged cow's milk elimination diets. Allergy 2006;61:370–4.
56. Cardones AR, Hall RP 3rd. Pathophysiology of dermatitis herpetiformis: a model for cutaneous manifestations of gastrointestinal inflammation. Dermatol Clin 2011;29:469–77.
57. Cardones AR, Hall RP 3rd. Management of dermatitis herpetiformis. Immunol Allergy Clin North Am 2012;32:275–81.
58. James JM, Bernhisel-Broadbent J, Sampson HA. Respiratory reactions provoked by double-blind food challenges in children. Am J Respir Crit Care Med 1994;149:59–64.
59. Kivity S, Dunner K, Marian Y. The pattern of food hypersensitivity in patients with onset after 10 years of age. Clin Exp Allergy 1994;24:19–22.
60. Novembre E, de Martino M, Vierucci A. Foods and respiratory allergy. J Allergy Clin Immunol 1988;81:1059–65.
61. James JM, Crespo JF. Allergic reactions to foods by inhalation. Curr Allergy Asthma Rep 2007;7:167–74.
62. Rudders SA, Arias SA, Camargo CA Jr. Trends in hospitalizations for food-induced anaphylaxis in US children, 2000–2009. J Allergy Clin Immunol 2014;134:960–2.
63. Sampson HA, Mendelson L, Rosen JP. Fatal and near-fatal anaphylactic reactions to food in children and adolescents. N Engl J Med 1992;327:380–4.
64. Bock SA, Munoz-Furlong A, Sampson HA. Fatalities due to anaphylactic reactions to foods. J Allergy Clin Immunol 2001;107:191–3.
65. *Muraro A, Werfel T, Hoffmann-Sommergruber K, et al. EAACI food allergy and anaphylaxis guidelines: diagnosis and management of food allergy. Allergy 2014;69:1008–25.
66. Commins SP, Platts-Mills TA. Delayed anaphylaxis to red meat in patients with IgE specific for galactose alpha-1,3-galactose (alpha-gal). Curr Allergy Asthma Rep 2013;13:72–7.
67. Boyce JA, Assa'ad A, Burks AW, et al. Guidelines for the Diagnosis and Management of Food Allergy in the United States: Summary of the NIAID-Sponsored Expert Panel Report. J Allergy Clin Immunol 2010;126:1105–18.
68. Sporik R, Hill DJ, Hosking CS. Specificity of allergen skin testing in predicting positive open food challenges to milk, egg and peanut in children. Clin Exp Allergy 2000;30:1540–6.
69. Mehl A, Rolinck-Werninghaus C, Staden U, et al. The atopy patch test in the diagnostic workup of suspected food-related symptoms in children. J Allergy Clin Immunol 2006;118:923–9.
70. Sicherer SH, Wood RA. Advances in diagnosing peanut allergy. J Allergy Clin Immunol Pract 2013;1:1–14.
71. Sicherer SH, Wood RA. American Academy of Pediatrics Section On A, Immunology. Allergy testing in childhood: using allergen-specific IgE tests. Pediatrics 2012;129:193–7.
72. Dang TD, Tang M, Choo S, et al. Increasing the accuracy of peanut allergy diagnosis by using Ara h 2. J Allergy Clin Immunol 2012;129:1056–63.
73. Masthoff LJ, Mattsson L, Zuidmeer-Jongejan L, et al. Sensitization to Cor a 9 and Cor a 14 is highly specific for a hazelnut allergy with objective symptoms in Dutch children and adults. J Allergy Clin Immunol 2013;132:393–9.
74. Masthoff LJ, Pasmans SG, van Hoffen E, et al. Diagnostic value of hazelnut allergy tests including rCor a 1 spiking in double-blind challenged children. Allergy 2012;67:521–7.
75. Ando H, Moverare R, Kondo Y, et al. Utility of ovomucoid-specific IgE concentrations in predicting symptomatic egg allergy. J Allergy Clin Immunol 2008;122:583–8.
76. Konstantinou GN, Ramon B, Grishin A, et al. The role of casein-specific IgA and TGF-beta in children with food protein-induced enterocolitis syndrome to milk. Pediatr Allergy Immunol 2014.
77. Sampson HA, Gerth van Wijk R, Bindslev-Jensen C, et al. Standardizing double-blind, placebo-controlled oral food challenges: American Academy of Allergy, Asthma & Immunology-European Academy of Allergy and Clinical Immunology PRACTALL consensus report. J Allergy Clin Immunol 2012;130:1260–74.
78. Nowak-Węgrzyn A, Assa'ad AH, Bahna SL, et al. Work Group report: oral food challenge testing. J Allergy Clin Immunol 2009;123:S365–83.
79. *Leonard SA, Caubet JC, Kim JS, et al. Baked milk- and egg-containing diet in the management of milk and egg allergy. J Allergy Clin Immunol Pract 2015;3:13–23.
80. Allen KJ, Turner PJ, Pawankar R, et al. Precautionary labelling of foods for allergen content: are we ready for a global framework? World Allergy Organ J 2014;7:10.
81. Simonte SJ, Ma S, Mofidi S, et al. Relevance of casual contact with peanut butter in children with peanut allergy. J Allergy Clin Immunol 2003;112:180–2.
82. Roberts G, Golder N, Lack G. Bronchial challenges with aerosolized food in asthmatic, food-allergic children. Allergy 2002;57:713–17.
83. Maloney JM, Chapman MD, Sicherer SH. Peanut allergen exposure through saliva: assessment and interventions to reduce exposure. J Allergy Clin Immunol 2006;118:719–24.
84. Comstock SS, DeMera R, Vega LC, et al. Allergic reactions to peanuts, tree nuts, and seeds aboard commercial airliners. Ann Allergy Asthma Immunol 2008;101:51–6.
85. Sicherer SH, Furlong TJ, DeSimone J, et al. Self-reported allergic reactions to peanut on commercial airliners. J Allergy Clin Immunol 1999;104:186–9.

86. Greenhawt M, MacGillivray F, Batty G, et al. International study of risk-mitigating factors and in-flight allergic reactions to peanut and tree nut. J Allergy Clin Immunol Pract 2013;1:186–94.

87. Young MC, Munoz-Furlong A, Sicherer SH. Management of food allergies in schools: a perspective for allergists. J Allergy Clin Immunol 2009;124:175–82, 82.

88. Groetch M, Nowak-Węgrzyn A. Practical approach to nutrition and dietary intervention in pediatric food allergy. Pediatr Allergy Immunol 2013;24:212–21.

89. *Groetch M, Henry M, Feuling MB, et al. Guidance for the nutrition management of gastrointestinal allergy in pediatrics. J Allergy Clin Immunol Pract 2013;1:323–31.

90. Gold MS, Sainsbury R. First aid anaphylaxis management in children who were prescribed an epinephrine autoinjector device (EpiPen). J Allergy Clin Immunol 2000;106:171–6.

91. Jarvinen KM, Sicherer SH, Sampson HA, et al. Use of multiple doses of epinephrine in food-induced anaphylaxis in children. J Allergy Clin Immunol 2008;122:133–8.

92. Ma S, Sicherer SH, Nowak-Węgrzyn A. A survey on the management of pollen-food allergy syndrome in allergy practices. J Allergy Clin Immunol 2003;112:784–8.

93. *Fleischer DM, Spergel JM, Assa'ad AH, et al. Primary prevention of allergic disease through nutritional interventions. J Allergy Clin Immunol Pract 2013;1:29–36.

94. de Silva D, Geromi M, Halken S, et al. Primary prevention of food allergy in children and adults: systematic review. Allergy 2014;69:581–9.

95. Du Toit G, Katz Y, Sasieni P, et al. Early consumption of peanuts in infancy is associated with a low prevalence of peanut allergy. J Allergy Clin Immunol 2008;122:984–91.

96. *Du Toit G, Roberts G, Sayre PH, et al. Randomized trial of peanut consumption in infants at risk for peanut allergy. N Engl J Med 2015;372:803–13.

97. Moran TP, Vickery BP, Burks AW. Oral and sublingual immunotherapy for food allergy: current progress and future directions. Curr Opin Immunol 2013;25:781–7.

98. *Nowak-Węgrzyn A, Albin S. Oral immunotherapy for food allergy: mechanisms and role in management. Clin Exp Allergy 2015;45:368–83.

99. Vickery BP, Scurlock AM, Kulis M, et al. Sustained unresponsiveness to peanut in subjects who have completed peanut oral immunotherapy. J Allergy Clin Immunol 2014;133:468–75.

100. *Kulis M, Burks AW. Effects of a pre-existing food allergy on the oral introduction of food proteins: findings from a murine model. Allergy 2015;70:120–3.

101. Varshney P, Steele PH, Vickery BP, et al. Adverse reactions during peanut oral immunotherapy home dosing. J Allergy Clin Immunol 2009;124:1351–2.

102. *Wood RA, Sampson HA. Oral immunotherapy for the treatment of peanut allergy: is it ready for prime time? J Allergy Clin Immunol Pract 2014;2:97–8.

103. Fleischer DM, Burks AW, Vickery BP, et al. Sublingual immunotherapy for peanut allergy: a randomized, double-blind, placebo-controlled multicenter trial. J Allergy Clin Immunol 2013;131:119–27.

104. Keet CA, Frischmeyer-Guerrerio PA, Thyagarajan A, et al. The safety and efficacy of sublingual and oral immunotherapy for milk allergy. J Allergy Clin Immunol 2012;129:448–55.

105. Dupont C, Kalach N, Soulaines P, et al. Cow's milk epicutaneous immunotherapy in children: a pilot trial of safety, acceptability, and impact on allergic reactivity. J Allergy Clin Immunol 2010;125:1165–7.

106. *Sampson HA, Agbotounou W, Thébault C, et al. Epicutaneous immunotherapy (EPIT) is effective and safe to treat peanut allergy: a multi-national double-blind placebo-controlled randomized Phase IIb trial. J Allergy Clin Immunol 2015;135:AB390.

Key references are preceded by an asterisk.

CHAPTER 13

Anaphylaxis

Simon G. A. Brown and Paul J. Turner

CHAPTER OUTLINE

INTRODUCTION
HISTORICAL PERSPECTIVE
EPIDEMIOLOGY
PATHOPHYSIOLOGY
Triggering
Biochemical Mediators and Effects
Mechanisms of Anaphylactic Shock
CLINICAL FEATURES (PHENOTYPES)
PATIENT EVALUATION, DIAGNOSIS, AND DIFFERENTIAL DIAGNOSIS
Laboratory Testing

TREATMENT
Epinephrine
Intravenous Fluid (Volume) Resuscitation
Other Measures
Monitoring
ONGOING MANAGEMENT AND REFERRAL
CONCLUSIONS

SUMMARY OF IMPORTANT CONCEPTS

- Drugs, foods, and insect stings are the most common triggers of anaphylaxis.
- Activation of multiple inflammatory pathways causes fluid extravasation (tissue edema, hypovolemia), vascular dilation (erythema, reduced venous return to the heart), bronchospasm, and smooth muscle contraction (bronchospasm, abdominal and pelvic cramps).
- The cornerstones of emergency management are support of the airway and/or ventilation, a supine position, epinephrine (also called adrenaline in some countries; usually intramuscular but occasionally intravenous), and volume expansion with intravenous isotonic crystalloid.
- Mortality risk from anaphylaxis may be increased in patients with a history of severe reactions, asthmatics (risk of severe bronchospasm), teenagers and young adults (possible risk-taking behaviors), and older people with comorbidities (limited cardiorespiratory reserve).
- Following an episode of anaphylaxis, prevention of further episodes requires identification of likely triggers and co-factors, optimizing the management of comorbidities, allergen avoidance strategies, and consideration for immunotherapy, if available.
- Patient education including an anaphylaxis action plan and an epinephrine auto-injector should be considered (e.g., food and insect sting anaphylaxis, exercise-induced anaphylaxis, idiopathic anaphylaxis).

INTRODUCTION

Anaphylaxis is a severe, immediate-type generalized hypersensitivity reaction affecting multiple organ systems and characterized at its most severe by bronchospasm, upper airway angioedema, hypotension, and collapse.[1] Immediate recognition and relatively simple emergency management will prevent death on most occasions, but lack of familiarity with the condition can lead to avoidable deaths through the lack of recognition of atypical presentations and/or inappropriate treatments. Once the acute episode has resolved, patients will also benefit from a careful assessment of likely causes and potential cross-reactivities, avoidance strategies, attention to relevant comorbidities, immunotherapy if available, and action management plans for future reactions including an assessment for provision of an epinephrine auto-injector.

HISTORICAL PERSPECTIVE

The term *anaphylaxis* (from the Greek words *ana*, 'contrary to,' and *phylaxis*, 'protection') was coined by Portier and Richet in 1902, after they observed the sudden cardio-respiratory collapse that occurred in dogs after repeated exposure to small amounts of jellyfish venom. This response was eventually attributed to an immunoglobulin E (IgE) to the venom, and so the term *anaphylaxis* was initially applied to systemic, immediate hypersensitivity reactions caused by IgE-mediated immunologic release of mediators from mast cells and basophils, and the term *anaphylactoid reaction* was later introduced to refer to a clinically similar event not mediated by IgE.

Recently, the World Allergy Organization proposed a change in terminology, such that anaphylaxis refers to a "*severe, life-threatening, generalized or systemic hypersensitivity reaction.*" The term *allergic anaphylaxis* should be used when this reaction is mediated by an immunologic mechanism (IgE, IgG, immune complex, complement related), and *non-allergic anaphylaxis* should be used to refer to a non-immunologic reaction. To avoid confusion, and making the point that for emergency management the mechanism by which anaphylaxis was triggered is irrelevant, this terminology eliminated the use of the term *anaphylactoid* (Fig. 13-1).

The difficulties producing a clinical definition of anaphylaxis have been highlighted in symposia jointly sponsored by the US National Institutes of Health (Allergy and Infectious Disease) and the Food Allergy and Anaphylaxis Network. A general consensus was reached with clinical criteria for diagnosis that recognized the generalized, potentially life-threatening and multiple organ system nature of anaphylaxis. This was in terms of both the 'typical' presentation of skin manifestations plus involvement of another major organ system, and also atypical clinical syndromes that occur in the right clinical context (Box 13-1). This approach has been subsequently adopted by the World Allergy Organization.[2]

EPIDEMIOLOGY

Although the exact incidence of anaphylaxis is unknown, estimates range from 50 to 2000 episodes per 100 000 person-years, with a 'lifetime' prevalence of 0.05–2%. The incidence of anaphylaxis appears to be increasing, at least in industrialized populations, although the uncertainties introduced by retrospective methodologies and changes in clinical practice (decision to admit) and coding can be hard to dissect. Despite this, the available data from the US, UK, and Australia indicate that fatal anaphylaxis is rare, with an annual incidence of around 0.05 cases per 100 000 population. Recent data from the UK found no increase in the rate of fatal anaphylaxis (of any cause) over the

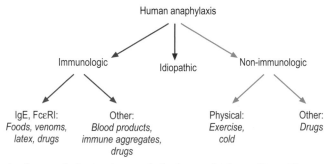

Figure 13-1 Visual schema of change in anaphylaxis terminology. *(From Simons FE. Anaphylaxis, killer allergy: long-term management in the community. J Allergy Clin Immunol 2006; 117:367–377.)*

Box 13-1 **Critical Criteria for Diagnosing Anaphylaxis**

Anaphylaxis is highly likely when any *one* of the following three criteria is fulfilled:

1. Acute onset of an illness (minutes to several hours) with involvement of the skin, mucosal tissues, or both (e.g., generalized hives, pruritus or flushing, swollen lips-tongue-uvula). And at least one of the following:
   a. Respiratory compromise (e.g., dyspnea, wheeze-bronchospasm, stridor, reduced PEF, hypoxemia)
   b. Reduced BP or associated symptoms of end-organ dysfunction (e.g., hypotonia [collapse], syncope, incontinence).

2. Two or more of the following that occur rapidly after exposure *to a likely allergen for that patient* (minutes to several hours):
   a. Involvement of skin-mucosal tissue (e.g., generalized hives, itch-flush, swollen lips-tongue-uvula)
   b. Respiratory compromise (e.g., dyspnea, wheeze-bronchospasm, stridor, reduced PEF, hypoxemia)
   c. Reduced BP or associated symptoms of end-organ dysfunction (e.g., hypotonia [collapse], syncope, incontinence)
   d. Persistent gastrointestinal symptoms (e.g., crampy abdominal pain, vomiting).

3. Reduced BP after exposure *to known allergen for that patient* (minutes to several hours):
   a. Infants and children: low systolic BP (age specific) or >30% decrease in systolic BP*
   b. Adults: systolic BP <90 mmHg or >30% decrease from their baseline.

PEF, peak expiratory flow; BP, blood pressure.
*Low systolic BP for children is defined as <70 mmHg from 1 month to 1 year; <70 mmHg + [2×age] from 1 to 10 years; and <90 mmHg from 11 to 17 years.
(From Sampson HA et al. Second symposium on the definition and management of anaphylaxis. J Allergy Clin Immunol 2006; 117:391–7.)

---

last two decades, despite a seven-fold increase in hospitalizations over the same time period. Iatrogenic causes (medication, blood products, contrast media) were the most common triggers in 55% cases, followed by food (26%) and insect stings (19%). Admission and fatality rates for drug- and insect sting–induced anaphylaxis increased with age. In contrast, younger adults appear to be most at risk of fatal food-triggered anaphylaxis, with a marked peak in the incidence of fatal reactions during the second and third decades of life.[3] These data are similar to that found in a smaller cohort of fatal anaphylaxis over 9 years in Australia, although in this latter study, an increase in drug-related fatal anaphylaxis but not food-induced anaphylaxis was observed.[4]

In the US and Australia, epinephrine auto-injector prescriptions and anaphylaxis admissions are fewer in states with warmer climates and more year-round sunlight, suggesting that that lower vitamin D levels might predispose to anaphylactic events. Anaphylaxis is more frequent in adults than children for some agents (radiocontrast media, plasma expanders, anesthetics, antibiotics, insect stings), which may be the function of exposure frequency. Random surveys have found anaphylaxis to be more frequent in females overall, although males are affected more frequently under the age of 15 years. Atopy has been identified as a risk factor for anaphylaxis as a result of food antigens, exercise anaphylaxis, idiopathic anaphylaxis, radiocontrast media reactions, and latex reactions, but it does not appear to be a risk factor for insulin, penicillin, and *Hymenoptera* sting reactions. UK and US studies have shown that asthma is a risk factor for anaphylactic events and that the more severe the asthma, the higher the risk.

PATHOPHYSIOLOGY

Triggering

Anaphylaxis can result from several triggers (Table 13-1). The classic *IgE-dependent* immunologic mechanism is best understood and characterized by allergen cross-linking of FcεRI receptors (high-affinity IgE receptors) on mast cells and basophils. Other immunologic mechanisms involving other types of antibody and various inflammatory pathways are referred to as *IgE-independent*. These are not as well understood and are possibly overlapping. For example, aspirin and other non-steroidal anti-inflammatory drugs (NSAIDs) can cause agent-specific reactivity or class reactivity. This suggests an immunoglobulin mechanism for the former and a metabolic mechanism (e.g., arachidonic acid metabolism) for the latter. Reactions to NSAIDs also tend to have delayed onset and protracted course, which suggests antibody-dependent reactivity to a

TABLE 13-1   Summary of Incidence for Common Triggers of Anaphylaxis

Agent	Comment/findings
Antibiotics[5]	Arguably most common cause of drug-induced anaphylaxis, most frequently β-lactams, accounting for as many as 22% of all drug-related episodes. Non-fatal drug-induced anaphylaxis to penicillin may affect 1.9–27.2 million Americans.
Latex[6]	Populations at risk experience multiple mucosal exposures to latex, e.g., healthcare workers, patients with multiple catheterizations/surgeries. Overall incidence of latex allergy in the US is 2.7–16 million. Although incidence of latex allergy has risen greatly over last 15 years, with reduced use of powdered gloves and substitution of non-latex gloves in hospitals, incidence appears to have stabilized.
Perioperative anaphylaxis[7,8]	Depending on the country, perioperative anaphylactic reactions represent 9–19% of complications of anesthesia. Fatality rate approximates 5–7%. Muscle relaxants account for 62% and latex 16%; the remainder of reactions result from hypnotics, antibiotics, plasma substitutes, and opioids. Serial data collected in France showed increased incidence of perioperative anaphylactic events. Muscle relaxants still remain the most common cause.
Radiocontrast media[9]	Adverse reactions to ionic contrast media (hyperosmolar agents) occur with a frequency of 4–12% and to non-ionic (lower osmolar agents) of 1–3%. Severe adverse reactions occur in 0.16% of ionic media administration and 0.03% with non-ionic media. Paradoxically, mortality rate (1–3 per 100 000 contrast administrations) appears similar for both ionic and non-ionic media.
Hymenoptera stings[10]	Potentially life-threatening systemic reactions to insect stings occur in an estimated 0.4–0.8% of children and 3% of adults.
Food[11,12]	As many as 6% of children and 3–4% of adults have food allergy. Based on incidence in Colorado, approximately 0.0004% of the US population, or 1080 Americans, have anaphylactic reactions to food each year. Shellfish is probably the most common source in adults and peanuts in children. Also, 1.1% of the US population may be allergic to tree nuts or peanuts.
Non-steroidal anti-inflammatory drugs[13]	Incidence varies depending on whether or not asthmatic patients are included. NSAIDs are probably the second most common medication offender after antibiotics.
Antisera	Once the most important cause of anaphylaxis, antisera have greatly diminished in importance with their decreased use as therapeutic agents, but antiserum is still used for snakebites and immunosuppression. Incidence in patients receiving antilymphocyte globulin may be as high as 2%, and incidence to antivenom 4.6–10%. Incidence may decline further with recent release of Crotalidae Polyvalent ImmunFab, a purified preparation of Fab fragment obtained from sheep immunized with venom. Although urticaria has been reported, no anaphylactic episodes have occurred with this agent.
Reactions associated with hemodialysis[14]	Incidence appears to be increasing. Drug administration data show 3.5 severe hypersensitivity reactions per 100 000 hollow-fiber dialyzers sold. In 260 000 dialysis treatments, 21 severe reactions occurred, including one fatality.
Idiopathic anaphylaxis[15]	Cause remains unidentified in as many as two thirds of adults presenting to allergist/immunologist for evaluation of anaphylaxis. Survey of 75 US allergists found 633 cases encountered. The authors extrapolated data to the US population and estimated as many as 20 592–47 024 cases.
Biologic agents[16,17]	With increased use of biologic agents, anaphylactic reactions to these products have also increased, including omalizumab, tumor necrosis factor antagonists, cetuximab, tocilizumab, and natalizumab.

metabolite. In animal models in mice, anaphylaxis can be triggered by the IgG FcγRIII receptor, requiring proportionately more antigen and antibody than the IgE-dependent pathway. IgG-dependent anaphylaxis has not been demonstrated in humans. However, human IgG receptors are capable of activating macrophages to release PAF, which can activate mast cells in-vitro. There are also emerging data from both human and animal studies that allergen-specific IgG can interfere with IgE-dependent anaphylaxis, modulating the response. Some agents can initiate degranulation of mast cells and basophils without help from immune pathways, and this is termed *non-immunologic* anaphylaxis. Examples include physical factors, such as heat or cold, and opioids and vancomycin, which directly activate mast cells. Importantly, anaphylaxis can also be *summative*, in which a combination of physical stimulus (usually exercise) in close proximity to allergen ingestion (to which the patient has allergen-specific IgE) results in a reaction.

Biochemical Mediators and Effects

Many of the pathophysiologic events that occur during anaphylaxis are easily explained by the actions of mediators, summarized in Table 13-2, all of which have overlapping actions of similar clinical importance. This results in the triad of smooth muscle

TABLE 13-2   Mast Cell and Basophil Mediators and Roles in Producing Anaphylactic Events

Mediators	Pathophysiologic activity	Clinical correlates
Histamine and products of arachidonic acid metabolism (leukotrienes, thromboxane, prostaglandins, platelet-activating factor)	Smooth muscle spasm, mucus secretion, vasodilation, increased vascular permeability, activation of nociceptive neurons, platelet adherence, eosinophil activation, eosinophil chemotaxis	Wheeze, urticaria, angioedema, flush, itch, diarrhea, abdominal pain, hypotension, rhinorrhea, bronchorrhea
Neutral proteases: tryptase, chymase, carboxypeptidase, cathepsin G	Cleavage of complement components, chemoattractants for eosinophils and neutrophils, further activation and degranulation of mast cells, cleavage of neuropeptides, conversion of angiotensin I to angiotensin II	May recruit complement by cleaving C3; may ameliorate symptoms by invoking hypertensive response through angiotensin I–II conversion and by inactivating neuropeptides, although angiotensin II also may cause deleterious coronary artery vasoconstriction. Also, proteases can magnify response because of further mast cell activation
Proteoglycans: heparin, chondroitin sulfate	Anticoagulation, inhibition of complement, phospholipase A_2 binding, chemoattractant for eosinophils, cytokine inhibition, kinin pathway activation	Can prevent intravascular coagulation and recruitment of complement. Can recruit kinins, increasing severity of reaction
Chemoattractants: chemokines, eosinophil chemotactic factors	Summons cells to site	May be partly responsible for recrudescence of symptoms in late phase reaction or extension and protraction of reaction
Tumor necrosis factor-α activates nuclear factor κB	Produces platelet-activating factor (PAF)	Vascular permeability and vasodilation; PAF synthesized and released late, involved in late phase reactions

contraction, vasodilation and increased vascular permeability that characterize clinical anaphylaxis. Rapid systemic spread of immune activation and mediator release appears to be required for the development of severe anaphylaxis.[18] This may be due to mediators released by triggering mast cells directly affecting other mast cells and/or a complex 'mast cell–leukocyte cytokine cascade' initially proposed in the context of allergic airway inflammation but now supported by studies using mouse models of anaphylaxis and a human study of leukocyte gene activation in the early phase of anaphylaxis.[19] Recent data also indicate an important role for basophil activation in systemic allergic reactions, with a dose–response between the degree of activation and symptom severity.

The activation of basophils and mast cells releases an array of biochemical mediators and chemotactic substances by degranulation of preformed mediators and *de novo* synthesis. Table 13-2 summarizes the main activities of these mediators and pathophysiologic consequences and clinical correlates. Additionally, low constitutional levels of regulatory enzymes such as PAF-AH may contribute to reaction severity in some patients.[18,20]

Mechanisms of Anaphylactic Shock

Box 13-2 summarizes likely key pathologic mechanisms of human anaphylactic shock. The balance of evidence from human observations and animal studies suggests that the main pathophysiologic features of anaphylactic shock are a profound reduction in venous tone and fluid extravasation. The resulting mixed hypovolemic and distributive shock involves reduction in blood volume (hypovolemia) from extravasation and distribution of blood to the wrong areas. Both of these combine to cause reduced venous return to the heart and an empty ventricle. Animal models and a few human case reports also suggest that depressed myocardial function can be a factor in some cases, introducing a component of temporary cardiogenic shock as well. Electrocardiographic (ECG) changes are seen in some cases, but it is not known if this represents a mediator effect on the myocardium and/or arrhythmia generation, a reduction in coronary perfusion caused by low diastolic blood pressure (blood flow through coronary arteries occurs during diastole when the heart relaxes), coronary spasm, or sometimes plaque rupture.

Arguably the most important human study to date is a series of 205 episodes of anaphylactic shock occurring under anesthesia, in which the treating anesthesiologist

---

Box 13-2   **Key Pathophysiologic Mechanisms of Human Anaphylactic Shock**

COMMON/CLEARLY DEMONSTRATED*

- Fluid extravasation causing hemoconcentration, hypovolemia, and reduced venous return to the heart manifested as low filling pressures and reduction in cardiac output

LIKELY[†]

- Venodilation and blood pooling, contributing to reduced venous return
- Impaired myocardial contractility contributing, along with reduced venous return, to reduced cardiac output
- Relative bradycardia (neurally mediated) in awake patients, contributing to reduced cardiac output
- Early transient increase in pulmonary vascular resistance, contributing to reduced cardiac output by obstructing venous return to left side of heart
- Early arteriolar dilation, manifested as a widened pulse pressure and contributing to hypotension. (However, an *increase* in systemic vascular resistance caused by increased arteriolar tone may predominate after this early phase.)

UNCOMMON/POSTULATED[‡]

- Severe global depression of myocardial contractility, with non-specific ST-segment electrocardiographic changes (unresponsive to adrenaline) possibly more likely in those with underlying cardiac disease or taking β-blockers
- Severe arteriolar dilation as well as venous dilation
- Coronary ischemia caused by coronary vasospasm and plaque ulceration.

---

*Supported by unambiguous observations of human anaphylaxis.
†Unproven but supported by animal studies, studies of histamine infusion in volunteers, known mediator actions, or indirect physiologic observations during human anaphylaxis.
‡Based on case reports, speculation, and plausible mechanisms.
(Modified from Brown SGA. The pathophysiology of shock in anaphylaxis. Immunol Allergy Clin North Am 2007; 27:165–175.)

was asked to provide detailed clinical and laboratory information immediately after the event.[21] Increases in hematocrit signaled extravasation of up to 35% of circulating blood volume within 10 min. A total of 46 patients with central or pulmonary artery catheters placed before or soon after onset of anaphylaxis had a significant fall in filling pressures, except in 9 of 11 patients with cardiac disease, who had elevated pressures. Even so, these patients appeared to need volume expansion to achieve a stable blood pressure. In all six patients with balloon pulmonary artery catheters, pulmonary pressure rose initially and then fell over the next 10 min.

A report of eight closely observed hypotensive anaphylactic reactions found that hypotension was preceded by a fall in diastolic blood pressure (suggesting reduced systemic vascular resistance) with tachycardia. Following this, in every case, the onset of hypotension was accompanied by a relative bradycardia. That is, rather than the heart rate further increasing to compensate for falling blood pressure, it fell as the blood pressure fell.[22] This may have been caused by a neurocardiogenic reflex, triggered by cardiac mechanoreceptors, and enhanced by increased levels of various mediators known to potentiate this reflex that are also elevated during anaphylaxis. However, bradycardia may also be a non-specific feature of severe hypovolemic/distributive shock in awake animals. Physiologic studies of awake mammals have identified two phases of response to hypovolemia, an initial phase of blood pressure maintenance by tachycardia and peripheral arteriolar constriction, followed by a second phase with more severe hypovolemia, characterized by bradycardia, reduced peripheral arteriolar tone, and a profound fall in blood pressure. However, bradycardia has not been reported as a feature of anaphylaxis under anesthesia, where tachycardia is the norm. This may be explained by the blunting of central reflexes that occurs under anesthesia and with different allergen routes and dosages.

Upright or semirecumbent (sitting upright) posture has been associated with fatal anaphylaxis. Movement from a supine to an upright or semi-upright position reduces venous return to the heart and is likely to exacerbate all the pathophysiologic processes involved in anaphylaxis (reduced venous return, profound bradycardia with further reduction in cardiac output myocardial ischemia). Keeping a patient flat to maximize venous return to the heart is therefore a key component of the initial response to anaphylaxis.

CLINICAL FEATURES (PHENOTYPES)

Allergic reactions occur across a broad spectrum, from localized and clinically mild systemic (skin only) allergic reactions to severe life-threatening anaphylaxis. The definition of anaphylaxis (Box 13-1) is based around the concept of a multisystem, severe reaction. This is helpful clinically, as it defines the need for urgent intervention, but is nevertheless somewhat artificial because essentially the same process (systemic effector cell activation triggered by allergen) may cause a mild reaction on one occasion but a life-threatening reaction on another occasion, even under controlled conditions in the same individual.

The main clinical manifestations of anaphylaxis are summarized in Table 13-3. Overall, the clinical similarities shared by patients in various published case series are striking. The most common manifestations are cutaneous, combined with respiratory, cardiovascular, and/or gastrointestinal features. Severe reactions tend to be either predominantly cardiovascular (hypotensive) or respiratory (hypoxemic/bronchospasm), although some (about 30%) display both. Food-triggered reactions tend to involve respiratory symptoms, which is consistent with data from the UK Fatal Anaphylaxis Registry in which the majority of food-triggered fatalities included respiratory involvement.[3] Older age and drug causation are risk factors for severe reactions; the latter may be related to administration via the parenteral route and/or the rapid absorption characteristics of oral drug formulations, causing rapid exposure to high doses of allergen.[18]

There are exceptions to the prototypical clinical presentation of skin features plus other organ involvement. For example, cardiovascular collapse with shock can occur immediately without any cutaneous or respiratory symptoms. The lack of cutaneous symptoms, specifically urticaria, in severe events was also noted in fatal reactions, and

TABLE 13-3   Signs and Symptoms of Anaphylaxis: Frequency of Occurrence*

Signs/symptoms	Percentage of cases[†]
Cutaneous	>90
Urticaria and angioedema	85–90
Flush	45–55
Pruritus without rash	2–5
Respiratory	40–60
Dyspnea, wheeze	45–50
Upper airway angioedema	50–60
Rhinitis	15–20
Dizziness, Syncope, Hypotension	30–35
Abdominal	
Nausea, vomiting, diarrhea, cramping pain	25–30
Miscellaneous	
Headache	5–8
Substernal pain	4–6
Seizure	1–2

*Based on a compilation of 1784 patients reviewed in Lieberman P. Anaphylaxis and anaphylactoid reactions. In: Middleton E. et al., eds. Allergy: principles and practice. 5th edn. St Louis: Mosby–Year Books; 1998:1079–1092.
[†]Percentages are approximations (see text).

may have contributed to delays in diagnosis and appropriate treatment. Even in food-triggered reactions, cutaneous symptoms are absent in up to 10% of reactions. Thus, in severe episodes, cutaneous features are not always clearly evident and/or may be overlooked. In some cases, the lack of cutaneous symptoms may have been caused by an inability to manifest them because of profound hypotension and reduced cutaneous blood flow. The signs and symptoms of anaphylaxis that occur during anesthesia may be different from those noted in episodes occurring outside the operating room (OR). Cardiovascular collapse appears to occur more often in operative events than those occurring outside the OR. During operative events, cardiovascular collapse and bronchospasm are significantly more common during IgE-mediated events than those that are not IgE-mediated.

Anaphylaxis presents with a different pattern of signs and symptoms in infants, with non-specific behavioral changes common, such as crying, fussing, irritability, and fright. Hoarseness and dysphonia with drooling and increased secretions, coughing, stridor, and choking can occur, as well as nasal congestion and gastrointestinal symptoms (e.g., regurgitation/vomiting within minutes of ingestion of an allergenic food, spitting up, loose stools, colicky pain). With severe reactions they may exhibit drowsiness and somnolence, followed by unresponsiveness and lethargy. Seizures can occur. Examination may show a weak pulse, pallor, and diaphoresis.

Characteristically, anaphylaxis is associated with a compensatory tachycardia that occurs in response to a decreased effective vascular volume. However, bradycardia can also occur, as described in the section above on mechanisms. In a study of 21 healthy adults with systemic allergic reactions to insect venom, hypotension was always accompanied by an initial tachycardia followed by a relative bradycardia, which occurred with the onset of hypotension. In two subjects, this was severe enough for atropine to be given.[22] Myocardial depression with decreased cardiac output as a result of contractile depression can also occur and persist for several days. ECG abnormalities include ST-segment elevation, flattened T waves, inverted T waves, and arrhythmias (e.g., from heart block); cardiac enzyme elevations also occur. The mechanisms are uncertain but may include mediator effects on the myocardium, coronary spasm, plaque ulceration (perhaps mediated by mast cells that are found in the coronary vasculature), and poor coronary blood flow secondary to hypotension and hypoxemia.

Anaphylaxis can present with unusual manifestations that make diagnosis difficult, especially when the episode has not been directly observed by a healthcare professional. Syncope without skin or respiratory manifestations can occur, sometimes with a seizure, especially if propped upright during hypotension, which further reduces cerebral blood flow and increases the risk of seizure from cerebral tissue hypoxia. This may be followed by a period of postictal confusion. In this situation, if a history of likely allergen exposure is missed, unnecessary cardiovascular and neurologic evaluations are often done before establishing the diagnosis of anaphylaxis.

Rarely, anaphylaxis can cause adrenal hemorrhage and thus prolonged hypotension. Profound anaphylactic episodes with hypotension can also result in clotting abnormalities. In some settings, it is also important to recognize coexistent coagulopathies, such as in anaphylactic reactions to snake venom and anti-venoms (associated with snake venom–induced consumption coagulopathy) and in anaphylaxis to leech bites (heparin-like anticoagulant effect from the leech contents if they are squeezed into the body on leech removal).

An anaphylactic episode can appear to abate and then exhibit a recrudescence several hours later. This is often termed 'biphasic anaphylaxis' but can also represent (and be difficult to distinguish from) protracted anaphylaxis with a temporary response to epinephrine. The exact incidence of biphasic reactions is uncertain, and probably depends on initial reaction severity. Events range from mild to severe, with fatalities reported. Reported biphasic reaction rates range from 1% in large inclusive studies with a range of initial reaction severities, to 20% in selected severe cases (patients admitted to hospital). In one large prospective study, such delayed deteriorations treated with epinephrine occurred in 29 of 315 anaphylaxis cases (9.2%) and were more common after initially hypotensive reactions and in people with pre-existing lung disease. In total, 22 of the 29 delayed deteriorations (76%) occurred within 4 hours of initial epinephrine treatment. Of the remaining seven cases, two were severe and occurred after initially severe reactions, within 10 hours.[18]

PATIENT EVALUATION, DIAGNOSIS, AND DIFFERENTIAL DIAGNOSIS

The diagnosis of anaphylaxis is a clinical one, based on the typical clinical features outlined above. However, for any episode of hypotension/shock or severe bronchospasm/hypoxemia in which the cause is not evident, a diagnosis of anaphylaxis should be considered and treatment with epinephrine initiated if there is an immediate threat to life.

The differential diagnosis of anaphylaxis is presented in Box 13-3. This first includes some consideration of the causes of anaphylaxis, then conditions that should be considered as potential alternate diagnoses. This process should start with the physician who sees the patient during the acute event, as careful contemporaneous documentation of all clinical features and patient recollection of potential exposures and timing is important in reaching a correct diagnosis.

The physician must first consider the likely cause and timing of exposure. While some exposures are obvious (e.g., a common allergenic food being ingested with immediate oral allergy symptoms followed by anaphylaxis, a drug injection, or an insect sting), some may not be. Anaphylaxis may not start for several hours after ingestion of an NSAID (possibly related to the generation of metabolites) and monoclonal antibody injections. A similar delay in symptom onset occurs for food allergic-reactions triggered by the alpha-gal allergen in mammalian meat. In the case of summative anaphylaxis, the triggering food alone does not result in anaphylaxis; anaphylaxis starts only when there is additional physical stress (typically physical exertion, although this can be moderate in activity). Sometimes, a very likely trigger (something known to frequently cause anaphylaxis, or a known allergen for that individual patient) may lead to a diagnosis of anaphylaxis even when the reaction is not typical (see Box 13-1, criteria 2 and 3). Where a likely trigger cannot be identified, where a trigger is known to be associated with non-anaphylaxis diagnoses (e.g., fish ingestion and scombroid poisoning, various

---

Box 13-3 Differential Diagnosis of Anaphylaxis

ANAPHYLAXIS

Anaphylaxis to exogenously administered agents
Physical factors
  Exercise
  Cold, heat, sunlight
Idiopathic

VASODEPRESSOR REACTIONS

Flush syndromes
  Carcinoid
  Menopause
  Chlorpropamide, alcohol
Medullary carcinoma thyroid
Autonomic epilepsy

RESTAURANT SYNDROMES

Monosodium glutamate (MSG)
Sulfites
Scombroidosis

OTHER FORMS OF SHOCK

Hemorrhagic
Cardiogenic
Endotoxic

EXCESS ENDOGENOUS PRODUCTION OF HISTAMINE SYNDROMES

Systemic mastocytosis
Urticaria pigmentosa
Basophilic leukemia
Acute promyelocytic leukemia (tretinoin)
Hydatid cyst

NON-ORGANIC DISEASE

Panic attacks
Munchausen stridor
Vocal cord dysfunction syndrome
Globus hystericus
Undifferentiated somatoform anaphylaxis

MISCELLANEOUS

Hereditary angioedema
Progesterone anaphylaxis
Urticarial vasculitis
Pheochromocytoma
Hyper-IgE, urticaria syndrome
Neurologic (seizure, stroke)
Pseudoanaphylaxis
Red man syndrome (vancomycin)
Capillary leak syndrome

drugs and flushing, ACE inhibitors, and angioedema), and/or when the reaction is atypical, then careful consideration of differential diagnoses is required.

Perhaps the most common condition mimicking anaphylaxis is the vasodepressor reaction (vasovagal syncope), which is associated with vasodilatation, bradycardia, hypotension, and loss of consciousness. It often results from a threatening event or emotional trauma. Bradycardia and the absence of cutaneous manifestations are often used to distinguish these episodes but, as previously noted, bradycardia is also a feature of hypotensive anaphylaxis and skin features may not be evident during anaphylaxis.

It is also important to recognize the entities that can produce flushing. Flushing is a common phenomenon and can result from a variety of agents, including niacin, nicotine, catecholamines, ACE inhibitors, and alcohol (with and without associated drugs). Flush is also seen in association with: ingestion of spicy foods containing capsaicin; carcinoid syndrome; pancreatic tumors; medullary carcinoma of the thyroid; hypoglycemia; rosacea; pheochromocytoma; menopause; autonomic epilepsy; panic attacks; and systemic mastocytosis. A group of postprandial syndromes (restaurant syndromes) resembling anaphylaxis have been attributed to the ingestion of monosodium glutamate (MSG), sulfites, or histamine. Ingestion of MSG can produce chest pain, facial burning, flushing, paresthesia, sweating, dizziness, headaches, palpitations, nausea, and vomiting. Children can experience shivering and chills, irritability, screaming, and delirium. The occurrence of these symptoms has been termed 'the Chinese restaurant syndrome.' The mechanism is unknown, but MSG is thought to cause a transient acetylcholinosis. About 15–20% of the general population appear to be sensitive to small doses of MSG, but reactions can occur in any individual if the dose is large enough. Scombroidosis poisoning caused by the ingestion of histamine and other biogenic amines accumulating in spoiled fish, also causes flushing plus other typical signs and symptoms that include urticaria, angioedema, nausea, vomiting, diarrhea, wheeze, and hypotension.

Non-organic disease can mimic anaphylaxis. Such episodes can be involuntary, such as in panic attacks, undifferentiated somatoform anaphylaxis, vocal cord dysfunction syndrome, and Munchausen stridor. Panic attacks are accompanied by tachycardia, flushing, GI symptoms, and shortness of breath. Vocal cord dysfunction syndrome is caused by an involuntary adduction of the vocal cords that occludes the glottal opening. A bunching together of the false vocal cords produces obstruction in both inspiration and expiration; the patient is unaware of the process. The term *Munchausen stridor* was coined to describe patients who intentionally adduct their vocal cords and present to the ED with self-induced manifestations of laryngeal edema. This entity occurs in psychologically disturbed individuals and can be distinguished from vocal cord dysfunction syndrome by laryngoscopy during the acute episode. Also, patients with Munchausen stridor can be distracted from their vocal cord adduction by asking them to perform maneuvers such as coughing. 'Undifferentiated somatoform anaphylaxis' is a term used to describe patients who present with manifestations that mimic idiopathic anaphylaxis but who lack objective confirmatory findings, do not respond to therapy, and exhibit psychologic signs of an undifferentiated somatoform disorder.

Other entities traditionally listed in the differential diagnosis of anaphylaxis include hereditary angioedema; progesterone anaphylaxis; anaphylaxis associated with recurrent and chronic urticaria; pheochromocytoma; neurologic disorders; tracheal foreign body; pseudoanaphylactic syndrome occurring after administration of procaine penicillin; and red man syndrome, often occurring after administration of vancomycin. Hereditary angioedema can cause laryngeal edema, abdominal pain, and an erythematous rash that can be confused with urticaria, although these two entities can usually be differentiated without difficulty.

Laboratory Testing

In some patients, laboratory evaluations can help establish a diagnosis of anaphylaxis or exclude other conditions. Serum mast cell tryptase (MCT) is the only widely available assay used to confirm the diagnosis of anaphylaxis. Almost all human mast cells contain preformed tryptases in their granules; small amounts are also found in human basophils.

Serum tryptase is specific to these cells, and released during anaphylaxis. The increase in serum concentrations of MCT levels seen during an anaphylactic event consists of the mature β-tryptase stored in mast cell granules, however the only widely available assay measures total tryptase. Total tryptase is affected by the baseline release of constitutively secreted tryptase (a mixture of α- and β-protryptase). MCT peaks 60 to 90 min after the onset of anaphylaxis and persists longer than plasma histamine levels do. In some cases, a very high MCT found on one sample taken during a reaction may confirm a diagnosis of anaphylaxis, but a repeat sample is required several weeks later to exclude a diagnosis of mastocytosis, which may cause very high MCT concentrations.

A single MCT sampling approach is less sensitive than a multiple sampling approach at three time points: first assessment, 1 hour later, and then 3 to 4 hours later (or the next day). MCT is relatively stable over time in an individual who is not experiencing anaphylaxis; serial sampling may detect a peak that would otherwise be missed by a single sample and also detects significant changes over time in an individual, sometimes within the normal range that applies to a single measurement. Various approaches to interpretation have been used and some caution is required because the specificity of serial MCT sampling (whether it is negative in other critical illnesses) has not been defined. Furthermore, this approach is expensive and is probably only required when there is clinical doubt about the diagnosis.[23]

It is sometimes also beneficial to obtain serum for the analysis of specific IgE against suspected antigens (specific IgE, sIgE). For example, confirming the presence of sIgE to an insect venom species implicated in an anaphylactic event may streamline the subsequent decision to commence venom immunotherapy and the choice of venom extract. However, in general sIgE testing is probably best left until follow-up after the acute event, when a careful history has identified potential allergens for appropriate testing, if needed. In some instances, skin testing is preferable and more sensitive for sIgE. However, skin responses to allergen are often suppressed following anaphylaxis, thus skin testing for sIgE should be deferred until several weeks after the acute reaction. Most importantly, sIgE testing is non-specific because many people have detectable sIgE without any history of anaphylaxis; test results should be interpreted in the proper context by an allergist before the result is used to inform subsequent treatments and allergen avoidance strategies.

TREATMENT

Life-threatening reactions often occur in response to accidental exposure or drug administration in a setting with practitioners who do not regularly treat this condition. The outcome of successful resuscitation will often be determined well before the patient reaches an emergency department or critical care environment staffed with highly experienced practitioners. A simple and easy-to-follow approach plus a one-page anaphylaxis emergency management plan (kept with resuscitation drugs) may assist. An example of this is the Australian Prescriber Anaphylaxis Wallchart, available at http://www.australianprescriber.com/magazine/34/4/artid/1210.

There is a paucity of high-level evidence to guide the emergency treatment of anaphylaxis, but there is a general consensus that the cornerstones are as follows[2]:

1. Basic life support (airway support, oxygen, ventilation support and external chest compressions if cardiac arrest occurs)
2. Supine posture to prevent a deleterious reduction in venous return to the heart
3. Early administration of epinephrine, which physiologically antagonizes most of the pathophysiologic manifestations of anaphylaxis
4. If the blood pressure is low, intravenous fluid (volume) resuscitation to improve venous return to the heart

Epinephrine

Intramuscular (IM) epinephrine in a dose of 0.01 mg/kg (max. 0.6 mg) is a sensible first-line option, even when the patient already has intravenous (IV) access. This dose can be repeated after 5 min if the response is inadequate. When given early before the onset of shock, the systemic absorption of IM epinephrine is rapid and an effect is seen within minutes, often negating the need for any further treatment. In this dose, it is also remarkably safe and relatively tolerant of dosing errors. Conversely, IV bolus dosing of epinephrine is less safe and, in inexperienced hands, incorrect dosing has been associated with serious adverse events, including acute pulmonary edema, ventricular arrhythmias, intracerebral hemorrhage, and death. Consequently, our preference is to reserve bolus IV dosing of epinephrine for cardiac arrest, in which case standard cardiac arrest dosing (1 mg IV bolus approximately every 3 min) is appropriate.

However, in severe anaphylaxis, poor muscle perfusion may result in slow absorption of epinephrine into the circulation. Furthermore, relative high serum concentrations of epinephrine may be required for an adequate therapeutic effect in severe anaphylaxis where there is marked vasodilation. When a patient is severely shocked or has not responded to an initial dose of epinephrine, an intravenous infusion of epinephrine may be required and can be titrated to achieve the desired balance between efficacy and adverse effects. In particular, as soon as an adequate blood pressure has been achieved, the infusion can be scaled back to avoid excessive blood pressure surges. There are several infusion regimens available that have been designed for a rapid response to anaphylaxis. One example for practitioners who do not have an infusion pump available, is given in the Australian Prescriber Wallchart, and uses 1 mg epinephrine in a 1 L bag of saline. In critical care environments, more concentrated infusions may be used. One approach is to use 1 mg in 100 mL, starting at 0.5 to 1 mL/kg per hour and titrated to response.[22] This provides a fairly rapid response and sufficient epinephrine to complete the treatment of most reactions, compared with more concentrated infusions, which are given at low infusion rates for longer periods of time.

Whatever protocol is followed, it is important to note that:

1. There is typically a time lag of 5 to 10 min between a change in the epinephrine infusion rate and a new 'steady state' serum concentration of epinephrine being achieved; therefore, if the infusion rate is rapidly escalated to counter life-threatening features, one must be aware of a delayed and rather sudden transition from therapeutic to toxic serum concentrations.

2. Increasing heart rate, pallor, sweating, and tachyarrhythmia in the setting of a normal or raised blood pressure are indicative of epinephrine toxicity, so the infusion rate should be reduced.

3. After 30 to 60 min, it is typical for a reaction to start resolving. It is appropriate to start turning the infusion down at this point (e.g., halving the rate) because as the reaction subsides, a previously therapeutic serum concentration can cause toxic effects.

4. Once the reaction has fully resolved clinically and remains so after halving the infusion rate, the infusion may need to be continued for another 1 to 2 hours (or longer) while the reaction continues to subside.

Intravenous Fluid (Volume) Resuscitation

If hypotension occurs, aggressive fluid (volume) resuscitation with isotonic crystalloid (normal saline or Hartman solution) is a critical component of therapy. Wide-bore intravenous access (16 gauge in adults) will facilitate this. Start with 20 mL/kg initially over 2 to 3 min, given under pressure. Repeat this dose again if necessary. As noted above, studies in humans monitoring changes in hematocrit have shown that extravasation of up to 35% of circulating blood volume can occur within the first 10 min; on rare occasions, large volumes of isotonic crystalloid in the order of 50 mL/kg over the first 30 min have been needed. One caveat is that volume resuscitation is used to treat distributive/hypovolemic shock; if the patient is not hypotensive or is overloaded (e.g., distended neck veins are present), aggressive fluid resuscitation may be harmful.

Other Measures

- *Upper airway obstruction*: in addition to parenteral epinephrine, give nebulized epinephrine (5 mg/5 mL by nebulizer with oxygen at highest flow rate). Intubation or a needle cricothyrotomy/surgical airway may, very rarely, be required.
- *Severe bronchospasm*: in addition to parenteral epinephrine, give salbutamol (albuterol) by nebulizer or inhaler puffed directly into a ventilation circuit (if intubated). Given the diagnostic overlap of severe bronchospasm in this setting with asthma and the known beneficial response of asthma to corticosteroids, corticosteroid therapy should also be considered.
- *Persisting hypotension/shock*: intravenous atropine may be required to treat profound bradycardia, but this will be of little use if fluid status is not corrected. Some patients may have profound vasodilation, so a trial of selective vasoconstrictor (e.g., metaraminol, vasopressin) may be warranted if blood pressure remains low despite the above measures. Also, because some patients have profound but reversible myocardial depression, urgent bedside echocardiographic assessment, glucagon/phosphodiesterase inhibitor inotropes (particularly if the patient is taking β-blockers) and mechanical circulatory support may be considered.
- *Persisting skin symptoms (itch)*: symptomatic treatment with an oral non-sedating antihistamine. There is no evidence for any beneficial effect of antihistamines other than relief of skin symptoms (which usually respond to epinephrine anyway). Conversely, there is evidence of potential harm from the use of parenteral antihistamines causing hypotension in patients who have not been given epinephrine.

Monitoring

Although the majority of reactions will respond promptly to a single dose of epinephrine, in severe reactions (hypotension or hypoxemia) around 40% will require multiple doses of epinephrine.[18] Therefore, close monitoring is required after the initial treatment. Patients with ongoing resuscitation requirements may require admission to intensive care. Because of the risk of a delayed deterioration/biphasic reaction, an extended period of observation should be considered. A period of 4 hours of observation after the last dose of epinephrine will detect the majority of significant delayed recurrences; however, for patients with initially severe reactions, a period of at least 10 hours of observation is recommended.[2] This may also be appropriate for children requiring more than one dose of IM epinephrine, as this has been found to be a risk factor for delayed biphasic reactions.

ONGOING MANAGEMENT AND REFERRAL

All individuals experiencing anaphylaxis that have a risk for repeat accidental exposure should be prescribed an epinephrine auto-injector device prior to discharge from hospital. Training in the use of the device is mandatory, due to a high incidence of misuse resulting in no injection being administered. There is a discussion in the literature as to how many devices should be prescribed, with some healthcare professionals recommending at least two devices, in the event of misfiring of the first device, or a suboptimal response to the first injection. However, perhaps the most important counseling involves the recommendation to contact Emergency Medical Services early, as refractory anaphylaxis will require intensive medical intervention, which cannot be delivered in the community. This recommendation is well-founded; around one third of fatalities occur despite a first dose of epinephrine being given in a timely manner.

Patients should be provided with a written management or action plan (e.g., from: http://www.allergy.org.au/health-professionals/anaphylaxis-resources/ascia-action-plan -for-anaphylaxis).

Fatal anaphylaxis is rare but also unpredictable. It is thus difficult to identify those individuals who are most at risk of severe reactions. Risk factors include:

- *Dose of exposure*: the greater the exposure, the more severe the resulting allergic reaction may be.
- *Risk-taking behaviors*: these are considered to be important in teenagers and young adults, in whom compliance with dietary avoidance and carriage of epinephrine auto-injectors can be an issue.
- *Asthma*: although asthma is so common (up to 50% of food-allergic children have asthma) the vast majority of asthmatics will never experience a severe anaphylaxis; the predictive value of asthma for severe anaphylaxis is thus poor. However, poorly controlled asthma may contribute to reaction severity and has been associated with pediatric deaths from anaphylaxis. Therefore, it is important to optimize asthma management/symptom control.
- *Delayed administration of rescue epinephrine or other medical treatments*: this highlights the need to contact emergency medical services early.
- *Presence of co-factors*: data from anaphylaxis registries and studies of immuno-therapy have found that allergen exposure occurring together with co-factors (such as exercise, alcohol intake, use of antihypertensive medication and/or non-steroidal anti-inflammatory drugs) can increase symptom severity. Where possible, exposure to these co-factors should be minimized where they have been identified as a risk factor in previous reactions. Although some medications such as β-blockers and ACE inhibitors have been anecdotally associated with severe anaphylaxis, these medications also have demonstrated mortality reduction benefits for hypertension, heart disease, and stroke. Therefore, any decision to stop them or to use a substitute requires very careful consideration of these competing risks and benefits.
- *Severity of previous reactions*: for insect venom allergy, prior reaction severity tends to predict maximum subsequent reaction severity. However as noted above, this does not appear to be reliable for other forms of allergy.

Where exercise may have contributed to a food-allergic event, affected individuals should be advised to avoid exercise for 4 hours after ingestion.

Importantly, the degree of sensitization (demonstrated through allergy skin testing or blood tests for allergen-specific IgE) does not reliably predict future severity of reactions, nor does a history of prior anaphylaxis. Evidence is emerging that individuals with specific IgE to certain lipid transfer proteins (both in food and pollen) may be more at risk of severe reactions. Testing for these should be guided by an allergy specialist.

To provide some guidance to healthcare professionals, the European Academy of Allergy and Clinical Immunology suggests six absolute indications for provision of epinephrine auto-injectors:

1. Previous anaphylaxis to food, latex, aeroallergens, e.g., animals or other unavoidable triggers
2. Exercise-induced anaphylaxis
3. Previous idiopathic anaphylaxis
4. Coexistent unstable or moderate to severe, persistent asthma with food allergy
5. Venom allergy in adults with previous systemic reactions, who are not receiving venom immunotherapy
6. Underlying mast cell disorder and any previous systemic reaction.

Where an episode occurs in someone with a known allergy, referral for specialist assessment and investigation may not be needed. Urgent referral is appropriate in the following situations:

- No clear trigger for the anaphylaxis exists
- First presentation of food allergy as anaphylaxis, so that appropriate dietary advice (including an assessment of potential cross-reactive allergens) can be provided, along with support strategies
- Features suggesting an underlying contributing pathology, such as mastocytosis.

Referral should also be expedited where immunotherapy to prevent subsequent ana-phylaxis is an option. This applies to most insect venom anaphylaxis and some drug anaphylaxis, where the agent is considered essential and an alternative drug is not available. For some food allergies, experimental immunotherapy research programs may be available locally as an option for the patient to consider.

CONCLUSIONS

Despite a significant increase in hospitalizations due to anaphylaxis over the past 20 years, the rate of fatal anaphylaxis has not increased and remains very low. However, while fatal anaphylaxis is rare at a population level, it is also unpredictable and in people at risk of severe anaphylaxis, the risk is higher and contributes to anxiety and social restrictions that impact significantly on quality of life measures. Management of acute anaphylaxis should follow a straightforward structured approach focusing on epinephrine, intravenous fluid (volume) resuscitation and standard life-support measures. Follow-up is important in reducing the risk of repeat episodes; family and general physicians play an important role in allergen identification and risk reduction through a careful history, epinephrine auto-injector and action plan provision, and patient education. Specialist referral can assist with these, particularly with allergen identification, avoidance strategies and assisting with the management of comorbidities, and by providing access to immunotherapy where appropriate. Our ability to predict those most at risk of severe reactions is limited, and this remains the greatest challenge in improving management and patient outcomes. Work is ongoing to understand the mechanisms that predispose to severe anaphylaxis, in the hope that risk stratification of patients will be a realistic management strategy in the future.

REFERENCES

1. *Johansson SG, Hourihane JO, Bousquet J, et al. A revised nomenclature for allergy. An EAACI position statement from the EAACI nomenclature task force. Allergy 2001;56(9):813–24.
2. *Simons FE, Ardusso LR, Bilò MB, et al. World allergy organization guidelines for the assessment and management of anaphylaxis. World Allergy Organ J 2011;4(2):13–37.
3. *Turner PJ, Gowland MH, Sharma V, et al. Increase in anaphylaxis-related hospitalizations but no increase in fatalities: an analysis of United Kingdom national anaphylaxis data, 1992–2012. J Allergy Clin Immunol 2015;135(4):956–63.
4. *Liew WK, Williamson E, Tang ML. Anaphylaxis fatalities and admissions in Australia. J Allergy Clin Immunol 2009;123(2):434–42.
5. Leone R, Conforti A, Venegoni M, et al. Drug induced anaphylaxis: case/non-case study based on Italian pharmacovigilance database. Drug Saf 2005;28:547–56.
6. Hetner D, Casdell SM. Latex allergy: an update. Anesth Analg 2003;96:1219–29.
7. Mertes P, Laxenaire M, Lienhart A, et al. Reducing the risk of anaphylaxis during anesthesia: guidelines for clinical practice. J Investig Allergol Clin Immunol 2005;15:91–101.
8. Mertes PM, Alla F, Trechot P, et al. Anaphylaxis during anesthesia in France: an 8-year national survey. J Allergy Clin Immunol 2011;128:366–73.
9. Cochran ST. Anaphylactoid reactions to radiocontrast media. Curr Allergy Asthma Rep 2005;5:28–31.
10. Moffitt JE, Golden D, Reisman R, et al. Stinging insect hypersensitivity: a practice parameter update. J Allergy Clin Immunol 2004;114:869–86.
11. Palmer K, Burks W. Current developments in peanut allergy. Curr Opin Allergy Clin Immunol 2006;6:202–6.
12. Sicherer SH, Sampson HA. Food allergy. J Allergy Clin Immunol 2006;117:S470–5.
13. Moneret-Vautrin DA, Kanny G, Morisset M, et al. The food anaphylaxis vigilance network in France. Allergy Clin Immunol Int 2003;15:155–9.
14. Ebo D, Bosmans J, Couttenye M, et al. Hemodialysis-associated anaphylaxis and anaphylactoid reactions. Allergy 2006;61:211–20.
15. Webb L, Lieberman P. Anaphylaxis: a review of 601 cases. Ann Allergy Asthma Immunol 2006;97:39–43.
16. Pichler WJ. Adverse side effects to biological agents. Allergy 2006;61:912–20.
17. Paoloa C, Mauriziob B, Mariangelec M, et al. Hypersensitivity reactions to biological agents with special emphasis on tumor necrosis factor alpha antagonists. Curr Opin Allergy Clin Immunol 2007;7:393–403.
18. *Brown SGA, Stone SF, Fatovich DM, et al. Anaphylaxis: clinical patterns, mediator release, and severity. J Allergy Clin Immunol 2013;132(5):1141–9.
19. *Stone SF, Bosco A, Jones A, et al. Genomic responses during acute human anaphylaxis are characterized by upregulation of innate inflammatory gene networks. PLoS ONE 2014;9(7):e101409.
20. *Vadas P, Gold M, Perelman B, et al. Platelet-activating factor, PAF acetylhydrolase, and severe anaphylaxis. N Engl J Med 2008;358(1):28–35.
21. *Fisher MM. Clinical observations on the pathophysiology and treatment of anaphylactic cardiovascular collapse. Anaesth Intensive Care 1986;14(1):17–21.

22. *Brown SGA, Blackman KE, Stenlake V, et al. Insect sting anaphylaxis; prospective evaluation of treatment with intravenous adrenaline and volume resuscitation. Emerg Med J 2004;21(2): 149–54.
23. *Brown SGA, Stone SF. Laboratory diagnosis of acute anaphylaxis. Clin Exp Allergy 2011;41(12): 1660–2.

Key references are preceded by an asterisk.

CHAPTER 14

Occupational Allergy

Catherine Lemière and Olivier Vandenplas

CHAPTER OUTLINE

INTRODUCTION AND DEFINITIONS
Occupational Asthma
Occupational Rhinitis
HISTORICAL PERSPECTIVES
EPIDEMIOLOGY
PATHOGENESIS AND ETIOLOGY
Agents Causing Occupational Asthma and Rhinitis
Pathophysiology
  Immunologic, IgE-Mediated
  Immunologic, Non-IgE-Mediated
Risk Factors
  Environmental Risk Factors
  Individual Risk Factors
CLINICAL FEATURES

PATIENT EVALUATION, DIAGNOSIS, AND DIFFERENTIAL DIAGNOSIS
Patient Evaluation and Diagnosis
  History
  Serial Peak Expiratory Flow Monitoring
  Immunologic Testing
  Non-invasive Measures of Airway Inflammation
Differential Diagnosis
OUTCOMES AND TREATMENT
PREVENTION
SOCIOECONOMIC IMPACT AND MEDICOLEGAL ASPECTS
WORK-RELATED ANAPHYLAXIS
CONCLUSIONS

SUMMARY OF IMPORTANT CONCEPTS

- Occupational allergic respiratory diseases represent a significant public health concern owing to their high prevalence and their long-term respiratory health consequences and socioeconomic costs for both the affected worker and society as a whole.
- Evaluation for occupational asthma (OA) and occupational rhinitis (OR) is indicated in all workers in whom asthma and/or rhinitis symptoms develop or worsen in relation to their work environment.
- The diagnosis of OA and OR should be established with the highest level of accuracy by performing a comprehensive investigation to avoid unwarranted socioeconomic costs.
- Complete avoidance of the causative agent remains the recommended management approach because available information indicates that reduction of exposure is a less beneficial management option.
- Continued exposure to the causative agent will result in substantial long-term respiratory morbidity because it is associated with a low rate of recovery, especially when the diagnosis is delayed.
- Primary prevention should be directed toward reducing exposure to levels below those known to induce the onset of asthma in all workers, irrespective of their individual susceptibility.

INTRODUCTION AND DEFINITIONS

Occupational Asthma

During the past decade, there has been growing recognition that work-related asthma is a major public health concern owing to its high prevalence and societal burden.

Work-related asthma is a broad term indicating that asthma is caused or worsened by the workplace. Work-related asthma encompasses both *occupational asthma* (OA), which is asthma caused by a specific agent in the workplace, and *work-exacerbated asthma* (WEA), which is asthma worsened by non-specific stimuli in the workplace but not caused by it.[1]

Occupational asthma is a disease characterized by airway inflammation, variable airflow limitation, and bronchial hyperresponsiveness due to causes and conditions attributable to a particular occupational environment and not to stimuli encountered outside the workplace.[2] *Sensitizer-induced OA* is characterized by the development—after a latency period—of immunologically mediated specific bronchial hyperresponsiveness to an agent present in the workplace. By contrast, irritant-induced asthma (IIA), also called 'OA without a latency period,' encompasses a wide spectrum of clinical presentations.[3] The most typical form is represented by *reactive airways dysfunction syndrome* (RADS), which refers to a type of OA without latency and immunologic sensitization, occurring after a single massive irritant exposure with subsequent severe airway injury, resulting in persistent airway inflammation and non-specific bronchial hyperresponsiveness (NSBHR). In many cases, the onset of asthma is gradual and follows repeated low-dose exposure to one or more bronchial irritants. In keeping with the focus of this book on allergic diseases, the scope of this chapter is restricted to sensitizer-induced OA.

Occupational Rhinitis

Occupational rhinitis (OR) has been defined as an inflammatory disease of the nose, which is characterized by intermittent or persistent symptoms (i.e. nasal congestion, sneezing, rhinorrhea, itching) and/or variable nasal airflow limitation and/or hypersecretion due to causes and conditions attributable to a particular work environment and not to stimuli encountered outside the workplace.[4]

As with work-related asthma (Fig. 14-1), the broad spectrum of rhinitis syndromes related to the work environment can be broken down into the following categories: (1) allergic OR; (2) non-allergic OR; and (3) work-exacerbated rhinitis.

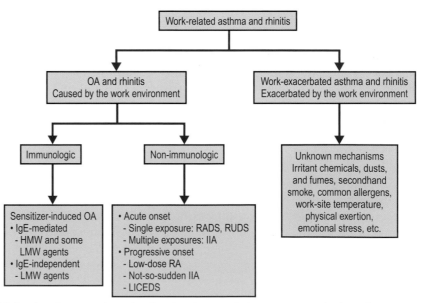

Figure 14-1 Classification of work-related asthma and rhinitis. HMW, high-molecular-weight; IIA, irritant-induced asthma; LICEDS, low-intensity chronic exposure dysfunction syndrome; LMW, low-molecular-weight; RADS, reactive airways dysfunction syndrome; RUDS, reactive upper airways dysfunction syndrome.

HISTORICAL PERSPECTIVES

In the early 18th century, for the first time, an entire chapter of a medical treatise—Bernardino Ramazzini's *De morbis artificum diatriba*—was devoted to the disease of *"sifters and measurers of grain."* It was not until the 19th and early 20th centuries, however, when progressive industrialization demanded that work be carried out indoors, often in insufficiently ventilated environments, that many asthmagenic agents handled in the workplace were described. From the very beginning, both proteinaceous substances and chemicals were incriminated. Diisocyanate-induced asthma was first described in 1951 by Fuchs and Valade. The interest in asthma in the workplace arose from the research, enthusiasm, and insight of the father of British clinical allergy, the late Jack Pepys, who, between 1960 and 1980, described numerous causes of OA and suggested experimental replication of the asthmatic reaction in a hospital laboratory as a means of confirming the diagnosis. This important work served to refocus attention on the *late asthmatic reaction* (frequent in OA), which is the cornerstone of the physiopathology of asthma.

EPIDEMIOLOGY

A pooled analysis of all epidemiologic studies published up to 2007 indicated that 17.6% of all cases of adult-onset asthma are attributable to workplace exposures.

Information on the incidence and prevalence of OR in the general population is largely lacking, although surveys of workforces exposed to sensitizing agents indicate that OR is 2 to 4 times more common than OA.

PATHOGENESIS AND ETIOLOGY

Agents Causing Occupational Asthma and Rhinitis

The workplace agents known to cause immunologically mediated OA and OR usually are categorized into high-molecular-weight (HMW; molecular mass >10 kDa) and low-molecular-weight (LMW; molecular mass <10 kDa) agents. HMW agents are (glyco) proteins of vegetable and animal origin, whereas LMW agents include reactive chemicals, transition metals, and wood dusts. The agents and occupations most commonly implicated are listed in Table 14-1. The main differences between HMW and LMW agents are summarized in Table 14-2. A very large number of substances (>400) used in the workplace have been documented as causing immunologic OA and OR (listed at www.asthme.csst.qc.ca). However, only a few agents—specifically, flour, isocyanates, latex, persulfate salts, aldehydes, animals, wood dusts, metals, and enzymes—account for the vast majority of reported cases in industrialized countries. Nevertheless, the distribution of causative agents may vary across geographic areas, depending on the pattern of industrial activities.

Workers in occupations with the highest incidence rates of OA are bakers and pastry makers, other food processors, spray painters, hairdressers, wood workers, healthcare workers, cleaners, farmers, laboratory technicians, and welders. In more recent years, population-based studies conducted in various countries worldwide have consistently found that cleaning activities were associated with an excess risk of asthma and work-related asthma symptoms. Industrial and domestic cleaners are exposed to a wide variety of products containing irritant chemicals (e.g., detergents, acids, alkali, solvents, chelating compounds) as well as some potentially sensitizing substances, including biocides (e.g., quaternary ammonium compounds, aldehydes, chloramine-T), ethanolamines, enzymes, and latex gloves.

Pathophysiology

The pathophysiology of sensitizer-induced OA and OR involves in most cases an immunoglobulin E (IgE)-dependent mechanism, especially for HMW agents, whereas in most

TABLE 14-1   Principal Agents Causing Immunologic Occupational Asthma

Agent		Workers/occupations at risk
High-molecular-weight agents		
Cereals (flour)	Wheat, rye, barley, buckwheat	Millers, bakers, pastry makers
Latex	Gloves	Healthcare workers, laboratory technicians
Animals	Mice, rats, cows, seafood	Laboratory workers, farmers, seafood processors
Enzymes	α-Amylase, maxatase, alcalase, papain, bromelain, pancreatin	Baking products manufacture, bakers, detergent production, pharmaceutical industry, food industry
Low-molecular-weight agents		
Isocyanates	Toluene diisocyanate (TDI), methylene diphenyl-diisocyanate (MDI), hexamethylene diisocyanate (HDI)	Polyurethane production, plastic industry, molding, spray painters, insulation installers
Metals	Chromium, nickel, cobalt, platinum	Metal refinery, metal alloy production, electroplaters, welders
Biocides	Aldehydes, quaternary ammonium compounds	Healthcare workers, cleaners
Persulfate salts	Hair bleach	Hairdressers
Acid anhydrides	Phthalic, trimellitic, maleic, tetrachlorophthalic acids	Epoxy resin workers
Reactive dyes	Reactive black 5, pyrazolone derivatives, vinyl sulfones, carmine	Textile workers, food industry workers
Acrylates	Cyanoacrylates, methacrylates, di- and triacrylates	Manufacture of adhesives, dental and orthopedic materials, sculptured fingernails, printing inks, paints and coatings
Wood dusts	Red cedar, iroko, obeche, oak	Sawmill workers, carpenters, cabinet and furniture makers

TABLE 14-2   Main Differences between High- and Low-Molecular-Weight Agents Causing Occupational Asthma

Feature	High-molecular-weight agents	Low-molecular-weight agents
Nature	(Glyco)proteins derived from plants and animals	Highly reactive chemicals, metals, and wood dusts
Immunologic mechanisms	IgE-mediated	Uncertain; specific IgE for some agents (e.g., platinum salts, reactive dyes, acid anhydrides)
Type of airway inflammation	Eosinophils	Eosinophils and sometimes neutrophils
Type of asthmatic reactions	Immediate and dual	Often isolated late and atypical
Associated disorders Rhinoconjunctivitis	Common (~90%)	Less common (~50%)
Contact dermatitis	Rare, but protein contact dermatitis may occur (e.g., flour, seafood)	May occur (e.g., epoxy resins, acrylates, metals)
Urticaria and, anaphylaxis	Frequent with some agents (e.g., latex)	Rare

IgE, immunoglobulin E.

cases of OA induced by LMW agents, the production of specific IgE antibodies or the upregulation of IgE receptors has not been identified.

Immunologic, IgE-Mediated

The pathophysiology of OA induced by IgE-dependent agents is similar to that of allergic asthma unrelated to work. High-molecular-weight agents (proteinaceous products such as animal proteins and flour) act as complete antigens and induce the production of specific IgE antibodies. Certain LMW occupational agents, including platinum salts, acid anhydrides, reactive dyes, and some wood species, also induce specific IgE antibodies, probably by acting as haptens and binding with proteins to form functional antigens.

Immunologic, Non-IgE-Mediated

Many LMW chemicals, including isocyanates and plicatic acid (the agent causing Western red cedar asthma), cause OA but do not consistently induce specific IgE antibodies. The absence of specific IgE antibodies to LMW compounds on appropriate testing may be due to a technical inability to identify those antibodies or to the existence of another immunologic mechanism such as cell-mediated reactions.

Risk Factors

Environmental Risk Factors

Occupational asthma and OR result from the complex interaction between environmental and individual factors (Fig. 14-2). The evidence supporting the role of potential risk factors is summarized in Table 14-3.

Level of Exposure. The intensity of exposure to sensitizing agents is currently the best characterized and the most important environmental risk factor for the development of OA (Table 14-3). The timing of exposure may also play a role because the prevalence of onset of work-related asthma symptoms is consistently higher within the early period of exposure to the occupational agents, and exposure–response gradients are more clearly documented in those workers who develop these outcomes soon after the onset of exposure.

Smoking and Exposure to Other Pollutants. A number of studies suggested that exposure to cigarette smoke can increase the risk of IgE-mediated sensitization to some HMW and LMW agents (Table 14-3), but the evidence supporting an association between smoking and the development of clinical OA is still very weak.

Growing evidence indicates that environmental pollutants, such as ozone, nitrogen dioxide, tobacco smoke, diesel exhaust particles, and endotoxin, can act as adjuvants

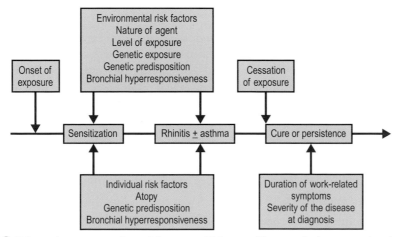

Figure 14-2 Schematic representation of the natural history of immunologic occupational asthma and rhinitis.

TABLE 14-3   Summary of Potential Risk Factors for Development of Occupational Asthma

Risk factor	Evidence	Agents/settings
High level of exposure	Strong	*HMW agents*: Wheat flour, α-amylase, laboratory animals, detergent enzymes, snow crab allergens *LMW agents*: Platinum salts, acid anhydrides
	Moderate	Diisocyanates
Skin exposure	Weak	Diisocyanates
Cigarette smoking	Moderate	*IgE sensitization*: laboratory animals, seafood, psyllium, green coffee, enzymes, acid anhydrides, platinum, reactive dyes
	Weak	*Clinical OA*: laboratory animals, enzymes
Atopy	Strong	*HMW agents*: flour, laboratory animals, latex; snow crab, detergent enzymes, α-amylase
	Weak	*LMW agents*: platinum, acid anhydrides
HLA class II alleles	Moderate	*LMW agents*: diisocyanate, red cedar, acid anhydrides, platinum salts *HMW agents*: laboratory animals, latex
IL-4RA (I50V) II variant	Weak	Diisocyanates
Antioxidant enzymes	Moderate	Diisocyanates
Pre-existing rhinitis	Weak	IgE sensitization to HMW agents
Work-related rhinitis	Strong	Development of asthma in workers with OR; development of OA in workers with OR related to laboratory animals
Pre-existing non-specific bronchial responsiveness	Weak	Apprentice workers exposed to HMW agents

HMW, high-molecular-weight; IgE, immunoglobulin E; IL4RA, interleukin-4 receptor α chain; LMW, low-molecular-weight; OR, occupational rhinitis; TLR4, Toll-like receptor 4; OA: Occupational asthma.

in allergic responses to common inhalant allergens. Only limited information, however, is available on the potential interactions between pollutants and sensitizing agents in the workplace.

Individual Risk Factors

Atopy. Atopy has consistently been demonstrated as an important host risk factor for the development of IgE-mediated sensitization, OA, and OR, due to HMW agents (Table 14-3), whereas this association remains controversial for some LMW agents and absent for most other LMW agents. Pre-exposure sensitization to common allergens that are structurally related to workplace allergens, such as pets in the case of laboratory animal workers, could be a stronger predictor of OA than atopy.

Genetic Susceptibility. A number of studies documented that certain major histocompatibility complex (MHC) class II molecules involved in the presentation of processed antigens to T lymphocytes are associated with either susceptibility to or protection against OA due to various and LMW and HMW occupational agents (Table 14-3). Some evidence suggests that genes associated with Th2 cell differentiation may play a role in the development of OA caused by isocyanates. Furthermore, some genetic variants in the MHC class I and class II genes may be associated with isocyanate-induced asthma (Table 14-3). Overall, the information currently available indicates that genetic testing is limited for both diagnostic and preventive purposes. In addition, there is convincing evidence that environmental factors can interact with genetic determinants to affect disease susceptibility.

Rhinitis. Epidemiologic evidence confirms that OR is associated with an increased risk for the subsequent development of asthma and OA. However, the proportion of subjects with OR who will develop OA remains uncertain. Among apprentices in animal health technology, the predictive value of work-related nasal symptoms on the subsequent development of probable OA was only 11.4% over a follow-up period of 30 to 42 months (Table 14-3). Prospective cohort studies of apprentices also have shown that rhinitis present before work exposure is an independent risk factor for IgE sensitization to HMW allergens.

Non-specific Bronchial Hyperresponsiveness. Prospective cohort studies have shown that the presence of non-specific bronchial hyperresponsiveness (NSBHR) and a physician's diagnosis of asthma before initiation of exposure to HMW occupational agents are associated with an increased risk of subsequent IgE sensitization and OA.

CLINICAL FEATURES

As in non-work-related asthma, the clinical features of OA include signs and symptoms of variable cough, wheezing, dyspnea associated with reversible airflow limitation, NSBHR, and airway inflammation. Some clinical features are more specifically related to OA. Typically, the affected worker initially complains of cough, wheeze, and dyspnea, either as soon as the work shift exposure starts or at the end of the work shift or even in the evening, after working hours, with remission during weekends and holidays. As the disease progresses, symptoms tend to occur earlier during the day and fail to remit during days off and long holidays. With further exposure, asthma symptoms may persist and become permanent, despite complete withdrawal from exposure. In these instances, even prolonged removal from exposure will result in only partial reversal of the asthma. It is therefore very important to establish the diagnosis of OA early and to remove the patient from exposure. Rhinitis is associated with respiratory symptoms in a majority of cases of OA and often precedes the occurrence of respiratory symptoms, especially with exposure to HMW agents. Identification of direct or even indirect exposure to a known respiratory sensitizer in the workplace is an important aspect of the history, but such exposure often is not readily apparent to the worker or the clinician.

PATIENT EVALUATION, DIAGNOSIS, AND DIFFERENTIAL DIAGNOSIS

Patient Evaluation and Diagnosis

History

Occupational asthma should be suspected in every adult patient with new-onset asthma. A substantial proportion of subjects evaluated for work-related respiratory symptoms fail to demonstrate any objective evidence of asthma. Therefore, the first diagnostic step is to confirm the presence of asthma and to exclude conditions with asthma-like manifestations such as vocal cord dysfunction, hyperventilation, and sick building syndrome.

A good occupational history, not only of the current job and exposure but also of past jobs and exposures, is essential. A scheme for addressing relevant points has been published and includes employment history (current and past jobs), symptoms (nature, temporal relationship to work, improvement while away from work), and potential risk factors. In many cases, the patient may not be aware of the exact chemical exposures at work; material safety data sheets (MSDSs) can be requested from the workplace and may be of help in clarifying the presence of a workplace sensitizer. If the content of the causative agent is <1%, it may not be listed in the MSDS. In such instances, the manufacturer must be contacted. It often is helpful to ask the worker to sketch the work site and the work process itself, and to indicate the locations where he or she works during the work shift. In addition to identifying potential high-risk agents, the exposure history should include the duration of exposure and the frequency and concentrations of exposure. The substances to which the worker is potentially exposed at work can be checked against a comprehensive list of agents recognized as causing OA, and the specific job for that worker checked against the list of at-risk occupations. These lists are available from various sources (websites and published tables). If available, the occupational health record and the industrial hygiene record from the company should be reviewed.

Figure 14-3 shows the algorithm to be used in evaluating a patient suspected of having OA. A methacholine or histamine challenge test to assess the degree of NSBHR should be carried out. A negative reaction to a histamine or methacholine challenge does not exclude OA if such testing is performed when the patient is off work and free of symptoms. However, if the challenge test is performed when the patient is working and

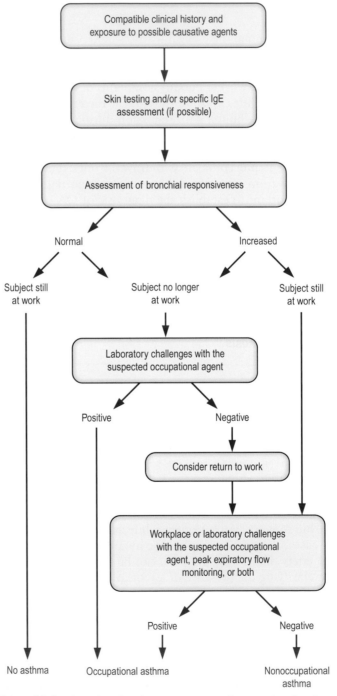

Figure 14-3 Algorithm for the investigation of occupational asthma.

symptomatic, the diagnosis of OA can reasonably be excluded. The relationship between work and asthma, if any, should then be evaluated using serial measurements of peak expiratory flow (PEF) and/or assessments of NSBHR at work and off work and/or specific inhalation challenge (SIC) tests in the laboratory or at the workplace.[5]

Serial Peak Expiratory Flow Monitoring

Serial measurement of PEF with the subject at work and away from work has been found to be useful in obtaining objective information for the confirmation of OA.

As with asthma in general, compliance with PEF monitoring has been shown to be poor, especially when patients were asked to record values four times per day. The optimal duration of recording of PEF has not been established, but monitoring should include a minimum period of 2 weeks at work and exposed to the suspected causative agent and a similar period away from work, unless significant changes are recorded earlier at work. If the patient is using inhaled corticosteroids, it is important to keep the same dose throughout the period of monitoring. Inhaled bronchodilators should be used only when necessary and the patient's self-dosing history should be recorded. PEF should be performed before use of bronchodilators.

No uniformly accepted criteria for the interpretation of PEF recordings have been established. Attempts have been made to develop such criteria, but the sensitivity and specificity of the diagnosis based on these objective criteria were no better than for the 'eyeballing' method of experienced physicians. A computer-assisted diagnostic aid, OASYS (observation and appraisal system), has been developed to distinguish occupational from nonoccupational causes of airflow obstruction. One version, OASYS-2, is based on discriminate analysis and has achieved a sensitivity of 75% and a specificity of at least 94%. In comparison with SIC tests, reported sensitivity of OASYS ranges between 35% and 73%, whereas specificity is between 65% and 100%. Accordingly, PEF monitoring examined with OASYS-2 analysis is better used to confirm than to exclude OA.

Serial Measurement of Non-specific Bronchial Hyperresponsiveness.

The lack of NSBHR after a period at work, at which time the worker experiences the usual symptoms, almost excludes OA and asthma. Although theoretically a decrease in NSBHR should occur after a period away from work, this has not been found to be a reliable means of confirming OA, probably because assessments are repeated after too short an interval of being away from work (usually 2 weeks).

Specific Inhalation Challenge Tests.

Specific inhalation challenge tests consist of exposing the subjects to the agent suspected to cause their asthma. These tests are considered to be the reference tests in investigation of OA.[6] Laboratory-specific challenge tests are time-consuming and require specialized facilities that are available in only a few clinical centers. Specific challenge tests are useful in the following circumstances: (1) when the diagnosis of OA remains in doubt after serial monitoring of PEF or airway responsiveness; (2) when a patient clearly has OA but it is necessary for management personnel to confirm or identify the causative agent at work; (3) when a new agent is suspected of causing OA; and (4) when the patient cannot be returned to the incriminated workplace.

Although SIC testing is still considered the gold standard for the diagnosis of OA, the potential for false-positive and false-negative responses is well recognized. A false-negative response may occur if the wrong agent is used (e.g., different types of diisocyanates), or if the exposure conditions are not comparable with those in the workplace. Specific inhalation challenge testing at the workplace consists of serial spirometric measurements performed by a respiratory technologist, whilst the worker is doing his or her usual tasks. It can be useful to perform an SIC at the workplace when the SIC result in the laboratory is negative. Specific inhalation challenge tests at the workplace have been shown to be positive in 22% of the subjects with a highly suggestive history and negative SIC reaction in the laboratory. However, they do not allow for the identification of the causative agent.

Immunologic Testing

Immunologic tests in the diagnosis of OA are limited by the lack of standardized commercially available reagents for skin and in-vitro tests. In a systematic review assessing the sensitivity and specificity of skin-prick testing in patients exposed to HMW agents in comparison with SIC, the pooled sensitivity was 80.6% (95% CI, 69.8–88.1), whereas the pooled specificity was 59.6% (95% CI, 41.7–75.3). In patients exposed to LMW agents, the pooled sensitivity was 72.9% (95% CI, 59.7–83.0), whereas the pooled specificity was 86.2% (95% CI, 77.4–91.9). The same review assessed the sensitivity and specificity of serum-specific IgE in comparison with SIC. Sensitivity was higher for the HMW agents studied (73.3%; 95% CI, 63.9–81.0), whereas the specificity was 79.0% (95% CI, 50.5–93.3). In subjects exposed to LMW agents, the pooled sensitivity was 31.2% (95% CI, 22.9–40.8) and the pooled specificity was 88.9% (95% CI, 84.7–92.1). Most in-vitro tests to assess specific sensitization to occupational chemicals remain research tools at present.

Non-invasive Measures of Airway Inflammation

Sputum Cell Counts. Similar to the airway inflammation found after common allergen inhalation challenges, an increase in sputum eosinophils has been observed after SICs to a number of HMW and LMW agents.[7] In subjects with OA, the increase in sputum eosinophils precedes the occurrence of functional changes occurring after exposure to the occupational agent responsible for OA. An increase in sputum eosinophil count greater than 3% after the first day of exposure during SIC seems to be an accurate parameter for predicting the development of an asthmatic response on subsequent exposures, with a sensitivity of 67% and a specificity of 97%. Therefore, a notable increase in the sputum eosinophil count in the absence of a fall in FEV_1 should incite pursuing the investigation.

The lack of increase in sputum eosinophil counts after exposure to occupational agents should not rule out the diagnosis of OA. Interfering factors that can modify the sputum cell response such as corticosteroid treatment should be considered in the interpretation.

Exhaled Nitric Oxide. Studies that assessed the usefulness of exhaled nitric oxide (eNO), measured as the fraction of exhaled gas (FeNO), in the investigation of OA have provided inconsistent results. FeNO levels seem to increase more consistently in subjects with OA due to HMW agents than in subjects with OA due to LMW after exposure to those agents.

Although the measurement of FeNO has some advantages over the analysis of induced sputum in OA, the interpretation of increased FeNO is more difficult than sputum differential cell counts, owing to its lack of specificity as well as the potential confounding factors that may influence the results. Further studies are needed to clarify the role and the interpretation of changes in FeNO in the investigation of occupational asthma.

Combination of Different Tests. A systematic review of studies on the diagnosis of OA assessed the sensitivity and specificity of the combination of various diagnostic tools: measure of NSBHR, skin-prick test (SPT) and serum IgE.[8] For OA due to HMW agents, the NSBHR, SPT, and serum-specific IgE had sensitivities >73% when compared with SIC, the reference test. High specificity was demonstrated for a positive result on NSBHR tests and SPTs alone (82.5%; 95% CI, 54.0–95.0) or in combination with specific IgE (74.3%; 95% CI, 45.0–91.0) versus SIC.

The highest sensitivity for the diagnosis of OA due to LMW agents occurred between combined NSBHR tests and SPTs versus SIC (100%; 95% CI, 74.1–100). When compared with SIC, specific IgE and SPT had similar specificities (88.9%; 95% CI, 84.7–92.1; and 86.2%; 95% CI, 77.4–91.9, respectively). Making an accurate diagnosis of OA is crucial because of the significant social and financial consequences associated with this diagnosis. The validity of the different diagnostic tests and their practical limitations and advantages are summarized in Tables 14-4 and 14-5.

TABLE 14-4   Validity of Objective Diagnostic Tests

Test	Sensitivity (%)	Specificity (%)
Single assessment of non-specific bronchial responsiveness*	84 (69–93)	48 (26–72)
Immunologic tests:		
HMW agents (SPT)*	81 (70–88)	60 (42–75)
LMW agents (specific IgE antibodies)*	31 (23–41)	89 (85–92)
Serial measurements of PEF*	64 (43–80)	77 (66–85)
Serial measurements of PEF and non-specific bronchial responsiveness[†]	84–92	61–67
Single assessment of sputum eosinophils[‡]		
≥1%	50	67
≥3%	22	91
Serial assessments of sputum eosinophils at and away from work[§]:		
Increase >1%	65 (45–81)	76 (57–88)
Increase >2%	52 (33–71)	80 (61–91)
Increase >6.4%	26 (13–46)	92 (75–98)
Serial assessment[§]	50 (24–76)	75 (51–90)

Sensitivity and specificity of diagnostic tests are expressed as a percentage, with 95% confidence interval in parentheses when available.
Sensitivity and specificity of combined diagnostic tests.
PEF, peak expiratory flow; HMW, high-molecular-weight; LMW, low-molecular-weight; SPT, skin-prick test.
*(Modified from Beach J, Russell K, Blitz S, et al. A systematic review of the diagnosis of occupational asthma. Chest 2007; 131:569–578.)
[†](Modified from Perrin B, Lagier F, L'Archevêque J, et al. Occupational asthma: validity of monitoring of peak expiratory flow rates and non-allergic bronchial responsiveness as compared to specific inhalation challenge. Eur Respir J 1992; 5:40–48; and Côté J, Kennedy S, Chan-Yeung M. Sensitivity and specificity of PC20 and peak expiratory flow rate in cedar asthma. J Allergy Clin Immunol 1990; 85:592–598.)
[‡](Modified from Malo JL, Cardinal S, Ghezzo H, et al. Association of bronchial reactivity to occupational agents with methacholine reactivity, sputum cells and immunoglobulin E-mediated reactivity. Clin Exp Allergy 2011; 41:497–504.)
[§]Difference between the percentage of eosinophils at work and away from work. (Modified from Girard F, Chaboillez S, Cartier A, et al. An effective strategy for diagnosing occupational asthma: use of induced sputum. Am J Respir Crit Care Med 2004; 170:845–850.)

Differential Diagnosis

The most challenging aspect of the differential diagnosis for OA is certainly the diagnosis of WEA.[1] In both conditions, the affected worker complains of a worsening of asthma symptoms when at work. Along with those symptoms, impairment of respiratory function, as evidenced by increased airflow limitation, increased NSBHR, and increased variability of serial PEF measurements, can be identified during periods at work, in comparison with periods away from work. Although workers with OA exhibited greater PEF variability during a period at work than workers with WEA, these differences in variability do not allow differentiation between the two conditions in clinical practice. The gold standard test to differentiate OA from WEA remains the SIC. Whereas the exposure to a specific occupational asthmagen induces a 15–20% fall in FEV_1 in workers with OA, no sustained fall in FEV_1 is observed in subjects with WEA. The occurrence of an eosinophilic inflammatory process on exposure to an occupational agent also favors the diagnosis of OA.

Eosinophilic bronchitis is a variant of asthma that represents 12% of the causes of chronic cough. It consists of cough or asthma-like symptoms related to an underlying eosinophilic inflammation without airflow obstruction or NSBHR. This condition is responsive to inhaled corticosteroids. Eosinophilic bronchitis can be caused by sensitization to occupational agents and has been labeled occupational eosinophilic bronchitis. The diagnostic criteria consist of the following: isolated chronic cough (lasting >3 weeks) that worsens at work; sputum eosinophilia with counts of ≥2.5% in either spontaneous

TABLE 14-5 Advantages and Limitations of Diagnostic Tests Used in the Investigation of Occupational Asthma (OA)

Diagnostic test(s)	Advantages/limitations
Assessment of bronchial responsiveness	Simple, low cost Allow to confirm the diagnosis of asthma Low specificity for diagnosis of OA. The lack of NSBHR does not allow discarding the diagnosis of OA in subjects who have been removed from the workplace.
Immunologic tests	Easy to perform, low cost Commercial extracts are available (SPT or specific IgE for HMW agents). Lack of standardization for a majority of occupational allergens except latex Measure of specific IgE available for some LMW agents (anhydrides, acids, isocyanates, aldehydes), but low sensitivity Identify the sensitization but not the disease itself
PEF monitoring	Low cost Requires the worker's collaboration Low adherence (<60%) Possible falsification of the results Requires 2 weeks at and away from work, which are not always possible for the workers Impossible to perform when the worker has already been removed from exposure No standardized method for interpreting the results Interpretation of the results requires experience.
Specific inhalation challenges in the laboratory	Confirmation of the diagnosis of OA when the test is positive False-negative tests are possible. Costly Available in a small number of centers worldwide
Specific inhalation challenges at the workplace	Exclude diagnosis if response is negative when performed in the usual work conditions Requires usual work condition Costly

Non-invasive measures of airway inflammation	Sputum cell counts
	    Impossible to falsify
	    Bring additional evidence to the diagnosis of OA
	    Costly
	    Not widely available
	    Does not allow to confirm or discard the diagnosis of OA by itself
	Exhaled NO measurement
	    Easy to perform
	    Inconsistent results
	    Difficult to interpret
	    Affected by many different factors

HMW, high-molecular-weight; IgE, immunoglobulin E; LMW, low-molecular-weight; NSBHR, non-specific bronchial hyperresponsiveness; NO, nitric oxide; PEF, peak expiratory flow.

or induced samples; increases in sputum eosinophilia related to exposure to the offending agent; spirometric parameters within normal limits and not significantly affected by exposure to the offending agent; absence of NSBHR to methacholine (provocative concentration of methacholine inducing a 20% fall in FEV1 [PC$_{20}$] >16 kDa mg/mL) both at work and away from work; other causes of chronic cough are ruled out.[9] Occupational eosinophilic bronchitis has been causally related to a number of occupational agents, including latex, wheat flour, α-amylase, egg lysozyme, isocyanates, acrylates, formaldehyde, chloramine-T, epoxy resin hardener, stainless steel welding fumes, and mushroom spores.

Exposure to specific occupational agents such as textile, grain dust, or aluminum can induce conditions that are considered as variants of occupational asthma (byssinosis, potroom asthma). Exposure to those agents can lead to partially reversible airflow obstruction with chronic airflow limitation.

OUTCOMES AND TREATMENT

Systematic reviews of existing data on the outcome of immunologic OA indicate that complete and definitive avoidance of exposure to the causative agent remains the optimal treatment for immunologic OA.[10] Workers with immunologic OA who continue to be exposed to the causative agent are at high risk for deterioration of asthma symptoms, airway obstruction, and NSBHR. Reduction of exposure to the agent causing OA has been acknowledged as an alternative option to complete avoidance when elimination of exposure or accommodation of affected workers to unexposed jobs is not possible. The limited available evidence, however, indicates that this option is less beneficial than cessation of exposure, because it is associated with a lower likelihood of asthma improvement and a higher risk of worsening. This management approach should therefore be restricted to selected patients, and careful medical monitoring is required to ensure early identification of asthma worsening.

A few case reports provided some suggestion that treatment with the anti-IgE omalizumab could improve asthma control in subjects with flour-induced OA who remain exposed to the causal work environment. Further prospective investigations, however, are required in subjects who choose to continue exposure.

Clinicians should be aware that OA is not always reversible after cessation of exposure to the sensitizing agent. Asthma symptoms and NSBHR persist in approximately 70% of the patients with OA several years after their removal from the offending environment. Besides environmental interventions, the pharmacologic treatment of OA should follow the clinical practice guidelines for asthma. Systematic treatment with high-dose inhaled corticosteroids in addition to exposure cessation provides only a slight additional benefit.

Follow-up studies consistently show that a better outcome of asthma after cessation of causal exposure is associated with a shorter symptomatic period before removal and with less severe disease at the time of diagnosis. These findings emphasize the need for early diagnosis and intervention.

The management of OR not only should aim at reducing nasal symptoms and their impact on quality of life but may also offer the opportunity to prevent the subsequent development of OA in keeping with the fact that OR is regarded as an early marker of OA. Complete cessation of exposure should be recommended to workers with OR. Only a few quantitative estimates of the risk of OA in workers with OR have been derived, however; accordingly, a reduction of exposure should be considered a reasonable option when complete avoidance would have important adverse socioeconomic consequences.

PREVENTION

Primary prevention aims at blocking, or at least limiting, the development of immunologic sensitization and OA by excluding susceptible workers from at-risk jobs and minimizing exposure to potentially sensitizing substances. Primary preventive strategies for OA and OR should focus on the control of workplace exposures because strong evidence supports a dose–response relationship between the level of exposure to sensitizing agents and the occurrence of OA (Table 14-3). Identifying susceptible persons at the time of pre-employment examination to exclude them from employment or from high-risk jobs is inefficient and unduly discriminating. The currently identified markers of individual susceptibility (Table 14-3) offer only a low positive predictive value for the development of OA, especially when these markers, such as atopy, are highly prevalent in the general population.

Secondary prevention of immunologic OA and OR involves detection of the disease process at an early (preferably preclinical) stage, to prevent the development of overt OA and to modify the disease process through appropriate interventions to eliminate exposure. The rationale underlying secondary prevention is the consistent finding that the outcome of OA is better with an early diagnosis and milder disease at the time of removal from exposure. Increasing awareness of the disease among workers and health-care professionals is a key step to enhance the recognition of OA because the condition still remains underdiagnosed and inappropriately investigated. Recent evidence suggests that appropriately designed surveillance programs are effective in identifying OA in subjects with less severe asthma and a more favorable outcome.

A few observational studies and historical data indicate that prevention is effective in reducing the incidence of OA and OR caused by natural rubber latex in healthcare workers, enzymes in the detergent industry, flour, laboratory animals, and isocyanates. However, available data do not distinguish among the relative effects of the diverse components of prevention strategies, because such strategies usually are implemented as multicomponent programs targeting education, control of exposure, and medical surveillance.

SOCIOECONOMIC IMPACT AND MEDICOLEGAL ASPECTS

In the US, it has been estimated that the total cost of OA was US$1.6 billion in 1996, including 76% in direct costs (healthcare expenditures) when assuming that 15% of adult asthma is attributable to workplace exposures. However, OA is likely to generate higher indirect costs than non-OA, because the former condition most often requires job changes to either avoid or reduce exposure to the causative agent or agents. Follow-up studies of workers with OA have consistently documented that the condition is associated with a high rate of prolonged unemployment, ranging from 18% to 69%, with a reduction in work-derived income in 44–74% of affected workers. Complete avoidance of exposure to the sensitizing agent, employment in smaller-sized companies, a lower level of education, older age, and lack of effective job retraining programs are associated with a worse socioeconomic outcome. Data derived from Quebec's Public Health Insurance Plan have shown that OA is associated with higher rates of physician visits, admission to an emergency department, and hospitalizations compared with asthma unrelated to work. Although medical resource utilization decreases after removal from exposure to the incriminated workplace, an excess rate of visits to physicians and emergency departments has been documented for such workers compared with other asthmatics. The socioeconomic impact of OR has rarely been investigated but is likely to be substantial.

Because bronchial hyperresponsiveness to occupational agents almost never completely disappears, workers with OA should be considered to be permanently and completely disabled for jobs involving exposure to the sensitizing agent that caused their OA. They should be thoroughly informed about the possibilities for compensation, and established cases should be reported to the appropriate public health authorities, in accordance with national regulations. Evaluation of physiologic impairment should take into account the characteristic features of asthma and should be based on the level of airway obstruction, the degree of NSBHR, the medication regimen required for controlling asthma, and the effects of asthma on quality of life.

WORK-RELATED ANAPHYLAXIS

The majority of work-related allergic symptoms are respiratory and cutaneous. Allergic symptoms are often reported in some occupations such as beauticians who are exposed to methacrylates by sculpting artificial nails, or healthcare workers exposed to chlorhexidine. Occupational agents can also induce anaphylactic reactions. Cases of anaphylaxis have been reported with several HMW and LMW agents encountered at the workplace. Beekeepers, gardeners, farmers, truck drivers, and masons are the occupations the most at risk of experiencing occupational venom allergy. Up to 32% of beekeepers and their family members had a history of insect sting anaphylaxis, which is much higher than in the general population (0.34–7.5%). Latex has been responsible for cases of anaphylaxis in healthcare workers. Laboratory animal workers are also at risk to develop anaphylactic reactions.

Several cases of occupational anaphylaxis to different chemicals have also been reported; for example, nurses have developed an anaphylactic reaction after exposure to antibiotics. Exposure to cobalt has been associated with an anaphylactic reaction in a ceramic decorator. Therefore, clinicians need to be aware that severe allergic life-threatening reactions may occur in workers sensitized to proteinaceous or chemical occupational agents.

CONCLUSIONS

During the past decade, it has become apparent that OA and OR are highly prevalent and underdiagnosed diseases that impose a large medical and socioeconomic burden on affected workers and society in general. Because a late diagnosis of OA is associated with a poor outcome, and because prevention programs have been shown to decrease the incidence of new cases of OA, efforts should be made to increase the awareness of OA and OR in primary care practice. Evaluating the cost-effectiveness of preventive measures and compensation systems should become a priority for assisting policy-makers in elaborating rational strategies.

Current understanding of the pathophysiology of OA is limited, especially regarding OA induced by LMW agents. More research is needed to identify biologic markers, allowing an easier and more accurate way of diagnosing OA and OR, as well as developing effective surveillance programs for use in high-risk workforces.

Although additional tools such as non-invasive measures of airway inflammation have been made available for the investigation of OA in the past decade, its diagnosis remains difficult and requires a comprehensive investigation in order to avoid any misdiagnosis. Access to centers that offer a comprehensive investigation is limited. Furthermore, no current standardized approach to the investigation of OA has yet been established. Development and standardization of diagnostic procedures and consensus diagnostic algorithms for OA and OR would be helpful in formulating a consistent approach to the management of OA and OR worldwide. Determining the cost-effectiveness of different management options requires further investigations using the outcomes that have been validated for the evaluation of asthma and rhinitis, such as the level of disease control, disease-specific quality of life, and measurements of airway inflammation. Although the majority of work-related allergic symptoms are respiratory and cutaneous, work-related anaphylaxis can occur in workers exposed to HMW or LMW agents.

REFERENCES

1. Henneberger PK, Redlich CA, Callahan DB, et al. An official American Thoracic Society statement: work-exacerbated asthma. Am J Respir Crit Care Med 2011;184(3):368–78.
2. Bernstein I, Bernstein D, Chan-Yeung M, et al. Definition and classification of asthma in the workplace. Asthma in the workplace. New York: Taylor & Francis; 2013. p. 1–8.
3. Vandenplas O, Wiszniewska M, Raulf M, et al. EAACI position paper: irritant-induced asthma. Allergy 2014;69(9):1141–53.
4. Moscato G, Vandenplas O, Van Wijk RG, et al. EAACI position paper on occupational rhinitis. Respir Res 2009;10:16.
5. Tarlo SM, Lemiere C. Occupational asthma. N Engl J Med 2014;370(7):640–9.
6. Vandenplas O, Suojalehto H, Aasen TB, et al. Specific inhalation challenge in the diagnosis of occupational asthma: consensus statement. Eur Respir J 2014;43(6):1573–87.
7. Quirce S, Lemiere C, de Blay F, et al. Non-invasive methods for assessment of airway inflammation in occupational settings. Allergy 2010;65(4):445–58.
8. Beach J, Russell K, Blitz S, et al. A systematic review of the diagnosis of occupational asthma. Chest 2007;131:569–78.
9. Quirce S. Eosinophilic bronchitis in the workplace. Curr Opin Allergy Clin Immunol 2004;4:87–91.
10. Vandenplas O, Dressel H, Wilken D, et al. Management of occupational asthma: cessation or reduction of exposure? A systematic review of available evidence. Eur Respir J 2011;38(4):804–11.

CHAPTER 15

Insect Allergy

David B. K. Golden

CHAPTER OUTLINE

STINGING INSECT ALLERGY
HISTORICAL PERSPECTIVE
EPIDEMIOLOGY
ETIOLOGY
Apidae
Vespidae
Formicidae
INSECT VENOMS
CLINICAL FEATURES AND CLASSIFICATION OF REACTIONS
PATIENT EVALUATION AND DIAGNOSIS
Clinical History
Skin Tests
In-vitro Tests
Sting Challenge Test
TREATMENT OF ACUTE REACTIONS
PREVENTION OF ACUTE REACTIONS
Epinephrine Kits
PREDICTORS OF RISK FOR STING ANAPHYLAXIS
Natural History
Markers of Risk for Sting Anaphylaxis

VENOM IMMUNOTHERAPY
Indications
Safety
Effectiveness
Venom Species and Dose
Schedules
Maintenance
Discontinuation
Fire Ant Immunotherapy
BITING INSECT ALLERGY
Triatoma (Kissing Bug, Cone-nose Bug)
Culicidae (Mosquito)
Tabanidae (Horsefly, Deerfly)
Allergic Reactions to Other Biting Insects
INHALANT INSECT ALLERGY
CONCLUSIONS

SUMMARY OF IMPORTANT CONCEPTS

- Anaphylaxis to insect stings occurs in 3% of adults and 1% of children, and even the first reaction can be fatal.
- Cutaneous systemic reactions are most common in children, hypotensive shock is most common in adults, and respiratory complaints occur equally in all age groups.
- The chance of a systemic reaction to a sting is low in those with large local reactions and in children with mild (cutaneous) systemic reactions; the rate varies from 25% to 70% among adults, depending on the severity of previous systemic sting reactions.
- Venom skin tests are most accurate for diagnosis, but the serum-specific immunoglobulin E (IgE) test is an important complementary test. The degree of sensitivity on skin or serum tests does not predict the severity of a sting reaction. The history is important because venom sensitization can be detected in up to 25% of adults.
- Patients discharged from emergency care for anaphylaxis should be well educated on how to use an epinephrine kit and should understand that using the kit is not a substitute for emergency medical attention. Allergy consultation and preventative treatment should be arranged.
- Venom immunotherapy is 75–98% effective in preventing sting anaphylaxis, and it is as safe as inhalant allergen immunotherapy. Most patients can discontinue treatment after 5 years with a low residual risk of a severe sting reaction.

- Better tests are needed for markers of susceptibility (e.g., determining who is at high risk for sting anaphylaxis) and markers of tolerance (e.g., determining who can safely discontinue venom immunotherapy).

STINGING INSECT ALLERGY

Insect stings are a common cause of allergic reactions, but also a common subject of misunderstanding. Both physicians and patients/carers often overestimate or underestimate the risk of sting anaphylaxis in patients with suspected insect allergy. Most primary care physicians are unaware that venom immunotherapy (VIT) is available, is rapidly protective, and is virtually curative for severe insect sting allergy. Current management is based on decades of epidemiologic, clinical, and laboratory research that have helped to characterize the natural history, risk factors, and mechanisms, and identify optimal treatment for insect sting allergy.[1,2]

HISTORICAL PERSPECTIVE

The potential for life-threatening allergic reactions to insect stings has been known since antiquity, but the first report of immunotherapy for insect sting allergy was in 1930. That study concluded falsely that body proteins were responsible for the allergy, and it was not until 50 years later that insect venoms were approved for clinical use in place of whole body extracts. Subsequent lengthy studies of large populations helped to clarify the natural history of the allergy in different groups and the risk factors for severe sting reactions.[1-3]

EPIDEMIOLOGY

Insect sting allergy can occur at any age, often after a number of uneventful stings, and is more common than once thought. In the US systemic allergic reactions are reported by up to 3% of adults, and almost 1% of children have a medical history of severe sting reactions. The frequency of large local reactions is less certain, but is estimated in the range of 5–15%.

At least 40 fatal stings occur each year in the US half of which occur in persons with no prior history of allergic reactions to stings. In postmortem blood samples, it has proved possible to document the presence of venom-specific immunoglobulin E (IgE) antibodies and elevated serum tryptase, suggesting a possible mechanism for some cases of unexplained sudden death. However, the presence of IgE antibodies to Hymenoptera venom is common even in those with no prior history of allergic reaction. More than 30% of adults who have been stung in the previous few months (with no abnormal reaction) will show venom-specific IgE antibodies on skin testing or immunoassay, and 10–20% of all adults demonstrate positive skin test or blood test results for yellow jacket or honeybee venom. Such asymptomatic sensitization is common with all known allergens.

Although insect sting allergy is sometimes familial, the vast majority of insect allergic individuals have no family history of insect allergy. There is only a weak concordance with other allergic conditions, but the frequency of venom sensitization (regardless of history) is higher among individuals with sensitization to inhalant allergens (with or without symptoms).

ETIOLOGY

Allergic reactions can occur after insect stings or bites, but insect-induced anaphylaxis is caused by stings and rarely by bites. Insect bite allergy is discussed at the end of this chapter. Stinging insects belong to the order Hymenoptera. The Hymenoptera of importance in allergy are from three families: Apidae, Vespidae, and Formicidae (Table 15-1).

TABLE 15-1   Taxonomy of the Hymenoptera Insect Order

Family and subfamily	Scientific name	Common name
Apidae	*Apis mellifera*	Honeybee
	Bombus spp.	Bumblebee
	Megabombus spp.	
	Halictus spp.	Sweatbee
	Dialictus spp.	
Vespidae		
Vespinae	*Vespula* spp.	Yellow jacket
	Dolichovespula arenaria	Yellow hornet
	Dolichovespula maculata	White-faced hornet
Polistinae	*Polistes* spp.	Paper wasp
Formicidae	*Solenopsis invicta*	Fire ant
	Myrmecia spp.	Jack Jumper ant
	Pogonomyrmex spp.	Harvester ant
	Pachycondyla spp.	

Selected representatives of these families are depicted in Figure 15-1. Yellow jackets are the most frequent culprits in northern North America and Europe, whereas the *Polistes* species are more commonly implicated in the Gulf Coast areas of the US and the Mediterranean coast of Europe. Common names in general usage can be misleading: the term *bee* can refer to honeybees only, or to all stinging insects. Similarly, *wasps* may refer to any of the social wasps (vespids) or only to the *Polistes* species. The stinging ants are an increasingly prevalent cause of anaphylaxis in the US, Asia, and Australia.

Apidae

Honeybees are relatively docile and rarely sting or swarm without considerable provocation. Africanized honeybees look the same as other honeybees and deliver the same venom when they sting, but they have an unusual tendency to swarm and sting in large numbers. Delivery of large numbers of stings at one time can cause toxic reactions that have been fatal to livestock and humans; this has earned these insects the common name of *killer bees*.

Bumblebees usually are not aggressive and do not usually sting. Allergic reactions to bumblebee stings (*Bombus* species) occur especially in greenhouse workers. Bumblebee venom shows very limited cross-reactivity with honeybee venom.

Vespidae

Vespids use a wood pulp to construct nests that contain one or more layers of comb, each of which contain a large number of cells. These comb layers are attached in a vertical arrangement and usually are enclosed in papier-mâché outer layers. The vespid sting apparatus usually has finer barbs than in the apids and does not commonly detach from the insect, so vespids are able to sting repeatedly. Some yellow jacket species do leave the sting apparatus in the skin, so this is not unique to the honeybee.

Yellow jackets (genus *Vespula*) are highly aggressive and may sting for no apparent reason, particularly in the autumn, when larger populations compete for limited food supplies. Yellow jacket nests are located in the ground or in cracks in buildings or residential landscape materials.

Yellow hornets and white-faced (bald-faced) hornets (genus *Dolichovespula*) are aerial nesting yellow jackets that are present in North America, but not in Europe. They often build their nests in shrubs and trees, and their sensitivity to vibration can initiate their defensive sting behavior.

Paper wasps are primarily of the genus *Polistes*. The coloring of wasps varies greatly, and they can be black, brown, red, or striped. *Polistes* wasps are somewhat less aggressive than yellow jackets and hornets, but they sting readily when disturbed and can sting repeatedly without losing their sting apparatus.

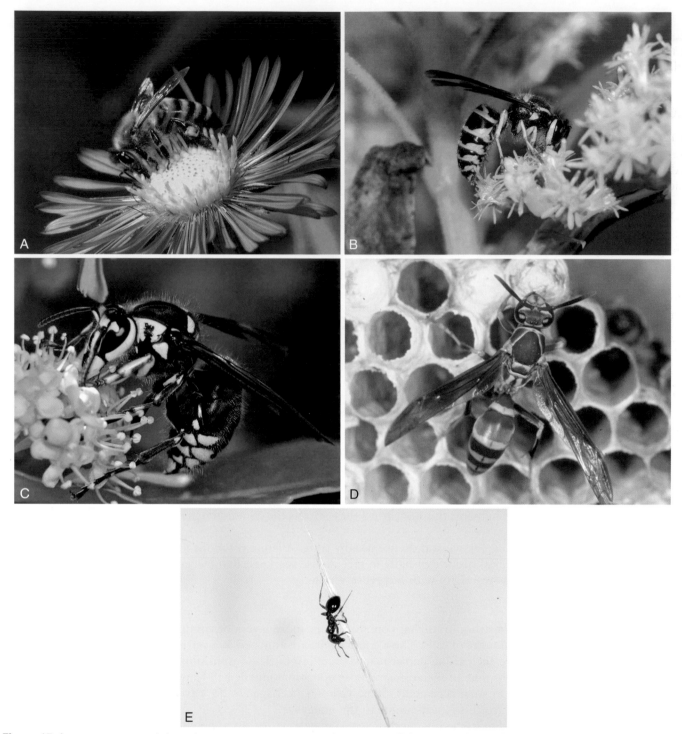

Figure 15-1 Stinging insects of the order Hymenoptera. **A.** Honeybee (*Apis mellifera*). **B.** Yellow jacket (*Vespula maculifrons*). **C.** White-faced hornet (*Dolichovespula maculata*). **D.** Paper wasp (*Polistes exclamans*). **E.** Imported fire ant (*Solenopsis invicta*). *(Reproduced by permission of ALK-Abelló A/S, Høsholm, Denmark© 2012, ALK.)*

Formicidae

The ants of the Formicidae family have a true sting apparatus. Ants of the genus *Solenopsis* are widespread in the southeastern US, and stings occur so frequently that in many areas, as much as 50% of the population is stung each year.[4] In most cases, multiple ants each administer multiple stings, although they are not painful. The unique lesions form sterile pustules that can become infected if excoriated or opened.

Other genera of the formicid ants include the harvester ants (*Pogonomyrmex* spp.) found in western areas of the US Canada, and Mexico; the Australian jack jumper ants (*Myrmecia* spp.); and Asian ants (*Pachycondyla* spp.), which have been reported to cause allergic reactions.

INSECT VENOMS

Commercial extracts are prepared from Hymenoptera venoms (honeybee, yellow jacket, yellow hornet, white-faced hornet, and *Polistes* wasp) and from imported fire ant bodies. Although imported fire ant venom is superior, their whole-body extracts contain sufficient quantities of venom allergens to be clinically useful.

Most of the native venoms contain vasoactive amines, acetylcholine, and kinins, which account for the localized burning, pain, and itching after a sting. Some venom components can cause toxic reactions, including neurologic complications. Within the Vespidae family, there is extensive cross-allergenicity of the venoms of different genera. This is not the case in the Apidae and Formicidae families. There is limited cross-reactivity of honeybee and bumblebee venoms, but most patients with bumblebee allergy do not show cross-reactivity to honeybee venom. There is significant cross-reactivity among the various fire ant (*Solenopsis*) species and among the harvester ant (*Pogonomyrmex*) species, but the two genera do not cross-react with each other. The venoms of different insect families have almost no cross-reactivity. There is limited and infrequent cross-reactivity between honeybee and vespid venoms, some of which may be related to cross-reacting carbohydrate determinants of uncertain clinical significance. Cross-reactivity can be distinguished from multiple sensitization by testing the serum in an inhibition immunoassay, or measuring specific IgE using recombinant venom allergens.

CLINICAL FEATURES AND CLASSIFICATION OF REACTIONS

Insect stings cause reactions that are classified as 'local' or 'systemic' in distribution. Most large local reactions represent a late-phase, IgE-dependent reaction that is mild initially but that develops after 12 to 24 hours to a diameter often exceeding 10 to 20 cm. These reactions may manifest with a lymphangitic streak toward the axilla or the inguinal region, but this represents the drainage of inflammatory mediators, rather than an infectious process. A large local reaction subsides after 5 to 10 days and is not dangerous except for potential local anatomic compression, especially on the head, neck, tongue, or throat.

A systemic reaction causes symptoms and signs in one or more anatomic systems distant from the site of the sting, usually representing IgE-mediated anaphylaxis. Patients may exhibit cutaneous signs (e.g., generalized urticaria, angioedema, flushing, pruritus); respiratory changes (e.g., throat tightness, dysphagia, dyspnea, stridor or dysphonia, chest tightness, wheezing); or a circulatory component (e.g., dizziness, hypotension, unconsciousness, shock). Less frequently, gastrointestinal complaints (e.g., cramps, diarrhea, nausea, vomiting) or uterine cramping occur. Cardiac anaphylaxis after insect stings can cause coronary vasospasm, tachyarrhythmias, or bradycardia, even with no underlying coronary or cardiac abnormality. The diagnosis of the acute reaction can be difficult when hypotension or cardiac manifestations occur with no other signs or symptoms. The absence of urticaria or angioedema is associated with more severe reactions to stings. Children have a higher frequency of isolated cutaneous reactions and a lower frequency of vascular symptoms or anaphylactic shock compared with adults.

Systemic reactions may be caused by underlying mast cell disorders in 1–2% of cases.[5] Up to 25% of patients with severe anaphylactic reactions to venom have elevated baseline serum tryptase. Hypotensive shock without urticaria after a sting is suggestive of mastocytosis. Systemic reactions may occasionally be caused by toxic effects from the vasoactive substances in a large number of stings. Massive envenomation from large numbers of stings can cause life-threatening reactions with renal failure, rhabdomyolysis, hemolysis, and acute respiratory distress syndrome or diffuse intravascular coagulation. Seizures have occurred, particularly after multiple fire ant stings. Unusual reactions of unknown mechanisms are usually delayed and include serum sickness-like reactions, encephalitis, peripheral and cranial neuropathies, glomerulonephritis, myocarditis, and Guillain–Barré syndrome.

PATIENT EVALUATION AND DIAGNOSIS

Diagnostic evaluation of patients for insect sting allergy includes historical inquiry as well as an array of laboratory tests that provide useful information about the diagnosis, the prognosis (relative risk of reaction), and long-term outcome with VIT (Table 15-2). The current approach to diagnosis of insect sting allergy is summarized in Box 15-1.[3] Diagnostic testing for venom-specific IgE antibodies by skin or serum tests is recommended in all individuals with a prior history of systemic reactions to insect stings, with the exception of children who had reactions limited to cutaneous manifestations. The rationale for diagnostic testing is to confirm the diagnosis in patients who are candidates for venom immunotherapy based on their clinical history and to identify the venoms to be included in treatment.

Clinical History

The diagnosis of insect sting allergy rests on the history as the primary evidence of allergic reactivity because venom-specific IgE antibodies are present in a large number of clinically nonreactive individuals. Physicians should inquire about severe reactions to insect stings when obtaining a complete medical history because most affected individuals fail to mention the event during a routine history. The history should be reviewed in detail with respect to the location and timing of the stings, the time course of the reaction, and all associated symptoms and treatments. Concurrent medications, such as

---

TABLE 15-2   Diagnostic Evaluation of Insect Sting Allergy

Variable	History	Skin test	Specific IgE	BAT	Recombinant allergen	RAST inhibition	Tryptase baseline
Diagnosis							
No reaction	X						
LLR	X						
Mild SR	X	X	X				
Anaphylaxis	X	X	X	X	X	X	X
Predict severe reaction (to stings or VIT)	X			X			X
Cross-reactivity (HB/YJ)					X	X	
Discontinue VIT	X			X			X

BAT, basophil activation test; HB, honeybee; LLR, large local reaction; SR, systemic reaction; VIT, venom immunotherapy; YJ, yellow jacket.
(From: Golden DBK. Advances in diagnosis and management of insect sting allergy. Ann Allergy Asthma Immunol 2013;111:84–89.)

Box 15-1   **Current Diagnosis**

- History of systemic allergic reaction to a sting
- Positive test for venom-specific IgE (by serum or skin tests)
- Degree of sensitivity (by serum IgE or skin test) correlates with frequency but not severity of sting reaction
- Low risk if previous large local reaction only
- Low risk in children with mild (cutaneous) systemic reactions
- Quality of life and frequency of exposure a consideration

β-adrenergic blocking agents and angiotensin-converting enzyme inhibitors (ACEIs), may contribute significantly to the severity of the anaphylactic reaction.

Skin Tests

The standard method of skin testing employs the well-validated intradermal technique, using the five commercial Hymenoptera venom protein extracts at concentrations in the range of 0.001 to 1.0 μg/mL. Fire ant sensitivity can be tested with reasonable diagnostic accuracy using whole-body extracts of imported fire ants.

Skin test results are clearly positive for most patients with a convincing history, but they can be negative in >20% of cases. In the days or weeks after a sting reaction, some patients have negative skin test results attributed to a refractory period of anergy (absence of the expected immune response); they should have skin tests repeated after 4 to 6 weeks. Negative skin test results for a history-positive patient may represent the loss of sensitivity in a person with a remote history of sting reaction. Some cases of sting anaphylaxis may be non-IgE-mediated or be attributable to subclinical (indolent) mastocytosis. Some persons with negative venom skin test results will have systemic reactions to subsequent stings. Most insect-allergic patients with negative venom skin test results have detectable venom-specific IgE antibodies in the serum. For these reasons, patients with negative skin test results and a convincing history of anaphylaxis should be further investigated with serologic testing, and if results remain negative, the skin tests should be repeated after 3 to 6 months.

Venom skin test sensitivities have different patterns. Because of cross-reactivity, almost all patients who have a positive skin test result in response to yellow jacket venom will also have positive skin tests to one or both of the hornet venoms, and approximately one half will have positive tests to *Polistes* wasp venom. The degree of skin test sensitivity does not correlate reliably with the degree of sting reaction. The most reactive skin tests may occur in patients who have had only large local reactions and have a very low risk of anaphylaxis, whereas some patients who have had near-fatal anaphylactic shock show only weak skin test reactivity.

In-Vitro Tests

The diagnosis of insect sting allergy by detection of allergen-specific IgE antibodies in serum has improved greatly over the past 10 years. A high level of venom-specific IgE is usually diagnostic, but low levels are more difficult to detect with reliability. Venom skin tests and venom-specific IgE assays correlate imperfectly. The latter produce negative results in up to 20% of skin test-positive subjects, and venom skin test results are negative for almost 10% of persons with elevated IgE antibodies. Neither test alone can detect all cases of insect sting allergy, and each test is useful as a supplement to the other. The clinical significance of a positive IgE antibody assay result with a negative skin test result is not known in all cases, but it is clearly associated with a risk of systemic reaction to a sting.

Sting Challenge Test

It has been assumed that the ultimate test of whether an individual will have a systemic reaction to a sting is to observe the outcome of a supervised live sting challenge. This procedure has been used as the gold standard in research studies of the efficacy of VIT and to determine the relapse rate after discontinuation of VIT. Sting challenge of untreated patients with a history of previous systemic reactions to stings and with positive venom skin test results has resulted in systemic reaction rates ranging between 30% and 65%. This variability in part reflects the variability of the culprit insect. The quantity of venom protein injected during a sting is relatively consistent for honeybees but varies greatly for vespids. The routine use of a live sting challenge as a diagnostic procedure for selection of patients for immunotherapy has been proposed, but there have been ethical and practical objections. Moreover, the lack of reaction to a single challenge sting has limited clinical significance, because a subsequent sting can still cause a systemic reaction in up to 20% of cases.

TREATMENT OF ACUTE REACTIONS

Large local reactions, if severe or involving the head and neck, are best treated with a brief burst of an oral corticosteroid (e.g., initial dose of 40–60 mg of prednisone, tapering to 0 in 4–6 days). For best results, steroids should be started within a few hours of the sting in patients with a known history of large local reactions to stings. Milder reactions may be treated conservatively, with cold compresses, and medication for pruritus or pain. Large local reactions can be mistaken for cellulitis, especially on the extremities, where intense inflammation can cause an apparent lymphangitis directed toward the axillary or inguinal nodes. When such a reaction presents 24 to 48 hours after the sting, infection is very unlikely, and treatment may include ice and moderate-dose oral steroids, but antibiotics are not necessary.

Systemic reactions require more urgent intervention and close monitoring. Urticaria may respond to H_1-antihistamines alone, but anaphylactic reactions require epinephrine injection. Any sign of hypotension or respiratory obstruction should be treated promptly with aqueous epinephrine intramuscularly into the anterolateral aspect of the thigh, and should have full emergency medical attention and observation for 3 to 6 hours. The recommended dose of epinephrine is 0.3 to 0.5 mg (0.3–0.5 mL of 1:1000 wt./vol. solution) for adults and 0.01 mg/kg for children to a maximum of 0.3 mg. After use of self-injectable epinephrine, the individual should be taken to an Emergency Department for observation and further treatment, if necessary. Some patients who have a history of rapid-onset or very severe systemic reactions may warrant treatment immediately after the sting. Delay in the use of epinephrine has contributed to fatal reactions, and some individuals with anaphylactic shock are resistant to epinephrine. Patients taking β-blocker medications may, for example, be resistant to the effects of epinephrine; glucagon injection can be beneficial in these cases. For a few patients, anaphylaxis is prolonged or recurrent for 6 to 24 hours, and it may require intensive medical care. The patient with hypotension should be kept supine with legs raised because upright posture has been associated with sudden death due to lack of venous return (i.e. empty ventricle syndrome).

Emergency treatment of anaphylaxis requires patient education before discharge. The risk of recurrence should be clearly described, and the use of self-injectable epinephrine requires consistent instruction and follow-up. Many patients are not specifically instructed about the need for self-injectable epinephrine, and they are not referred for an allergy consultation and preventive treatment. This is important because affected individuals often think the reaction was a chance occurrence and fail to inform their personal physicians about it.

PREVENTION OF ACUTE REACTIONS

Patients should avoid high-risk exposures such as yard and garden work, trash containers, and outdoor areas where food and drink are exposed. Food and flavored drinks in cans, bottles, and straws can be an unsuspected source of a sting to the tongue or throat (Box 15-2). Avoidance of wearing brightly colored clothes is of uncertain benefit, and insect repellants have little or no effect.

Epinephrine Kits

Epinephrine auto-injectors (as used in the US: 0.3 mg EpiPen and 0.15 mg EpiPen Jr, Dey Labs, Napa, CA; 0.3 mg Twinject and 0.15 mg Adrenaclick, Shionogi Pharma, Atlanta, GA; 0.3 mg and 0.15 mg Auvi-Q, Sanofi, Bridgewater, NJ) should be prescribed and explained to all patients at risk for anaphylaxis. The age at which to prescribe an adult-dose instead of pediatric-dose auto-injector is uncertain, but the question may be considered when the child reaches a weight of 25 to 30 kg. Even when epinephrine kits are prescribed, patients often fail to carry the injector with them and delay or defer using them when they have a reaction. Patients, caretakers in homes and schools, and physicians need initial and follow-up education about the correct use of the device and how to recognize the expiration date on the unit and replace outdated units promptly.

Box 15-2   **Patient Information to Limit the Risk of Insect Stings**

- Avoid drinking outdoors from cans or straws that may harbor stinging insects.
- Exercise caution when doing yard work, handling garbage, picnicking, swimming, cycling, riding in open-air vehicles, boating, camping, or other outdoor activity.
- Always wear shoes outdoors.
- Avoid loose-fitting clothing that may entrap insects. Insects are attracted to bright colors and floral patterns. Wear light-colored clothing: white, green, tan, and khaki.
- Avoid scented perfumes, lotions, soaps, colognes, or hair preparations.
- Look for insects in vehicles before driving, and keep vehicle windows closed.
- Avoid rapid or jerking movement around insects. Remain still. Most insects will not sting unless provoked.
- All nests or hives in the vicinity of the home should be removed by a professional exterminator and not by the insect-sensitive patient.
- Insect repellents do not deter stinging insects. Immunotherapy does not lessen the need for other measures of prevention.
- Wear an identification tag or bracelet at all times.
- Have an epinephrine injection kit available at all times, especially if at greater risk; instruct family members and companions in its use.
- Seek medical attention immediately after emergency treatment is given.

(From: Golden DBK: Insect allergy. In: Manual of Allergy and Immunology, 5th edition. (Eds: DC Adelman, T Casale, J Corren), Lippincott Williams & Wilkins, Baltimore, 2012, pp. 278–291.)

Box 15-3   **Patients with Low Risk for Anaphylaxis**

- General population
- Asymptomatic sensitization
- Patients on venom immunotherapy
- Children with cutaneous systemic reactions
- Large local reactors
- Patients who completed 5 years of venom immunotherapy

The prescription of an epinephrine injector should always be considered when there is a known risk of anaphylaxis. However, the prescription itself creates fear in some people and reassurance in others. Studies have described the burden of epinephrine prescriptions, and the frequent negative impact on quality of life (cf VIT, which improves quality of life).[6] When VIT is indicated, epinephrine prescription is clearly indicated. In individuals at low risk for sting anaphylaxis (Box 15-3), the prescription of an epinephrine injector is a matter of clinical judgment and may be discussed with the patient. There is some disagreement about whether epinephrine prescription is necessary when the chance it will be needed is relatively small, but once the risk is identified, it is reasonable to offer the epinephrine prescription and discuss it with the patient.

PREDICTORS OF RISK FOR STING ANAPHYLAXIS

Natural History

The prognosis for affected patients is based on the understanding of the natural history of the condition (Table 15-3), and on specific clinical factors and biologic markers (Table 15-4). The chance that a future sting will cause an allergic reaction depends on the history and immunologic status of the patient. Because one in five healthy adults has detectable venom-specific IgE antibodies, testing of asymptomatic individuals is not recommended.

In patients with positive venom skin test results and previous systemic reactions, the outcome of the next sting is somewhat unpredictable because systemic reactions may occur on some occasions but not on others. The average frequency of systemic reaction to a subsequent sting has been 45% (range 30–65%). Even among patients who have no reaction to one challenge sting, 20% will have a systemic reaction to a subsequent sting.

The risk of recurrence is higher for those who are allergic to honeybee stings than for those with vespid allergies, higher for adults than for children, and higher for patients

TABLE 15-3   Risk of Systemic Reactions and Clinical Recommendations Based on Reaction to Previous Stings and Venom Skin Test or Serum IgE Test Results

Previous sting reaction	Skin and/or serum IgE test	Chance of future systemic sting reaction		Clinical recommendation
		Any	Severe	
None	Positive	10–15%	5%	Avoidance
Large local	Positive	5–10%	2%	Avoidance
Cutaneous systemic				
Child	Positive	1–10%	<3%	Avoidance
Adult	Positive	10–20%	<5%	Venom immunotherapy
Moderate systemic	Positive	30–50%	10%	Venom immunotherapy
Anaphylaxis	Positive	50–75%	30%	Venom immunotherapy
Anaphylaxis	Negative	5–10%	30%	Repeat skin/serum venom-IgE test

(From: Golden DBK. Allergic reactions to hymenoptera. ACP Medicine 2011. DOI 10.2310/7900.1129.)

TABLE 15-4   Predictors of Risk of Systemic Reaction to Insect Stings

Natural history	Screening tests and markers
Severity of previous reaction	Venom skin test
Insect species	Venom-specific IgE
Age, gender	Basophil activation test
No urticaria or angioedema	Baseline serum tryptase value
Medications	Platelet-activating factor (PAF) acetylhydrolase
Multiple or sequential stings	Angiotensin-converting enzyme (ACE)

who had more severe systemic reactions previously than for those with milder systemic reactions. Contrary to popular belief, it is uncommon for patients to have more severe reactions with each subsequent sting.

There are a number of subtypes of people with positive tests for venom-IgE who are at low risk for sting anaphylaxis (Box 15-3). Most large local reactors consistently have similar reactions with repeated stings. The risk of systemic reactions (not all of which are severe) in those with large local reactions is 4–10%. The level of sensitivity shown by a venom skin test or specific IgE level does not predict future occurrences, and no known clinical or laboratory characteristics differentiate patients who will progress to systemic reactions from those who will continue to have only large local sting reactions. Evaluation and treatment for large local reactions is summarized in Figure 15-2.

In children with a history of systemic reactions to stings, the skin tests or specific IgE level became negative in 25–50% after an average of 10 years of follow-up without VIT. During 10 to 20 years of follow-up, children who had had strictly cutaneous systemic reactions had a 10–15% chance of subsequent systemic reactions (mostly milder than the previous reaction) and only about a 3% chance of more severe reactions with respiratory or circulatory symptoms. Those who had moderate or severe reactions in childhood had a significantly higher risk of reaction in adulthood, estimated to be 30%.[7]

The chance of progression from a mild (cutaneous) reaction to a more severe reaction has not been conclusively determined in adults. Some retrospective studies showed more frequent progression, but prospective sting challenge studies found a very low risk of progression (<5%).

Markers of Risk for Sting Anaphylaxis

Risk factors for severe reactions to insect stings, based on natural history and in-vitro tests, are shown in Table 15-4. The history (i.e. severity and pattern of previous sting

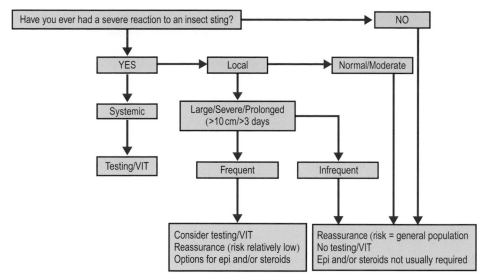

Figure 15-2 Algorithm for large local reactions. *(From: Golden DBK. Large local reactions to insect stings. J Allergy Clin Immunol: In Pract 2015;3(3):331–334.)*

reactions) has been the most reliable predictor of the severity of subsequent sting reactions. Absence of urticaria or angioedema during anaphylaxis, and rapid onset, were associated with a higher frequency of severe reaction. Measurable markers that predict the risk of systemic reaction to a sting are summarized in Table 15-4. Results of skin tests and specific IgE tests correlate better with the frequency of sting reactions than with the severity of reactions. The baseline serum tryptase level correlates closely with the risk of severe anaphylaxis from a sting. It is likely that abnormal measurements of other mast cell mediators will be found to reflect an increased risk of severe anaphylaxis. This is true for platelet-activating factor (PAF). The level of PAF correlates with the serum activity of PAF acetylhydrolase.

Another growing concern has been the effect of medications on the risk of reaction. β-Blockers can increase the risk of anaphylaxis primarily by interfering with the effects of epinephrine. β-Blockers should be avoided in all patients who are at risk for anaphylaxis, including those with insect sting allergy and those receiving allergen immunotherapy. However, risk analysis has suggested that in many patients with cardiovascular disease, stopping β-blockers can create greater risk than not stopping the drug during VIT. It is therefore acceptable, when necessary, to proceed with VIT in patients receiving β-blockers. Another concern has been the risk of anaphylaxis in patients taking ACEIs. Some reports have suggested a significant risk of more severe anaphylaxis, while others do not.

Baseline serum tryptase activity can predict severe sting anaphylaxis, and it has been useful as a predictor of systemic reactions during VIT, failure of VIT, and relapse of sting anaphylaxis after discontinuing VIT. Elevated baseline tryptase levels often indicate underlying mastocytosis, which occurs in approximately 1–2% of patients with sting anaphylaxis. Sting anaphylaxis is the most common cause of anaphylaxis in patients with indolent mastocytosis, and it can be the presenting sign of the disease.[5]

VENOM IMMUNOTHERAPY

Indications

VIT is the treatment of choice for prevention of systemic allergic reactions to insect stings, but it requires careful selection of patients (Table 15-3).[3] VIT is indicated in patients with a history of previous systemic allergic reaction to a sting and positive results on venom skin test or venom specific IgE test. Those with recent and severe anaphylaxis are at highest risk (40–70%) and require VIT. The lowest risk (<10%) has been found for children and adults with a history of large local reactions and for children with systemic reactions limited to cutaneous signs and symptoms but with no respiratory or vascular manifestations. VIT is generally not required for patients with the lowest risk of anaphylaxis. Some low-risk patients request treatment because of their fear of reaction and its impact on their lifestyle. Quality of life is impaired in patients with a history of systemic reactions and is improved by VIT but not by prescription of self-injectable epinephrine.

The risk of severe anaphylactic reaction to a later sting in adults with a history of mild systemic reactions is uncertain because there are inconsistent results in published reports. For this reason, VIT is recommended to adults with cutaneous systemic reactions. There is no test that predicts which patients will progress from large local or cutaneous systemic reactions to more severe anaphylactic reactions. There is evidence that VIT inhibits large local reactions to stings, which can benefit patients who have frequent and severe local reactions.

Safety

Adverse reactions to VIT are no more common than reactions during inhalant allergen immunotherapy. Systemic symptoms occur in 5–15% of patients during initial updosing, regardless of which of the two standard schedules is used. There is an association between severe or repeated systemic reactions to injections and underlying mast cell disease (e.g., mastocytosis, urticaria pigmentosa, elevated baseline serum tryptase levels).

Systemic reactions to venom injections occur more frequently in patients treated with honeybee venom than in those treated with yellow jacket venom. Most systemic reactions are mild, and <5% of patients receiving VIT ever require epinephrine treatment for a reaction to an injection.

Pretreatment with antihistamines or a leukotriene modifier reduces the local reactions to injections. Antihistamines also reduce the frequency of systemic reactions to VIT and to subsequent stings. In the unusual case of recurrent systemic reactions to injections, therapy may be streamlined to a single venom and given in divided doses 30 min apart. In patients with recurrent systemic reactions to VIT, rush VIT, or omalizumab treatment have been successful. Large local reactions to venom injections occur in up to 50% of patients, but it may be necessary to advance the dose in the face of moderately severe local reactions in order to achieve the full maintenance dose. Although large local reactions to venom injections have not predicted systemic reactions to subsequent doses, an association has been reported for fire ant immunotherapy. As with inhalant immunotherapy, maintenance VIT is considered acceptable during pregnancy.

Effectiveness

VIT with vespid venoms is 85–95% effective in preventing systemic reactions to stings, but honeybee VIT is only 75–85% effective. VIT with Jack Jumper ant venom was associated with complete protection from sting challenge in >95% of patients. Even in cases considered to be treatment failures, the repeat sting reactions are usually milder than pretreatment reactions. Treatment failure can be overcome with higher treatment doses (e.g., 200 μg). Failure of VIT occurs in 25% of patients with underlying mastocytosis.

VIT has been a model for the study of the mechanism of immunotherapy. Evidence supports the role of IgG in intercepting allergen and in facilitating lymphocyte responses. Immunotherapy induces suppression of venom skin test and specific IgE antibodies, and it reduces basophil release of histamine or leukotrienes. Studies of VIT have elucidated an important role for interleukin 10 (IL-10) in the suppression of the Th2 cytokines during VIT and suggest a role for regulatory T cells in the protective effects of VIT.[8] Additional investigation has identified more specific pathways of T cell regulation and identified a role for dendritic cells. Another novel pathway involves the role of IgG4 antibodies in facilitated antigen presentation to T cells and B cells that regulate the allergic response to venom.

Venom Species and Dose

The selection of venom extracts to be used for immunotherapy depends on the venom skin test reaction or venom-specific IgE antibody level to each venom. Therapy should include all venoms that elicit a positive response, because anaphylaxis to one venom may predispose to anaphylaxis to another venom. For this reason, the most common therapy for vespid sensitivities in the US is with the mixed vespid venoms preparation: 100 μg each of yellow jacket, yellow hornet, and white-faced hornet venoms. Although therapy with yellow jacket venom alone can protect against hornet stings because of the marked cross-reactivity of the *Vespula* venoms, treatment with mixed vespid venoms gives a more robust immune response and more reliable clinical protection. The skin test result is also positive to *Polistes* wasp venoms in at least 50% of vespid allergic patients, and treatment is usually given as a separate injection. Therapy with yellow jacket or mixed vespid venoms can protect against wasp stings, but this has been established only for patients whose wasp IgE showed complete cross-reactivity with yellow jacket venom as assessed by inhibition immunoassays. In patients with dual positivity to honeybee and yellow jacket venoms, serologic testing using recombinant venom allergens can distinguish those with cross-reactivity (which may be due to the cross-reacting carbohydrate determinants on the native venoms) from those with true dual sensitization.

The recommended maintenance dose for VIT is 100 μg of each venom. Data on the use of lower doses are limited, with various degrees of efficacy reported for adults. Patients who are not adequately protected with the 100 μg dose usually can be protected with higher doses. The treatment recommendations for children ≥3 years of age are the same as for adults. However, some studies have shown similar efficacy and long-term outcomes using a 50 μg maintenance dose in children.

Schedules

Initial VIT follows a schedule that can vary according to the recommendations of the source laboratory that prepared the allergen extract and the level of caution preferred by the clinician. Table 15-5 shows the recommended schedules for the two products available in the US. The modified rush regimen (ALK-Abelló, Round Rock, TX) is more rapid than the traditional regimen (Hollister-Stier Laboratories, Spokane, WA), achieving maintenance dose in 8 weekly injections instead of 15 weeks, respectively. These regimens show equal efficacy and safety. Once the full dose is achieved, it is usually repeated in 1 week, again after another 2 weeks, and then after another 3 weeks before beginning maintenance treatment every 4 weeks.

Rush VIT regimens administered over 2 to 3 days have been equally effective and safe, with adverse reactions occurring no more often than with traditional regimens. Ultra-rush regimens, given over a period of hours, are associated with an increased risk of severe reactions.[9] Rush VIT has been used successfully in patients unable to achieve maintenance doses due to repeated systemic reactions using standard schedules. Use of rush regimens has become routine in Europe due to the regional availability of specialized treatment, and in the US military to hasten return to duty.

Maintenance

Maintenance VIT is administered every 4 weeks for at least the first year. There are few studies on longer maintenance intervals, but clinical experience supports the practice of extending the maintenance interval to every 6 to 8 weeks over several years in most cases. A few patients require maintenance doses every 2 to 3 weeks to avoid systemic reactions. VIT with a 12-week interval has been shown to be effective for extended maintenance treatment after several years of routine therapy. Maintenance evaluation should include a review of the dose and frequency of injections, all adverse reactions, any intervening stings, and all current medications. Repeat skin tests or immunoassays may be performed every 2 to 3 years. Venom skin test results become negative in at least 20% of patients after 5 years of treatment, but 50–60% had negative results after

TABLE 15-5 Examples of Conventional Dosing Schedules for Venom Immunotherapy

Schedule 1*			Schedule 2*		
Week No.	Concentration (µg/mL)	Volume (mL)	Week No.	Concentration (µg/mL)	Volume (mL)
1	1.0	0.05	1a	0.01	0.1
			1b	0.1	0.1
			1c	1.0	0.1
2	1.0	0.1	2a	1.0	0.1
			2b	1.0	0.5
			2c	10	0.1
3	1.0	0.2	3a	10	0.1
			3b	10	0.5
			3c	10	1.0
4	1.0	0.4	4a	100	0.1
			4b	100	0.2
5	10	0.05	5a	100	0.2
			5b	100	0.3
6	10	0.1	6a	100	0.3
			6b	100	0.3
7	10	0.2	7a	100	0.4
			7b	100	0.4
8	10	0.4	8a	100	0.5
			8b	100	0.5
9	100	0.05	9	100	1.0
10	100	0.1	Monthly	100	1.0
11	100	0.2			
12	100	0.4			
13	100	0.6			
14	100	0.8			
15	100	1.0			
16	100	1.0			
18	100	1.0			
21	100	1.0			
Monthly	100	1.0			

*Injections are usually given weekly. Schedule 2 prescribes two or three doses, at 30-min intervals for the first 8 weeks. When the maintenance dose is achieved, the interval may be advanced from weekly to monthly. Schedule 1 is based on the package insert for Hollister–Stier venom extracts (Spokane, WA). Schedule 2 is based on the package insert for ALK-Abelló venom extracts (Round Rock, TX).

7 to 10 years. Venom-specific IgE antibody levels usually remain detectable, even after many years of treatment and even when skin tests become negative.

The level of venom-specific IgG antibodies can be used to confirm protective levels after initial therapy (especially with honeybee VIT because it has a greater frequency of incomplete protection) and then to determine whether the venom IgG level is adequately maintained at longer maintenance intervals. Some argue that this is unnecessary because of the high degree of overall efficacy of the treatment. In the assay clinically validated by one laboratory, the venom IgG level was more consistently associated with protection when it was >3 µg/mL during the first 4 years of maintenance therapy.

Discontinuation

Although the product package inserts recommend VIT indefinitely, the question is no longer whether VIT can be discontinued, but when and in which patients. Stopping VIT

Box 15-4   **Considerations in Discontinuing Venom Immunotherapy**

- Severity of systemic reaction to stings
- Elevated baseline serum tryptase
- Honeybee sting allergy (beekeepers)
- Duration of venom immunotherapy
- Systemic reaction during VIT (to injection or sting)
- Frequency of exposure
- Persistent strong serum or skin test for venom IgE
- Age (child, adult, senior)
- Quality of life

---

when venom skin test results or specific IgE antibody levels become negative has been successful, but only a small number of patients develop negative test results in the first 5 years of therapy.

Several studies have shown that 5 years of treatment was associated with better suppression of allergic sensitivity and lower risk of relapse than 3 years of VIT.[1,2,10] The chance of relapse was minimal initially, but increased 3 to 5 years after discontinuation and did not disappear during up to at least 13 years observation. There is an approximately 10% chance of systemic reaction with each sting after stopping treatment, with a cumulative risk of relapse of 15–20% after 10 years off treatment (because repeat stings increase the chance of reaction). Fortunately, most reactions are mild and much less severe than the pretreatment reaction, but patients who had very severe reactions before VIT can have severe reactions again if they do relapse after stopping treatment. Reactions have occurred even in patients who developed negative venom skin test or specific serum IgE test results.

Collectively, the published studies on discontinuing VIT suggest that treatment may be stopped after 5 years for most patients, with the exception of those treated for honeybee allergy, those who had systemic reactions to an injection or sting during VIT, those with elevated baseline serum tryptase levels, and those who had very severe sting reactions before treatment (Box 15-4). Mastocytosis has been associated with fatal reactions to stings after a course of immunotherapy. Long-term extension of treatment may also be considered for patients who are not willing to accept the 10–20% chance of reaction to a subsequent sting, particularly if they have frequent exposures, which increases the cumulative risk of systemic reaction. In these cases, treatment at 12-week intervals can maintain protection.

Fire Ant Immunotherapy

The natural history of fire ant allergy is not as well described as for other Hymenoptera, but there is a clear need for effective immunotherapy. Although immunotherapy using whole-body extracts of imported fire ants has been reported to be effective in preventing systemic reactions to fire ant stings, there have been no placebo-controlled trials. The suggested materials, methods, regimens, and doses for fire ant immunotherapy have been reviewed.[4] The duration of fire ant immunotherapy is still uncertain, because attempts at discontinuation led to relapse within several years in a significant minority of cases.

BITING INSECT ALLERGY

There are few credible reports of allergic reactions to biting insects. Sensitization to salivary proteins may cause abnormal local swelling following insect bites, but anaphylaxis is rarely reported.

Triatoma (Kissing Bug, Cone-Nose Bug)

The most common confirmed cause of systemic reactions to insect bites is the kissing bug (*Triatoma* spp.). The relevant species in the US are found throughout the arid areas of the southwest states and California. The allergens are salivary gland proteins, and they have little cross-reactivity between species. Immunotherapy with a salivary gland extract was effective in preventing anaphylaxis from *Triatoma* bites in a small number of patients.

Culicidae (Mosquito)

Considering the widespread exposure to mosquitoes and the frequency of mosquito bites, it is remarkable that so few cases of anaphylaxis have been reported. There has been increased recognition of the clinical impact of large local reactions to mosquito bites in children (i.e. Skeeter syndrome).[11] Unfortunately, the mosquito extracts commercially available in the US are of unreliable composition and activity and are not approved for therapeutic use.

The major allergens in mosquito extracts have been identified and recombinant allergens have been prepared. These studies demonstrated significant cross-reactivity of the major worldwide mosquito species. Immunotherapy with whole-body extracts has not been proven effective, and there have been no studies of immunotherapy with purified or recombinant allergens.

Tabanidae (Horsefly, Deerfly)

The tabanid species are large flies that suck blood and inflict painful bites. They have widespread distribution in rural and suburban areas. Allergic reactions to insect bites from horseflies and deerflies have been reported. The possibility of immunotherapy has been little studied.

Allergic Reactions to Other Biting Insects

There have been anecdotal reports of allergic reactions to a number of other biting insects. Fleas (order Siphonaptera) are an uncommon cause of allergy in humans. The most commonly encountered reaction to flea bites in humans is papular urticaria, a form of persistent papular inflammation. The reaction usually begins about the ankles and becomes generalized over a period of weeks, often persisting for months, and resolving spontaneously.

INHALANT INSECT ALLERGY

Respiratory exposures to antigens from outdoor insects (e.g., caddis flies, midges, lake flies) or indoor insects (e.g., cockroaches, lady bugs) may cause allergic respiratory symptoms. In other cases, airborne insect antigens produce occupational disease. Respiratory allergy to insects is discussed in other chapters.

CONCLUSIONS

Stinging insects are a common cause of allergic reactions ranging from large local reactions to life-threatening anaphylaxis. Clinical and immunologic features can predict the risk of future severe reactions to stings. Skin or serum tests for venom-specific IgE antibodies are useful to confirm sensitization to venom allergens. VIT is recommended for patients at moderate to high risk for systemic reactions to future stings, but it is not required for low-risk patients despite positive venom-IgE test results. VIT can rapidly achieve complete clinical protection from systemic reactions to stings in 75–95% of patients. VIT can be discontinued after 5 years in most patients but may be continued indefinitely in those at high risk for relapse. An elevated baseline serum tryptase level predicts the severity of reactions to stings, systemic reactions to VIT, limited protection with VIT, and chance of relapse if VIT is stopped after 5 years. Anaphylaxis is rare from biting insects, but large local reactions can be severe, especially with mosquito bites.

Clinical Pearls Summary

- Large local reactions are not due to infection or cellulitis and do not require antibiotics.
- Absence of hives is associated with more severe anaphylaxis.
- Hypotension without hives suggests mastocytosis.
- Patients with symptoms and signs of hypotension should remain supine until recovered (upright posture is associated with sudden death).
- Avoid drinking from beverage containers or straws; a hidden yellow jacket can cause a sting on the tongue or throat.
- Honeybees always lose their stinger in the skin, but so do some common yellow jackets.
- Children do not always outgrow insect sting allergy. Those with mild (cutaneous) systemic reactions have only 3% chance of anaphylaxis to a future sting, but children who had more severe reactions have up to 30% chance of another reaction even 10–20 years later.
- The strength of the venom allergy test (skin test or serum test) does not reliably predict the severity of a sting reaction.
- Do not test people who have no history of systemic reaction to a sting because more than 20% of normal adults have positive tests for venom-IgE but do not have a high risk of anaphylaxis to future stings.
- VIT gives complete protection in a matter of weeks.
- VIT gives a lasting tolerance in most patients after 5 years of treatment.
- VIT improves quality of life, epinephrine injectors do not.

REFERENCES

1. Golden DBK. Advances in diagnosis and management of insect sting allergy. Ann Allergy Asthma Immunol 2013;111:84–9.
2. Golden DBK. Insect allergy. In: Adkinson NF Jr, Bochner BS, Burks W, et al., editors. Middleton's allergy: principles and practice. 8th ed. Philadelphia: Elsevier; 2014. p. 1260–73.
3. Golden DBK, Moffitt J, Nicklas RA, Joint Task Force on Practice Parameters, et al. Stinging insect hypersensitivity: a practice parameter update 2011. J Allergy Clin Immunol 2011;127:852–4.
4. Steigelman DA, Freeman TM. Imported fire ant allergy: case presentation and review of incidence, prevalence, diagnosis and current treatment. Ann Allergy Asthma Immunol 2013;111:242–5.
5. Golden DBK, Kagey-Sobotka A, Norman PS, et al. Outcomes of allergy to insect stings in children with and without venom immunotherapy. N Engl J Med 2004;351:668–74.
6. Niedoszytko M, deMonchy JGR, van Doormaal JJ, et al. Mastocytosis and insect venom allergy: diagnosis, safety and efficacy of venom immunotherapy. Allergy 2009;64:1237–45.
7. Lerch E, Muller U. Long-term protection after stopping venom immunotherapy. J Allergy Clin Immunol 1998;101:606–12.
8. Oude-Elberink JNG, deMonchy JGR, vanderHeide S, et al. Venom immunotherapy improves health-related quality of life in yellow jacket allergic patients. J Allergy Clin Immunol 2002;110:174–82.
9. Brown SG, Wiese MD, van Eeden P, et al. Ultrarush versus semirush initiation of insect venom immunotherapy: a randomized controlled trial. J Allergy Clin Immunol 2012;139:162–8.
10. Ozdemir C, Kucuksezer UC, Akdis M, et al. Mechanisms of immunotherapy to wasp and bee venom. Clin Exp Allergy 2011;41:1226–34.
11. Simons FER, Peng Z. Skeeter syndrome. J Allergy Clin Immunol 1999;104:705–7.

Internet Resources

Organization/Resource	Internet address
Professional organizations	
Allergy Academy	www.allergyacademy.org
American Academy of Allergy Asthma & Immunology	www.aaaai.org
American Academy of Pediatrics	www.aap.org
American Association of Immunologists	www.aai.org
American College of Allergy, Asthma & Immunology	www.acaai.org
American College of Chest Physicians	www.chestnet.org
American College of Physicians	www.acponline.org
American College of Rheumatology	www.rheumatology.org
American Medical Association	www.ama-assn.org
American Thoracic Society	www.thoracic.org
Asia Pacific Association of Allergy, Asthma and Clinical Immunology (APAAACI)	www.apaaaci.org
Australasian Society of Clinical Immunology and Allergy (ASCIA)	www.allergy.org.au
British Society for Allergy & Clinical Immunology (BSACI)	www.bsaci.org
British Thoracic Society	www.brit-thoracic.org.uk
Canadian Society of Allergy & Clinical Immunology	http://csaci.ca/
Clinical Immunology Society	www.clinimmsoc.org
European Academy of Allergy and Clinical Immunology (EAACI)	www.eaaci.net
Global Asthma Association	www.interasma.org
International Eosinophil Society, Inc.	www.eosinophil-society.org
Scottish Allergy and Respiratory Academy	http://scottishallergyrespiratoryacademy.org
World Allergy Organization	www.worldallergy.org
Government agencies	
Centers for Disease Control and Prevention (USA)	www.cdc.gov
Clinical Trials registry	www.clinicaltrials.gov
Global Initiative for Asthma	www.ginasthma.com
National Institute of Allergy and Infectious Diseases (USA)	www3.niaid.nih.gov
National Heart, Lung, and Blood Institute (USA)	www.nhlbi.nih.gov
National Institutes of Health (USA)	www.nih.gov
National Institute of Health Research (UK)	www.nihr.ac.uk/research/
U.S. Food and Drug Administration	www.fda.gov
World Health Organization	www.who.org
Lay support organizations	
Allergy & Asthma Network/Mothers of Asthmatics	www.aanma.org
Allergy UK	www.allergyuk.org
American Partnership for Eosinophilic Disorders (APFED)	www.apfed.org

Continued on following page

Organization/Resource	Internet address
American Latex Allergy Association (ALAA) (A.L.E.R.T., Inc.)	www.latexallergyresources.org
American Lung Association	www.lung.org
Anaphylaxis Campaign (UK)	www.anaphylaxis.org.uk
Asthma and Allergy Foundation of America	www.aafa.org
Asthma UK	www.asthma.org.uk
European Federation of Allergy and Airways Diseases Patients Associations (EFA)	www.efanet.org
Food Allergy Research & Education (FARE)	www.foodallergy.org
Immune Deficiency Foundation	www.primaryimmune.org
The Mastocytosis Society, Inc. (TMS)	www.tmsforacure.org
Medical resources	
Allergic Rhinitis and its Impact on Asthma (ARIA)	www.whiar.org
American Partnership for Eosinophilic Disorders	http://apfed.org
Asthma and Allergic Disease Management Center	www.aaaai.org
Asthma Prevention Program and Guidelines	www.nhlbi.nih.gov/about/naepp/index.htm
British Thoracic Society/Scottish Intercollegiate Guidelines Network Asthma Guideline	www.brit-thoracic.org.uk/document-library/clinical-information/asthma/btssign-asthma-guideline-2014/
Clinical Trials	https://clinicaltrials.gov
European Academy of Allergy and Clinical Immunology Food Allergy and Anaphylaxis Guidelines	www.eaaci.org/resources/scientific-output/guidelines/2533-food-allergy-and-anaphylaxis-guideline.html
International Food Information Council Foundation	www.ific.org
MedWatch: The FDA Safety Information and Adverse Event Reporting Program (USFDA)	www.fda.gov/medwatch
NLM Literature Searches (PubMed)	www.ncbi.nlm.nih.gov/sites/entrez?db=PubMed
Scientific resources	
Allergome Database (allergenic molecules)	www.allergome.org
Biocompare Buyer's Guide for Antibodies	www.biocompare.com/antibodies/
Cytokines and Cells Online Pathfinder Encyclopedia (COPE)	www.copewithcytokines.de/cope.cgi
Genetic Association Database	http://geneticassociationdb.nih.gov
Human Cell Differentiation Molecules	http://hcdm.org
IUIS Allergen Nomenclature Subcommittee	www.allergen.org/Allergen.aspx
Mouse Genomic Informatics	www.informatics.jax.org
National Center for Biotechnology Information	www.ncbi.nlm.nih.gov
The Cytokines Web	http://cmbi.bjmu.edu.cn/cmbidata/cgf/CGF_Database/cytweb
The International Cell Death Society (ICDS)	www.celldeath-apoptosis.org
Web-based Protein Resources (NCBI)	www.ncbi.nlm.nih.gov/guide/proteins/
Credentialing organizations (USA)	
Accreditation Council for Graduate Medical Education	www.acgme.org
American Board of Allergy and Immunology	www.abai.org
American Board of Internal Medicine	www.abim.org
American Board of Medical Specialties	www.abms.org
American Board of Pediatrics	www.abp.org

Page numbers followed by '*f*' indicate figures, '*b*' indicate boxes, and '*t*' indicate tables.

A

Acaridae, 97–101, 101*f*
Acarids, house dust allergens, 97*b*
Acceptable macronutrient distribution range (AMDR), 330–331
ACE-I induced angioedema (AAE), 242, 242*f*
Aceprometazine + Acepromazine + Clorazepate, 228*t*
Acid anhydrides, asthma due to, 364*t*
ACQ. *see* Asthma Control Questionnaire (ACQ)
Acrylates, asthma due to, 364*t*
ACSS. *see* Asthma Control Scoring System (ACSS)
ACT. *see* Asthma Control Test (ACT)
Activator protein 1 (AP-1), 6–7
Acute asthma, 189–197
 emergency department care for, 193–196
  in children, 196–197
  heliox in, 196
  inhaled, short-acting β₂ agonists in, 194
  inhaled anticholinergic agents in, 194–195
  leukotriene modifiers in, 196
  magnesium sulfate in, 196
  other therapies in, 196
  oxygen in, 193
  systemic (injected) β₂-agonists, 191*t*–192*t*
  systemic corticosteroids in, 195–196
 evaluation of, 190
 home management for, 191–193, 193*f*–194*f*
  in children, 196
 hospital management for, in children, 197
 office management for, in children, 196–197
 post-hospital care for, 197
 treatment for, 191–196, 191*t*–192*t*
Acute bronchospasm, 318*t*
Acute generalized exanthematous pustulosis (AGEP), 233, 236*f*
Acute infusion-related reactions (IRR), in biologicals, 244
Acute respiratory symptoms, 317
Acute urticaria (AU), 250
ADAM33, 158–164
Adaptive immune responses
 in allergic disease, 4–5
 features of, 5–6
 innate instruction of, 4
Adaptive immune system, components of, 5
Adaptive immunity, 4–6
 mechanisms of diseases, 6
ADR. *see* Adverse drug reactions (ADR)
ADRB2. *see* β2-adrenergic receptor gene (ADRB2)
β2-adrenergic receptor gene (ADRB2), 38–39

Adult asthma, 60
 diagnosis of, 166–169, 168*b*
  assessment of airway inflammation, 169
  bronchial hyperreactivity, 168
  determination of allergic status, 168–169
  history and examination, 166
  imaging, 169
  lung function, 166–168, 168*b*
  risk factors, 166, 167*b*
 long-term management in, 177
 pharmacologic treatment in, 177–181, 179*b*
 phenotypes of, 164, 165*b*, 165*t*
Adults, food allergy in, 305, 308
Advair. *see* Fluticasone/salmeterol (Advair)
Adverse drug reactions (ADR), 225–226
 classifications of, 226, 226*f*
 nomenclature for, 226*f*
 safety concern from, 227, 228*t*
Aeroallergen sensitization, 185
Aeroallergens, in atopic dermatitis, 275
Agammaglobulinemia, 7–8
β₂-Agonists, skin tests and, 124*t*, 125–126
Air pollution, 65, 108–111
 sources of, 109–111
  biomass, 110
Airway epithelial cells, 22–23, 22*f*
Airway function, neuronal control of, 23
Airway inflammation, 153
 assessment of, 169
 non-invasive measures of, 370
Airway remodeling, 156–157
Airway smooth muscle (ASM), 23
Airway smooth muscle cells, 23
Albuterol, for asthma, acute, 191*t*–192*t*
Alcohol, adverse reactions to food due to, 303*t*–304*t*
Alder, allergen and, 88*t*–89*t*
Alleles, 32
Allergen avoidance, in select circumstances, 327*t*
Allergen avoidance diets, 330
Allergen extracts, 120–121
 modes/routes of administration, 147, 148*b*
 modifications of, 147–149, 148*b*
 and adjuvants, 147–149
Allergen immunotherapy
 for atopic dermatitis, 290–291
 specificity of, 137
Allergen Nomenclature Subcommittee, 80–81
Allergen prediction software, 82*t*
Allergen-derived peptides, 149
Allergenic, 74–75
Allergenicity, 74–75, 105–106
 environmental modifiers, 112*t*
Allergens, 65–66, 74–75, 75*f*, 105–106
 in atopic dermatitis, 274–275, 281–282
  aero, 275
  autoantigens, 276

 foods, 275
 microbial agents, 275–276
 cell wall modifying, 86
 chemical nature of, 78–80
 databases of, 80–81
  information on structure and function, 82*t*
 environmental modifiers, 112*t*
 exposure concentration, 79*t*
 indoor, 73–116
  avoidance measures for, 106–108
  monitoring, 77–78
  pollen, 81–85
  sources, 75–76, 103*f*
 involved in defense, 86–89
 ligand binding PR-10, 89–90
 modified, 149
 molecular structure of, 105
 multiple mixtures of, specific immunotherapy for, 137
 nomenclature of, 80–81
 outdoor, 73–116
  fungi, 90–96
  monitoring, 77, 78*f*
  sources, 75–76
 pollution effects on, 111–114
 specific, clinical efficacy with, 136–137
 tested, 128
 unmodified, 148
Allergen-specific IgE, production of, 74
Allergen-specific immunotherapy, 133–150. *see also* Specific immunotherapy (SIT)
Allergen-triggered urticaria, 252
Allergic anaphylaxis, 346
Allergic asthma, 156
Allergic disease
 adaptive immune response in, 4–5
 chemokines in, 15–18, 16*f*–17*f*
 definitions of, 52–55
 effects of indoor/outdoor pollutants on, 109*b*
 epidemiology of, 51–72
 epigenetics and, 39–40, 39*f*
 finding genes for, 32–33
 genetics of, 31–33, 31*b*
  approaches to the study of, 32–33
  current understanding of, 33–36
  evidence for, 31–32
  potential for clinical application of, 40–41, 40*b*
 Genome-wide association studies (GWAS) for, 160*t*–164*t*
 maternal environmental of, 42–46
  exposures during pregnancy, 43–46, 44*f*, 45*t*
 mechanisms of, 1–27
 origins of, 29–50, 30*f*
  developmental, 41–49, 41*f*
 pharmacogenetics of, 38–39
 postnatal immune development and, 46–49, 47*t*

Allergic disease *(Continued)*
  risk factors for, 63–67
    air pollution, 65
    allergens, 65–66
    environmental exposures and genetic
       predisposition, 66–67, 66*f*
    hygiene hypothesis, 64
    rural areas, protective exposures in,
       64–65
    timing of exposure, 65
    urban lifestyle, 65
  risk in offspring, 43–46, 44*f*, 45*t*
  team science for, 67–68
  in-utero programming of, 42–46
Allergic eosinophilic gastroenteritis, 312*t*
Allergic infants, ontogeny of immune
   responses in, 47*t*
Allergic inflammation, 1–2
  cytokines in, 12–15
    networks, 24–25, 24*f*
  major pathways, 26
  resolution of, 26
Allergic proctocolitis, 312*t*
Allergic rhinitis, 205–224
  associated diseases in, 207–208
  and asthma, 207
  atopic dermatitis and, 266
  classification of, 211, 211*b*
  clinical features of, 209, 213*t*
  definitions of, 53–54
  and dental malocclusion, 209
  diagnosis of, 209–210
  differential diagnosis of, 211–214,
     211*b*
  epidemiology of, 206–208
  etiology of, 208–215
  factors influencing development of,
     207*b*
  historic perspective of, 206
  incidence and prevalence of, 206–207,
     207*b*
  laboratory testing of, 210–211
  local, 210, 212
  otitis media with effusion, 207–208
  pathogenesis of, 208–215, 208*f*
  during pregnancy, 213
  prevalence of, 60, 67
    trends in, 61–63
  quality of life and economic impact of,
     207
  and rhinosinusitis, 207
  seasonal, diagnosis of, 209
  specific immunotherapy (SIT) for, 134
  stepped therapy for, 219*f*
  treatment of, 215–221
    allergen avoidance, 215–216
    allergen immunotherapy, 218
    overall approach to, 219–220, 219*f*
    pharmacotherapy in, 216–218
    surgery in, 219
Allergic rhinoconjunctivitis, 318*t*
  and atopic dermatitis, 269–270
  definition of, 60
Allergic sensitization, 108–111, 123–124
  pollution effects on, 111–114
'Allergoids,' 148
Allergy, 74
  diagnosis, principles of, 117–131
    clinical features of, 120
    epidemiology of, 119
    historical perspectives on, 118–119
    pathogenesis and etiology of, 119
    in patient, 126–130
    referral, 130

inflammation in, 24*f*
  to specific foods, prevalence of, 305*t*
  tests, positive, 54
Alternaria, 91–96, 92*t*–94*t*, 95*f*
AMDR. *see* Acceptable macronutrient
   distribution range (AMDR)
American Thoracic Society (ATS), asthma
   definitions of, 53*t*
Aminophylline, for acute asthma, 196
Ammonium lactate emulsion, for atopic
   dermatitis, 283
Anaphylactic degranulation, of basophils
   and mast cells, 349*t*
Anaphylactic shock, mechanisms of,
   349–351, 350*b*
Anaphylaxis, 345–360
  allergic, 346
  asthma and, 184
  biomechanical mediators and effects,
     348–349, 349*t*
  biphasic, 352–353
  clinical features of, 347*b*, 351–353, 351*t*
  clinical manifestations of, 351, 351*t*
  criteria for diagnosing, 347*b*
  delayed, caused by mammalian meat, 320
  diagnosis of, 353, 353*b*
  differential diagnosis of, 353–355, 353*b*
  due to antibiotics, 348*t*
  due to antisera, 348*t*
  due to biologic agents, 348*t*
  due to food allergy, 348*t*
    sign and symptoms of, 351–352
  due to hemodialysis, 348*t*
  due to hymenoptera stings, 348*t*
  due to latex, 348*t*
  due to Non-steroidal anti-inflammatory
     drugs NSAIDs, 348*t*
  due to radiocontrast media, 348*t*
  emergency management for, 331–335
  epidemiology of, 346–347
  exercise-induced, 319
  generalized, 319
  genetics, 36
  historical perspective of, 346
  idiopathic, 348*t*
  incidence of, 346–347
    conclusions regarding, 359
  in infants, 352
  management of, 321*t*–322*t*
  non-allergic, 346
  non-organic disease in, 354
  ongoing management and referral,
     357–359
  pathophysiology of, 347–351, 350*b*
    basophils in, 349, 349*t*
    idiopathic, 348*t*
    IgE-dependent, 347–348
    IgE-independent, 347–348
    mast cells in, 349, 349*t*
  perioperative, 348*t*
  prevention and management of
    epinephrine as, 355–356
    laboratory testing, 354–355
  pseudo-, 354
  sign and symptoms of, 351–352, 351*t*
    during anesthesia, 351–352
  from stinging insect allergy
    clinical features of, 381–382
    emergency treatment of, 384
    patients with low risk for, 385*b*
    predictors of risk of, 385–387
  terminology for, 346, 346*f*
  treatment in, 355–357
  undifferentiated somatoform, 354

Angioedema, 233, 234*f*, 249–263
  in children, 263
  definition of, 250
  physical examination for, 256, 258*f*
Angiotensin-converting enzyme inhibitor
   (ACEI), 241–242
  skin tests and, 126
Angle closure glaucoma, 215
Animal-derived indoor allergens, 100*t*–101*t*
Animal-induced asthma, 364*t*
Ant bites, 380
Antibiotics, anaphylaxis due to, 348*t*
Anticholinergics
  for allergic rhinitis, 217–218
  for asthma, 177
    acute, 191*t*–192*t*
    inhaled, 194–195
Antigen, 74–75
Antigen presenting cells (APCs), 5
Antigenic, 74–75
Antigenic determinants, 78–79. *see also*
   Epitopes
Antigenicity, 74–75
Antigen-presenting dendritic cells, in immune
   cells, 20
Antihistamines, 332
  for allergic rhinitis, 216
  for atopic dermatitis, 288
  H$_1$. *see* H$_1$ antihistamines
  H$_2$, 124*t*, 125
  and skin tests, 124*t*, 125
Anti-infective therapy, for atopic dermatitis,
   287–289
Antimicrobial peptides (AMPs), in innate
   immune system, 2, 3*t*, 4*f*
Antioxidant, and occupational asthma, 366*t*
Anti-pruritic agents, for atopic dermatitis,
   288
Antisera, anaphylaxis due to, 348*t*
Anxiolytics, for atopic dermatitis, 288
Apidae stings, 379, 379*t*
Apis mellifera, 380*f*
Apoptotic cells, phagocytosis of, 26
Aquagenic urticaria, 251*t*, 260
Arthropod-derived indoor allergens, 98*t*–99*t*
Arthropods, phylogenetic relationships
   between, 101*f*
Ash, allergen and, 88*t*–89*t*
Aspergillus, 91–96, 92*t*–94*t*, 95*f*
Asthma, 15–16, 16*f*, 151–204, 318
  acute. *see* Acute asthma
  adult, 60
    diagnosis of, 166–169, 168*b*
      assessment of airway inflammation,
         169
      bronchial hyperreactivity, 168
      determination of allergic status,
         168–169
      history and examination, 166
      imaging, 169
      lung function, 166–168, 168*b*
      risk factors, 166, 167*b*
    long-term management in, 177
    pharmacologic treatment in, 177–181,
       179*b*
    phenotypes of, 164, 165*b*, 165*t*
  airway inflammation and, 153, 156, 156*f*
  airway remodeling and, 156–157,
     157*f*–158*f*
  airway smooth muscle (ASM), 23
  allergic rhinitis and, 207
  in athlete, 171
  atopic dermatitis and, 266
  attacks, 152, 189

background of, 152–153
childhood, 57–60
children
  diagnosis in, 171–173
    history and examination, 171, 172b, 173t
    laboratory evaluation, 173
    pulmonary function tests, 172
    radiographic studies, 172
  management in, 184–185, 185f–187f
  non-pharmacologic management in, 185–186
  pharmacologic therapy in, 187–189
  phenotypes in, 165–166
clinical features of, 164–166
comorbidities related, 165t, 177
conditions that mimic, 171
control levels of, 174t
definition of, 52–53, 53t
  by Global Initiative in Asthma (GINA), 152
diagnosis of, 153, 166–177, 197–198
  in specific settings, 169–171
differential diagnosis of, 171b
  in infants and children, 172b
early life development and, 35–36
education on, 186–189
in elderly, 170
environmental control of, 177
epidemiology of, 67–68, 154–156, 155f
etiology of, 156–164
evaluation of, 166–177
exacerbations, 175, 195f
genetics of, 34–36
  and epigenetics, 158–164
Genome-wide association studies for, 158–164, 160t–164t
historical perspective on, 154
immunologic factors of, 157–158, 159f
impact of, 153–154
incidence of, 154
management of, 177–189
  sample action plan for, 188f
  step care approach to, 181–184, 181f
medication in
  inhaler technique, 176
  long-term control, 179–181
  quick-relief, 177
  regular, adherence with, 176
  rescue, 176
mild/intermittent, 175
monitoring, 173–177, 174t, 197–198
  lung function, 176
occupational, 169
overview of, 152–154
pathogenesis of, 156–164
  genetic studies of, 34–35
personal action plan in, 176–177, 178f
phenotypes of, 164–166, 165b
pollution effects on, 111–114
prevalence of, 56, 57f, 67, 153–155
  geographical variations in, 57–60
  symptoms, 58f
  trends in, 61–63, 62f
  World Health Survey, 59f
prevention in, 199
quality of life related, 176
in respiratory food-allergic disorders, 318t
risk factors for, 63–67
  air pollution, 65
  allergens, 65–66
  death from, 190b

environmental exposures and genetic predisposition, 66–67, 66f
hygiene hypothesis, 64
rural areas, protective exposures in, 64–65
timing of exposure, 65
urban lifestyle, 65
severity of, 175, 175b, 182t
specific immunotherapy for, 134–135
sublingual immunotherapy for, 145
symptom control in, 175
team science for, 67–68
treatment for, 153, 198–199
  current, 198
  new, 198–199, 199f
trends in, 155–156
Asthma Control Questionnaire (ACQ), 175
Asthma Control Scoring System (ACSS), 175
Asthma Control Test (ACT), 175
Atopic dermatitis (AD), 16–18, 265–300
acute, 272
allergens in, 274–275
  aero-, 275
  autoantigen as, 276
  avoidance of, 280
  foods, 275
  microbial agents as, 275–276
allergic rhinoconjunctivitis and, 269–270
and asthma, 266
chronic, 272
clinical features of, 272–274, 272b
complicating features of, 273–274
cytokine expression in, 277–279
differential diagnosis of, 270t, 274–280
due to food allergy, 307t, 316
epidemiology of, 267–268
epidermal barrier in, 269f, 271–272
experimental and unproven therapies for, 291–293
genetics of, 36, 268, 269f
historical perspective on, 266–267, 266f
immunopathologic features of, 277, 278f
immunoregulatory abnormalities, 276–277, 276b, 279f
in infancy, 272–273
intrinsic vs. extrinsic forms of, 276–277
management for
  conventional therapy for, 280–287, 281f
    anti-infective therapy, 287–289
    anti-pruritic agents in, 288
    corticosteroids in, 283–286
    hydration in, 282–283
    irritants avoidance, 280–281
    moisturizers and occlusives in, 283
    patient education in, 282
    psychosocial factors in, 282
    tar preparations in, 287
    topical calcineurin inhibitors, 286–287
    wet dressings in, 287
  experimental and unproven therapies for
    dupilumab, 293
    intravenous immune globulin as, 291
    omalizumab as, 291–292
    other, 293
    probiotics as, 292
    recombinant human interferon-γ, 292
    rituximab, 293
natural history of, 270–271, 270t
pathophysiology of, 17, 17f
predisposition to, 268–269
psychosocial implications of, 274

skin inflammation in
  and atopic diathesis, 268–270
  role of IgE in, 279–280
  Th2-like cell response in, 280
subacute, 272
Atopic diathesis, 268–270
Atopic keratoconjunctivitis, and atopic dermatitis, 273
Atopic predisposition, food allergy as, 308
Atopic sensitization
  definitions of, 54–55
  prevalence of, 55–61, 67
  trends in, 61–63
Atopy
  and asthma, occupational, 366
  definitions of, 54–55
  genetics of, 33–34
  prevalence of, 55–61, 67
  trends in, 61–63
  stratification of, 54–55, 56f
Atrophic rhinitis, 212
Augmentation factors, in food allergy, 311
Autoantigens, in atopic dermatitis, 276
Autoimmunity, urticaria and, 251–252
Autologous serum skin test (ASST), 253
Avoidance
  general approach, 326–327
  for schools and camp, 329–330
Azathioprine, for atopic dermatitis, 289

B
B cell epitope, 79, 80f
B cell receptor (BCR), 6–7, 19
B cells, 12t
  in atopic dermatitis, 276–277
B lymphocytes, 6–7
  in immune cells, 19
'Baboon syndrome,' 233
Baker's asthma, 328–329
Baking products, occupational asthma due to, 364t
Basidiomycota, 92t–94t
Basophil activation test (BAT), 241
Basophil degranulation, in anaphylaxis, 349, 349t
Basophils
  activation of, in chronic urticaria, 255
  in immune cells, 20
  in stinging insect allergy, 388
Beclomethasone, for asthma, 179t
Bee sting, 378–379, 379t
Benfluorex, 228t
Beta-lactams, 242–243, 243f
BHR. see Bronchial hyperreactivity (BHR)
Bifidobacteria, for atopic dermatitis, 292
Biocides, asthma due to, 364t
Biologic agents, anaphylaxis due to, 348t
Biologicals drug, drug allergy and, 243–244
Biomass, air pollution sources, 110
Biopharmaceuticals drug, drug allergy and, 243–244
Biphasic anaphylaxis, 352–353
Birch, allergen and, 88t–89t
Birch pollen grains, scanning electron microscopy of, 106f
Biting insect allergy, 391–392
  to Culicidae (mosquito), 392
  other, 392
  to Tabanidae (horsefly, deerfly), 392
  to Triatoma (kissing bug, cone-nose bug), 391–392
Bitolterol, for asthma, acute, 191t–192t
Blackley, Charles, 77

Bleach baths, for atopic dermatitis, 283
Blepharitis, 214
Bombus species, 379
Bronchial hyperreactivity (BHR), 168
Bronchial hyperresponsiveness, non-specific, 367
  serial measurement of, 369
Bronchial provocation tests, 168
Budesonide, for asthma, 179*t*
Budesonide-formoterol (Symbicort), for asthma, 180*t*
Bufexamac, 228*t*
Buflomedil, 228*t*
Bumblebees, 379
  venom, 381

C

Caffeine, adverse reactions to food due to, 303*t*–304*t*
Calcineurin inhibitors, topical, 286–287
Candida, 96
Candida albicans/boidinii, 92*t*–94*t*
Candidate gene association studies, 32
Carisoprodol, 228*t*
Cat-allergic patient, symptoms of, 103
Cathelicidin (LL-37), in innate immune system, 3*t*
Cats
  allergens, avoidance measures for, 108*b*
  hair, antigen in, 103*f*
  indoor allergens sources, 100*t*–101*t*, 103–104
CCDs. *see* Cross-reacting carbohydrate determinants (CCDs)
CD4+ helper T lymphocytes, types of, 140
CD14, in innate immune system, 3*t*
CD19, 6–7
CD25+ Tregs, 12*t*
CD81, 6–7
CDHR3, 35
Celiac disease, 312*t*, 315
Cell wall modifying allergens, 86
Cellular response, to immunotherapy, 139*b*
Central tolerance, 9–11
Cereals, occupational asthma due to, 364*t*
Cetuximab, 79–80
Chemical additives, in food allergy, 309–310, 310*b*
Chemical nature, of allergens, 78–80
Chemokines, 12–18, 21*t*
  in allergic diseases, 15–18, 16*f*–17*f*
Chenopodium album, allergen and, 87*t*–88*t*
Chestnut, allergen and, 88*t*–89*t*
Childhood asthma, 57–60
Children
  cow's milk allergy in, 306
  food allergy in, 304–305
  peanut allergy in, 306–308
  sensitization to egg white in, 308
  urticaria and angioedema in, 263
Chinese restaurant syndrome, 354
Cholinergic urticaria, 251*t*, 257*f*, 259
Chronic autoimmune urticaria (CAU), 250
Chronic idiopathic urticaria (CIU), 250
Chronic rhinosinusitis (CRS), 211
Chronic spontaneous urticaria (CSU), 250
  skin lesions in, 257*f*
Chronic urticaria (CU), 250
Chymase mediator, 21*t*
CIBA Foundation, asthma definitions of, 53*t*
Ciclesonide, for asthma, 179*t*
Ciclosporin, for urticaria, 262

Cladosporium, 91–96, 92*t*–94*t*, 95*f*
Claudin-1 (CLDN1), in atopic dermatitis, 271
Clobutinol, 228*t*
Clonidine, skin tests and, 124*t*, 126
CNVs. *see* Copy number variations (CNVs)
Cockroach sensitivity, specific therapy for, 136
Cockroaches
  allergen and, 91*t*
  avoidance measures for, 108
Cold contact urticaria, 251*t*, 259
Colic, infantile, 313–314
Collectins, in innate immune system, 3*t*
Commonest test, 168
Complementary foods, 330–331
Component-resolved diagnosis (CRD), 324
Concha bullosa, 213–214
Cone-nose bug bites, systemic reactions to, 391–392
Conidiophores, photographs of clinically important, 95*f*
Conjunctivitis, 205–224
  differential diagnosis of, 214–215
  infectious, 214
  toxic, 214–215
Constant region (C), 7
Contact dermatitis, 274
  allergic, 265–300
Contact urticaria, acute, 316
Copenhagen Prospective Study for Asthma in Childhood, 272–273
Coprinus comatus, 92*t*–94*t*
Copy number variations (CNVs), 32
Corticosteroids
  for asthma, 179, 179*t*
    acute, systemic, 195–196
  oral
    for atopic dermatitis, 286
    for urticaria, 262
  skin tests and, 124*t*, 125
  topical, for atopic dermatitis, 283–286, 284*t*
Costimulatory receptors, 11
Cow, indoor allergens and, 100*t*–101*t*
Cow's milk allergy, in children, 306
CR2, 6–7
C-reactive protein (CRP), in innate immune system, 3*t*
Cromolyn, skin tests and, 124*t*, 126
Cromolyn sodium
  for allergic rhinitis, 217
  for asthma, 181
  education on, 189
Cross-contact, 328
Cross-contamination, 328
Cross-reacting carbohydrate determinants (CCDs), 79, 128
Cross-reactive allergens, 75
Cross-reactivity, 310
  of insect venoms, 381
Cryopyrin-associated periodic syndrome (CAPS), 260–261
CTLRs. *see* C-type lectin receptors (CTLRs)
C-type lectin receptors (CTLRs), 106
  in innate immune system, 2, 3*t*
Culicidae bites, systemic reactions to, 392
Cupressus spp., 84–85
Curvularia lunata, 92*t*–94*t*
Cutaneous food allergy, 315–317, 316*t*
Cutaneous IgE-mediated food allergy, 315–316, 316*t*
Cutaneous lymphocyte antigen (CLA), in atopic dermatitis, 280

Cyclosporin A, for atopic dermatitis, 288–289
Cypress, allergen and, 88*t*–89*t*
Cytokines, 1, 12–19, 21*t*
  allergic rhinitis in, 208
  atopic dermatitis in, 277–279
  epithelium-derived, 15*f*
Cytosolic, in innate immune system, 3*t*

D

Dapsone, for urticaria, 262
DC-SIGN, in innate immune system, 3*t*
Decongestants, for allergic rhinitis, 216
DECTIN-2, in innate immune system, 3*t*
Deerfly bites, systemic reaction to, 392
α-Defensins, innate immune system, 3*t*
β-Defensins, innate immune system, 3*t*
Delayed pressure urticaria, 251*t*, 259–260
Delayed type reactions, drug allergy and, 226, 230, 231*f*, 241
  drugs eliciting, 237*t*
  exfoliative dermatitis, 234–238, 237*f*
  fixed drug eruptions, 234
  isolated drug-induced organ damage, 239
  maculopapular exanthem, 233, 235*f*
  systemic drug reactions, 238–239
  warning signs of, 232, 232*t*
Dendritic cells (DCs), 12*t*, 20
  in atopic dermatitis, 278*f*
Dermatitis
  atopic, 36, 316
  exfoliative, 234–238, 237*f*
Dermatitis herpetiformis
  diagnosis of, 317
  due to food allergy, 317
Dermatophagoides farinae, 103*f*
Dermatophagoides pteronyssinus, 96
Dermatophytosis, with atopic dermatitis, 273
Dermcidin, in innate immune system, 3*t*
Dermographism, symptomatic, 251*t*, 256*f*, 259–260
Desensitization, 335, 336*b*
  for atopic dermatitis, 290–291
Developmental programming, in allergic disease, 42–43
Dextropropoxyphene, 228*t*
DHS. *see* Drug hypersensitivity syndrome (DHS)
Diagnosed current asthma, 60
Diesel exhaust particles, in immune development and allergy risk, 45*t*
Diet diaries, 320
  for food allergy, 320
Dietary factors, in immune development and allergy risk, 44*f*, 45*t*
Dietary protein-induced enteropathy, 312*t*, 314–315
Differential blood count, delayed type reaction and, 240
Diisocyanates, occupational asthma due to, 366*t*, 369
DILI. *see* Drug induced liver injury (DILI)
Dipeptidyl peptidase, 96
Disease modification, evidence of, 137–138, 137*b*
Dogs, indoor allergens sources, 100*t*–101*t*, 103–104
Dolichovespula spp. stings, 379, 380*f*
Domestic animals, avoidance measures for, 108, 108*b*
Domestic pets allergens, specific therapy for, 136

Dopamine, skin tests and, 124*t*, 126
Doxepin, for urticaria, 262
DRESS. *see* Drug rash with eosinophilia and systemic symptoms (DRESS)
Drug, classes of, of special interest, 241–244
Drug allergy, 225–247
  clinical features of, 232–239
  common elicitors of, 233*t*
  definition of, 225–226
  diagnosis of, 239–241, 239*t*
  epidemiology of, 229, 229*t*
  etiology of, 230–232, 230*t*
  historical perspective of, 227–228
  pathogenesis of, 230–232, 230*t*
  patient evaluation for, 239–241
  pediatric aspects in, 239
  referral for, 245–246
  risk of sensitization in, 226, 227*t*
  treatment of, 244–246
Drug hypersensitivity syndrome (DHS), 238
Drug induced liver injury (DILI), delayed type reaction and, 232
Drug intake, chronologic documentation of, 239*t*
Drug rash with eosinophilia and systemic symptoms (DRESS), 238
Dry eye syndrome, 214
Dual-allergen-exposure hypothesis, for food allergy, 335*f*
Dulera. *see* Mometasone/formoterol (Dulera)
Dupilumab, for atopic dermatitis, 293
Dust mite, 103*f*
Dysbiosis, 49*f*

E

EAACI. *see* European Academy of Allergy and Clinical Immunology (EAACI)
EASI. *see* Eczema area and severity index (EASI)
ECRHS. *see* European Community Respiratory Health Survey (ECRHS)
Eczema, 18
Eczema area and severity index (EASI), 272
Eczema herpeticum (EH), 273
Eczema vaccinatum, 273
Effector cell *vs.* naive T cell, 19
Effector T cell responses, 43*t*
Egg allergy, extensively heated egg protein for, 338
Elder patient, allergic rhinitis treatment considerations for, 220–221
Elimination diets, in food allergy, 322
Emergency department (ED) care, for acute asthma, 193–196
  after hospitalization, 196
  in children, 196–197
  heliox in, 196
  inhaled, short acting β₂-agonists in, 194
  inhaled anticholinergic in, 194–195
  leukotriene modifiers in, 196
  magnesium sulfate in, 196
  other therapies in, 196
  oxygen in, 193
  systemic (injected) β₂-agonists in, 191*t*–192*t*
  systemic corticosteroids in, 191*t*–192*t*, 195–196
Emollient, for atopic dermatitis, 283, 285
End-organ response, to immunotherapy, 139*b*

Endotype, 164
English plantain, pollen producing plant, 83*f*
Environmental exposures, 66*f*
Environmental modifiers, of allergic sensitization and disease, 106–108, 112*t*
Environmental pollutants, in immune development and allergy risk, 44*f*, 45*t*
Environmental tobacco smoke (ETS), air pollution sources, 111
Enzyme-induced asthma, 364*t*
EoE. *see* Eosinophilic esophagitis (EoE)
Eosinophilic bronchitis, 371–372
Eosinophilic esophagitis (EoE), due to food allergy, 312*t*, 313
Eosinophils
  in allergic rhinitis, 210
  in atopic dermatitis, 277–278
  in immune cells, 12*t*, 20–22, 21*t*
Eotaxin, in atopic dermatitis, 270
Epicutaneous immunotherapy (EPIT), for food allergy, 339
Epidemiology
  in 21st century, 67–68
  of allergic diseases, 51–72
    definitions of, 52–55
    risk factors for, 63–67
  of allergic rhinitis
    definitions of, 53–54
    prevalence of, 60, 67
  of asthma
    adult, 60
    childhood, 57–60
    definitions of, 52–53, 53*t*
    prevalence of, 56, 57*f*
    risk factors, 63–67
    definition of, 51
  of food allergy
    definitions of, 55
    prevalence of, 60–61, 67
Epidermal barrier, in atopic dermatitis, 269*f*, 271–272
Epigenetics, 164
  and allergic disease, 39–40, 39*f*, 41*f*
Epinephrine
  for anaphylaxis, 355–356
  monitoring for, 357
  in stinging insect allergy, 384–385
Epinephrine auto-injector, 384
EPIT (epicutaneous immunotherapy), for food allergy, 339
Epithelial cell-derived cytokines, 22*f*
Epithelial tight junctions (TJ), 23
Epitopes, 78–79
Erythema exsudativum multiforme (EEM), 236–238
ETS. *see* Environmental tobacco smoke (ETS)
Eucapnic voluntary hyperpnea (EVH), 168
European Academy of Allergy and Clinical Immunology (EAACI), 240–241
European Community Respiratory Health Survey (ECRHS), 55–56, 60
European Respiratory Society (ERS), in asthma phenotypes, 166
EuroPrevall study, 61
Evaluation, of patient, with allergic rhinitis, 209–210
Exacerbations, asthma, 175, 189
  drugs for, 191*t*–192*t*
  management of, in children, 196
Exercise-induced urticaria, 251*t*
Exfoliative dermatitis, 234–238

Exhaled nitric oxide (NO), 370
Exotoxins, in atopic dermatitis, 275–276
Exposure
  manner of, 328–331
  timing of, 65
Extrinsic asthma, 156

F

Fagales tree pollen, allergen and, 91*t*
Familial cold autoinflammatory syndrome, 260–261
Fatal food anaphylaxis and comorbid conditions, risk for, 332*b*
Favism, 226
FDEIA. *see* Food-dependent, exercise-induced anaphylaxis (FDEIA)
FEV₁. *see* Forced expiratory volume in 1 second (FEV₁)
Feverfew, allergen and, 87*t*–88*t*
Fiberoptic rhinoscopy, 210
Filaggrin *(FLG)* gene, 36
  in atopic dermatitis, 271
Fingertip unit (FTU), for topical corticosteroids, 285
Fire ant immunotherapy, 391
Fire ant venom, 381
Fixed drug eruptions, 234
Flea bites, systemic reaction to, 392
Flour, occupational asthma due to, 366*t*
Flunisolide, for asthma, 179*t*
Fluorescent immunoassay (FEIA), 119
Fluticasone, for asthma, 179*t*
Fluticasone/salmeterol (Advair), for asthma, 180*t*
Folate, in immune development and allergy risk, 44*f*, 45*t*
Food additives and colorings, 309–310
  categories of, 310*b*
Food allergen(s), 309–310
  anaphylaxis, emergency management of, 331–335
  avoidance of
    nutritional issues, 330–331
    in restaurant, food establishments, travel, 329
    in school and camp, 329–330, 330*t*
  plant derived, 309
  timing of, 307*t*
Food allergen, in atopic dermatitis, 275
Food allergen avoidance strategies, 326–328
Food Allergen Labeling and Consumer Protection Act (FALCPA), 327
Food allergy, 301–343
  in adults, 305, 308
  allergen-specific, epicutaneous immunotherapy, 339
  anaphylaxis due to, 348*t*
    emergency management of, 331–335
    emergency plans and special considerations for school, 332–333
    epinephrine and antihistamines for, 332
    generalized, 319
  asthma and, 184
  augmentation factors, 311
  clinical features of, 311–320
  cross-reactivity, 310
  cutaneous, 315–317
  definition of, 55, 302*b*
  diagnosis of, 320–325, 323*f*
  differential diagnosis of, 303*t*–304*t*, 320–325
  epidemiology of, 304–311
    in children, 304–305, 305*t*

Food allergy *(Continued)*
  future therapeutic strategies for, 335–339, 335f, 336t, 337f
    sublingual immunotherapy (SLIT) as, 338–339, 339t
  gastrointestinal, 311–315
  gastrointestinal IgE-mediated, 311–313
  genetics of, 36
  guidelines, 320, 321t–322t
  historical perspective on, 302–304
  IgE-mediated, 310–311, 311t
  management of, 323f
  as marker of atopic predisposition, 308
  natural history of, 306–308
  oral food challenges, 325, 325b, 326f
  pathogenesis and etiology of, 308
    oral tolerance in, 333–335, 334b
  pathophysiologic mechanisms of, 310
  patient evaluation, 320–325
  practical management for, 325–326
  prevalence of, 60–61, 67, 305–306, 305t
    trends in, 63
  prevention of, 333, 334t
  risk factor for, 307t
  treatment of, 325–331
  unproven tests for, 325
Food aversions, 302b
Food cross-reactivity syndrome, in indoor/outdoor allergens, 91t
Food hypersensitivity, prevalence of, 306
Food intolerances, 302b
Food odors, 328–329
Food protein-induced enterocolitis syndrome (FPIES), 312t, 314
Food protein-induced proctocolitis, 314
Food-allergic disorders, classification of, 311t
Food-dependent, exercise-induced anaphylaxis (FDEIA), 319
Food-induced anaphylaxis, 306
  emergency management of, 331
Food-induced contact dermatitis, 317
Food-induced generalized anaphylaxis, 319
Food-induced hypersensitivity reactions, 320
Food-induced pulmonary hemosiderosis, 319
Food-induced respiratory disease, diagnosis of, 318
Forced expiratory volume in 1 second (FEV$_1$), in asthma, 166–168
Forced expiratory volume in 1 second to forced vital capacity (FEV$_1$/FVC) ratio, in asthma, 166–168
Formicidae bites, 379t, 380–381
Formoterol, for asthma, 180t
FPIES. *see* Food protein-induced enterocolitis syndrome (FPIES)
Frey syndrome, adverse reactions to food due to, 303t–304t
Fructose intolerance, 303t–304t
Fructose malabsorption, 303t–304t
Fungal spore
  equipment used in monitoring, 78f
  photographs of clinically important, 95f
Fungi
  house dust allergens, 97b
  specific therapy for, 136
Fungi-derived aeroallergens, 92t–94t

G

Galactose-α-1, 3-galactose (α-gal), 320
Gallbladder disease, adverse reactions to food due to, 303t–304t

Gaseous pollutants, 113–114
Gastroesophageal reflux disease (GERD), adverse reactions to food due to, 303t–304t
Gastrointestinal anaphylaxis, 313
Gastrointestinal food allergy, 311–315, 312t
  immediate, 313
Gastrointestinal IgE-mediated food allergy, 311–313
Gastrointestinal syndromes, 301–343
  normal immune response to ingested food antigens, 308–309
Gene-environment interaction, 37–38, 37f
  in pathogenesis of allergic disease, 44f
Genetic polymorphism, in food allergy, 307t
Genetic predisposition, 66f
Genetic studies
  for asthma pathogenesis, 34–35
  interpreting results of, 33
Genetics, of allergic disease, 31–33, 31b
Genome-wide association studies (GWAS), 32–33, 158–164
GINA. *see* Global Initiative in Asthma (GINA)
Glaucoma, angle closure, 215
Gleich syndrome, 260
Global Initiative in Asthma (GINA), 152, 183
Glucose-6-phosphate dehydrogenase (G6PD) deficiency, 226
Glutathione S-transferase (GST), 35
Gluten-sensitive enteropathy, 312t
GM-CSF. *see* Granulocyte-macrophage colony-stimulating factor (GM-CSF)
Granule proteins, 21t
Granulocyte-macrophage colony-stimulating factor (GM-CSF), 153
Grass pollen aeroallergens, 86t, 102f
Grass pollens, specific therapy for, 136
Guinea pig, indoor allergens and, 100t–101t
Gustatory rhinitis, adverse reactions to food due to, 303t–304t
Gut microbiome, 48–49
GWAS. *see* Genome-wide association studies (GWAS)

H

H$_1$ antihistamines
  for allergic rhinitis, 216
  skin tests and, 124t, 125
H$_2$ antihistamines, skin tests and, 124t, 125
Hand, atopic dermatitis of, 273
Haptens, 78–79
Hazel, allergen and, 88t–89t
HDM. *see* House-dust mite (HDM)
Heat contact urticaria, 251t
Heiner syndrome, 318t, 319
Helicobacter pylori, 252
Heliox, for acute asthma, 196
Helper T (Th) cells, 5–6
Helper T type 1 (TH1) cells, 18–19, 18f
Helper T type 2 (TH2) cells, 18–19, 18f
  in atopic dermatitis, 268–269, 277, 280
Helper T type 17 (TH17) cells, 18–19, 18f
Hemodialysis, anaphylaxis due to, 348t
Hemosiderin-laden macrophages, 319
Heparin mediator, 21t
Herbaceous dicotyledon species, pollen-derived aeroallergens from, 87t–88t
Heritability studies, in allergic disease, 31–32

Herpes simplex virus (HSV), with atopic dermatitis, 273
Hiatal hernia, adverse reactions to food due to, 303t–304t
Hirschsprung disease, adverse reactions to food due to, 303t–304t
Histamine, adverse reactions to food due to, 303t–304t
Histamine mediator, 21t
Histamine receptors 1 (H$_1$) antihistamines, 125. *see also* H$_1$ antihistamines
Histamine receptors 2 (H$_2$) antihistamines, skin tests and, 124t, 125
Honeybee stings, 379
Honeybee venom, 381
Hormonal rhinitis, 213
Hornbeam, allergen and, 88t–89t
Hornet stings, 379, 380f
Horse, indoor allergens and, 100t–101t
Horsefly bites, systemic reaction to, 392
Hospitalization, for atopic dermatitis, 288
House dust, 96, 97b
House-dust mite (HDM), 96, 102f, 136, 215
  asthma and, 136
  avoidance measures for, 107, 107b
  fecal pellets, aerodynamic properties of, 104
Human immunoglobulin isotypes, 9t
Human leukocyte antigen (HLA), interaction of, 5f
Human papillomavirus (HPV), with atopic dermatitis, 273
Humeral response, to immunotherapy, 139b
Humoral immune response, 6–7, 19
Hydration, for atopic dermatitis, 282–283
Hygiene hypothesis, 48, 64, 157–158, 307t
Hymenoptera
  sting, 378–379, 379t, 380f
    anaphylaxis due to, 347, 348t
  venom, 135, 140, 381
Hyper-IgE syndrome (HIE), 274
Hyper-IgM syndromes, 7–8
Hypereosinophilic syndrome, urticaria and, 260

I

Icatibant, for ACE-I induced angioedema, 242
Ichthyosis vulgaris, 36
ICS-LABA. *see* Inhaled corticosteroid-long acting β$_2$-agonist (ICS-LABA)
Idiopathic non-allergic rhinitis, 212–213
Idiosyncrasy, 226
IFN-γ. *see* Interferon-γ (IFN-γ)
Ige antibody, production of, 2
IgE-mediated allergic diseases, 118f
IgE-mediated food allergy, 310–311, 312t
  immunologic changes in, 337t
IgE-mediated reactions, 230
IgE-mediated respiratory food allergy, 318t
IIA (irritant-induced asthma), 362
IL-3. *see* Interleukin-3 (IL-3)
IL-10. *see* Interleukin-10 (IL-10)
IL-12. *see* Interleukin-12 (IL-12)
Imipramines, skin tests and, 124t, 125
Immediate gastrointestinal food allergy, 313
Immediate type reactions, drug allergy and, 226, 240
  angioedema and, 233, 234f
  urticaria and, 233, 234f

Immune cells, biology of, 18–22
Immune development, 42
  postnatal, 46–49
    T regulatory cells, 47–48
Immune dysregulation, polyendocrinopathy,
    enteropathy, and X-linked (IPEX)
    syndrome, *vs.* atopic dermatitis,
    274
Immune effector cells, 11–12
Immune stimulation, risk of, 227t
Immune tolerance, 6, 9–12
  central tolerance, 9–11
  mechanisms of, 9, 10f
  peripheral tolerance, 10f, 11
  physiopathology of, 9
Immunodominant, 79
Immunoglobulin
  function, 6–7
  gene rearrangement, 7
  and human disease, 7–8
  structure, 6–7, 8f
Immunoglobulin A (IgA), 7
Immunoglobulin D (IgD), 7
Immunoglobulin E (IgE), 7, 12t
  in atopic dermatitis, 279–280
  in occupational asthma and rhinitis,
    365
  specific, in allergic rhinitis, 210
  total serum, 210
Immunoglobulin E (IgE)-dependent
    anaphylaxis, 347–348
Immunoglobulin E (IgE)-independent
    anaphylaxis, 347–348
Immunoglobulin G (IgG), 7
Immunoglobulin M (IgM), 7
Immunohistochemical staining, of atopic
    dermatitis, 277, 278f
Immunomodulation
  for asthma, 180–181
  education on, 189
Immunomodulators, skin tests and,
    125
Immunomodulatory drugs, for urticaria,
    262–263
Immunopathologic penicillin reactions,
    230t
Immunotherapy
  allergen-specific, 133–150
  cessation of, clinical improvement after,
    137–138, 138f
  education on, 189
  follow-up for, 129
  immunologic response to, 139b
    overview of, 139–140
  sublingual, 142–147
  venom, for stinging insect allergy,
    387–391
    discontinuation of, 390–391
      considerations in, 391b
    effectiveness of, 388
    fire ant, 391
    indications for, 387–388
    maintenance in, 389–390
    safety of, 388
    schedules for, 389, 390t
    venom species and dose for, 389
Impairment, 175, 184
In-vitro tests, for stinging insect allergy,
    383
Indoor allergens, 96–105
  animal-derived, 100t–101t
  arthropod-derived, 98t–99t
  avoidance measures for, 106–108
  monitoring, 77–78

oral allergy/food cross-reactivity
    syndromes, 91t
pollen, 81–85, 83f–84f
sources, 75–76
  aerobiology of, 76–77
  mammalian, 103–105
  non-mammalian, 97–102
  photomicrographs of clinically
    important, 103f
Indoor pollutants, effects of allergic disease,
    109b
Inducible urticaria, 250, 251t, 259–260
Infant(s)
  anaphylaxis in, 352
  atopic dermatitis in, 272–273
  with non-IgE-mediated CM allergy,
    304–305
Infantile colic, 313–314
Infections
  with atopic dermatitis, 273–274
  urticaria and, 252
Infectious agents, adverse reactions to food
    due to, 303t–304t
Infectious conjunctivitis, 214
Inflammation, in allergy, 24f
Inflammation resolution, 26, 26f
Ingested food antigens, normal immune
    response to, 308–309, 309t
Inhalant insect allergy, 392
Inhaled corticosteroid-long acting β2-agonist
    (ICS-LABA), 180t
Inhaled corticosteroids (ICS), 153
  for asthma, 179t
  education on, 187
Innate immune system, 48
Innate immunity, 2–4
  and allergy, 4
  cellular responses of, 3–4
  microbial pattern recognition in, 2
  pattern-recognition receptors, 2, 3t, 4f
Innate lymphoid cells (ILC), 19
Innate responses, 43t
Insect allergy, 377–393, 393b
  biting, 391–392
  inhalant, 392
  stinging, 378
    acute reactions to
      prevention of, 384–385, 385b
      treatment of, 384
    anaphylaxis from
      clinical features of, 381–382
      emergency treatment of, 384
      predictors of risk of, 385–387,
        386t
    classification of reaction to, 381–382
    clinical features of, 381–382
    epidemiology of, 378
    etiology of, 378–381, 379t, 380f
    historical perspective on, 378
    insect venoms from, 381
    local reaction to
      algorithm for, 387f
      clinical features of, 381
      treatment of, 384
    patient evaluation and diagnosis for,
      382–383, 382b, 382t
    systemic reactions to
      clinical features of, 381–382
      treatment of, 384
    venom immunotherapy for. *see* Venom
      immunotherapy
Insect venoms, 381
Insecta, 102
Insects, house dust allergens, 97b

Interferon-γ (IFN-γ), 140
  in atopic dermatitis, 292
Interleukin-3 (IL-3), 153
Interleukin-4 (IL-4)
  in allergic inflammation, 12–13, 13f, 13t
  in atopic dermatitis, 277
Interleukin-5 (IL-5), in allergic inflammation,
  13
Interleukin-6 (IL-6), 5–6
Interleukin-9 (IL-9), in allergic inflammation,
  13–14
Interleukin-10 (IL-10), 140
  in immune tolerance, 11–12, 12t
Interleukin-12 (IL-12), 140
  in atopic dermatitis, 278
Interleukin-13 (IL-13)
  in allergic inflammation, 13f, 13t, 14, 25
  in atopic dermatitis, 278
Interleukin-23 (IL-23), in allergic
    inflammation, 5–6
Interleukin-25 (IL-25), in allergic
    inflammation, 14, 25
Interleukin-31 (IL-31), in atopic dermatitis,
    278–279
Interleukin-33 (IL-33), in allergic
    inflammation, 14
International Study of Asthma and Allergies
    in Childhood (ISAAC), 57–60,
    154–155, 206–207, 268
  phase one, 57–60
  phase three, 61–62
  phase two, 57–60
International Study of Life with Atopic
    Eczema (ISOLATE), 282
International Union against Tuberculosis and
    Lung Disease (IUATLD), 55–56
International Union of Immunologic
    Societies (IUIS) allergen
    nomenclature criteria, 76b
Intradermal skin test, 240f
Intradermal test, 121–122, 121f
  advantages of, 123t
  errors in, 122b
  risk factor in, 127
Intralymphatic route, for allergen
    immunotherapy, 147
Intranasal corticosteroids, for allergic
    rhinitis, 216–217
Intranasal steroids (INSs), for allergic
    rhinitis, 216–217
Intravenous fluid resuscitation, 356
Intravenous immune globulin (IVIG), for
    atopic dermatitis, 291
Intrinsic asthma, 156
In-vitro allergen-specific IgE tests, 324, 324t
Involucrin, in atopic dermatitis, 268
Ipratropium/albuterol, for asthma, acute,
    191t–192t
Ipratropium bromide
  for allergic rhinitis, 217–218
  for asthma, acute, 191t–192t
Irritant avoidance, for atopic dermatitis,
    280–281
Irritant-induced asthma (IIA), 362
ISAAC. *see* International Study of Asthma
    and Allergies in Childhood (ISAAC)
Isoallergen, 81
Isocyanate-induced asthma, 364t
Isolated drug-induced organ damage, 239
Isolated wheezing, 318
Itch-scratch cycle, in atopic dermatitis, 274
IUATLD. *see* International Union against
    Tuberculosis and Lung Disease
    (IUATLD)

J

Japanese cedar, allergen and, 88t–89t, 91t
Juniper species, allergen and, 88t–89t
Juniperus spp., 84–85

K

Kaposi varicelliform eruption, 288
Keratinocytes, in atopic dermatitis, 277
Keratitis, 215
Keratoconjunctivitis, atopic, and atopic
        dermatitis, 273
Keratoconus, and atopic dermatitis, 273
Killer bees, 379
Kissing bug bites, systemic reaction to,
        391–392
Klebsiella ozaenae, 212

L

LABA. *see* Long-acting β2-adrenoceptor
        agonists (LABA)
LABAs. *see* Long-acting β₂-agonists (LABAs)
Lactobacillus, for atopic dermatitis, 292
Lactobacillus plantarum, 149
Lactose intolerance, 303t–304t
LAMA. *see* Long-acting antimuscarinic
        cholinergic antagonists (LAMA)
Late phase reaction (LPR), 119, 126
Latex, anaphylaxis due to, 348t
Latex allergy, 310
LEKTI-1, in atopic dermatitis, 268
Leukotriene inhibitors, for allergic rhinitis,
        217
Leukotriene modifiers
        for asthma, 179
            acute, 196
            education on, 189
Leukotriene pathway inhibitors, for
        urticaria, 261–262
Leukotriene receptor antagonists (LTRA),
        153
Levalbuterol (R-albuterol), for asthma,
        acute, 191t–192t
Ligand binding PR-10 allergens, 89–90
Lilac, allergen and, 88t–89t
Linkage disequilibrium (LD), 33
Lipid mediators, 21t
Lipid rafts, 6–7
Lipids, 79
Lipocalins, 104–105
Lipopolysaccharide (LPS), air pollution
        sources, 111
Liposomes, 148
Liver disease, adverse reactions to food due
        to, 303t–304t
London plane tree, allergen and, 88t–89t
Long-acting antimuscarinic cholinergic
        antagonists (LAMA), 153
Long-acting β2-adrenoceptor agonists
        (LABA), 38–39
Long-acting β₂-agonists (LABAs)
        for asthma, 153, 180, 180t
        education on, 187–189
Loricrin, in atopic dermatitis, 268
LPS. *see* Lipopolysaccharide (LPS)
LPS binding protein, in innate immune
        system, 3t
LTC₄/LTD₄ mediator, 21t
LTRA. *see* Leukotriene receptor antagonists
        (LTRA)
Lumiracoxib, 228t
Lung hyperinflation, 169
Lymphocyte antigen (LY98) 96, 3t

Lymphocyte transformation test (LTT), 241
LYN tyrosine kinase, 6–7

M

Macrophages, 12t
Maculopapular exanthem (MPE), 233,
        235f
Magnesium sulfate, for acute asthma, 196
Major allergens, 76
Malassezia furfur, 92t–94t
Malassezia sympodialis, 92t–94t
        in atopic dermatitis, 275
Malignancy, urticaria and, 252
Mammalian, indoor allergens sources,
        103–105
        cats, 100t–101t, 103–104
        dogs, 100t–101t, 103–104
        rabbits, 100t–101t, 103–104
        rodents, 105
Mammalian allergens, 96–97
Mammalian meat, delayed anaphylaxis
        caused by, 320
Mammals, house dust allergens, 97b
Manner of exposure, 328–331
Mannose receptor (CD206), in innate
        immune system, 3t
Mannose-binding lectin, in innate immune
        system, 3t
Manufactured products, labeling of,
        327–328
Mas-related g-protein coupled receptor
        member b2 (Mrgprb2), 231–232
Mas-Related G-Protein Coupled Receptor
        Member X2 (MRGPRX2),
        231–232
Mast cell-leukocyte cytokine cascade,
        348–349
Mast cells (MC)
        activation of, in chronic urticaria, 254,
            254f
        in anaphylaxis, 348–349, 349t
        in immune cells, 12t, 20, 21t
Maternal antioxidant intake, in immune
        development and allergy risk, 45t
Maternal environmental
        of allergic disease, 42–46
            risk in offspring, 43–46, 44f
        exposures during pregnancy, 43–46, 44f
Maternal microbial exposure, in immune
        development and allergy risk, 45t
Maternal n-3 PUFA intake, in immune
        development and allergy risk, 44f,
        45t
Maternal obesity, 43–44
Maternal smoking, during pregnancy, 44,
        44f, 45t
MD-2 (myeloid differentiation factor 2), in
        innate immune system, 3t
MDA5, in innate immune system, 3t
Mechanically-induced urticaria, 259–260
Medications
        associated with, chronic nasal symptoms,
            213t
        combination of, 218
        for ocular symptoms, 218
Mercurialis annua, allergen and, 87t–88t
Metals, asthma due to, 364t
Methotrexate, for atopic dermatitis, 289
Methylxanthines, for asthma, 181
Microbial agents, in atopic dermatitis,
        275–276
Microbial factors, in immune development
        and allergy risk, 44f, 45t

Microbial pattern recognition, in innate
        immune system, 2
Milk allergy, extensively heated milk
        products for, 338
Minor allergens, 76
        criteria for defining a, 76b
Mite species, 101–102, 102f
Mixed IgE-mediated cutaneous food allergy,
        316–317
Mixed IgE-mediated gastrointestinal food
        allergy, 313–314
Modified allergens, 149
Moisturizers, for atopic dermatitis, 283
Molecules, 11–12
Molluscum contagiosum, with atopic
        dermatitis, 273
Mometasone, for asthma, 179t
Mometasone/formoterol (Dulera), for
        asthma, 180t
Monocyte chemotactic protein 4 (MCP-4),
        in atopic dermatitis, 270
Monocytes, 12t
Monophosphoryl lipid A (MPL), 148
Monosodium glutamate, adverse reactions to
        food due to, 303t–304t
Montelukast, skin tests and, 124t, 126
Mosquito bites, systemic reaction to, 392
Mouse, indoor allergens and, 100t–101t
MPE. *see* Maculopapular exanthem (MPE)
Muckle-Wells syndrome (MWS), 260–261
Mucosal immune system, 48–49
Mugwort, allergen and, 87t–88t, 91t
Multicenter Allergy Study, 271
Multiple allergen mixtures, 137
Multiple early atopy subtype, 54–55
Multiple late atopy subtype, 54–55
Munchausen stridor, 354
Mupirocin (Bactroban), for atopic
        dermatitis, 287–288
Mycophenolate mofetil (MMF), for atopic
        dermatitis, 289
Myeloid differentiation factor 2 (MD-2), in
        innate immune system, 3t

N

Naive T cell *vs.* effector cell, 19
Nasal congestion, allergic rhinitis and, 209
Nasal symptoms, chronic, medications
        associated with, 213t
National Ambient Air Quality Standards of
        the USA, 110t
National Cooperative Inner-City Asthma
        Study (NCICAS), 105
National Eczema Association, 282
National Heart, Lung, and Blood Institute
        (NHLBI), asthma definitions of,
        53t
National Institutes of Health (NIH), asthma
        definitions of, 53t
Natural history, of food allergy, 306–308
Natural rubber latex (NRL), occupational
        asthma due to, 364t
NCDs. *see* Non-communicable diseases
        (NCDs)
NCICAS. *see* National Cooperative
        Inner-City Asthma Study (NCICAS)
Nedocromil, skin tests and, 126
Nedocromil sodium
        for asthma, 181
        education on, 189
Nefazodone, 228t
Neonatal immune function, on allergic risk/
        outcomes, 43t

Neonates, with allergic predisposition, 42–43, 43t
Neutrophilic urticaria, 253
Neutrophils, 12t
NHLBI. *see* National Heart, Lung, and Blood Institute (NHLBI)
Nifedipine, skin tests and, 126
NIH. *see* National Institutes of Health (NIH)
Nikolsky sign, 238
Nitrogen dioxide (NO$_2$), 113
NNT. *see* Number needed to treat (NNT)
NOD-like receptors, in innate immune system, 3t
Non-dust mite atopy subtype, 54–55
Non-allergic anaphylaxis, 346
Non-allergic asthma, 156
Non-allergic infants, ontogeny of immune responses in, 47t
Non-allergic rhinitis, 219–220
Non-communicable diseases (NCDs), 41, 42f
    risk factors for, 159f
Non-food items, examples of food allergens in, 328t
Non-IgE-mediated cutaneous food allergy, 316–317, 316t
Non-IgE-mediated gastrointestinal food allergy, 312t, 313–315
Non-IgE-mediated respiratory food allergy, 318t, 319
Non-immunologic anaphylaxis, 347–348
Non-mammalian, indoor allergen sources, 97–102
    acaridae, 97–101
    insecta, 102
Non-PR defense-related pollen allergens, 90
Non-specific lipid transfer proteins (PR-14), 90
Non-steroidal anti-inflammatory drugs (NSAIDs), 241
    anaphylaxis due to, 348t
    urticaria and, 252
N-3-polyunsaturated fatty acids, in food allergy, 307t
Nuclear factor-κB (NF-κB), 6–7
Nuclear factor of activated T cells (NFAT), 6–7
Number needed to treat (NNT), 195–196
Nutritional issues, in food avoidance, 330–331, 331t

O

OA. *see* Occupational asthma (OA)
Oak, allergen and, 88t–89t
OAS. *see* Oral allergy syndrome (OAS)
Occlusives, for atopic dermatitis, 283
Occupational allergy, 361–375
Occupational asthma (OA), 169, 170f, 170t, 361–362
    agents causing, 364t
        high-molecular-weight, 364t
            baking products as, 364t
            latex as, 364t
        low-molecular-weight, 364t
            diisocyanates as, 366t
            wood dust as, 364t
    algorithm for investigation of, 368f, 372t
    classification of, 362f
    clinical features, 367
    conclusions, 375
    defined, 362
    diagnosis of, 367–372, 371t
    differential diagnosis of, 367–372

environmental risk factor, 365–366
epidemiology of, 363, 364t
evaluation of, 367–372, 368f
historical perspectives on, 363
immunologic
    IgE-mediated, 365
    non-IgE-mediated, 365
immunologic testing for, 370
irritant-induced, 362
outcomes and treatment for, 373
overview of, 361–362
pathophysiology of, 363–365
prevention of, 373–374
risk factors, 365–367, 365f
sensitizer-induced, 362
socioeconomic impact and medicolegal aspects for, 374
without latency period, 362
work-exacerbated, 361–362
work-related, 361–362, 362f
Occupational rhinitis (OR)
    agents causing, 364t
    classification of, 362f
    defined, 362
    pathophysiology of, 363–365
    prevalence and incidence of, 363
Occupations, work-related rhinitis and, 212t
Ocular complications, of atopic dermatitis, 273
Ocular rosacea, 215
Olive, allergen and, 88t–89t
Omalizumab (Xolair®)
    for asthma, 180–181
    for atopic dermatitis, 291–292
    skin tests and, 125
    for urticaria, 263
Oral allergy syndrome (OAS), 75, 311
    in indoor/outdoor allergens, 91t
Oral corticosteroids, for atopic dermatitis, 286
Oral food challenges, 325, 326f
Oral immunotherapy, 335–338
    side effects of, 338b
Orciprenaline, 228t
Otitis media with effusion (OME), allergic rhinitis and, 207–208
Outdoor allergens, 81–96
    allergic reactions to, 81
    fungi, 90–96
    monitoring, 77, 78f
    sources, 75–76
        aerobiology of, 76–77
Outdoor pollutants, effects of allergic disease, 109b
Oxidative products, 21t
Oxidative stress, 109–110
Oxygen, for acute asthma, 193
Ozone (O$_3$), 113–114

P

PAMPs. *see* Pathogen-associated molecular patterns (PAMPs)
Pan-allergens, 75
Pancreatic insufficiency, 303t–304t
Panic disorder, adverse reactions to food due to, 303t–304t
Paper wasp stings, 379, 380f
Paraneoplastic pemphigus, 238
Parenchyma-airway interdependence, 158f
Parental allergic disease, 43–44
Parental mental status, 186
Particulates pollutant, 111–113, 112f

Pathogen-associated molecular patterns (PAMPs), in innate immune system, 2
    postnatal, 48
Patient, evaluation of, in allergic rhinitis, 209–210
Patient education, for atopic dermatitis, 282
Pattern-recognition receptors (PRRs), 105–106
    in innate immune system, 2, 3t, 4f
        secreted, 2, 3t
        transmembrane, 2
Peak expiratory flow (PEF), in asthma, 168
Peanut allergy
    in children, 306–308
    prevalence of, 60–61
PEF. *see* Peak expiratory flow (PEF)
Penicillin reactions, immunopathologic, 230t
Penicillium, 96
Penicillium chrysogenum/notatum, 92t–94t, 95f
Penicillium citrinum, 92t–94t, 95f
Penicillium oxalicum, 92t–94t, 95f
Pentraxins, in innate immune system, 3t
Pepsin digestion, of immunoglobulin, 8f
Peptic ulcer disease, adverse reactions to food due to, 303t–304t
Perioperative anaphylaxis, 348t
Peripheral blood mononuclear cells (PBMCs), in atopic dermatitis, 276–277
Peripheral tolerance, 10f, 11
Persistent organic pollutants, in immune development and allergy risk, 45t
Personal asthma action plan, 176–177, 178f
Persulfate salts, asthma due to, 364t
PGD$_2$ mediator, 21t
Pharmacogenetics, 164
    of allergic disease, 38–39
    definition of, 38–39
Phenothiazines, skin tests and, 124t, 125
Phenotype, 164
    definition of, 33
    of drug allergy, 232–239
Photochemotherapy, for atopic dermatitis, 290–291
Phototherapy, for atopic dermatitis, 290–291
Physical examination, allergic rhinitis and, 209–210
Physical urticaria, classification of, 250, 251t
P-i concept, 227–228, 230–231
Pimecrolimus, for atopic dermatitis, 286
Pirbuterol, for asthma, acute, 191t–192t
Pitrakinra, 38–39
Plant-derived food allergens, 309
Platelet-activating factor (PAF), 311
PLCγ2, 6–7
Plicatic acid-induced asthma, 365
Polcalcins, 90
Polistes spp. stings, 378–379, 380f
Polistinae, 379t
Pollen, 81–85, 83f
    allergen release, 83–85, 84f
    house dust allergens, 97b
    and particulate interactions, 106f
    structure, 83–85, 84f
Pollen allergens, 85–90, 85t
Pollen proteins, 86–89
Pollen-food allergy syndrome, 311, 312t
Pollen-food syndrome, 75. *see also* Oral allergy syndrome (OAS)

Pollutants
  indoor, 73–116
  interactions between, and allergen
    exposures, 109t
  outdoor, 73–116
  types of, 111–114
Polymorphisms, 32
  ILRA, 38f
Postnatal immune development
  and allergic disease, 44f, 46–49, 47t
  gut microbiome and, 48–49
  innate immune system, 48
  T regulatory cells, 47–48
Postnatal/perinatal microbial exposure, in
    immune development and allergy
    risk, 45t
P-particles, 83
Prebiotics, in immune development and
    allergy risk, 45t
Predominantly dust mite atopy subtype,
    54–55
Pregnancy
  allergic rhinitis treatment considerations
    for, 220
  urticaria during, 263
Prenatal factors, in asthma risk factors, 65
Prick-puncture method, allergy skin testing
    and, 210
Prick-puncture test, 121, 121f
  risk factors in, 126
Privet, allergen and, 88t–89t
Probiotics, for atopic dermatitis, 292
Profilins, 90
PRRs. see Pattern-recognition receptors
    (PRRs)
Pruritus, due to atopic dermatitis, 278–279,
    288
Psilocybe cubensis, 92t–94t
Psoralen and ultraviolet A (PUVA) therapy,
    for atopic dermatitis, 290
Psychosocial factors, in atopic dermatitis,
    282
Pulmonary function tests, 172
Pulmonary hemosiderosis, 318t
Pyloric stenosis, adverse reactions to food
    due to, 303t–304t

Q

QALY. see Quality-adjusted life year
    (QALY)
QoL. see Quality of life (QoL)
Quality-adjusted life year (QALY), 147
Quality of life (QoL), 176

R

Rabbits, indoor allergens and, 100t–101t,
    103–104
RAD (reactive airways dysfunction
    syndrome), 362
Radio contrast media (RCM), 243
Radioallergosorbent test (RAST), 119
Radiocontrast media, anaphylaxis due to,
    348t
Radiographic imaging, for allergic rhinitis,
    211
Ragweed pollen, allergen and, 91t
Ragweed-allergic patients, 313
R-albuterol. see Levalbuterol (R-albuterol)
Rat, indoor allergens and, 100t–101t
Reactive airways dysfunction syndrome
    (RAD), 362
Reactive dyes, asthma due to, 364t

Recombinant (rAllergens), 119
Recombinant allergen vaccines, 148
Recombinant human interferon-γ (rhIFN-γ),
    for atopic dermatitis, 292
Recombinant venom allergens, 389
Red cedar-induced asthma, 364t
Red flags, for delayed type drug
    hypersensitivity, 232t
Referral, indications for, 221
RefIIIγ, in innate immune system, 3t
Regulatory function, on allergic risk/
    outcomes, 43t
Regulatory T cells, 6f, 11
Remodeling, 156
Respiratory food allergy, 317–319, 318t
Restaurants, food establishments, travel, in
    food allergy, 329
Rhinitis
  allergic, 205–224
    associated diseases in, 207–208
    and asthma, 207
    atopic dermatitis and, 266
    classification of, 211, 211b
    clinical features of, 209, 213t
    definitions of, 53–54
    and dental malocclusion, 209
    diagnosis of, 209–210
    differential diagnosis of, 211–214,
      211b
    epidemiology of, 206–208
    etiology of, 208–215
    factors influencing development of,
      207b
    historic perspective of, 206
    incidence and prevalence of, 206–207,
      207b
    laboratory testing of, 210–211
    local, 210, 212
    and otitis media with effusion, 207–208
    pathogenesis of, 208–215, 208f
    during pregnancy, 213
    prevalence of, 60, 67
      trends in, 61–63
    quality of life and economic impact of,
      207
    and rhinosinusitis, 207
    seasonal, diagnosis of, 209
    specific immunotherapy (SIT) for, 134
    stepped therapy for, 219f
    treatment of, 215–221
      allergen avoidance, 215–216
      allergen immunotherapy, 218
      overall approach to, 219–220, 219f
      pharmacotherapy in, 216–218
      surgery in, 219
  associated with drugs, 212–213, 213t
  atrophic, 212
  chronic, 206
    classification of, 211b
    differential diagnosis in, 214b
    genetics of, 36
    hormonal, 213
    idiopathic non-allergic, 212–213
    non-allergic, 219–220
    occupational
      pathophysiology, 363–365
      prevalence and incidence of, 363
    related to systemic disease, 213
    vasomotor, 212
    work-related, 211, 212t
Rhinitis medicamentosa, 212–213
Rhinoconjunctivitis, 317
  allergic, and atopic dermatitis, 269–270
Rhinoscopy, fiberoptic, 210

Rhinosinusitis
  allergic rhinitis and, 207
  chronic, 211
RIG-1, in innate immune system, 3t
Rimonabant, 228t
Rituximab, for atopic dermatitis, 293
Rodents, indoor allergens sources, 105
Rofecoxib, 228t
Rosiglitazone, 228t
Rural areas, protective exposures in, 64–65
Russian thistle, allergen and, 87t–88t
Rye grass, pollen producing plant, 83f

S

Salmeterol, for asthma, 180t
Salmeterol Multicenter Asthma Research
    Trial (SMART), 183
Scabies, vs. atopic dermatitis, 274
SCFA. see Short chain fatty acids (SCFA)
Schnitzler syndrome, 260
Schools and camp, avoidance for, 329–330
SCIT. see Subcutaneous injection
    immunotherapy (SCIT)
Secreted PRRs, 2
Sensitization
  definitions of, 54–55
  of food allergens, 301
  risk of, 227t
Serial measurement, of non-specific
    bronchial hyperresponsiveness, 369
Serial peak expiratory flow monitoring, 369
Serine proteases, 96
Serotonin, adverse reactions to food due to,
    303t–304t
Serum mast cell tryptase (MCT), 354–355
Severe drug hypersensitivity syndromes,
    238–239
Severity scoring of atopic dermatitis
    (SCORAD), 272
Short chain fatty acids (SCFA), 46
Short ragweed
  allergen and, 87t–88t
  pollen producing plant, 83f
Short-acting β2-adrenoceptor agonists,
    38–39
Short-acting β2-agonists (SABAs)
  for asthma, 177
    acute, inhaled, 194
    skin tests and, 124t, 125–126
Short-acting inhaled bronchodilators, 153
Sibutramine, 228t
Siglecs, in innate immune system, 3t
SIT. see Specific immunotherapy (SIT)
Sitaxentan, 228t
Skin biopsy, for urticarial vasculitis,
    258–259
Skin hydration, for atopic dermatitis,
    282–283
Skin inflammation, in atopic dermatitis
  and atopic diathesis, 268–270
  keratinocytes in, 277
  role of IgE in, 279–280
  Th2-like cell response in, 280
Skin rashes, drug allergy and, 232
Skin test(s) and testing, 120–121
  allergen quantity in, 122
  allergic profile, 128–129
  allergic sensitization, 123–124
  anti-histaminic treatment and, 127
  areas of, 128
  in clinical practice, 121
  component resolved diagnosis in, 129
  drug allergy and, 240–241

drug interference with, 124–126, 124t
immediate-reading on, 126
in infancy, 127
limitation of, 118
methods of, 121f
positivity of, 123
precautions in, 122b
regular, 127
reliability of, 130
risk in, 126–127
skin reactivity in, 122–123
for specific food, 120–121
for stinging insect allergy, 383
technique in, 121–126
tested allergens, 128
Skin-prick test (SPT), 121–122
advantages of, 123t
errors in, 122b
for food allergy, 322
SLIT. see Sublingual immunotherapy (SLIT)
SMART. see Salmeterol Multicenter Asthma Research Trial (SMART)
Sodium metabisulfite, adverse reactions to food due to, 303t–304t
Solar urticaria, 251t, 260
Solenopsis species bites, 381
Somatoform anaphylaxis, undifferentiated, 354
Specific immunotherapy (SIT), 134
adherence to, 142
adverse reactions to, 141–142
for asthma, 134–135
conventional, disadvantage of, 147–148
effect of, on cellular inflammation, 139
end-organ changes and, 138–139
evidence of disease modification and, 137–138, 137b
historical perspective on, 134
immunologic mechanisms of, 139–140
indications for, 134–135, 134b, 135f, 140–142
inhalant, immunologic response to, 138, 139b
injection schedules of, 140–141, 141b, 141t
persistence of effect of, 138f
pharmacoeconomics of, 138
in pregnancy, 142
sublingual. see Sublingual immunotherapy (SLIT)
Specific inhalation challenge test, 369
Sphingomyelin (SM) deacylase, in atopic dermatitis, 283
SPINK5 gene, in atopic dermatitis, 268
Spirometry, 166–168
Sputum cell count, for occupational asthma, 370
Staphylococcus aureus, in atopic dermatitis, 266–267, 273
Starch granules, 83
Step care approach to asthma, 181–184
food allergy and anaphylaxis, 184
immunotherapy, 184
for intermittent asthma, 181–182
for mild persistent asthma, 181f, 182
for moderate persistent asthma, 182–183
for severe persistent asthma, 181f, 182t, 183
step-up and step-down considerations, 184
vaccination, 184
Stevens-Johnson Syndrome (SJS), 234–238, 237f

Sting challenge test, 383
Stinging insect allergy, 378
acute reactions to
prevention of, 384–385
treatment of, 384
anaphylaxis from
clinical features of, 381–382
emergency treatment of, 384
predictors of risk of, 385–387, 386t
classification of reactions to, 381–382
clinical features of, 381–382
epidemiology of, 378
etiology of, 378–381, 379t, 380f
historical perspective on, 378
insect venoms from, 381
local reactions to
algorithm for, 387f
clinical features of, 381
treatment of, 384
patient evaluation and diagnosis for, 382–383
systemic reactions to
clinical features of, 381
treatment of, 384
venom immunotherapy for, 387–391
discontinuation of, 390–391
considerations in, 391b
effectiveness of, 388
fire ant, 391
indications for, 387–388
maintenance in, 389–390
safety of, 388
schedules for, 389, 390t
venom species and dose for, 389
Strict avoidance, 326–327, 327t
Structural cells, 22–23
Subcutaneous injection immunotherapy (SCIT), 142
for asthma, 189
Sublingual immunotherapy (SLIT), 142–147
for asthma, 145
cost-effectiveness of, 146–147
durability of, 146
effects on natural history of allergic disease of, 146, 146f
efficacy of, 145, 145f
future of, 149
mechanisms of, 143f, 144, 144b
safety of, 146–147
side-effects of, 144–145
Sulfites, in food allergy, 309–310, 310b
Sulfur dioxide (SO₂), 113
Sulphasalazine, for urticaria, 262
Sunflower, allergen and, 87t–88t
Superantigens, in atopic dermatitis, 275–276
Surfactant proteins A, in innate immune system, 3t
Surfactant proteins D, in innate immune system, 3t
Symbicort. see Budesonide-formoterol (Symbicort)
Symmetrical drug-related intertriginous and flexural exanthema (SDRIFE), 233
Symptomatic dermographism, 251t, 256f, 259–260
Systemic allergic reaction, follow-up for, 129
Systemic (injected) β₂-agonists, for asthma, acute, 191t–192t
Systemic corticosteroids
for allergic rhinitis, 217
for asthma, acute, 191t–192t
Systemic drug reactions, 238–239
Systemic lupus erythematosus (SLE), 258–259

T
T cell anergy, 11
T cell epitope, 79
T cell-mediated reaction, 230
T cells, 12t
in atopic dermatitis, 276–278, 278f
T lymphocytes, in immune cells, 18–19
T regulatory cells, in postnatal immune development, 47–48
Tabanidae bites, systemic reaction to, 392
Tacrolimus, for atopic dermatitis, 286
Tar preparations, for atopic dermatitis, 287
TCRS. see Tucson Children's Respiratory Study (TCRS)
TDI (toluene diisocyanate) asthma, occupational, 364t
Telephone survey, 60–61
TGF-β. see Transforming growth factor beta (TGF-β)
Th1 cells, 140
Th1 response, 5–6
Th2 cells, 140
Th2 response, 5–6
Th17 response, 5–6
Theobromine, adverse reactions to food due to, 303t–304t
Theophylline
education on, 189
skin tests and, 124t, 125
Thermally-induced urticarias, 259
Thioridazine, 228t
Thymic stromal lymphopoietin (TSLP), in allergic inflammation, 14–15, 25
Thyroid autoantibodies, in chronic urticaria, 258
Tight junctions (TJs), in atopic dermatitis, 271
Tiotropium, for asthma, 177
TLRs. see Toll-like receptors (TLRs)
Tolerance, 335, 336b
Toll-like receptors (TLRs), 148
in innate immune system, 2, 3t
Toluene diisocyanate (TDI) asthma, occupational, 364t
Topical calcineurin inhibitors (TCIs), for atopic dermatitis, 286–287
Toxic epidermal necrolysis (TEN), 234–238, 237f
Tracheoesophageal fistula, adverse reactions to food due to, 303t–304t
Tranquilizers, skin tests and, 124t, 125
Transforming growth factor beta (TGF-β), 5–6, 140
in immune tolerance, 11, 12t
Transmembrane PRRs, 2
Tree pollen aeroallergens, physicochemical and biochemical characteristics of, 88t–89t
Tree pollens, specific therapy for, 136
Triamcinolone acetonide, for asthma, 179t
Triatoma spp bites, systemic reactions to, 391–392
Trichophyton, 96
Trichophyton rubrum, 92t–94t
in atopic dermatitis, 275
Trichophyton tonsurans, 92t–94t
Tryptase, 239
Tryptase mediator, 21t
Tucson Children's Respiratory Study (TCRS), 165–166
Type 2 innate lymphoid cells, in immune cells, 19
Type A reactions, adverse drug reaction and, 226

Type B reactions, adverse drug reaction and, 226, 230
Tyramine, adverse reactions to food due to, 303*t*–304*t*

U

Ultraviolet (UV) light therapy, for atopic dermatitis, 290
'Under-perceivers,' 176
Unmodified allergens, 148
Unproven test, for food allergy, 325–331
Urban lifestyle, 65
Urticaria, 233, 234*f*
    acute, 250
    allergen-triggered, 252
    aquagenic, 251*t*, 260
    cholinergic, 251*t*, 257*f*, 259
    chronic, 250
        autoimmune, 250
        classification of, 250, 251*t*
        definition of, 250
        diagnostic approach of, 255–261
            history in, 255–256, 255*f*
            laboratory assessment in, 256–260
            physical examination in, 256, 256*f*–258*f*
        disease associated with, 251–252
        diseases resembling, 260
        epidemiology of, 251
        etiology of, 252–255
        historical perspective on, 250
        idiopathic, 250
        malignancy and, 252
        natural history and prognosis for, 251
        pathogenesis of, 252–255
            autoimmune hypothesis in, 253, 254*f*
            blood basophils in, 255
            skin mast cells in, 254
    physical, classification, 250, 251*t*
    skin histopathologic features of, 252–253
    spontaneous, 250
        skin lesions in, 257*f*
    treatment of, 261–263
        in children, 263
        general principles for, 261

in pregnancy, 263
    special considerations in, 263
contact, 250
    cold, 251*t*, 259
    heat, 251*t*
    definition of, 250
    delayed pressure, 251*t*, 259–260
    exercise-induced, 251*t*
    factitia, 251*t*
    inducible, 250, 251*t*, 259–260
    neutrophilic, 253
    solar, 251*t*, 260
    systemic diseases and, 260–261
    vibratory, 251*t*
    without wheals, 249–263
Urticarial vasculitis, 259*f*
    skin biopsy for, 258–259
Utero programming, of allergic disease, 42–46

V

Vaccination, for asthma, 184
Vaccines, recombinant allergen, 148
Valdecoxib, 228*t*
Variable region (V), 7
Vasculitis, urticarial, 259*f*
Vasomotor rhinitis, 212
Venom immunotherapy (VIT), for stinging insect allergy, 387–391
    discontinuation of, 390–391
        considerations in, 391*b*
    effectiveness of, 388
    fire ant, 391
    indications for, 387–388
    maintenance in, 389–390
    safety of, 388
    schedules for, 389, 390*t*
    venom species and dose for, 389
Venom skin test, 383
Venoms, insect, 381
Veralipride, 228*t*
Vespid venoms, 381
Vespidae stings, 379, 379*t*
Vespinae, 379*t*
Vespula, 379, 380*f*
Vibratory urticaria, 251*t*

Viral infections, with atopic dermatitis, 273
Vitamin D, in immune development and allergy risk, 44*f*, 45*t*, 46
Vocal cord dysfunction syndrome, 354

W

Wall pellitory, allergen and, 87*t*–88*t*
Wasp stings, 378–379, 380*f*
WEA. *see* Work-exacerbated asthma (WEA)
Weed pollens, specific therapy for, 136
Western red cedar asthma, 365
Wet dressings, for atopic dermatitis, 287
Wet-wrap dressings, for atopic dermatitis, 287
Wheezing, 154
    age-related differential diagnosis for, 173*t*
    'episodic,' 166
    'multi-trigger,' 166
    non-atopic persistent, 166
    transient, 165–166
    'viral,' 166
WHO. *see* World Health Organization (WHO)
Wiskott-Aldrich syndrome, *vs.* atopic dermatitis, 274
Wood dust, occupational asthma due to, 364*t*
Work-exacerbated asthma (WEA), 169, 170*f*, 361–362
Work-related anaphylaxis, 374–375
Work-related asthma, 169, 170*f*, 361–362, 362*f*
Work-related rhinitis, 211, 212*t*
World Health Organization (WHO), asthma definitions of, 53*t*

X

Ximelagatran/melagatran, 228*t*
Xolair®. *see* Omalizumab (Xolair®)

Y

Yellow jacket stings, 379, 380*f*
Yellow jacket venom, 381